Praise for Better Livir ||||||||||||||||||| ls

"This may be one of the most useful, com| of its
kind. It gives you practical ideas that you ca   .d feel
fantastic without counting calories, feeling hu   _ j, _. .cciing deprived. It's about time
something like this was written!"
— **Dr. Jack Singh, N.D., H.M.D., Founder/CEO Organic Food Bar**

"Al's course is based in science and is the foundation for sustainable nutrition in
America. His work teaches a "whole foods revolution" that is your key to vibrant
health. Better Living With Whole Foods is a long overdue manifesto for the whole
foods movement!"
— **Mark McAfee, Founder/CEO Organic Pastures Dairy Company**

"This is amazing! I have studied nutrition and weight loss for over 15 years and
have yet to come across a better tool. This is not your typical diet book; it's a simple
guide that takes you step-by-step, so you can easily learn its principles. Al Morentin
presents the information in a sensible and easy to follow method that will bring greater
wellness. He is direct and to the point and the course is loaded with incredibly valuable
information."
— **Dr. Brandy McCans, D.C., CEO Quantum Success Training, Inc.**

"Stunning and amazing. Alexander Morentin has broken down complex principles
into easy to use actionable steps that will dramatically improve your life. You've got
to read this book!"
— **Dr. Neil Anjan Chatterjee, M.D.**

"Better Living With Whole Foods takes the mystery out of what to do and what to look
for in choosing and eating the right food. Al Morentin knows more about whole foods
than anyone I have ever met. In fact, I have personally been working with Al for more
than a year and I have never felt or looked better."
— **Dr Ron Murase, D.C., North Orange County Wellness**

"I have known Al Morentin on a professional basis for more than 15 years. His new
course, Better Living With Whole Foods, takes you by the hand on a virtual supermarket
tour clearly explaining what foods you should put in your shopping basket and what
foods should stay on the shelves at your local grocery store, so there is no confusion. If
you are looking to lose weight and improve your health without the use of crazy diets
and harmful supplements, you need this course."
— **Dr. John Quackenboss, D.C., Boss Chiropractic**

"The information is phenomenal. This is the best explanation of the foods you need
to eat to achieve optimal health. Al has broken down this vital information into easily
usable bite sized chunks. This book will change your life!"
— **Dr. Tommy Chau, D.C., QME, Advanced Care Sports Rehab**

"I've known Al Morentin close to twenty years. This is an individual that I trust with my health, my family's health, and the health of my patients. Al is one of the most dedicated practitioners in helping people shape their lives in being healthier and happier. The man's mission in life is about growth and improving himself and everybody that knows him, meets him, or is associated with him. This recommendation is my word that Mr. Morentin should be believed and followed."
— **Dr. Paul P. Alderete, D.C., QME, IME**

"Alexander Morentin has dedicated his life to helping people safely lose weight and achieve vibrant health. His new program, Better Living With Whole Foods, provides you with the tools needed to lose weight and keep it off for life. It's a fantastic program."
— **Dr. Scott Lifschitz, D.C.**

"Better Living With Whole Foods is the bible for healthy eating in the 21st century."
— **Dr. David Jacob, D.C., Advanced Care Sports Rehab**

"Alexander Morentin's insights into eating a natural diet are valuable to me as a personal trainer and a formerly obese person. I lost over 120 lbs. over six years ago and know the importance of proper nutrition for myself as well as my clients. Al's treatment of whole food nutrition is crisp and fresh…explaining in raw detail how to implement change into your diet today!"
— **Brandon Locatell, CPT, PES, CES, Fitness Manger, 24 Hour Fitness**

"Better Living with Whole Foods is a must read for anyone who is serious about building a healthy body and changing to a healthy lifestyle. This is not a "fad diet"! Al's program is designed to teach you how to be healthy and lean for life. As a trainer, I'm constantly looking for new, healthy ways of eating. Well, the search is over, all the answers are in Al's book! I encourage you to read this and unveil the secrets that will change your life forever!"
— **Kimberly Manzo, Certified Personal Trainer**

"Al Morentin's Better Living With Whole Foods offers the reader an important, easily-usable Reference Guide to the supermarket; helping us find our way thru the abundance of choices and the dazzle of the slick packaging, to find the truly healthiest foods available. Thank you Al for this helpful guide."
— **Marsha Youde, Certified Nutritional Therapist**

"Alexander Morentin exposes the fake denatured foods that fill your local grocery store and gives a much better solution; delicious nutritious foods that can be easily woven into your every day life. The sections on meat and dairy are especially eye opening. You will never look at your supermarket in the same light. This new course contains valuable information that everyone must have."
— **Ray Bonaventura, Account Executive, Balchem Corporation**

"Al's program for Better Living With Whole Foods offers you an incredible tool to begin your journey to health and vitality. For those of you lucky enough to come across this program sooner than later, count yourself as blessed with good timing and go for it."
— **Renee Terese Plasky, Healing Arts Practitioner**

Better Living With
Whole Foods

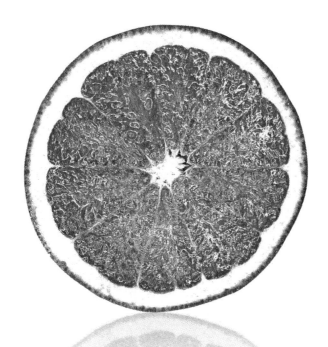

**The Delicious and Nutritious Guide
To Looking Great and Feeling Younger**

Alexander Morentin, C.E.S.

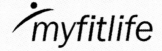

Better Living With Whole Foods, 1ˢᵗ Edition: The Delicious And Nutritious Guide To Looking Great And Feeling Younger.

Visit our website at www.BetterLivingWithWholeFoods.com for more information and resources on better living.

ISBN: 978-0-9799766-0-5
LCCN: 2007908878

Edited by: Pam Jacob & Jessica Wendel
Cover by: Kenneth Ussenko Productions

ATTENTION CORPORATIONS, CHURCHES, UNIVERSITIES, COLLEGES, AND PROFESSIONAL ORGANIZATIONS: Quantity discounts are available on bulk purchases of this book for wellness programs, educational, gift purposes, or as premiums for increasing sales, subscriptions, or renewals. Special books or book excerpts can also be created to fit specific needs. For information, please contact My Fit Life, P.O. Box 1462, Brea, CA 92822; ph: (877) 941-9922.

ACKNOWLEDGMENTS

I would like to express my most sincere gratitude and appreciation to all those who have contributed to the realization of this book, allowing me to share my message with the world.

To my parents Alex and Amy, thank you for encouraging me to follow my dreams.

To Pam Jacob, thank you for your continued support and encouragement. You bring out the best of who I am.

To my family and friends, thank you for believing in me, you hold a special place in my heart.

To all of my beloved clients whose commitment to excellence is truly inspiring. Thank you for trusting me with your health and wellness.

Finally, I want to thank God for giving me the courage and inspiration to see this book to completion.

Thank you all.

TABLE OF CONTENTS

DAIRY

NUTS

OILS

SUGAR & SWEETENERS

PACKAGED FOODS

BABY FOOD

BEVERAGES

SPORT NUTRITION

PUTTING IT ALL TOGETHER

AFTERWORD:

MY PERSONAL JOURNEY

"We were born to succeed, not fail."
— Henry David Thoreau

Alexander Morentin, Clinical Exercise Specialist and owner of My Fit Life, is well known in Southern California as an expert in fitness and whole foods nutrition. He is a nationally certified Clinical Exercise Specialist, Personal Trainer, and Lifestyle and Weight Management Consultant. Over the past 20 years Al has helped a wide variety of individuals achieve their health and fitness best. His clients, who have ranged in age from 10 to 86, have improved their levels of health and fitness while dealing with a wide variety of medical issues including obesity, pregnancy, osteoporosis, diabetes, high blood pressure, low back problems, and many more.

If you are like most people you are probably saying to yourself: "This guy may have a lot of credentials and a lot of experience, but he doesn't know what it's like to be out of shape. There is no way he can relate to me." Well, I am here to tell you that I know exactly what it's like to be out of shape and overweight. I also know exactly what it takes for you to take control of your life and get into the best shape possible.

MY STORY

I have been interested in health and fitness as long as I can remember. It's almost as if I was born to exercise. One of my greatest influences was my mother. As a little boy, I remember my mother taking me to the Vic Tanny & Jack La Lane Health Spas. I didn't know exactly what she was doing in there, but it sure looked like fun. My mother and my aunt were always exercising... either at home or at the health spa. I would always try and imitate the exercises that they did. In fact, I remember doing my first yoga pose, the lotus position, when I was five years old. That was way back in 1970.

While in grade school I would wake up early to go jogging before school. In high school I joined the football team just to have access to the weight room. And in college I competed in powerlifting at the state and national levels.

In 1996 I opened a membership gym in downtown Los Angeles. My dream had come true. The gym was fantastic. It was featured in fitness magazines as well as local magazines and newspapers. I was on top of the world. And then tragedy struck...

Due to unfaithful business partners I had to close the gym. As a result, I turned my back on everything I knew to be true about fitness and nutrition. I stopped exercising and started eating poorly due to grieving over the loss of my gym.

One day I woke up from a horrible nights sleep and took a good look in the mirror. What I saw horrified me. I didn't even know who I was. It was as if I hadn't looked in the mirror for two years. I was so out of shape that I would start breathing hard from just tying my shoes.

IT WAS MY OWN PERSONAL "SUPER SIZE ME"

I decided right then and there that it was time to quit feeling sorry for myself. I called my best friend and told him to go to the store, buy a disposable camera and come directly over to my house. The image on the right is the picture that he took that day.

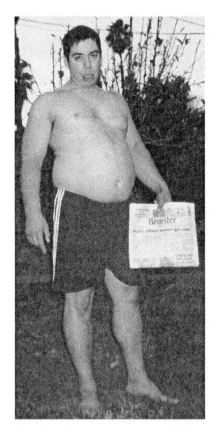

The long road back... I knew it was going to be a challenge, but I didn't realize how much determination it was really going to take to get into optimal shape. I had become so accustomed to eating processed and refined foods that I craved them at every meal. It seemed as though I was addicted to all of the processed and refined grains, sugars and fats. I knew from prior experience with clients that it would be impossible to stop eating the way I had been all at once, cold turkey. I would feel deprived. Also, when I would fall off the wagon and eat something that was "bad" for me, I would feel like a failure. I knew that I would have to change over my diet in gradual progressions, forming beneficial habits in little bits and pieces.

I HAD ABOUT A HUNDRED POUNDS TO LOSE!

I used my experience & expertise to lose body fat and gain muscle in the most efficient way possible, **without the use of protein powders or harmful diet pills. I had about a hundred pounds to lose and I didn't want to have the loose hanging skin that so many people get when they lose weight inefficiently.**

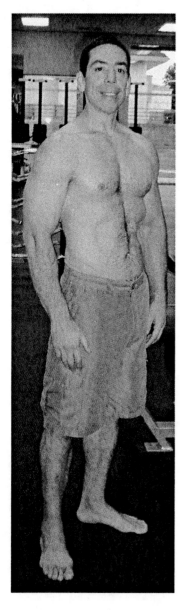

I decided I was going to be one of my best before and after success stories. In the end **I lost a total of 101 pounds and over 12 inches in my waist**. As you can see from the picture, left, I was able to keep my skin tight and my body balanced. I achieved these amazing results with delicious whole foods and a basic exercise routine.

The point of this story is to let you know that I realize what it's like to be out of shape. I'm not just some health nut who has been in shape his entire life. I know what it's like to be addicted to the processed, refined, and denatured foods that have become an integral part of the Standard American Diet (SAD). I know what it's like to dread going to the gym... hoping to God that I will be able to make a positive physical change.

I also know what it's like to be in great physical and mental shape. I know what it's like to feel great, to be healthy, and to have a zest for life. I know what it's like to be totally happy with the person staring back at me in the mirror.

I learned a lot of things on my journey back towards health & wellness. I found out what it is truly like to walk in the shoes of one of my clients. In fact, most of the individuals who come to me for guidance aren't as bad off as I was. I learned what a daunting task it is to attempt to lose such a dramatic amount of weight. I also discovered how absolutely wonderful it is to set realistic goals and achieve them. There is nothing like the personal satisfaction you receive when you make a noticeable physical change. Each positive change that you make will bring a greater sense of accomplishment.

THE SECRET TO LASTING WEIGHT LOSS AND FITNESS SUCCESS

At the beginning of 2001 I changed the name of my company to My Fit Life. I decided that I would create a health and wellness company that will truly make a difference in the world. In order to realize this goal I would have to create weight loss solutions that get dramatic results every single time. I utilized my education, my 20 years of in the trenches experience and my personal experience with the battle of the bulge to create health and wellness programs that do just that; get results every single time.

Often times a person will lose weight when she is following any of a number of diets or weight management programs, but as soon as she returns to her normal eating habits, she will gain all of her weight back and probably more. In essence she has wasted her time and money. Why? Because she didn't learn a thing.

COMMITTED TO YOUR SUCCESS!

I want you to achieve the best results possible and keep them. By following the principles outlined in this course your life will completely change. *Better Living With Whole Foods* is more than a diet; it's a sensible guide to healthful eating that will help you achieve lasting weight loss a fitness success.

WHY DID I WRITE THIS BOOK?

Everybody has heard at one time or another that they need to eat right and exercise, but what exactly does this mean?

For more than twenty years I have been teaching women and men how to achieve lasting weight loss and fitness success. My most successful program is the 16 Week Total Body Makeover. It's a wonderful program that gets fantastic results, but there was something missing.

Although I was teaching people how to recognize their current behavior and make beneficial adjustments in regards to exercise and nutrition, they still had questions. They wanted to know exactly what foods they should be eating and what foods they should avoid in order to achieve and maintain lasting weight loss and fitness success.

Though my clients understood the basics of nutrition I soon discovered that most of them were confused when it came to selecting the exact foods that they should place in their shopping cart at their local grocery store.

Consequently, I came to one simple conclusion: Although most of us have the interest and desire to eat healthy, we lack the basic knowledge and information on how to make the most informed decisions when it comes to selecting and eating the most healthful foods. Indeed, shopping for and selecting the right foods to eat can be a daunting task. (Note: I have found that most people have the determination to achieve vibrant health, but they are lacking the vehicle that will get them there.)

In response to this growing need, I developed a program that I called the Supermarket Tour. The Supermarket Tour involved taking a group of people to a local grocery store and going on a tour along the perimeter of the store, as well as up and down every aisle, explaining exactly which foods are bad, which foods are disguised, which foods are beneficial, and why.

When I held my first class in the local grocery store I didn't know how it would be received. However, 100 percent of the people who attended the Supermarket Tour loved it. More importantly, results skyrocketed. **Clients reported that they were able to achieve lasting weight loss and fitness success faster, easier, and with less effort than they ever imagined possible.**

The Supermarket Tour became a huge success, but there were two problems:

1. Because of limited space there was only enough room for a maximum of seven students.

2. There was such a large volume of information in the class that students were asking to attend a second and third time.

Better Living With Whole Foods was born out of the necessity to enlighten a growing number of people and give them a reference manual that they can refer to again and again. This manual contains everything that I teach in a live Supermarket Tour and more.

My goal is to empower you with the knowledge to make the most informed, most healthful choices for yourself and your loved ones. Knowledge is power. With this power comes freedom. Freedom to live the way that God intended. Vibrant, healthy, and full of life. Free of sickness and disease. It is with this freedom that we can truly make a difference.

TAKE CONTROL OF
YOUR OWN DESTINY

CONGRATULATIONS!

My name is Alexander Morentin. I want to congratulate you for taking an active interest in your health and fitness. The fact that you're reading this introduction shows me that you have what it takes to achieve lasting weight loss and fitness success.

I am very happy that you have found *Better Living With Whole Foods*. You hold in your hands your key to vibrant health and wellness. It has taken me over twenty years of research and experimentation to discover exactly what works and more importantly, what doesn't. You will soon discover how to easily choose the healthiest foods to eat and why.

WHO CAN BENEFIT FROM THIS COURSE?

If you've found yourself confused by the onslaught of diet books, magazine articles, advertisements, and infomercials, this course is for you. You will soon learn that there is a vast amount of deceptive marketing in the food industry. From ambiguities to outright lies, large corporations will do anything to get you to buy their wares. Believe me; these companies do not have your best interests at heart.

Because of this I have made it my mission in life to educate you with the truth in fitness and nutrition. *Better Living With Whole Foods* will clear up your confusion and provide you with the information needed to take control of your own destiny

WHAT YOU WILL FIND IN THIS MANUAL

This manual has been split into 4 sections:

- Whole Foods Nutrition
- Supermarket Tour
- Putting it all Together
- Appendices

WHOLE FOODS NUTRITION:

Included in this section are definitions, descriptions, and concepts that are essential for you to understand the principles and practices outlined in this course.

SUPERMARKET TOUR:

The next section of this manual shows you how to easily choose the healthiest foods to eat and why. You will also discover which foods are detrimental to your weight loss and fitness success and why you should avoid them.

PUTTING IT ALL TOGETHER:

This section provides you with an action plan for incorporating the principles of this course into your every day life. In addition, you are given precise guidelines of how I incorporate whole foods living into my life. From shopping for food, to eating well on the road, I give you detailed examples that guarantee your success with this program.

APPENDICES:

Finally, the last section contains concise outlines of all the principles contained in this course as well as complete lists of the healthiest foods to eat and recommended resources for locating everything you need to live a healthy vibrant life.

A BETTER WAY OF LIVING

GETTING THE MOST FROM THIS BOOK

This book is not about a fad or a trend, it's about a beneficial way of eating that will help you look better, feel better, and live better than you ever imagined possible. It's your complete reference for healthy living in the 21st century that you will refer to again and again.

This informative guide is divided into 38 chapters; do not rush through them. As you read each chapter, take the time to absorb its information before moving on to the next. Underline or highlight key points, jot down notes, and dog ear special pages of interest.

Take special note of the Putting It All Together section. Use the examples to develop a plan of action for implementing whole foods living into your life. Utilize the 8 Principles for Success as well as the outlines and food lists in the Appendices. Review this book often to keep its principles fresh in your mind.

This is your personal journey. Do the best that you can and be proud of yourself for making the effort to better your life. Do not try to be perfect from day 1. The best thing to do is to think of how you ate last week and eat a little better this week.

Always strive for constant improvement, but don't worry about perfection.

Because I know its many benefits, I encourage you to make *Better Living With Whole Foods* an integral part of your everyday life. I wish you the absolute best in your journey towards vibrant health and wellness.

Sincerely,

Alexander Morentin, C.E.S.
Health & Fitness Consultant
Owner / My Fit Life

1

AMERICA AT RISK!

Although we are enjoying economic prosperity greater than any other time in history, Americans are still getting fatter. A research study released by the *Trust for America's Health* in the latter part of 2007 reported that obesity rates climbed in 31 states across the nation, with no decline in any states.

Two-thirds of American adults and approximately 25 million American children are overweight or obese. It is estimated that 50% of the American population may become obese in less than a decade!

The increase in overweight and obesity is having a dramatic effect on us as a nation. When a person is overweight, the risk of obesity related diseases, such as diabetes, heart disease, high blood pressure, and stroke are dramatically increased. Most people in America, even those of normal weight, are unhealthy, but they don't know it. Symptoms such as poor digestion, fatigue, headaches, body aches, arthritis, and dozens of other minor and major ailments are commonplace. We are led to believe that these ailments are unavoidable symptoms of an aging population. However, these ailments, along with the incidence of overweight and obesity, are the direct result of a terrible diet.

"Economics is largely to blame for this state of affairs. A powerful trillion dollar food industry bombards us with messages calculated to make us eat more and more of the worst possible foods. Moreover, many of the emotional and medical challenges some people face today, from controlling one's temper to depression to cancer, are as much products of these junk food companies as are frozen pizza and low-fat cookies.

In the twentieth century, U.S. tobacco companies altered the chemical composition of their products to increase consumption – creating lifelong customers by getting children addicted to specific brands of processed tobacco. Recent legislation has forced Big Tobacco to curb some of these activities when it comes to promoting cigarettes, but they are not letting their acquired expertise go to waste – they have been purchasing the major brands of addictive processed foods. Phillip Morris, the world's largest tobacco company, now owns some of the most popular children's processed food brands, including Oreo cookies, Ritz crackers, and Life Savers candies. This makes Phillip Morris, which produces everything from Oscar Mayer bacon to Post cereals to Philadelphia cream cheese, the world's second largest food company after Nestle, Inc. In 2003, Philip Morris changed its name to Altria to keep consumers from finding out that Kraft Foods and its other children's food brands are from the same company that is bringing their children Marlboros and Virginia Slims."

— Source: *The New Wellness Revolution*, Paul Zane Pilzer (Wiley & Sons)

Knowing what you now know, it is easy to see that the obesity crisis in America is not an accident, but a cleverly calculated plan set in place by the trillion dollar food industry. These food giants burden our lives through sickness, disease, and financial hardship all in the name of higher profits and a bigger return on investments. However, there is good news. We have the power to take control of our health and wellness with natural whole foods. But first, it is imperative that you completely understand the epidemic we are facing in this country.

OBESITY RATES ARE SOARING IN THE UNITED STATES

According to the Center for Disease Control (CDC), between 1980 and 2000, obesity rates doubled among adults. Additionally, the incidence of overweight children in America has increased from 4% overweight in 1982 to more than 30% overweight in 2001 – increasing the number of years they are exposed to health risks of obesity. In fact, children account for 45% of all new cases of Type II diabetes.

According to the National Institute of Health, obesity and overweight together are the second leading cause of preventable death in the United States, close behind tobacco use. An estimated 400,000 deaths per year are due to the obesity epidemic.

Currently, more than 65% of Americans are overweight and more than 30% are clinically obese. This translates into 195 million Americans overweight and 90 million clinically obese. This is truly an epidemic of mammoth proportions.

OVER FED & UNDER NOURISHED

Although we are overfed as a nation, we are vastly under-nourished to the point of severe malnutrition. Much of the food we eat is denatured to•the point that it is stripped of all of its vital nutrients while containing large amounts of refined sugars, processed fats, and harmful chemicals. In other words, our modern food supply is abundant in calories, but deficient in essential nutrients.

Most of us remember the late night T.V. shows in the 80's and 90's depicting starving malnourished children in Africa. These children were skin and bones, but they had grossly distended bellies. This is the result of severe malnourishment due to a lack of food and vital nutrients.

Well, the same type of epidemic is occurring in the United States. It is a common occurrence to see men and women, both skinny and fat, who have distended bellies similar to those of the children in the late night T.V. shows. These men and women are not lacking food, but they are lacking vital nutrients. They are over fed and under nourished. These Americans are malnourished to the point that they live with constant headaches, body aches, gastrointestinal problems, heartburn, fatigue, arthritis, fibromyalgia, and dozens of other disorders that modern medicine tells them to accept as inevitable symptoms of advancing age. Pharmaceutical companies sell Americans billions of dollars worth of drugs, such as pain killers and antacids, that only treat their symptoms while ignoring the cause, a poor diet.

However, this is about to change, *Better Living With Whole Foods* is at the forefront of a whole foods revolution that will completely change the way you think about food, empowering you with the skills needed for healthy living in the 21st century. The principles outlined in this course will make a significant difference in your life. You will discover what's wrong with the commercial food industry and how to easily choose delicious whole foods that are your key to optimal health and wellness. Let's get started!

2

BASICS OF NUTRITION

Included in this section are definitions, descriptions, and concepts that are essential for you to understand the principles and practices outlined in this course.

NUTRIENTS

Your body requires water, macronutrients and micronutrients. The macronutrients are known as protein, carbohydrate, and fat. The micronutrients are known as vitamins, minerals, enzymes, and phytonutrients. These nutrients supply your body with the raw materials it needs for maintenance and repair, as well as the energy it needs to perform its daily functions.

WATER

Water is truly the most essential element of life. We can survive several weeks without food (I have seen people do this), but we cannot survive more than a few days without water. Water is discussed in greater detail in the Beverages section of this course, but it is worth mentioning here.

CARBOHYDRATES

Four calories per gram (4cal/g). Mainly used to provide your body with the energy it needs to perform basic bodily functions (also known as your basal metabolism), as well as immediate energy needed to perform the tasks of every day life.

Raw vegetables and fruits should be your major source of carbohydrates.

PROTEIN

Four calories per gram (4cal/g). Mainly used for building, maintenance, and repair of organs and muscle tissue, as well as the production and formation of vital enzymes. Proteins are chains of amino acids bonded together in varying lengths. Amino acids, the building blocks of protein, can be synthesized by your body or derived from the food that you eat. There are 20 different amino acids. 11 of them are considered non-essential amino acids because they can be made (synthesized) by your body. Nine of them are called essential amino acids because your body cannot make them and you must obtain them from the food that you eat.

FAT

Nine calories per gram (9cal/g). Your body's main source of energy storage. Fat is a calorie dense nutrient. Each gram of fat contains more than double the calories of either a gram of carbohydrate or protein. In other words, just one pound of fat has the same amount of calories as 2 ¼ pounds of protein or carbohydrate. Fats are one of the nutrients that people are most confused about. For this reason, we will look at fats a little more in depth.

WHY DO WE NEED FATS?

Fats perform a variety of important functions including:

- Absorption of fat soluble vitamins A, D, E, and K
- Stored energy
- Integrity of every cell wall
- Enhanced immune system
- Hormonal balance
- Proper brain function

GOOD FATS (ESSENTIAL FATTY ACIDS)

The omega-3 and omega-6 fatty acids are essential fatty acids (EFA) because they cannot be produced by your body. Both of these essential fatty acids are crucial to normal cell function as well as brain and body function.

Omega-3 fatty acids have anti-inflammatory responses in your body. They are crucial to the prevention of blood clots and are thought to be a key player in the prevention of strokes and heart disease.

Omega-6 fatty acids have pro-inflammatory responses. They tend to thicken the blood causing the formation of blood clots.

We need to consume equal amounts, a 1:1 ratio, of these two fatty acids in order to receive the vast benefits which they contain. **Here's the problem**: The Standard American Diet (SAD) contains a ratio of approximately 30:1 omega-6 to omega-3 fatty acids. This unhealthy ratio of essential fatty acids is thought to be a major contributor to heart disease, stroke, depression, eczema, cancer, autoimmune disorders and inflammation just to name a few.

Throughout this course, you will discover which foods you need to eat and which foods you need to avoid in order to obtain a beneficial ratio of these essential fatty acids.

BAD FATS

The refinement of fats and oils turn once healthy fats into bad fats. Some of the most dangerous fats are the *trans fatty acids* (Trans Fats). Trans Fats are contained in vegetable oils that are solid at room temperature such as margarine. Trans fats have been linked to cancer, heart disease, immune depression, and a whole host of other symptoms. Basically, fats found in processed and refined foods are very harmful to you and should be avoided at all costs.

WHAT ARE VITAMINS AND MINERALS?

Simply put, vitamins & minerals make your body work properly. Vitamins and minerals boost the immune system, support normal growth and development, and help your cells and all of the systems in your body do their jobs.

Vitamins: Vitamins fall into two categories: fat soluble and water soluble. The fat soluble vitamins (A, D, E, and K) can be obtained from the beneficial fats that we eat in our diet. These vitamins dissolve in fat and can be stored in the body. The water soluble vitamins (C and the B-complex of vitamins) dissolve in water. Because of this, your body cannot store these vitamins. Any water soluble vitamin that your body does not utilize as it passes through your system will be excreted, mostly in your urine. Therefore, you need a fresh supply of these vitamins every day.

Minerals: Your body requires larger amounts of some minerals, such as calcium and magnesium, for proper growth and maintenance. There are other minerals, such as copper, iron, and zinc that are called trace minerals because you only need very small amounts of them each day. I have found that minerals are an extremely vital part of your health and fitness. Do not underestimate their importance, especially that of the trace minerals. As Robert Williams, owner of Ultimate Raw Foods says, "It's all about the minerals". They help to balance and maintain an alkaline pH in your body

The best place for you to obtain your vitamins and minerals is through a variety of whole foods including raw organic fruits and vegetables and some fermented foods.

Phytonutrients: Plants also contain *thousands* of secondary nutrients, called phytonutrients, that have been shown to be of great benefit to your health and well being and organic foods have been shown to have a much higher content of these secondary nutrients than their commercially grown counterparts. This is one of the many reasons we need to eat whole organic fruits and vegetables.

ENZYMES

Enzymes are protein structures that are the catalyst to every chemical reaction in your body. In other words, they are the spark plug, the energy source needed for every action and reaction that occurs inside of you. Without them life would literally cease to exist.

There are three types of enzymes:

- Metabolic Enzymes
- Digestive Enzymes
- Food Enzymes

Metabolic Enzymes are responsible for almost every activity in your body. Breathing, swallowing, circulating blood,

11

FOOD FOR THOUGHT

When you eat vegetable soup, make sure to drink the broth as well. The water soluble nutrients will leach out of the vegetables and into the broth, making it extremely nutritious.

---

walking, talking, and fighting off infection and disease... you get the picture.

Digestive Enzymes are responsible for digesting food. It doesn't get any more simple than that, right? Digestive enzymes are created by your body in response to the foods that you eat and the available enzymes contained in these foods.

Which leads us to **Food Enzymes.** All whole foods grown in the ground contain all of the enzymes necessary to break them down in the body for digestion. Hence the name food enzymes.

The more food enzymes that you can get from the food you eat; the less digestive enzymes your body has to create. This takes a tremendous burden off of your body. However, food enzymes are very fragile. They are completely destroyed through processing and refining. Also, food enzymes are destroyed when subjected to temperatures above 118 degrees. This is far below the temperature required to cook foods. In addition, many vitamins, delicate proteins, essential fatty acids, and other vital nutrients are destroyed or denatured through processing and cooking.

This is one of the main reasons I encourage everybody that I come in contact with to eat raw organic vegetables and fruits. These are vital, living, enzyme rich foods. If the enzymes in your food are destroyed through cooking or processing, your body has to use its stores of minerals and other vital nutrients to produce digestive enzymes. This is a great burden on your body. These vital nutrient stores are meant to be used for maintenance, repair, and the building of a strong immune system. If you are constantly forcing your body to produce digestive enzymes, you are robbing your body of its vital nutrient stores and creating an environment for sickness and disease to flourish inside of you.

Listen, I am not saying that you should become a raw foodist. However, if your goal is weight loss and vibrant health, I am saying that your eating regimen should consist of about 70% raw foods. This is not something that should be done all at once, but it should be a goal of yours.

ALKALINE ENVIRONMENT

Throughout this course you will hear me mention foods that are alkaline forming and foods that are acid forming to your body. I have found that it is best to eat foods that are alkaline forming. The reason for this is that your body functions at its optimal level when it is slightly alkaline. But first...

Let's take a look at the acid alkaline pH scale:

The pH scale runs from 0 to 14. Seven is neutral. Anything below 7 is acidic. Anything above seven is alkaline or basic.

Your blood pH is slightly alkaline. It has a pH of between 7.35 and 7.45. If it deviates from this range you will die. If you eat acid forming foods and drink acid forming drinks, your body will have to use its mineral stores to keep your blood alkaline. These mineral stores and other nutrient stores are part of your body's defense mechanism. As mentioned above,

---

FIT FACT

An alkaline rich environment has been shown to carry as much as 20% more oxygen in your blood cells. Cancer cells cannot live in an oxygen rich environment. In other words, cancer cells die when they are introduced into an alkaline rich environment. And, you guessed it, cancer cells thrive when they are introduced into an acidic environment.

if you rob your body of these vital nutrient stores, you will be more susceptible to sickness disease, cancer and, ultimately, premature death.

Here's where it gets tricky. When your body is at an imbalance, you do not drop dead right then and there. On the contrary, your body is very resilient. If your body is forced to live in an acidic environment you will develop warning signs, such as dry skin, inflammatory responses, diabetes, lupus, and hypertension, just to name a few. These are all warning signs. These are signs that you need to take charge of your health by eating alkaline forming foods and exercising effectively.

There is much debate over this, but I have found that when people eat foods and drink water that promotes alkalinity in their bodies, they are much healthier. They look healthier, they have more energy, they appear more vibrant, and they do not get sick easily, if at all. People whose bodies are more alkaline tend to have that special glow. I personally do everything I can to keep my body alkaline and I do not get sick.

REMEMBER

- Drink plenty of good clean water.
- Eat foods that provide you with the most beneficial macronutrients and micronutrients.
- Enzymes are the key to life.
- Do your best to keep your body in an alkaline environment.
- Small changes taken one step at a time will produce dramatic results.

3

PROCESSED & REFINED FOODS

What you will learn in this section:

- What are processed and refined foods?
- Why are foods processed and refined?
- Why are they bad?

WHAT IS ALL THE FUSS ABOUT?

Processed and refined foods are one of the great mysteries of our modern culture. We've all heard at one time or another that we need to stay away from these "bad" foods, but few of us know why. Really, what's all the fuss about?

Processed & refined foods are dead foods devoid of all beneficial nutrition. They are basically a "Non-Food", a poison to your body. It's imperative that you know what the dangers are of processed foods. You need to learn how to recognize and avoid these non-foods at all costs.

Processed and refined foods are the major culprits in today's battle with the bulge. Dr. Joseph Mercola in his book *Dr. Mercola's Total Health Program* says:

> *"Today over 90% of grains are processed, making the negative consequences of grains far worse. The physiology of contemporary humans has not changed much from our distant ancestors, and our bodies have never adapted to the excessive amount of carbohydrates from grains and sweets in our present day diet. In fact, in a nation whose diet is still largely based on the severely misguided USDA Food Pyramid, which recommends an atrocious 6-11 servings of breads, cereals, rice, and pasta per day, this surplus of insulin-spiking carbohydrates is the main reason for the overweight epidemic and the scourge of related chronic diseases like diabetes."*

OUR GRANDPARENTS DIDN'T HAVE TO WORRY ABOUT THIS

You hear a lot of stories from people who will tell you that their grandparents ate whatever they wanted to and they lived long healthy lives. Well, the fact of the matter is that our grandparents were not exposed to the kinds of foods that we are exposed to today. Our grandparents ate healthy whole foods by default because that is what was available to them. They didn't have access to Twinkies, Pop Tarts, Captain Crunch, and Lunchables.

FORGET ABOUT THE FADS

Many of the so called health and fitness experts tell you to count calories, count points, limit carbs, limit fat, check the glycemic index, and get into the zone, just to name a few. In fact, many weight loss centers will sell you pre-packaged highly processed non-food items as their solution. These so called *convenience meals* are nothing more than false hope in a box.

Well, you can forget about all of these gimmicks and concentrate on three things:

1. Eat whole foods.
2. Avoid all processed & refined foods.
3. Perform a moderate amount of effective exercise.

Most health and fitness programs tell you to "eat right and exercise", but none show you exactly how this is accomplished, until now. *Better Living With Whole Foods* and the *16 Week Total Body Makeover* are your step by step guides towards truly achieving vibrant health.

WHAT ARE PROCESSED & REFINED FOODS?

When talking about processed and refined foods we generally think of processed and refined flour, sugar, and salt (these are known as the "White Devils"). However, as you will soon discover, there are many other types of foods that undergo harmful refining processes. It's estimated that more than 90% of all foods available today are processed.

When a food has been processed and refined it's stripped of all of its vital nutrients including the vitamins, minerals, and enzymes that help your body break down and utilize them. In most cases, processed foods will also be treated with a variety of harmful chemicals. **Processed and refined foods are basically a poison to your body.**

WHY ARE FOODS PROCESSED & REFINED?

There are a variety of reasons that the big corporations process foods. On the top of the list is money. Take a look at the food advertisements that the media subjects us to. Almost all of these ads are promoting processed foods. Yes, there's a ton of money being made off of processed and refined foods.

Other reasons for processing foods include:

- Longer Shelf Life
- Texture
- Flavor
- Color
- Odor

Longer Shelf Life: It's interesting to note that whole foods will spoil much quicker than processed and refined foods. A loaf of sprouted whole grain bread will have a shelf life of approximately one week. A loaf of your typical processed and refined bread will have a shelf life of approximately two to three weeks or longer.

Texture & Flavor: The texture and flavor of processed and refined grains, sugars, and fats are very unique. The way these "foods" feel on your tongue and taste in your mouth light up pleasure centers in your brain. This makes them very addictive. The problem with this is the fact that the pleasure that these comfort foods give you is short lived. This causes a vicious cycle that leaves you unsatisfied and wanting more. Sound familiar?

> **Note:** When you start eating healthy whole foods your tastebuds will change. Foods once thought of as delicious will start to taste strange. Your body will start to crave the nutrients contained in the whole foods you are giving it. At first it won't seem like this is possible, but given a chance, the transformation always happens. When it does, you'll be on your way to living a healthy vibrant life.

Color: Almost all processed and refined foods will have their color altered in order to make them more appealing to the human eye. These non-foods have an undesirable appearance after they have gone through their processing, so they are either bleached or treated with food coloring or both.

Odor: The processing of foods will often times cause them to turn rancid and foul smelling. These denatured foods must go through further deodorizing processes, such as bleaching, to give them a more pleasant odor.

WHAT ARE THE MAIN CULPRITS IN PROCESSED FOODS?

- Processed & Refined Grains
- Processed and Refined Sugars
- Processed & Refined Vegetable & Plant Oils
- Pasteurization
- Chemical Additives (Preservatives)

We'll discuss each of these in detail throughout this course.

WILL YOU STILL NEED A MORTICIAN WHEN YOU DIE?

A friend of mine, who was going through mortician school at the time, told me that morticians today use very little, if any, embalming fluid on their deceased clients when preparing them for their funerals. Reason being: They're already preserved from all of the chemical preservatives in the foods that they've eaten!

I don't know about you, but the statement above is more than enough reason for me to avoid processed and refined foods at all costs.

Which leads us into our next discussion...

4

GRAINS & FLOURS

GRAINS

The first types of processed and refined foods that you'll learn about are processed and refined grains. After you grasp the concept of what these foods are and why they're bad, it will be easy for you to understand why the other processed and refined foods are harmful to you and your loved ones.

When a plant (grain) is first harvested it has all the beneficial nutrients in it to help your body break down and utilize it. In other words, these plants are very nutritious. They are known as whole grains or sprouted grains. However, over 90% of grains today are processed and refined.

PROCESSED GRAINS ROB YOUR BODY OF VITAL NUTRIENTS

When a plant (grain) is processed & refined it is stripped of all of its vital nutrients, including its fiber, enzymes, vitamins, minerals, amino acids and fats, until just the pure carbohydrate remains. Now, instead of being beneficial, the grain is very hazardous to your body. When you eat these pure carbohydrates your body must use its reserves of vital minerals and vitamins to metabolize (breakdown and utilize) this incomplete food.

These vitamins, minerals and other nutrients are stored in your body to help it repair itself and fight off infection and disease. When your body is robbed of these vital nutrients your body's defense mechanism is put at risk. You are now more susceptible to sickness and disease. **In other words, eating processed and refined foods lowers your immune system.**

INSULIN AND FAT STORAGE

When you eat refined carbohydrates in the form of flour and sugar a mechanism in your body is triggered that produces a large amount of insulin. Insulin is your body's storage device. You always think of insulin as storing carbohydrates, right? Well, insulin doesn't just store carbohydrates it also stores fat. Here's where it gets tricky. You can only store a limited amount of carbohydrates as glycogen, a limited amount in your muscles (muscle glycogen), and a limited amount in your liver (liver glycogen). That's it. However, you can store an unlimited amount of fat in your body. Also, it's very easy for your body to convert carbohydrates to fat. Simply put, if you have an excess amount of carbohydrates and insulin in your blood stream, you are going to store a large amount of fat. This is not what you want!

FLOUR MAKES YOU FAT

When it comes to weight management, breads and flours are your enemy. The reason that flours are so dangerous is the fact that they are a very condensed form of carbohydrates. It

FOOD FOR THOUGHT

Many years ago I found a quarter pounder with cheese under the passenger seat of my car. It had been in my car for more than a month. I noticed two very interesting points right away.

1. The quarter pounder did not smell. Usually when food spoils it gives off a foul odor. Which leads us to our next point...

2. The quarter pounder did not spoil. It looked almost exactly like it did the day I bought it. The bread did not have any mold, nor did the hamburger meat or onions. It was basically petrified.

Many people I have told this story to are amazed. There are so many preservatives contained inside of the food at McDonalds that it isn't even a food any more. And millions of people eat this stuff everyday! Needless to say that I have not eaten at a fast food restaurant since that day.

takes approximately six to eight cups of whole grains to make one cup of flour. This means that one cup of flour has the same amount of calories as the six to eight cups of whole grains that it was derived from. Flour is very calorie dense. Also, the wholeness (nutrients) of the grain has been stripped away, which means that there is nothing to slow the absorption of their carbohydrates into your system.

In other words, when you eat flour you are putting a large amount of condensed carbohydrates in your blood stream all at once. This causes a spike in your insulin levels which we now know will cause you to create and store a large amount of body fat. This is the main reason you want to keep the consumption of flours, especially breads and all pastries, to a minimum.

DID YOU KNOW?

White flour is a natural insecticide. It's true. Pure white flour is so devoid of nutrients that any insect that tries to live off of it will die.

REMEMBER

If your goal is weight loss and vibrant health you will want to either eliminate processed foods from your diet or severely limit their intake, especially processed grains and sugars.

5

BREADS & TORTILLAS

Most breads are unhealthy, but there are some that are better than others. When it comes to these types of foods it is best to make the most informed decision. **In many cases you will be choosing the lesser of the evils.**

BEWARE THE WHITE DEVIL

It is widely known that white bread made from enriched white flour is the worst of all your choices on the bread aisle. This is one of the "white devils". Avoid these breads at all costs; they are like poisons to your body.

THE "WHOLE WHEAT" MYTH

Most people believe bread that is brown in color and says "whole wheat" on the label is good for them. Nothing could be further from the truth.

Slick marketers try to lead us into believing that 100% whole wheat means 100% whole grains. All wheat flour is 100%

whole wheat whether it is white, brown, or any other color. If breads say whole wheat or 100% whole wheat on the label it is usually bad for you. The brown color fools us into believing that these products are more beneficial, but they are just as bad as their white counterparts. In order for something to be 100% whole grain it has to say 100% whole grain on the label.

LET'S LOOK AT THE LABEL OF A TYPICAL 100% WHOLE WHEAT & WHOLE GRAIN BREAD:

Headline:

"Healthy People Healthy Planet"
100% Whole Wheat
Whole Grains
No Trans Fat

Sounds good doesn't it? Kinda makes you feel warm all over, as if by buying this bread you are providing yourself and your loved ones with a nutrient rich beneficial product. Yeah Right!

NOW, LET'S LOOK AT THE INGREDIENTS LIST

- Whole Wheat Flour
- Honey
- Yeast
- Salt
- Calcium Carbonate
- Sodium Stearoyl Lactylate
- Calcium Propionate
- Artificial Flavor
- Azodicarbonimide
- Sugar
- Wheat Gluten
- Soybean Oil
- Butter Cream
- Mono and Diglyceride
- Calcium Sulfate
- Soy Lecithin
- Dough Conditioner
- Caramel Color

Does this list of ingredients look healthy to you?

Let me break it down just for clarification:

Whole Wheat Flour: We've already learned that these types of flour will cause a spike in your insulin levels and cause you to store fat.

Sugar & Honey: These are both refined and processed forms of carbohydrates that result in a spike in your insulin levels. Along with the flour, these three items are a triple whammy in regards to fat storage.

Wheat Gluten, Yeast, Soybean Oil, Salt, and Butter Cream: Although these ingredients are not the most beneficial in regards to your health and well being, they are the least of your worries in regards to the above mentioned ingredients list.

Caramel Color: This is food coloring that gives the bread its brown color. That's right, the bread isn't naturally brown; food coloring is added to make you think that you are eating something healthy.

Dough Conditioners: Dough conditioners turn a food into a non-food substance. They give bread its mushy texture.

Artificial Flavor: Artificial flavor is MSG. MSG has been called edible nicotine because of it addictive properties. We will talk more about MSG later in the course.

Sodium Stearoyl Lactylate, Calcium Sulfate, Calcium Propionate, & Azodicarbonimide:

- **Question:** What in the world are these substances? And what are they doing in a loaf of bread?

- **Answer:** These are preservatives that are typical to processed and refined foods. Their main purpose is to repel insects, strengthen the dough, and provide a longer shelf life. Obviously, you do not want to feed these substances to yourself or anybody that you care about.

LEARN TO READ LABELS

It should be obvious to you by now that you need to read the labels of the foods that you buy. You should be able to recognize and pronounce every ingredient.

As a rule of thumb, if you cannot pronounce an ingredient, you do not want to eat it.

BEWARE THE HIDDEN FATS

The fat that we are most familiar with is the triglyceride, which has 9 calories per gram. This is the only fat that the FDA requires food manufacturers to report, in fat grams, on food labels. However, there are also other forms of **hidden fats** that you will see listed on ingredients lists. These fats are **monoglycerides, diglycerides, and soy lecithin**. There are more, but these are the most common.

Let me break it down for you:

A **triglyceride** is a glycerol molecule with three fatty acids attached.

A **diglyceride** is a glycerol molecule with two fatty acids attached.

A **monoglyceride** is a glycerol molecule with one fatty acid attached.

Mono and diglycerides are fats just like triglycerides and also have 9 calories per gram. Also, mono and diglycerides are treated by the body in the same way as triglycerides. However, due to an FDA loophole these *other* fats do not have to be included on the nutrient facts section of food labels.

Soy lecithin is a highly processed emulsifier that holds the "other" fats together. Soy lecithin itself is a fat which also has 9 calories per gram. This fat does not have to be included on the nutrient facts section of food labels either.

Let me make this perfectly clear: The nutrient facts section of a food label is the place where grams of fat, protein, carbohydrates, and other nutrients are listed. Food manufacturers do not have to list the fat grams on their label that come from monoglycerides, diglycerides, and soy lecithin; they are only required to list the fat grams from the triglycerides. However, food manufacturers *are* required to list these hidden fats in their ingredients list.

> **Note:** Many of the so called low fat and non fat products on grocery store shelves will contain these hidden fats in their ingredients. This is one of the reasons low fat diets do not work.

I hope that you are now starting to understand that the FDA and the big corporations do not have your best interests at heart. You have to take your health and fitness into your own hands. Study and put into use the principles in *Better Living With Whole Foods* for your own health and the health of the ones that you love.

IS THERE A BETTER CHOICE OF BREADS?

I realize that we live in a busy world and sometimes you need to make a quick meal such as a sandwich. Although I try to stay away from grains, there is one type of bread that I recommend; sprouted grain flourless bread. Sprouting grains activates their enzymes, making sprouted grain bread nutrient rich. Sprouted grain breads are more dense than other breads, but they are naturally lower in fat and overall calories

My favorite sprouted grain bread is Ezekiel by Food for Life. Ezekiel bread is great because it's organic and it's flourless. One look at the ingredient list and you'll understand why this is my bread of choice:

EZEKIEL 4:9 SPROUTED GRAIN BREAD

INGREDIENTS:

Organic Sprouted Wheat, Organic Sprouted Barley, Organic Sprouted Millet, Malted Barley, Organic Sprouted Lentils, Organic Sprouted Soybeans, Organic Spelt, Filtered Water, Fresh Yeast, Sea Salt.

I will let the makers of this delicious whole food describe its many benefits:

THE LIVE GRAIN DIFFERENCE

Ezekiel 4:9 Organic Sprouted Whole Grain Products are inspired by the Holy Scripture verse: *"Take also unto thee Wheat, and Barley, and beans, and lentils, and millet, and Spelt, and put them in one vessel, and make bread of it..."* Ez 4:9

We discovered when these six grains and legumes are sprouted and combined, an amazing thing happens. A complete protein is created that closely parallels the protein found in milk and eggs. In fact, the protein quality is so high, that it is 84.3% as efficient as the highest recognized source of protein, containing all 9 essential amino acids. There are 18 amino acids present in this unique bread — from all vegetable sources — naturally balanced in nature.

Ezekiel bread, made from freshly sprouted organically grown grains, is naturally flavorful and bursting with nutrients. Rich in protein, vitamins, minerals and natural fiber and contain **absolutely no flour and no added fat**.

THE SECRET IS IN THE SPROUTS!

We believe in sprouting the grains we use in our breads because sprouting is the only way to release all of the vital nutrients stored in whole grains. To unlock this dormant food energy, maximize nutrition and flavor, we add just the right amount of water to healthy whole organically grown grains which are already bursting with nutrients. Beneficial enzymes are activated which cause the grains to sprout and become a living food, so they're better for you.

TORTILLAS & WRAPS

To clear up any confusion, tortillas and wraps are basically the same thing. Wrap is simply a modern way of saying tortilla. Because of clever marketing, wraps are usually thought of as a healthier alternative to tortillas. Nothing could be further from the truth.

TORTILLAS & BREADS HAVE
VERY SIMILAR INGREDIENTS

Since tortillas and breads have similar ingredients, their nutrient values are also very similar. In other words, most of the tortillas on the market are non-foods that are detrimental to your health.

As with breads there are three levels of tortillas on the market today:

- The Bad
- The Disguised
- The Alternative

THE BAD

Since white flour is one of the "white devils" it should be obvious to you that white flour tortillas are a no-no.

31

THE DISGUISED

Nowadays, you see whole wheat tortillas on the supermarket shelves. These tortillas and wraps are brown in color, which leads many people to believe that they are healthier than white flour tortillas. *Wrong!* Marketers are playing the same games with tortillas as they are with breads. The labels have the same ambiguous headlines: 100% Whole Wheat, Whole Grains, etc.

Take one look at the ingredients list and you will learn the truth:

- Whole wheat flour
- Hydrogenated soybean oil
- Mono & di-glycerides
- Calcium propionate
- Dough conditioners
- Preservatives

And the list goes on and on. The whole wheat tortilla ingredient list is almost identical to the whole wheat bread ingredient list; it is just as long and just as bad.

> **I will say this one more time. Always read the ingredient list of all packaged foods that you're considering for purchase.**

THE ALTERNATIVE

There are two alternatives to consider:

- Corn Tortillas
- Sprouted Grain Tortillas

Corn tortillas are safe, but you have to buy the right kind. Some corn tortillas are similar to whole wheat tortillas. Look at their ingredient list to discover which ones are which.

The safest corn tortillas only have three ingredients on their ingredients list:

- Corn
- Water
- Lime

That's it. Nothing else. There is no need to add any other ingredients to a corn tortilla.

Sprouted grain tortillas are your best bet when selecting tortillas for the same reasons that sprouted grain bread is your best bet when selecting bread.

Food for Life makes Ezekiel organic sprouted grain tortillas which taste very good.

REMEMBER

It is best to stay away from breads and flours altogether; especially if your goal is weight loss. If you must eat bread, choose an option that is organic, sprouted grain, and flourless.

FOOD FOR THOUGHT

Buy organic whenever possible, especially when it comes to corn based products. Corn is one of the most genetically modified substances on the planet (more on this subject in the produce section). Also, stone ground corn is preferable over corn flour. Reason being, stone ground corn contains more nutrients than highly processed corn flour.

6

INTRODUCTION TO PRODUCE

What you will learn in this section:

- Why you need fruits and vegetables.
- Is organic really better?
- What are genetic modifications?
- What type of produce should you eat?
- What's going on with America's farmland?
- Think Global... Buy Local.

VEGETABLES & FRUITS

If you currently eat lots of vegetables and fruits, Great! If you don't presently eat many vegetables and fruits you need to start. Yes, your mother was right; you need to eat your fruits and veggies. As with every other aspect of your health and fitness, add them in slowly. Think of how you ate last week and try to eat a little better this week.

WHY DO I NEED VEGETABLES AND FRUITS?

Vegetables and Fruits are the most nutrient dense foods available, packed with vitamins, minerals, and thousands of phytonutrients. We have learned that these micronutrients are extremely beneficial for our health and well being, but it is worth mentioning again.

MY FIT LIFE

Look, I know first hand how hard it can be to incorporate vegetables and fruits into your daily routine. In fact, when I first started buying produce (notice that I said buying produce and not eating produce), I would have to throw most of it away because it would spoil before I ate it. A six ounce bag of spinach would spoil in my refrigerator before I was half way done with it.

If you are in a similar situation… keep on buying produce. You will eventually eat more and more of the green stuff as time goes by. I always get the same reaction from people when they hear me say this: "But I don't want to waste food or money."

Let me tell you something, if you don't have produce available for you and your family to eat in your home, you will never develop the habit of eating it. You have to make small sacrifices in the beginning in order to receive big rewards down the line.

Today, a six ounce bag of spinach will be gone in one day. I now eat about 4 pounds of spinach per week, plus a variety of other fruits and vegetables that are in season. And I have never felt better in my entire life!

The point I'm trying to make is this: I would never have gotten to this point in my life if I hadn't taken the steps to make sure that I always had produce available in my home.

In order to get in the habit of *eating* produce, you have to first get in the habit of *buying* produce.

Also, the macronutrients (protein, carbohydrates, & fat) in produce are the most bioavailable of all of the food groups. There are so many benefits to eating whole vegetables and fruits that I could write a whole book on this subject alone.

However, that is not the purpose of this course. My purpose here is to help you understand that a major portion of your diet should in fact come from these vital living foods. They will not only give you energy and vitality, but also help you to lose weight and get that "healthy glow" that is so often seen in the people who follow the principles of *Better Living With Whole Foods* and the *16 Week Total Body Makeover*.

YOU NEED THE HIGHEST QUALITY PRODUCE THAT YOU CAN FIND

As with every other food source, there are good and bad sources of vegetables and fruits. The bad sources of produce contain a limited amount of nutrients, while containing high amounts of substances that are detrimental to your health.

Which leads us to our next subject of discussion...

7

IS ORGANIC REALLY BETTER?

What's the big deal? Is organic produce really better than conventionally grown produce?

The answer is YES!

Most of us realize that organically grown produce is free of pesticides. However, organic goes beyond this basic concept.

Organic produce is free of a variety of harmful practices including:

- Pesticides
- Genetic Modifications
- Irradiation

Let's look at these harmful practices in depth, so you will have a better understanding of why you want to avoid them:

PESTICIDES

You might be under the impression that you can remove pesticide residues on your produce by simply washing them.

FIT FACT

According to Ana Lappe, co-author of *Grub* (www.eatgrub.org), "We're even born with them (toxic chemicals). In one study, an average of 200 chemicals and pollutants, including a number of pesticides — many known to be carcinogens or developmental toxins — were found in the blood of umbilical cords. There's now no place untouched; no child born chemical free. Thanks, guys."

However, numerous studies have shown that pesticides actually penetrate the skin of whatever it comes in contact with. If the produce has no skin, like strawberries, the concentration of pesticides is dramatically increased. Strawberries are like a sponge; they soak up everything they come in contact with.

To make matters worse, eating pesticide laden produce causes us to soak up the pesticides and store them in our muscle and fat. Not very good!

GENETIC MODIFICATIONS

Genetic modifications are a big deal. They are something that you should be concerned with. Most people are unaware of the fact that there are more than 50 different genetically modified fruits, vegetables, and grains that have been okayed by the FDA for human consumption.

WHAT ARE GENETIC MODIFICATIONS?

Genetic modifications are an alteration in the genetic makeup of a vegetable, fruit, or grain, which is accomplished through a process known as Genetic Engineering (GE). According to The True Food Network (www.truefoodnow.org), Genetic Engineering is a radical new technology that manipulates the genes and DNA – the building blocks of all living things.

Unlike traditional breeding, genetic engineering creates new life forms that would never occur in nature, creating new and unpredictable health and environmental risks. To create GE crops, genes from bacteria, viruses, plants, animals, and even humans have been inserted into plants like soybeans, corn, canola, and cotton. This is accomplished by injecting a foreign gene into the DNA strand of the plant.

ARE GENETIC MODIFICATIONS HARMFUL TO US?

Genetic modifications were not okayed by the FDA until the 1990's. Because of this, it is not known exactly what consequences genetic modifications will have on us. However, food allergies, along with the incidence of all major diseases, such as Type II Diabetes, Heart Disease, and Cancer, have escalated in dramatic proportions since the period of time that genetic modifications were okayed for human consumption.

WHY DO THEY GENETICALLY MODIFY OUR FOOD?

Multinational chemical companies such as Monsanto genetically modify our food for a variety of reasons. For instance, tomatoes are genetically modified with the gene from a clam shell in order to make its skin tougher. This way, the tomatoes can survive a two to three week trip across the country without getting damaged.

FOOD FOR THOUGHT

For years, scientists have been trying to make engineered foods in their labs which mimic the benefits of whole vegetables and fruits grown in nature. However, they're not able to do it. Reason being, the phytonutrients. This is a classic example of the whole being greater than the sum of all its parts. Thus the term "Whole Foods". Simply put, scientists cannot duplicate what Mother Nature has already provided for us.

A few years ago a woman was eating a bowl of corn flakes and almost died. It turned out that she was having severe allergic reactions to the bowl of cornflakes. Here's the only problem, she is not allergic to corn, she is allergic to peanuts. Upon further investigation, it was determined that the corn in the box of cornflakes the woman had purchased was genetically modified with the gene from a peanut. Isn't that terrible?

IT'S ALL ABOUT MONEY

When it comes right down to it, genetic modifications are all about money. In the 1990's the U.S. government made it possible for large corporations to patent genetically modified substances. In other words, a large corporation, such as Monsanto, can actually own the rights to a particular type of genetically engineered produce. Any farmer caught with a patented strain of any type of produce on his farm can be shut down or face heavy fines; even if the patented strain was introduced through cross pollination unbeknownst to the farmer himself. **These large multinational corporations are gaining control over farmers and the food chain itself.**

In a sense, these corporations are playing God. What was once a wonderful gift from God is now owned through a patent in the U.S Patent & Trademark Office. What a shame.

HOW CAN YOU BE SURE THAT YOUR FOOD IS FREE OF GENETIC MODIFICATIONS?

The FDA does not require food manufacturers to label food that is genetically modified. However, organically grown foods must be free of genetic modifications. This is just one of the many reasons you should buy organic.

It is interesting to note that all European countries require all food that is genetically modified to be labeled as such. For this reason, many European countries do not import American produce.

I AM HERE TO HELP

I hope that it's becoming clear that the U.S. Government and the big corporations do not have our best interests at heart when it comes to our health and fitness. It's because of this that I have dedicated my life to helping people such as yourself make the most informed and ethical decisions that you possibly can. You and your loved ones deserve it.

ROUNDUP READY & PHARMA CROPS

There are 2 more areas of concern in regards to genetically modified foods:

- Roundup Ready Crops.
- Pharma Crops.

Let's take a look at each of these individually:

ROUNDUP READY CROPS

Crops such as canola, soybeans, corn, and cotton have been genetically engineered to be impervious to Roundup. Roundup is the most widely used weed killer (herbicide) in the world.

According to Andrew Pollack of the New York Times, farmers like the genetically engineered crops, which are sold under the brand name Roundup Ready, because they can spray Roundup herbicide directly over those fields, killing the weeds while leaving the crops intact. He goes on to state that Roundup Ready soybeans now account for more than three-quarters of all soybeans grown in the United States. This fact should be very shocking to you. Farmers literally soak their crops with this harmful herbicide.

In case you are wondering, Roundup revenues in 2002 exceeded $470 million. So again, these genetic modifications are all about money with blatant disregard for our health, safety, and welfare. Roundup is a poison; you do not want to eat foods that have been soaked in this harmful substance.

PHARMA CROPS

Soy and corn are the most genetically modified substances on the planet. In fact, pharmaceutical drugs are grown from corn and soy. Yes, you read that right, pharmaceutical grade prescription drugs are grown from corn and soy. They are called **Pharma Crops** and the method used for growing these harmful crops has been called **pharming**. This is a real concern that you need to be aware of.

> *"A Growing Concern addresses the challenge of protecting the U.S. food supply from contamination by crops genetically engineered to produce drugs and industrial substances ("pharma" crops). Six experts commissioned by the Union of Concerned Scientists (UCS) to analyze this problem concluded that corn and soybean cannot be used as pharma crops while preventing contamination of the food supply —unless substantial changes are made to the commodity production and management practices applied to pharma crops.*
>
> *Because changes on this scale have yet to be implemented, UCS has concluded that contamination of the food system by pharma crops may have already occurred and may become more likely in the future. We therefore recommend that the U.S. Department of Agriculture halt the outdoor production of genetically engineered pharmaceutical and industrial crops immediately,*

> *until a new system for producing drugs and industrial substances without endangering the food system can be put in place."*
>
> — Source: Union of Concerned Scientists (www.ucsusa.org)

Pharming is a real concern for us as a nation. I hope you are beginning to understand why I encourage you to choose ethically grown organic foods. Look, I am not trying to scare you. All I am doing is giving you the information necessary to make the most informed decisions for yourself and your loved ones.

The main point that you need to take from this: If you are going to buy corn, soy, or products which contain these ingredients, **buy organic**. It really does make a difference. Really, I can go on and on, but hopefully you get the point by now: **Genetically modified foods are bad.**

IRRADIATION

Irradiation of commercial produce and meats has been approved by the FDA. The reasoning behind this harmful practice is to kill harmful bacteria and other unwelcome pests. In reality, food irradiation gives food manufacturers the ability to extend the shelf life of produce so that it can be stored for weeks on trucks, ships, or trains until it reaches your supermarket.

WHAT DOES FOOD IRRADIATION DO?

Irradiation of produce has been shown to deplete their vital nutrient stores, especially vitamin A, B-complex, C, and beta-carotene. Beneficial bacteria are also destroyed which indicate when food is spoiled. For instance, although they appear fresh, commercially grown apples on supermarket shelves will often have a mushy feel and taste bland. These apples look fresh, but they are actually spoiled and depleted of their vital nutrients.

A quote from Public Citizen regarding irradiation of produce:

> *"We, along with thousands of other consumers, opposed these regulations from the time they were originally proposed during the Clinton administration because of their effects on food, farmers and health," said a Public Citizen spokesman. "Until the irradiation of food is shown to be safe, this technology should not be used to 'treat' imported fruits and vegetables or any other food, for that matter. APHIS acknowledged receiving thousands of comments from citizens who raised safety concerns, but the agency apparently chose to ignore them."*

— Source: Public Citizen (www.publiccitizen.org)

Food irradiation is a real concern which not only affects our produce, but also our meat products, including beef, chicken, fish, and pork.

Now, let's change gears and talk about...

NUTRIENT DENSITY

Organic produce is definitely more nutritious than commercially grown produce. The amounts of vitamins, minerals, and phytonutrients found in organic produce far exceeds that of commercial produce. Don't let anybody tell you otherwise. There are numerous studies proving this fact. And this is what we need to eat; vital nutrient dense whole foods.

WHAT ABOUT THE COST?

One of the arguments against the consumption of organic produce is the cost. Many people are under the impression that organic produce costs two or three times as much as commercially grown produce. This is not true.

I recently went to Henry's Market to check the price of baby spinach:

* Organic Baby Spinach: $2.69 for 5 ounces
* Commercial Baby Spinach: $2.99 for 6 ounces
* Ounce for Ounce they cost about the same.

The price difference between organic produce and commercial produce is usually very marginal. However, organic produce is definitely worth the buy. The cost to benefit ratio for purchasing organic produce is off the charts.

FOOD FOR THOUGHT

Organic packaged and processed foods will often times cost more than commercial packaged foods. However, the purpose of this course is to encourage a positive life change, so you will eat more organic whole foods while severely limiting your consumption of packaged and processed foods... whether they are organic or not.

WHAT IF ORGANIC PRODUCE IS NOT AVAILABLE?

Do your best to eat as organic as you can. As always, do the best you can for the situation you are in. If you can't find organic, if it is not available, do not stop eating vegetables and fruits.

Let's face it, organic is readily available for most of us here in the United States, especially those of us who live in California. When you are first starting out, it may seem like a hassle to buy organic. Once you locate beneficial sources for your organic produce it's no hassle at all. In fact, it will become enjoyable. You'll revel in the fact that you are providing your family and yourself with wholesome goodness.

However, there will be times that you won't have access to organic produce. You may miss a farmer's market, be on vacation, or a whole host of other scenarios. In these situations you should still purchase and eat fruits and vegetables, even if they are from commercial sources. Let's face it, the alternative (packaged food) isn't any better. It's always more beneficial to eat foods that contain *some* nutrition as opposed to eating processed denatured garbage that isn't even a food any more.

8

THE DESTRUCTION OF AMERICA'S FARMLAND

Commercial produce, the kind found in supermarkets, are subjected to ungodly amounts of pesticides. It's just not necessary. These pesticides not only wreak havoc on our bodies, they also destroy our precious farmland.

The pesticides and herbicides used to kill insects and prevent plants from getting diseases also kill all of the life contained in the soil, such as earth worms. Earth worms are what oxygenate the soil. They keep it healthy. If they are gone then the soil dies. If the soil dies, then it loses all of its vital nutrients. And that's where all of the erosion comes from.

EROSION (TOP SOIL DEPLETION) FACTS

- Historic cause of demise of many great civilizations: Topsoil depletion

- Percentage of original U.S. topsoil lost to date: 75%

- Amount of U.S. cropland lost each year to soil erosion: 4,000,000 acres, the size of Connecticut

  — Source: Diet for a New America, John Robbins

The soil in commercial farms is dead, which means that it has been depleted of all of its beneficial nutrients. That is why commercial farms have to fortify their soil with fertilizers. You are probably familiar with fertilizers containing NPK (nitrogen, phosphorous, and potassium). These are minerals that are needed to grow most plants. However, our soil and our bodies need many more nutrients than NPK to remain healthy and vital.

Remember, a lot of the fruits and vegetables found in local supermarkets come from different parts of the country. So they could've been picked two, three, or four weeks prior to arrival. They come from huge agricultural farms that spray tons of pesticides on their crops for no good reason.

ORGANIC FARMS ARE BIODIVERSE

The farming methods used on organic farms promotes bio-diversity. Nutrients transfer from the soil, to the plant, and back to the soil. The soil is living, breathing, and full of life.

You see, **erosion does not occur on organic farms**. Harmful pesticides and herbicides are not used on organic farms, which mean that the soil has beneficial properties which make it nutrient rich. It is full of a diverse array of beneficial life that is transferred into the produce that it produces. This is why organically grown produce is much more nutritious than commercial produce.

FOOD FOR THOUGHT
Organic produce purchased at farmer's markets is generally more cost effective than produce purchased at supermarkets.

FARMER'S MARKETS

Do your best to obtain fruits and vegetables as much as you can from farmer's markets. Many of the farmers selling their produce at farmer's markets grow organically these days. Just ask them and they'll tell you whether they grow organically or not. But regardless of whether they grow organically or not, the produce from local farmers will be grown in much better conditions than the produce grown on the huge commercial agricultural farms. For the most part, smaller local farms are more conscious to the world than the large agricultural farms. Also, the fruits and vegetables found at farmer's markets are fresh. A lot of times, the fruits and vegetables will have been picked that day and, if not that day, then within the past couple of days.

Consumers are demanding more and more organically grown produce and local farmers are responding to this. For this reason it is becoming easier and easier to find locally grown organic produce at farmers markets and CSA's (Community Supported Agriculture).

MAKE SURE YOUR PRODUCE IS LOCALLY GROWN

Some farmer's markets allow resellers to sell produce at their markets. Resellers do not grow their own produce. On the contrary, they buy their produce from the same commercial sources that are found in your local grocery store.

If you are unsure about the origins of the produce at your farmer's market, simply ask the market coordinator. There is always a market coordinator present at every farmer's market.

He or she will be more than happy to tell you if the produce available is from local sources or resellers.

CSA: COMMUNITY SUPPORTED AGRICULTURE

What is Community Supported Agriculture (CSA)? A step above farmer's markets, the CSA model connects eaters to growers in a way no other distribution system can. Many markets don't have a reputation for providing organic produce, which has a circular effect of not attracting organic buyers, so when the organic farmers do show up, they get discouraged.

Many small farms are responding with going directly to the local food supporter in the form of a weekly subscription basket. Customer's get truly local, "just harvested" freshness. Produce in a grocery store is often 14 days old and has, on average traveled 1500 (unsustainable) miles, losing nutrition and flavor along the way. Having your fruit and vegetables harvested and delivered directly from the farm provides a fresher, tastier alternative.

The reasons for buying locally-produced food are compelling. These include the benefits of eating fresher, tastier, and more nutritionally intact food, greater variety, preserving farmland and open space, and keeping money within the local economy. Grocery store food from half-way around the world can never compete with the benefits of locally grown produce!

— *Source: Morning Song Farm Rainbow, CA*

SUPPORT YOUR LOCAL FARMER

One thing I'll mention about organic is that it's becoming a big buzzword, so it's getting extremely commercialized. This means that you have to be careful who you buy your organic produce from. This is another reason why I encourage you to go to the farmer's markets as much as you can for your produce. They are a small community of farmers. You are helping to support them and you are helping them to keep on doing what they are doing. If you don't, these small biodiverse local farms will become extinct and you'll lose your freedom of choice, as well as an excellent source of nutrient rich whole foods.

FOOD FOR THOUGHT

Local farmers will only have produce that is in season. For example, during the hot summer months there is an abundance of fruit available, as opposed to the colder months in the fall and winter where the produce available is predominantly vegetables. Mother Nature knows exactly what our bodies need during different times of the year in order to keep us healthy and full of life.

LOCAL IS THE NEW ORGANIC!
THE FUTURE OF FOOD

If you get a chance, watch the movie "The Future of Food". This movie exposes all of the horrible things that are going on with commercial farming and our food supply. It really is amazing. The point of the matter is this: **Support your local farmers, by doing so, you are voting with your dollars** and letting the big corporations and the government know that we have the power to make a choice.

WHAT TYPE OR VARIETY OF
PRODUCE SHOULD YOU EAT?

Generally, almost all whole fruits and vegetables are very beneficial for you. Your main concern should be to increase your consumption of these beneficial foods, especially in their raw form. Remember to eat a variety, so you'll obtain a wide range of nutrients.

Colorful vegetables are especially nutrient dense. The darker the color the more nutrient dense the vegetable will be. For example, spinach is much more nutrient dense than iceberg lettuce, even though they are both green in color.

You should eat leafy greens, such as spinach and kale, on a daily basis, along with a variety of other vegetables and fruits that are in season.

WHAT ABOUT SPROUTS?

Sprouts are awesome. Try and include them in your diet whenever possible. Most people are not aware of the immense variety of sprouts that are available: Alfalfa sprouts, broccoli sprouts, bean sprouts, sprouted sunflower seeds, sprouted almonds, and the list goes on.

Sprouts are young plants; they are just like a kid; they have a lot of nutrition inside of them; they are extremely nutrient dense.

EAT YOUR FRUITS & VEGGIES IN THE RAW!

Raw fruits and vegetables have all of the enzymes and nutrients inside of them that your body requires in order to break down and digest them. Vegetables and fruits eaten in their raw form add nutrients to your body, making it better able for you to maintain a healthy weight and fight off sickness and disease. As you learned earlier, cooking destroys vital enzymes, which can put a huge burden on your body. **Remember, its all about the enzymes!**

I have included with this manual a sample list of beneficial foods to eat. You truly do have all of the information you need to achieve vibrant health within this course.

REMEMBER

If you can take away one thing today, know that organic really is a big deal and do your best to get it from locally grown sources. It sounds a little activist like, but you have to be aware of what is going on with our food supply, because it's for your health and the health of your family. You have to lead by example, and then others will catch on and join in. It really is that important.

9

INTRODUCTION TO MEAT

OVERVIEW

There are many schools of thought when it comes to meat. Some groups claim that meat is the best source of protein on the planet. Other groups claim that the protein in meat is not bioavailable and the best source of protein is obtained from plant sources which have a much higher rate of bioavailability.

The purpose of *Better Living With Whole Foods* and the *16 Week Total Body Makeover* is not to turn you into a meat eater, vegetarian, or vegan. The purpose of these programs is to help you look and feel your absolute best. These programs work for vegetarians, vegans, and meat eaters alike.

Which leads us to...

DO YOU NEED TO EAT MEAT TO BE HEALTHY?

The answer is no, you don't need to eat meat in order to be healthy. As a matter of fact, eating commercial meat is very unhealthy. Good clean healthy meats eaten in moderation can be nutritious, but they are not essential to optimal health.

Take a look at the *Before* and *After* pictures of myself. The B*efore* picture is me eating processed and refined foods as well as a ton of commercial meat; mostly beef and chicken. The *After* picture is me on a healthy diet of vegetables, fruits, and some raw dairy. I have never felt more vibrant and full of life since adopting my vegetarian lifestyle in January of 2004.

MY FIT LIFE

I became a vegetarian for three main reasons:

1. You have to basically be a detective when it comes to eating meat. It is so hard to find quality beef, chicken, and fish that I came to the conclusion that it would be much easier to be healthy as a vegetarian.

2. I believe that it is easier to obtain good quality protein, that my body can actually absorb, from vegetables and raw dairy.

3. If I had to kill an animal, skin it, and clean it, I would not be a meat eater.

This is my personal choice. I do not expect everyone to become a vegetarian just because I am. However, the one thing I do suggest is that you limit your consumption of meat; 2 to 3 times per week is plenty for most people.

That being said, the one principal that I believe everybody can agree on is the fact that it is crucial to your health and well being to make the most informed and healthful decisions when choosing the types of food that you eat; and meat is no exception.

Reason being, commercial meats are subjected to a whole myriad of unhealthful practices that are detrimental to your health, including:

- Unnatural Diet
- Crowded and Contaminated Living Conditions
- Pesticides
- Hormones and Antibiotics
- Irradiation
- Virus Injections
- Dyes
- Cloning

We will discuss each of these harmful practices in detail throughout this section.

PESTICIDES IN MEAT?

Studies have shown that commercial meat and dairy products contain higher levels of pesticides than commercial vegetables or fruits. Reason being, grains which commercial animals are fed are subjected to higher levels of pesticide contamination than the vegetables, fruits, and grains that are grown for human consumption. And the animals soak these pesticides into their fat and muscle.

This is a key indicator that we need to eat foods that are free of pesticides and herbicides. If commercial farm animals contain high levels of pesticides in their muscle and fat from eating contaminated food, then, if we eat foods (meat, dairy, vegetables, fruits, etc.) that are contaminated with high levels of pesticides, we will absorb these harmful substances into our muscle and fat cells as well.

ARE YOU EATING CLONED MEAT?

Cloning is the most recent in an ever growing list of concerns in our food supply.

FDA Alert:

FDA announced on Thursday December 28th, 2006 preliminary approval of milk and meat from cloned animals and their offspring to enter the human food supply. Despite public outcry, FDA has not recommended these products be labeled if approved.

In other words, in the near future, the meat and dairy products found on the shelves of your local grocery stores may come from that of cloned animals. To make matters worse, these meat and dairy products will not be labeled as such.

Nobody knows the effect that consuming cloned animal products will have on our health and well being... not the FDA or anyone else. The consequences could be severe. This is further proof that the FDA does not have our best interests at heart and why you need to be as informed as you possibly can when it comes to the food that you and your loved ones will be eating.

MEAT CONTAMINATION

I want to make sure that you have a clear understanding of the impact that unhealthy meat has on our society. The following is an excerpt from a pamphlet distributed by Earth Save International, which is titled *Our Food Our Future: Making A Difference With Every Bite:*

> Eating a meat-centered diet is not only linked to lethargy, obesity, and the development of certain diseases, but also to life-threatening cases of food poisoning, antibiotic resistance, and

other problems. **Every year in the U.S., there are 75 million cases of food poisoning, with 5,000 of these cases being fatal. According to the USDA, 70 percent of food poisoning is caused by contaminated animal flesh.**

Explains Dr. Michael Greger, Director of Public Health and Animal Agriculture at The Humane Society of the United States, **"Farmed animals today are sick, these are sick and diseased chickens, pigs, fish, and cows, producing diseased and bacteria-laden flesh and pus-filled milk that even industry standards call 'unhealthful.'"**

Fecal matter in meat is a matter of grave concern. Not only are the cow's hides covered in manure when taken to the slaughterhouse, but their digestive tracts are often cut open and spill onto the contents during slaughter. Due to fast line speeds, workers cut so fast they have little time to examine each carcass, and can carve up 60 cows an hour. Food that comes in contact with fecal material can result in the dangerous pathogenic bacteria, E. coli.

—Our Food Our Future, Earth Save International
(www.vegpledge.com)

Let's put this information into perspective: Every year there are approximately 55 million reported cases of food poisoning due to contaminated meat, resulting in thousands of deaths every year. These statistics are alarming to me and they should be to you too, especially if you have children.

That being said, let's take a look at the bad and the good of individual meat products including beef, fish, chicken, and pork...

10

BEEF

The two main points of this section:

1. Commercial beef is bad for you.

2. Grass fed free range beef can be good for you.

THE COMMERCIAL BEEF INDUSTRY

The commercial beef industry is a huge lobbying force in Washington D.C. They are very influential in the FDA as well as with individual politicians including congressmen all the way up to the president of the United States.

WHY IS COMMERCIAL BEEF BAD FOR ME?

- Commercial cattle live in deplorable conditions.
- Commercial cattle are subjected to high amounts of growth hormones, antibiotics, and pesticides.
- Commercial cattle are grain fed.

- Commercial beef is subjected to irradiation, virus injections, and harmful dyes.

- Commercial beef may be cloned.

Most of the beef found in your local grocery store and almost all of the beef found in restaurants is not beneficial for you to eat. This commercial beef is derived from very unhealthy cattle.

Commercial feed lots commonly house 10,000 or more head of cattle. These cattle are forced to live in crowded conditions in their own mud and feces; ideal conditions for sickness and disease to proliferate. Additionally, these cattle are injected with growth hormones and steroids, so they will grow at a more rapid rate.

In addition, these cattle are given massive amounts of antibiotics in order to fight off the sickness and disease they are subjected to from the hormones they are forced to ingest, as well as the horrid conditions they are forced to live in. **Antibiotics and hormones soak into the muscle and fat of the beef, which we end up eating and absorbing into our systems.**

WHAT IS A FEED LOT OR A HEAD OF CATTLE?

- A commercial feed lot is the confined quarters in which cattle are forced to live. As mentioned above, commercial feed lots house thousands of cattle in an unnatural environment.

- A head of cattle is simply one cow or bull.

WHY ARE COMMERCIAL CATTLE SUBJECTED TO THESE HARMFUL PRACTICES?

Commercial cattle are subjected to these harmful practices in order to get them to slaughter quicker. In other words, **it's all about money**. Never mind the fact that their finished product is harmful for human consumption!

A head of cattle raised on a commercial feed lot that is given hormones and antibiotics will be ready for slaughter as young as 14 months. Grass fed free range cattle that are not subjected to antibiotics and hormones will be ready for slaughter after about 3 years. In other words, it takes twice as long to raise a healthy head of cattle for slaughter, which translates into more overhead and less profit. This is not conducive to big business.

IRRADIATION, VIRUS INJECTIONS, & HARMFUL DYES

Despite the use of massive amounts of antibiotics in cattle, sickness and disease proliferate in commercial feedlots and slaughter houses. Because of this, commercial beef is often

FIT FACT

The hormones, antibiotics, and pesticides that cattle are subjected to affects us as a population. Many of the children in the U.S. are much bigger than they were just a few decades ago. Part of the reason for this is the hormones that are contained in the meat that they eat.

Another interesting fact to consider is the average age of a girl's first menstrual cycle. During the 1970's, the average age of a girl's first menstrual cycle was 14 years old. Today, the average age of a girl's first menstrual cycle is 8 years old. This really is crazy, and it's directly correlated to the hormones in the meat and dairy products that we as a nation consume on a daily basis.

irradiated in order to kill harmful bacteria that remain. However, these high levels of radiation do not kill all of the harmful bacteria that are present in the beef.

You would think that the FDA would require the beef industry to clean up its act in order to prevent the spread of these harmful bacteria, but this is not the case. In the latter part of 2006 the FDA okayed the use of virus injections in commercial beef to kill harmful bacteria. I don't know about you, but it doesn't make sense to me to inject our food supply with a virus in order to kill harmful bacteria. It is not known what this virus will do to the human population, but the FDA has okayed its use anyway.

To make matters worse, commercial beef is often injected with harmful dyes. These harmful dyes are injected into beef for two main reasons:

1. To give beef a more pleasing appearance.

2. To give beef a longer shelf life.

These types of unhealthful practices are a common theme with the FDA. It is obvious that the commercial agri-business and the FDA do not have our best interests at heart. They are clearly more concerned with making money than with human welfare.

Hopefully, you are beginning to see a common theme with the food available for your consumption:

1. **Most of the food readily available for human consumption is unhealthy; it has the ability to promote sickness and disease.**

2. **There *are* healthy food choices; you just have to know what they are.**

The above two statements highlight the reasons that you are reading this course; to make the most informed and healthful choices for you and your loved ones. Which leads us to...

IS THERE A BETTER CHOICE?

Yes, there is. Unfortunately it's hard to find, although it's becoming more accessible as demand grows. The type of beef I'm referring to comes from grass fed free-range cattle that have not been subjected to antibiotics, hormones, and pesticide laden grains. In order to fully understand the benefits of grass fed beef, I conducted an interview with a local cattle rancher in Trabuco Canyon, California (South Orange County).

Frank Fitzpatrick has been raising grass fed cattle for 30 years. He raises his cattle as simple and pure as he possibly can:

* Free Range
* Grass Fed
* No Antibiotics
* No Hormones
* No Pesticides or Herbicides

He has not bred an outside bull into his cattle in the entire 30 years. He has owned every single mother, father, grandmother, grandfather, and so on... of every head of cattle on his ranch for 14 ½ generations.

WHY GRASS FED CATTLE?

Over 30 years ago when he was working towards his animal science degree at Cal Poly San Luis Obispo, Frank discovered that it takes 32 pounds of grain to make one pound of beef protein.

His thinking: "With millions of people starving all over the world, why would you harvest 32 pounds of grain and put it in an animal that can feed off of marginal ground that cannot be used for farming? Why not change the species of what you plant (the crop) to grow 25 pounds of human food? It seemed ridiculous."

Frank started out with the concept of raising his cattle from conception to the plate entirely on grass. He has been doing this for 30 years. He believes that his meat is "health food", makes you feel better, and having it in your diet is a benefit to your life.

I have personally visited Frank Fitzpatrick's cattle ranch as well as a variety of commercial feed-lots throughout California. Frank's cattle look much healthier than the sickly cattle housed at commercial feed lots. There is no doubt in my mind that his beef is immensely healthier than commercial grain fed beef.

WHAT ARE THE BENEFITS OF GRASS FED FREE RANGE CATTLE?

The most apparent benefits are the fact that these cattle are free of pesticides, herbicides, antibiotics, and hormones. Also, the beef from these cattle are not subjected to irradiation, virus injections, or harmful dyes.

HEALTHY FATS

One of the biggest benefits to grass fed cattle as opposed to grain fed cattle are the beneficial omega-3 fatty acids contained in grass fed cattle. Remember that the Standard American Diet (SAD) has an unhealthy omega-3 to omega-6 fatty acid ratio of as high as 1:50. The suggested ratio is 1:1. Grass fed cattle has an omega-3 to omega-6 fatty acid ratio of 1 to .16, which is 7 or 8 times the amount of omega-3 fatty acids compared to omega-6. Grain fed cattle has an unhealthy omega-3 to omega-6 fatty acid ratio of 1 to 20. In other words, there are 800 times more omega-3 fatty acids in grass fed cattle than in grain fed cattle.

> *"From a health food standpoint, the grain fed animal*
> *doesn't stand a chance. It produces fats that will clog*
> *your arteries and stop your heart"*
>
> — Frank Fitzpatrick

Another health benefit of grass fed beef is its CLA content. CLA is a fatty acid that is claimed to help prevent you from getting cancer or reduce it if you have it.

HISTORY CHANNEL FACTOID

The history channel aired a segment on American feed lots. They were filming from a feed lot that housed 600,000 head of cattle. Can you believe that? 600,000 head of cattle!

During this segment they posted a factoid stating, "God intended cows to eat grass not grain; fully 50% of the bicarbonate of soda produced in America is fed to feed lot cattle to cure chronic indigestion."

I find it interesting that the two most common over the counter drugs sold in the United States are antacids and pain relievers to relieve chronic indigestion and body aches and pains. Now, here's the point that should be of interest to you: Chronic indigestion and body aches and pains are a direct result of eating processed grains, sugars, plant oils, and meat that is fed an unnatural grain fed diet.

People are convinced that they can eat whatever they want; when they become ill, all they have to do is go to the doctor and he will fix you.

> *"People have to be responsible for their own health; a cow is, why shouldn't you? The only way to get a cow to eat something wrong is to put a fence around it and feed it something unnatural. Cattle that eat unnatural feed are like humans that sit at home and eat M&M's; they are not happy, they are not healthy."*
>
> — Frank Fitzpatrick

Taking the time to learn how to eat well and exercise effectively not only makes you look better, but you will feel better, and ultimately live better. This is the underlying principal of what I teach and the tagline for my company: *Look Better. Feel Better. Live Better™*.

SUPPORT LOCAL FARMERS

If you eat beef, purchase it from local sources, as opposed to buying beef from other countries. Buying from farmers such as Frank Fitzpatrick is great because it sustains local farmers. It allows them to keep doing what they are doing. Without your support they will slowly disappear and so will your freedom of choice.

REMEMBER, LOCAL IS THE NEW ORGANIC!

WHAT DOES ALL OF THIS MEAN TO ME?

There are 4 main points that you need to take from this section:

1. Find a local source of healthy grass fed beef.

2. Avoid commercial grain fed beef at all costs.

3. Eat beef in moderation.

4. Your beef should not contain any of the following:
   - Antibiotics
   - Hormones
   - Pesticides
   - Irradiation
   - Virus Injections
   - Dyes

11

CHICKEN

Many people have turned to chicken as a healthy alternative to conventional red meat. However, most chickens are raised in horrid conditions.

HOW THEY LIVE

I recently viewed a documentary on the Internet which showed the horrible conditions in which chickens are forced to live. In fact, chickens are quite possibly subjected to the most inhumane conditions of all livestock. For instance, it is common practice to clip off the beaks of chickens in order to prevent them from pecking each other and the people who raise them.

Most of the chickens available on our grocery store shelves were raised in huge warehouse like pens which house as many as 30,000 chickens. They live in very crowded conditions where they can barely move throughout their entire lives. This is a very unhealthy situation in which sickness and disease run rampant. Because of this, large doses of antibiotics are administered to the chickens. Many times the antibiotics are sprayed on the chickens at timed intervals throughout the day. They literally live in a cloud of antibiotics that soak into every part of them. To make matters worse, antibiotic resistant bacteria have been found on chicken bought from the grocery store.

Moreover, these chickens are given high doses of growth hormones in order to get them to market faster. In the 1950's it took 84 days to raise a five pound chicken. Today, due to growth promoting drugs, it takes only 45 days. Many times the chickens' muscles grow faster than their joints can handle, which causes them to be very feeble. These poor chickens are unable to support their own body weight.

Also, the chickens' diet consists of genetically modified grains that are subjected to high amounts of pesticides. All of these substances, antibiotics, hormones, and pesticides, soak into their muscle and fat, which we eat.

DIRTY BIRDS

In January of 2007, Consumer Reports released a study in which they analyzed fresh, whole chickens bought in grocery stores across the nation. 83% of the chickens they tested harbored campylobacter or salmonella, which are the leading causes of food born illness. I will say that again, 83% of the chickens they tested harbored bacteria that are the leading causes of food born illness! This is a dramatic increase from their last study in 2003 where they found that 49% of the chickens were positive for one or both of those bacteria.

WHAT SHOULD YOU DO?

Be very careful when selecting chickens at the supermarket. Today, most chickens are factory raised. You may have to do some investigating to find chickens that are raised on smaller farms in healthy and humane conditions.

Although it does not guarantee that chickens will be free of harmful bacteria, purchase chickens that are organically raised, pasture raised or free range, and free of antibiotics and hormones. Smaller local farms that follow these guidelines are a little more conscious to the world. And they will usually be your best bet. **Note:** Look at the glossary in the back of this course to understand the differences between pasture raised and free range chickens.

Make sure to check the Recommended Resources section in the back of this manual to locate beneficial sources of pasture raised organic chickens.

12

FISH

Fish are an excellent source of protein and the omega 3 fatty acids EPA and DHA, which are essential to our bodies. As mentioned earlier, the omega 3 fatty acids EPA and DHA are essential to proper brain function, the integrity of your cell walls, and a whole host of other functions. However, all fish are not created equal. The type of fish, as well as the environment in which they are raised, will determine their nutritional benefits, if any.

WHAT ABOUT MERCURY?

There has been a lot of coverage in the media regarding high levels of mercury found in fish. The oceans and many lakes have become polluted with mercury, which the fish then ingest. Mercury is extremely toxic to your body. It is best to avoid contact with mercury at all costs. Note: Because of their longer life span, larger fish, such as tuna, accumulate more mercury than smaller fish.

WHAT SHOULD I DO?

It is best to eat coldwater fish raised in the wild. Remember, smaller fish are preferred over larger fish.

According to Dr. Joseph Mercola, the following six fish are the safest to choose from:

- Wild Pacific Salmon
- Tilapia
- Croaker
- Sardines
- Haddock
- Summer Flounder

Make sure the fish that you eat comes from the wild. Wild Pacific Salmon is the type of fish that I recommend the most.

WHAT ABOUT FARM RAISED FISH?

The concept of farm raised fish sounds nice, but it's not. **Never eat farm raised fish.**

6 reasons to stay away from farm raised fish:

1. They live in crowded conditions that promote sickness and disease.

2. They are subjected to large amounts of antibiotics and other drugs.

3. For economical reasons fish are fed a diet, such as grains, that they would not normally eat in the wild.

4. The abnormal diet of farm raised fish does not form the beneficial omega 3 fatty acids EPA and DHA.

5. Farm raised fish may contain high levels of pesticides due to their diet and contaminated water ways.

6. **Harmful dyes are added to make the fish more appealing to the eye. Farm raised fish are usually grey in color. Yuck!**

Grocery stores usually have signs next to each type of fish that they sell stating whether they are farm raised or wild. If you're in doubt as to the origin of the fish, simply ask the butcher, he will be more than happy to tell you its origins.

Wild fish is usually available in most supermarkets. If they don't have it, then don't get it; it's that important. There really is a world of difference.

LIVING GREEN

More than 90 percent of the world's swordfish, marlin, giant tuna, and other large predatory fishes have been caught by far roaming industrial fishing fleets. In other words, these fish are in danger of becoming extinct. Case in point: Atlantic swordfish filets now come from fish that average 90 pounds, down from 400 pounds a century ago. 90 pounds sounds big for a fish, until you hear that females can't reproduce until they weigh at least 150 pounds. If fish are caught before they are able to reproduce, they will cease to exist.

— "Green Living," by the editors of *E*/The Environmental Magazine.

FOOD FOR THOUGHT

Stay away from shellfish. They are bottom feeders that are the most toxic of all fish. Environmental agencies use the levels of toxic substances found in shellfish as a gauge for reporting the levels of toxicity in the waters in which the shellfish are found.

REMEMBER

- It is best to eat coldwater fish caught in the wild.
- Stay away from farm raised fish.
- Smaller fish are preferred over larger fish.
- Eliminate or severely limit your intake of shellfish.

13

PORK

In my twenty years of professional experience I have found that it is best to stay away from pork and pork products, especially if your goal is weight loss.

You will be able to find arguments both in favor and against the consumption of pork, but I have never seen anybody achieve lasting weight loss success while pork remained a part of their diet. There are plenty of other foods available that we *know* are healthy.

HERE'S MY REASONING

Pigs and swine are filthy animals. They live in horrid conditions. Pigs are bottom feeders just like shellfish. They eat whatever slop that is put in front of them. They'll even eat their young. It's just wrong.

Additionally, from conception to the shelves of your local supermarket, more than 90% of the pigs raised in America are subjected to the most horrible conditions imaginable; conditions that are not only inhumane, but also promote sickness and disease on a massive scale.

14

DELI MEATS

Deli meats are generally not beneficial for achieving lasting weight loss success. They are generally high in fat and contain preservatives such as nitrates, sulfides, and MSG, all of which are detrimental to your health and fitness.

Although I do not recommend eating deli meats, I do realize that there may be times that you do use them. Picnics, a day at the beach, kids' birthday party, etc. As always, do the best you can for the situation you are in. Look for sources that are free of preservatives. Whole turkey or chicken breast will generally be better for you than salami. If at all possible, buy freshly sliced deli meats that are prepared in the supermarket and free of MSG. If nothing else, you can be sure that the turkey meat came from a real turkey.

FOOD FOR THOUGHT

MSG is found in almost every type of packaged food including deli meats, potato chips, soups, and salad dressing. Fast food restaurants, including McDonalds and KFC, are notorious for their use of MSG. Also known as hydrolyzed vegetable protein, MSG is very detrimental to your health; it has been shown to cause obesity, migraines, and is thought to contribute to Alzheimer's. In his book, The Slow Poisoning of America (www.spofamerica. com), John Erb states that MSG is added to food for the addictive effect it has on the human body... the reason they add it to food is to make people eat more. No wonder we crave junk food!

MSG is often hidden under a variety of names on labels such as:

- Hydrolyzed Vegetable Protein
- Hydrolyzed Protein
- Hydrolyzed Plant Protein
- Plant Protein Extract
- Sodium Caseinate
- Calcium Caseinate
- Yeast Extract
- Textured Protein
- Autolyzed Yeast
- Hydrolyzed Oat Flour
- Flavoring
- Natural Flavoring
- Natural Beef or Chicken Flavoring

15

DAIRY

Milk and other dairy products are another of the categories of foods where there is a lot of misinformation and scare tactics used to fool you into drinking and eating products that are detrimental to your health.

The two main points of this section:

* Commercial Pasteurized milk is bad (unhealthy) for you.

* Organic Raw milk is good (healthy) for you.

It is the intension of this discussion to give you a clear understanding of exactly why the above two points are true.

GOT MILK?

The "Got Milk" campaign is one of the most successful marketing campaigns ever. With the onslaught of celebrity advertisements in every type of media, it is hard to accept the fact that commercial pasteurized milk could actually be bad for us.

Well, I'm here to tell you that not only is commercial pasteurized milk bad for you, but you should do everything you can to avoid it.

WHY IS COMMERCIAL DAIRY BAD FOR YOU?

- Commercial cows live in deplorable conditions.
- Commercial cows are subjected to high amounts of growth hormones, antibiotics, and pesticides.
- Commercial cows are grain fed.
- Commercial dairy is pasteurized.
- Commercial milk is comingled in central creameries.

I will expand on these points in a moment, but first...

WHAT ABOUT ORGANIC MILK?

Organic milk is still going to be bad for you. It sounds better, but it's not. Organic milk is free of antibiotics and hormones, so it *is* healthier than conventional milk in that respect. However, organic milk is subjected to the same unhealthful practices as conventional commercial milk.

Organic commercial milk comes from cows that live in deplorable conditions and are grain fed. Organic milk is also comingled in central creameries and pasteurized. You will soon learn the dramatic effect these unhealthful practices have on milk and dairy products whether they are organic or not.

> *"Organic dairies in the United States did not start out as organic dairies; they started out as conventional dairies in deep financial distress."*

> —Mark McAfee, Organic Pastures

WHY IS ORGANIC RAW MILK FROM GRASS FED COWS GOOD FOR YOU?

- Pasture (grass) fed cows live in much better conditions than their commercial counterparts.
- Organic cows are not subjected to growth hormones, antibiotics, or pesticides.
- Grass is a cow's natural diet.
- Organic raw milk is not pasteurized.
- Organic raw milk contains a broad spectrum of beneficial bacteria.

ORGANIC PASTURES

The following information was derived from interviews and discussions with Mark McAfee, founder/owner of Organic Pastures (www.organicpastures.com), an organic raw dairy farm in Central California.

According to Mark McAfee, all organic foods start out alive, but many of them are murdered along the way; milk and milk products are probably the most murdered of them all.

WHAT IS PASTEURIZATION?

Pasteurization is a process by which a substance, such as milk, is subjected to high amounts of heat for a short period

---

FIT FACT

Negative Phosphatase Test: The test that determines whether milk is pasteurized or not is called the negative phosphatase test. Milk is not considered pasteurized until this vital substance is destroyed. So, what is phosphatase? Phosphatase is the enzyme in milk that enables you to absorb calcium. Without phosphatase you cannot absorb the calcium contained in the milk. Isn't that a shame?

---

of time. This harmful process basically kills everything inside the milk. Vital enzymes, beneficial bacteria, and delicate vitamins and minerals are all destroyed through the process of pasteurization.

HISTORY

In the early 1900's the United States was in the process of converting from an agricultural (farm) based economy to an economy based on industry (factories).

In New York and Boston, large factories, such as breweries, were developing large amounts of waste that they didn't know what to do with. There were no good sources of sanitation at this time.

Well, somewhere along the way, these breweries figured out that cows would eat this "brewer's mash". The factory owners brought in cows to live in pens directly outside of the breweries. This seemed like a wonderful idea. The factory owners didn't have to lose money disposing of the brewer's mash and they could make money from the milk of the cows. However, the cows now lived in deplorable conditions. They lived in tight quarters, with no sunlight. These poor cows lived in mud and their own feces; much like commercial cows do today (It's strange how history repeats itself).

In those days, harmful bacteria and viruses were not yet understood. In fact, doctors were still arguing over the need to wash their hands before surgery. Needless to say that sickness and disease flourished among these factory cows. People, especially children, were becoming violently ill and many were dying from this bad milk. Meanwhile, grass fed, hill raised cows did not have these problems.

When Louis Pasteur discovered pasteurization, it seemingly solved everybody's problems. Pasteurization basically sterilized the milk, thus killing all of the harmful bacteria. Pasteurization was a good thing back then, but we now know the importance of cleanliness and proper hygiene. Pasteurization is not necessary in our modern world.

But the fact of the matter is, commercial cows today still live in horrid conditions, in mud and their own feces. Sickness and disease proliferate in these conditions. These same cows are also subjected to growth hormones to make them produce more milk than they normally would, they are fed high amounts of antibiotics to keep them alive while they are living in sickness and disease, and they are subjected to an unnatural grain fed diet that is contaminated with high amounts of pesticides and genetic modifications.

Remember what we just learned in the beef section of this manual: Cows that ingest growth hormones, antibiotics, and pesticide laden grain transfer all of these substances into their meat and dairy. We, in turn, ingest these same harmful substances. What a shame.

Also, remember that grain is unnatural for cows to eat because of the biology of their stomachs. The fats in the milk from a grain fed diet will be high in omega-6 and have very little omega-3 fatty acids. These unhealthy ratios wreak havoc on your body.

The fats in the milk from a grass fed cow will be high in omega-3 fatty acids and contain very little omega-6 fatty acids; which is what you want.

WHY IS MILK STILL PASTEURIZED?

You are probably asking yourself these questions by now:

1. Why is milk still pasteurized?

2. Why doesn't our government do anything about these harmful practices?

3. Why can't I find organic raw milk on the shelves of my local grocery store?

PASTEURIZATION COMES DOWN TO MONEY, MEDIA, AND GOVERNMENT

If raw milk were to become readily accepted, the commercial dairy industry would lose a ton of money (once again, it's all about money).

In order for a commercial dairy farm to convert over to an organic, grass fed, raw dairy farm, there would be a huge clean-up expense. Also, a 10,000 cow dairy farm would become a 1,000 or 500 cow dairy farm. This is bad news for the commercial dairy industry, but it's great news for individual farmers and consumers. It's bad news for the commercial dairy industry because it's not in line with their current practices. These powerful corporations have built their entire businesses around pasteurization and they make a ton of money in the process.

The National Dairy Council has a very strong lobby. They are extremely powerful. They are in bed with state and national governments. For instance, "Got Milk" is part of the California Milk Advisory Board (CMAB) which is a government appointed board.

RAW MILK IS ILLEGAL IN MOST STATES

In California, where I live, I am privileged to be able obtain raw milk legally. It's illegal in most states. If it were up to the National Dairy Council, raw milk would be illegal in every state. In fact the FDA is constantly doing everything they can to shut down raw milk operations in California. Thankfully, California's largest raw dairy farm, Organic Pastures, is willing to fight the FDA and the National Dairy Council for the right to provide raw milk to an ever growing legion of consumers.

MILK FROM 1,000 DIFFERENT COWS

A national news report once stated that a McDonald's hamburger could contain the beef from 1,000 different cows. Well, the same principle applies with milk. A carton of milk could contain milk from 1,000 different cows! Yes, you read that right.

Here's the deal. Individual commercial farms do not have their own creameries. Milk from many different farms is taken to a central creamery where it's processed, pasteurized, and bottled. Because of this, it doesn't matter if one farm uses good farming practices. If the other farms use standard (bad) farming practices, the milk from the one good farm is comingled with the other bad milk at the central creamery. Get the picture?

STANDARDS AND PRACTICES

In order for milk or dairy products to be considered safe for human consumption the bacteria count has to be below 15,000. Commercial milk routinely has a bacteria count of 75,000 up to 150,000. Some of this is harmful bacteria which contain pathogens that can make us very sick. They pasteurize the milk until the bacteria count is below a 15,000 count. However, the dead bacteria cells are still present in the milk. To make matters worse, these dead cells break open and release histamines.

The histamines released in the milk causes kids and adults to have allergic reactions, kids more so than adults, because kids tend to drink more milk than adults.

Well meaning parents tend to feed their children a lot of milk because they figure that it will give their children strong bones. However, we learned previously that the phosphatase in pasteurized milk is killed off. And we cannot absorb the calcium in milk if the phosphatase is not present. So it's just a big lie.

A VERY SPECIAL FARM

Organic Pastures is a very special farm. The cows are grass fed, so the fat contained in their milk is going to have high amounts of omega-3 fatty acids. The Organic Pastures cows live on green organic pastures. They change pastures on a regular basis, so there is never a huge buildup of feces and other contaminants. The grass that they eat is fresh. They eat the grass. The saliva from their mouths goes back in the earth, and it replenishes the earth. It's an extremely biodiverse environment.

One of the qualities I like best about Organic Pastures is the fact that you can visit their farm. They will actually give you a tour of their facilities. They have nothing to hide. Try doing that at a commercial dairy farm!

THEY BRING THE BARN TO THE COWS

Usually, cows that are grass fed have to walk through mud and feces to get to the barn for milking, which can be very unsanitary.

Because of this, Organic Pastures invented a portable milking station. They actually drive the milking station to the pasture that the cows happen to be on on that particular week. This makes the conditions as clean as they possibly can be.

There has never been a pathogen found in Organic Pastures milk and they check on a regular basis.

The Organic Pastures raw milk has a bacteria count of about 2,500. Way below the 15,000 requirement. **And, it is all beneficial bacteria.**

ISN'T BACTERIA BAD FOR YOU?

We don't understand our immune system. We have over 750 trillion bacterial cells in our body, more bacterial cells than mammalian cells by count. In fact, 75-80% of your immune system is made up of the biological diversity of beneficial bacteria in your intestines. Today, beneficial bacteria are more commonly known as **probiotics**.

IMMUNE DEPRESSION IS RAMPANT IN AMERICA

The American consumer by definition is immune depressed. This is why you are susceptible to sickness, disease, and cancer.

Antibiotics are immune depressants. They kill off the diversity of biological living bacteria in your intestines. In other words, antibiotics not only kill the bad bacteria in your body, but also the beneficial bacteria, which are needed for the proper digestion and absorption of the foods that you eat.

Preservatives kill bacteria in our food, which means that they also kill bacteria in our gut. Look at preservatives in our food. What do they do? They kill bacteria. They extend shelf life; they keep things from breaking down. Precisely what needs to happen when food enters your body; it needs to break down immediately, so it can become completely bioavailable. This is critical to absorption and utilization of nutrients.

Radiated foods are absolutely sterile. There is no good source of additional probiotic bacteria in our sterile food diet. It's an astronaut's diet. The astronauts no longer eat a sterile food diet because they become immune depressed in space.

> **Pasteurized dairy is sterilized. In other words, pasteurized dairy leads to immune depression.**

The Standard American Diet (SAD) is devoid of beneficial bacteria; it's literally sterilized.

Some of the problems associated with immune depression include:

- Inflammation
- Asthma
- Irritable Bowel Syndrome (IBS)
- Colitis
- Candida
- Lactose Intolerance
- Eczema (skin disorders)

PROBIOTICS

Today, people want beneficial bacteria in their foods. Consumers are seeking out whole living foods in order to take care of their sterile immune system. There is a lot of work that needs to be done in this country to give people a better understanding of how this all works. This is why raw milk is so important.

> *"Raw milk is Mother Nature's original probiotic food."*
>
> — Mark McAfee

WHAT ABOUT YOGURT?

Yogurt found on grocery store shelves is made from pasteurized dairy. It usually contains 4 types of beneficial bacteria. Raw milk contains about 24 different types of beneficial bacteria. This means that raw milk contains beneficial bacteria at levels 800 times greater in diversity than the very best commercial yogurts.

However, if you do decide to eat yogurt, make sure there are no artificial sweeteners contained in it. No sucralose, no aspartame, and no cane sugar. Your best bet when it comes to yogurt would be to eat plain organic yogurt and put in your own organic fruit to sweeten it up.

BUTTER VS. MARGARINE

Always choose natural organic butter over margarine. Butter from commercial sources has the same problems as commercial meat and dairy. Most notably: hormones, antibiotics, and pesticides. Organic butter, especially raw organic butter, is an excellent source of beneficial fats as well as the fat soluble vitamins A, D, E, and K. Basically, beneficial sources of organic raw butter have the same benefits as organic raw milk.

On the other hand, margarine is made from highly refined and processed vegetable oils. The refining process causes margarine to turn grey in color and have a foul rancid odor. Margarine must be bleached, dyed, and flavored in order to make it more appealing to consumers. For this reason, margarine should be avoided at all costs. It does not matter if they are trans-fat free or not. All margarines are detrimental to your health. You will learn more about processed and refined vegetable oils in the oils section of this manual.

WHAT ABOUT ICE CREAM?

Ice cream is something best to leave for your "cheat day". **Note**: the concept of the "cheat day" is discussed in detail in the Putting It All Together section of this course. Every once in a while it's okay to eat some bad stuff. Just know that that is what you're doing. As far as digestion is concerned, drinking raw milk inoculates your intestines with beneficial bacteria. So, when you do eat something like ice cream, you will be able to process through it because of the beneficial bacteria which remains in your small intestines.

When you eat something like ice cream just know that it's bad, and that's what it is. Don't try to fool yourself into thinking that it's something that's good for you, it's not. Every once in a while it's okay to eat some bad stuff; we are all human. Just enjoy it for that day and don't eat it every day.

REMEMBER

- Drink organic grass fed raw milk if it is available.
- Don't drink pasteurized milk; avoid it at all costs.
- If raw milk is not available; don't drink milk.

16

EGGS

Eggs are similar to chickens. The quality of your eggs is directly related to the quality of the chickens that lay them.

Qualities to look for in your eggs:

- Contain the omega-3 fatty acids (DHA & EPA).
- Pastured or pasture raised on smaller (local) farms.
- Organically fed.

It is definitely very beneficial to purchase organic omega-3 eggs with DHA and EPA.

Some egg cartons will even say, DHA and EPA omega-3 on them. With omega-3 eggs you definitely want to eat the yolks, because that is where the fat is, which is where the omega-3 fatty acids are.

A free range, organically raised chicken will produce eggs with an optimal omega-3:omega-6 fatty acid ratio of 1:1 to 1:4. However, a commercially raised chicken will produce eggs with an omega-3:omega-6 ratio of as high as 1:30. Remember, an excess of omega-6 fatty acids will cause inflammatory responses in your body.

A recent study conducted by *Mother Earth News* showed that true free range eggs are far more nutritious than commercially raised eggs. Compared to official U.S. Department of Agriculture nutrient data for commercial eggs, eggs from chickens raised on pasture may contain:

- 1/3 less cholesterol
- 1/4 less saturated fat
- 2/3 more vitamin A
- 2 times more omega-3 fatty acids
- 3 times more vitamin E
- 7 times more beta carotene

The diet of an organic pasture raised chicken is dramatically different than that of a commercially raised chicken. The key here is in obtaining eggs from truly free range or pasture raised chickens.

WHICH EGGS SHOULD YOU BUY?

Let me make this perfectly clear, the most important factor when choosing eggs is that they be organic and free range from a verifiable source. Smaller local farms are preferable. Omega 3 DHA and EPA eggs are preferred if they are organic and pasture raised, but they should be avoided if they are from commercial sources. If they don't say organic free range or cage free on the carton, do not buy them.

As with every other food choice, the type of egg that you choose to eat can be the difference between optimal health and poor health.

WHAT ABOUT THE YOLKS?

Two questions that women always ask me when I say it's okay to eat the yolks of the egg:

1. What about the cholesterol in the yolks?

2. What about the amount of fat in the yolks?

The cholesterol found in the yolks of the omega-3 eggs is beneficial cholesterol. There is good cholesterol, and bad cholesterol. If you didn't have any cholesterol in your system you would die. Cholesterol has gotten a bad rap just like saturated fat has. There are good saturated fats, and there is good cholesterol, but there are many more sources of bad ones. If you are eating fat and cholesterol from a beneficial source, then it is going to be beneficial for you. If it's from a commercial source or bad source then it's going to be bad for you. However, if you are the type of person that likes to take the yolks out and only eat the egg whites, this is what I suggest:

If you are going to eat three eggs, take out two of the yolks and leave one of the yolks in. Doing this will provide you with a low fat alternative to obtaining your omega-3's.

WHAT IS THE BEST WAY TO EAT EGGS?

It is best to eat eggs raw to obtain maximum benefit. Cooking destroys the delicate nutrients contained in highly nutritious eggs. Your next best solution is soft boiled eggs. The more you cook an egg, as in scrambling or frying, the more you will denature it.

REMEMBER

Your eggs should be organic, pasture raised, omega-3 eggs obtained from chickens that are free of antibiotics, hormones, and pesticides.

17

NUT MILKS
(NON-DAIRY)

Nut milks are another area that has created a lot of confusion amongst consumers. Many well meaning people drink nut milks, especially soy milk, in lieu of cow's milk. As I stated earlier, you need to avoid pasteurized cow's milk at all costs. However, most of the nut milks available in your local grocery store are not a much better choice.

Let's take a look at the three most popular nut milks on the market: soy milk, almond milk, and rice milk.

SOY MILK

I don't recommend drinking soy milk on a daily basis. Soy is one of the most genetically modified substances on the planet. If you do drink soy milk make sure that it's organic. Also, soy contains plant sterols called phytoestrogens which have been reported to mimic the hormone estrogen in humans. For this reason, you should do your best not to feed soy to children, especially young boys. We will discuss soy, in detail, in the baby food section of this book.

So, make the best decision for the situation you are in when purchasing soy milk. Always read the label. Some soymilk will contain evaporated cane juice, preservatives, xanthan gum, malted wheat, barley, and fortified vitamins and minerals; all of which are not beneficial for you.

Your soy milk should contain filtered water and whole organic soybeans, that's it. Westsoy makes organic unsweetened soy milk which contains only these two ingredients. It tastes good too.

ALMOND MILK

Almond milk is really good for you... if you make it yourself. However, most of the almond milk that you find in the supermarket or in the health food store is going to have a ton of added preservatives and sweeteners that you do not need and are not beneficial for you. In fact, **I have never seen almond milk sold in stores that I can recommend.**

WHAT SHOULD YOU DO?

The good news is: Almond milk is very easy to make at home. If you make it yourself, you will know exactly what is going into the almond milk. And, if you sprout the almonds, you will make a very nutritious, enzyme rich nut milk. Directions for sprouting almonds are contained in the Nuts & Seeds section of this course.

Many of my clients enjoy making their own almond milk; they love it. They'll use it in their coffee, in their smoothies, in their oatmeal, etc. It is very delicious and very nutritious.

THE LAZY PERSON'S GUIDE TO ALMOND MILK

Often times I will add sprouted almonds to my smoothie along with some purified water. This has a similar effect as using almond milk in the smoothie without making the almond milk separately.

RICE MILK

If I was you, I would stay away from rice milk. I know, I know, rice milk sounds like a good idea. In fact, I know plenty of women who drink rice milk as a healthier alternative to soy milk.

Here's the deal. All of the rice milk that I have seen on the shelves of supermarkets has oil added to it. The oil is added as an emulsifier. Often times, the added oil is canola oil, which is not good. To make matters worse, **manufacturers add harmful preservatives and sweeteners to rice milk that directly contribute to weight gain and disease.** Knowing this, it is easy to see why I suggest that you stay away from rice milk.

REMEMBER

* Keep your intake of soy milk to a minimum.

* It is better to make your own almond milk.

* Do not buy or use store bought almond milk or rice milk.

18

NUTS & SEEDS

It is best to avoid roasted nuts and seeds. Nuts and seeds that have been subjected to high heat, such as cooking or roasting, are not good for you. Reason being, the high temperatures denature the oils (fats) that they contain. What was once beneficial will now wreak havoc on your body.

EAT YOUR NUTS IN THE RAW

Raw nuts and seeds are a much better choice than their roasted counterparts. It really does make a difference. If you decide to make raw nuts and seeds a part of your diet, do so sparingly; they have the potential to make you gain body fat.

SPROUTING IS BEST

Most seeds and nuts can and should be sprouted. Sprouting activates the enzymes inside of them, which turns them into living organisms. This means that they contain everything you need to process through them. Because of this, sprouted nuts and seeds have to be refrigerated and will spoil in about a week or two as opposed to raw unsprouted nuts and seeds that you can keep on your shelf for long periods of time.

MOTHER NATURE INSTALLED A DEFENSE MECHANISM

Seeds and nuts have enzyme inhibitors inside of them which keep them dormant. This is a protective mechanism which allows them to be stored for long periods of time. Farmers must be able to store seeds in their dormant state until they are ready to use them. If this was not possible, farmers would lose all of their seed.

When they come in contact with moisture, the seeds will sprout and the enzymes will be activated. They become a living food again. This means that they will completely breakdown in your body, providing you with a ton of nutrition. Sprouted nuts and seeds are very delicious and are very beneficial. There is no comparison between sprouted nuts and seeds and their dormant unsprouted counterparts. **Once again: It's all about the enzymes!**

FOOD FOR THOUGHT (SPROUTING ALMONDS)

Almonds are the easiest of all of the nuts and seeds to sprout. Simply soak them in purified water for 8 to 12 hours. This will sprout them. Make sure to rinse them off thoroughly afterwards in a colander. You will see a brown film come off of them. You will say to yourself, "Man, I was eating that?" Sprouted almonds taste much different than regular raw almonds. They have to be refrigerated and they only stay good for about a week. Only sprout as many as you think you will eat in about three to five days.

Note: I am often asked if it's necessary to peel the almonds after they're sprouted. The answer is no.

WHAT ABOUT FLAXSEEDS?

Many well meaning people add ground flaxseeds or flaxseed oil to their food in order to supplement their diet with omega-3 fatty acids. As with every other aspect of food selection, the manner in which you prepare and ingest flaxseeds determines the amount of benefit you'll receive from the product, if any.

Let me break it down for you...

FLAX IS READILY AVAILABLE IN 3 FORMS

1. Flax Oil
2. Ground Flaxseed
3. Whole Flaxseed

Flaxseed Oils: Omega-3 fatty acids, especially the alpha linolenic acid (ALA) source of omega-3 found in flaxseeds, are very fragile. They start to denature as soon as they are exposed to the air. Because of this, flaxseed oils will start to lose their beneficial properties before they are bottled.

Ground Flaxseed: Ground flaxseeds will denature while they're sitting in their bag or whatever other type of container they may be kept in for the same reasons that were mentioned above with flaxseed oil.

Whole Flaxseeds: Whole flaxseeds are your best bet. However, you will not get their full benefit by eating them whole. They will not completely break down in your digestive system.

Here's the trick: Grind the whole flaxseeds yourself with a coffee grinder just prior to eating them, but only grind enough for you to eat at one sitting. In other words, grind them as you use them. Do not grind them and store them, they will denature.

REMEMBER

- Eat your nuts and seeds in the raw.
- Go organic.
- Sprouted nuts and seeds are best.

19

OILS

Oils are another area where there's a great amount of confusion and deception. I'll first explain which oils you need to stay away from. Then, I'll explain which oils are more beneficial for you to consume.

CANOLA OIL

There's a lot of hype surrounding canola oil. It's touted by many experts as the "healthy oil". Because of this, many health food restaurants proudly advertise the fact that they cook exclusively with canola oil. Hopefully, these well meaning establishments will read this course.

> **I have researched canola oil extensively and have come to one conclusion... Canola oil is bad for you!**

You'll hear certain industries say that oils which contain saturated fats are bad for you and vegetable oils are good for you, including canola oil. Nothing could be further from the truth. It is a fabrication made by the big corporations.

WHAT'S WRONG WITH CANOLA OIL?

Canola oil is derived from the rape seed plant. Oil from the rape seed plant is not suitable for human consumption. We cannot digest it properly; we get really sick when we eat it. A genetic modification was made to the rape seed plant so that humans can eat it and not get violently ill. We don't know exactly what effects this genetically modified oil will have on our bodies, but we don't immediately get sick after we eat it.

I stated earlier that in order for something to be considered organic it has to be free of genetic modifications. Because of the FDA and the big food lobbies, food manufacturers are allowed to say that canola oil is organic, even though it's a genetically modified version of the rape seed plant. There is no way it could be organic. In Europe they don't call it canola oil; they call it rape seed oil. Canola oil was first developed in Canada. Hence the name "can-o-la", which means "Canadian Oil, Low Acid". *Canola Oil* is much easier to market to American consumers than *Genetically Modified Rape Seed Oil*.

THE EXTRACTION PROCESS & THE OMEGA-3 MYTH

But there is more to canola oil than genetic modifications. The process by which canola oil is extracted from the genetically modified rapeseed plant is very harmful.

> **One of the supposed attributes to canola oil is the fact that it is high in omega-3 fatty acids. As you will soon see, this is all smoke and mirrors.**

Canola oil is removed from the genetically modified rapeseed plant through a combination of high temperature expeller pressing and hexane extraction. Hexane is a harmful solvent that is used to obtain maximum extraction of the oil from the plant.

"Hexane is the extraction medium used for most canola oil sold into the commodity grocery chain market as well as to the food industry. Hexane extraction reduces the oil content of the press cake to very low levels. Oil recovery from canola seed is approximately 96% when this form of extraction is used. This is accomplished by maximizing contact of the hexane with the press cake through a series of soakings or washings. All residual hexane in the extracted press cake and oil is removed through low temperature evaporation."

— Source: Canola Council
(wwww.canola-council.org)

This quote was taken directly from the Canola Council website! In other words, the canola seed is soaked and washed with hexane in order to obtain maximum extraction. Then, they extract the hexane from the canola oil through evaporation.

FOOD FOR THOUGHT

In Europe and other parts of the world if a food product contains a genetically modified substance, it has to be listed on its label. In the U.S., food manufacturers are not required to list genetically modified substances on their labels. By the way, Europe is not in favor of genetic modifications to food crops; they highly oppose it.

Do you really think that 100% of the hexane is removed from the canola oil through evaporation? I don't.

Hexane is proven to be harmful to us. According to the Environmental Protection Agency (EPA), hexane causes side effects including dizziness, nausea, headache, blurred vision, numbness, and fatigue. In other words, you don't want to eat anything that has come in contact with hexane.

To make matters worse, omega-3 fatty acids become rancid and foul smelling and the canola oil becomes discolored when subjected to these harsh refining processes. Because of this, canola oil goes through a deodorizing process that involves refining, bleaching, and degumming. The omega-3 fatty acids are basically destroyed in this process.

Let me make this absolutely clear. Canola oil has to be bleached and degummed in order to have an acceptable odor and appearance before it's bottled. I can go on and on, but hopefully you get the point by now. Canola oil is bad (unhealthy) for you.

Canola oil is everywhere. Read labels to insure that the food that you buy does not contain this harmful oil.

SAFFLOWER, CORN, SUNFLOWER, SOYBEAN, & COTTONSEED OILS

These vegetable oils are subjected to the same harmful high heat refining processes that canola oil is subjected to. These oils do not handle high heats very well and turn rancid very easily. Just like canola oil, these oils have to be bleached and degummed in order to have an acceptable odor and appearance.

Also, Safflower, Corn, Sunflower, Soybean, and Cottonseed Oils are extremely high in omega-6 fatty acids. Each of these oils consists of more than 50% omega-6 fatty acids and very low amounts of omega-3 fatty acids, if any. Safflower oil tops the list; it contains 80% omega-6 fatty acids.

As you already know, the Standard American Diet (SAD) is extremely high in omega-6 fatty acids. The omega-3:omega-6 fatty acid ratio is as high as 1:50. The preferable omega-3: omega-6 ratio is 1:1.

You need to avoid foods, such as vegetable oils, that are high in omega-6 fatty acids and concentrate on eating foods that are high in omega-3 fatty acids. Avoid vegetable oils at all cost.

SESAME OIL & PEANUT OIL

These oils are unique in the fact that they handle high heat much better than vegetable oils. However, they are also very high in omega-6 fatty acids. Because of this, it is best to avoid or severely limit these oils, as well.

WHAT OILS SHOULD YOU USE?

The two oils that I suggest you use are olive oil and coconut oil. As with everything else, you need to make an educated decision when selecting these oils for your consumption. Let's take a look at these two beneficial oils in detail.

OLIVE OIL

The type of olive oil that you want to purchase is organic, extra virgin, first cold pressed olive oil; **not just cold pressed, but**

first cold pressed. Some bottles of olive oil will say cold pressed, others will say first cold pressed, even from the same manufacturer. If it is just cold pressed, then it may have gone through a hot press first and a cold press afterwards.

The hot press enables manufacturers to extract more oil out of the olive, but when it's subjected to heat, it starts to denature right away; before the oil goes into the bottle, and while it is in the bottle. So you want first cold pressed extra virgin olive oil, also organic, if available.

Olive oil is high in oleic acid, which is an omega-9 fatty acid. Olive oil is not high in omega-6 or omega-3, so it doesn't put your ratios out of whack. Olive oil is a really good choice. It will say organic and first cold pressed right on the label.

Also, stay away from large containers of olive oil which are typical of the big warehouse stores. Exposing the oil to the air by continually opening and closing the bottle will cause the oil to denature. All of its beneficial properties will disappear. The solution is to purchase a bottle that you will use in a month or two, and not something that's going to be around your house for a year. You always want to get the most nutrition out of the foods that you're eating. **Olive oil does not handle high heat well. It is best used in salads, but not for cooking. In other words, olive oil is best used in its raw state.** You *can* cook with olive oil, but there *is* something better.

COCONUT OIL

Coconut oil handles high heat very well, so it is perfect for cooking. Coconut oil is a beneficial saturated fat. About two thirds of the saturated fats are medium chain triglycerides, which are very beneficial for you. Coconut oil is also high in lauric acid, which has anti-fungal and anti-microbial properties.

Unlike vegetable oils, medium chain triglycerides (MCTs) are not stored in

your body's fat cells. Rather, MCTs are immediately converted into energy. In other words, when you eat coconut oil, your body immediately uses it as energy and does not store it as body fat.

Remember that you need saturated fat in your diet. It just has to be from beneficial sources. Saturated fats are beneficial for brain activity as well as the integrity of your cell walls, hair skin nails etc. However, you have to be careful which coconut oil you do use. Some will be refined, mechanically expeller pressed, and exposed to high heat, which may denature the beneficial properties that this precious oil contains.

Coconut oil should be raw, unrefined, organic, extra virgin, and cold pressed. This has all the pluses. It's not refined, it's 100% raw, which means all of the nutritional activity is still inside of it, and it was cold pressed.

Coconut oil goes a long way. A small jar will last you a long time. In temperatures below 76°F, coconut oil will be solid and white in color. In temperatures above 76°F, coconut oil will be liquid and clear in color. It's okay either way. You don't have to refrigerate it.

Coconut oil has a wonderful nutty/buttery flavor, it's really nutritious, and it handles high heats, so you can cook with it. Basically, it's really good for you and it enhances the flavor of your food.

REMEMBER

- Stay away from processed and refined oils including hydrogenated oils. These include canola oil, safflower oil, corn oil, sunflower oil, soybean oil, and cottonseed oil.

- There are two types of oils that I recommend; first cold pressed extra virgin olive oil and raw unrefined coconut oil.

20

SUGAR & SWEETENERS

You've already learned that processed and refined grains are extremely bad for you. Well, the same principles apply to sugars as they do to grains.

Two key principles associated with sugar:

1. The sugar naturally found in organic whole foods, such as fruits and vegetables, are extremely beneficial and necessary for optimal health and wellness.

2. The processed sugars found in most foods and flavored drinks, including sport drinks, are extremely detrimental to your health.

What you will learn in this section:

* Why your body needs sugar.
* Beneficial sources of sugar.
* The evils of processed and refined sugar.
* The truth about fructose.

- Sources of disguised sugar.

- Health risks associated with processed sugar.

- The dangers of artificial sweeteners.

- The best alternative sweetener.

YOUR BODY NEEDS SUGAR

Sugar, in the form of glucose, is you body's only source of usable energy. When fat or protein is broken down to be utilized as energy, your body has to first convert it into glucose.

It is important to understand that sugars and carbohydrates are the same thing. This is where a lot of confusion comes into play. Many of us have been led to believe that carbohydrates are bad for us. Nothing could be further from the truth. We need good sources of carbohydrates in order to maintain a desirable body weight.

Your best sources of carbohydrates are organic vegetables and fruits

THE LOW CARB MYTH

In recent years we have been bombarded with low carb and no carb diets. These diets are very dangerous for two main reasons:

- Many people used these diets as an excuse to eat an abundance of high fat, artery clogging foods.

- Your body needs carbohydrate rich foods from beneficial sources.

I know a ton of people who went on the Atkins Diet mainly because it gave them an excuse to eat tons of bacon, sausage, pasteurized cheese, and every other imaginable type of high fat processed food. The fact is that these foods always have been and always will be detrimental to your health and cause you to store body fat.

Also, as mentioned above, your body needs carbohydrate rich foods. The trick is to get your carbohydrates from healthy sources. Beneficial carbohydrate rich foods are packed with nutrients including vitamins, minerals, phytonutrients, and enzymes.

Every person that I know that followed the Atkins Diet, or something similar, gained all of their weight back and more. Even worse, they lost muscle and gained a ton of fat. They took their body's fat burning ability and crippled it. Luckily some of these individuals sought my help and I was able to show them a simple effective plan of action to lose weight and keep it off.

We *do* need to avoid processed and refined carbohydrates at all costs. These types of foods are devitalized and denatured to the point that they are poisons to your body.

> **All of the foods that you eat, fat, protein, or carbohydrate, must come from beneficial sources. This is the only way that you can achieve lasting weight loss and fitness success.**

BENEFICIAL SOURCES OF SUGAR (CARBOHYDRATES)

The most beneficial sources of sugar are organic fruits and vegetables. Fruits and vegetables are your body's preferred sources of carbohydrates.

WHAT'S THE DEAL WITH FRUCTOSE?

Fructose, the carbohydrate found in fruits is very beneficial for you. It is easily absorbed and easily stored by your body. Also, when you obtain fructose from eating whole fruits, it is

---

FOOD FOR THOUGHT

High fructose corn syrup is now the most widely used sweetener in America. Because of this, corn is the number one crop in our country. The corn industry has grown to mammoth proportions in recent years. High fructose corn syrup is one of the most genetically modified and unhealthy foods available today.

You need to avoid any food that contains this harmful substance.

---

absorbed slowly into your blood stream because of the fiber and other nutrients contained in the whole fruit. Confusion sets in because of deceptive marketing from the big corporations.

The fructose found in fruit drinks, sport drinks, and packaged foods is much different than the fructose found in natural whole fruits. **The fructose found in packaged foods and drinks is processed and refined. It is just as bad as table sugar.**

Which leads us to our next point of interest...

SUGAR CULPRITS IN OUR FOOD

Processed and refined sugars take on many different forms. They are just as confusing and just as deceptive as the processed and refined grains that we discussed in the breads section of this book. We need to avoid these deadly foods at all costs. These include:

- Sucrose (from sugarcane and sugar beets)
- Fructose
- High Fructose Corn Syrup
- Corn Syrup
- Dextrose
- Turbinado Sugar

- Sugar in the Raw
- Brown Sugar
- Molasses

"Almost all nutritionists finger high fructose corn syrup consumption as a major culprit in the nation's obesity crisis. The inexpensive sweetener flooded the American food supply in the early 1980s, just about the time the nation's obesity rate started its unprecedented climb."

> — Source: "Sugar Coated- We're drowning in high fructose corn syrup." by Kim Severson, *San Francisco Chronicle* Staff Writer

HEALTH RISKS ASSOCIATED WITH PROCESSED SUGAR

There are many health risks associated with processed sugar. Too many to discuss here. However, processed sugar *is* a major contributor to the epidemic of overweight and obesity in our world.

Health risks of interest to women:

- Diabetes
- Heart Disease (the number one killer of women in America)
- Osteoporosis
- Breast and Ovarian Cancer
- Yeast Infections
- Depression

DID YOU KNOW?

It is estimated that the average American ingests 150 pounds of sugar each year! This figure includes children as well as adults.

> *"Obesity claims more lives and drains more of the healthcare budget than smoking. Obesity is linked to diabetes, arthritis, heart disease, stroke and certain cancers. It inflates healthcare costs by 36 percent and medication costs by 77 percent. Not only are people suffering from the negative effects of sugar; they're paying big money to be treated for these debilitating diseases that result from it."*

> —Source: "The Politics of Sugar" by Dani Veracity
> (www.newstarget.com)

The major culprit in this onslaught of sugar consumption is soft drinks. However, sport drinks and fruit drinks are also loaded with sugar. You will learn more about these drinks in the beverage section of this manual.

OUR CHILDREN ARE SUFFERING

It is interesting to note that, as of the writing of this manual, schools are beginning to restrict and in some cases remove, soft drinks from vending machines on their campuses. However, what these soft drinks are being replaced with is not much better. Harmful, sugar laden, sports drinks are taking their place. Unsuspecting parents and faculty members are gaining a false sense of satisfaction by providing their children with these drinks.

HOW MUCH SUGAR IS IN THAT DRINK (SODA)?

- One 12 oz. can = 11 teaspoons of sugar and 150 calories
- One 20 oz. bottle = 18 teaspoons of sugar and 250 calories
- One 32 oz. Big Gulp (no ice) = 29 teaspoons of sugar and 400 calories
- One 44 oz. cup = 40 teaspoons of sugar and 550 calories
- One 64 oz. Double Big Gulp = 59 teaspoons of sugar and 800 calories

Fruit on the bottom yogurt = 9 teaspoons of sugar. Almost as much as a can of soda!

One 32 oz. bottle of Gatorade = 14 teaspoons (56 grams) of sugar

Most of the sugar in these drinks comes from high fructose corn syrup, which we've already learned is a major cause of obesity and diabetes in this country.

WHAT SHOULD YOU DO?

I can go on and on, but you get the picture:

1. Stay away from soft drinks and sport drinks at all costs.
2. Drink plenty of good clean water

WHAT ABOUT ARTIFICIAL SWEETENERS?

Artificial Sweeteners should be avoided. These include Equal, Splenda, and Sweet-N-Low, also known as Aspartame, Sucralose, and Saccharine. Many experts believe that these artificial sweeteners are more dangerous than the sugars that they replace.

Many women use one or more of these artificial sweeteners on a daily basis and they have become very much attached to them. I am met with much resistance when I inform these women that they need to give up these dangerous sugar substitutes.

The fact of the matter is we as a society need to curb our addiction to sweets. We do not need to maintain the addiction by using artificial sweeteners. We simply need to overcome our addiction for sweets by eating foods that are beneficial for us and are going to get us closer to our ultimate weight loss and fitness goals.

A WORD ON ASPARTAME

I often hear reports from my clients regarding the adverse effects of aspartame either on themselves or someone that is close to them. The most common symptom that I hear is severe (migraine) headaches.

It seems that these people suffered from severe headaches; they went to doctors to try and find the cause or alleviate the symptoms with no positive results. Finally, it was suggested that they should stop using aspartame or products which contain aspartame, such as diet sodas. After cutting this harmful substance from their diet, their headaches completely went away. This is very interesting to me.

But don't take my word for it; let's take a look at excerpts from a debate on artificial sweeteners which took place in the U.K. in 2005:

"I am grateful for the opportunity to have this debate. For almost a year, I have been looking into the safety of the artificial sweetener, aspartame, and I was truly horrified by what I discovered. When I began my research, I was unconvinced by the off-the-wall internet conspiracy theories. I am a man of science, not of the internet. However, a number of eminent academics from the UK and further afield have persuaded me beyond doubt that aspartame represents a serious health problem.

There is strong scientific evidence that the components of aspartame and their metabolites can cause very serious toxic effects in humans. There is also a wealth of subjective evidence that suggests a range of adverse neurological reactions to aspartame.

The toxicity of aspartame's individual components is surely sufficient for us to be alarmed about its widespread use in the products that we and our children consume every day. But consumers and scientists alike have shown there is cause for concern from the regular consumption of products containing aspartame. The US Food and Drug Administration website lists more than 9,000 aspartame-related health complaints, but this could be just the tip of the iceberg.

Health professionals are often unable to diagnose a case of aspartame toxicity when they see one—after all, doctors are not currently trained to recognise it—and a number of cases have been misdiagnosed. A number of independent studies have shown that aspartame toxicity mimics conditions such as multiple sclerosis, Parkinson's disease, Alzheimer's disease, arthritis, chronic fatigue syndrome, panic disorder, lupus, diabetes, lymphoma, depression and other psychological disorders. It is perhaps not so surprising therefore that, frustrated by repeated flawed diagnosis, some people have turned to support groups as a method of sharing case history and exchanging information."

— Source: Roger Williams MP
(Member of Parliament, U.K.)
Westminster Hall Debates
www.TheyWorkForYou.com

DO YOU EXPECT ME TO AVOID SUGAR FOR THE REST OF MY LIFE?

Look, I am not asking you to avoid processed sugar for the rest of your life. In our modern world it would be virtually impossible.

However, you do need to be aware of the harmful effects of all processed sweeteners, including artificial sweeteners. Knowing what you now know, you should do your best to avoid and severely limit your intake of these refined sweeteners. Eat a piece of organic fruit if you crave something sweet.

Note: If I was you, I would avoid artificial sweeteners at all costs; it really is that important.

WHAT ABOUT HONEY?

There are two basic schools of thought in regards to honey:

1. Proponents of honey: Those who think that honey is one of the most beneficial foods on the planet.

2. Opponents of Honey: Those who think that honey and its derivatives are the biggest scam to ever be placed upon the health food industry.

Personally I do not recommend honey to my clients. There are three main reasons for my aversion to honey:

1. Honey is regurgitated pollen. Bees ingest pollen from flowers, go back to their bee hive, and regurgitate it. I don't know about you, but the whole process seems disgusting to me.

2. Honey has a high glycemic index of 83.

3. There is a healthier natural sweetener.

For those of you that absolutely have to have a sweetener in your life, there is a better sweetener. However, if you decide that you want to make honey a part of your diet, make sure that it is organic, raw, and unrefined.

THE BETTER SWEETENER

Raw Agave Nectar is a natural sweetener indigenous of Mexico. It is 75% sweeter than sugar, which means that you only need to use ¼ the amount that you would normally use. Raw Agave can be used anywhere that you would normally use sugar, including cooking and baking. Raw Agave is also low in calories and tastes great.

Raw Agave has a very low glycemic index rating. I have found different reports ranging between 11 and 27 on the glycemic index. White bread has a glycemic index of 112, while honey registers 83 on the glycemic index.

Raw Agave is the preferred alternative to processed sugars and artificial sweeteners.

REMEMBER

1. Avoid all processed and refined sugar.
2. Do not use artificial sweeteners... ever!
3. Eat a piece of fruit if you crave something sweet.
4. Raw Agave is the better sweetener.

21

INTRODUCTION TO PACKAGED FOODS

Packaged food is the area where people get themselves in the most trouble. Remember, if your goal is weight loss and optimal health, it is highly recommended that you eliminate or restrict your intake of grains and sugars, especially those that are processed and refined.

WHAT YOU WILL LEARN

- At least 90% of packaged foods are processed and refined.
- Processed grains, sugars, and oils are your worst enemy.
- Stay away from gluten.
- **Most processed foods contain genetic modifications.**
- Make the best choice for the situation you are in.

GLUTEN: WHAT'S THE BIG DEAL?

Gluten is the protein part of wheat, rye, and barley. Gluten is found in a wide variety of foods; especially processed foods. Here's the problem: Many people are allergic to gluten and don't know it.

In our society, we are bombarded with grains. They are everywhere. Grains, especially processed grains, have become the main staple in our diet. Many people don't even eat fruits and vegetables on a regular basis anymore.

The major allergic reactions to gluten are inflammatory responses. Symptoms such as arthritis and fibromyalgia, as well as aggressive behavior are common. Wheat and gluten can also cause irritability, lethargy, **and is a major contributor in the epidemic of obesity.**

MY FIT LIFE

When I eat wheat, especially processed wheat, it makes me feel extremely tired. At times, I will notice that I become more aggressive. I will get irritated at situations that normally wouldn't affect me. Many of my clients and friends have reported similar reactions to eating wheat.

As mentioned above, grains are used in many processed foods. The following terms found in food labels may mean that there is gluten in the product:

- Hydrolyzed Vegetable Protein, Hydrolyzed Plant Protein, or Vegetable Protein
- Flour or Cereal Products
- Malt or Malt Flavoring
- Modified Starch or Modified Food Starch
- Vegetable Gum

- Soy Sauce
- Malt Vinegar

Also, any of the following words on food labels usually means that a grain containing gluten has been used:

- Stabilizer
- Starch
- Flavoring
- Emulsifier

I have seen many people come off of gluten and they have experienced radical changes in their lives. They act, look, and feel remarkably better. People that were once bed ridden now lead healthy vibrant lives.

Some of the positive effects of a gluten free diet include:

- Relief of body aches and pains
- Relief from depression
- Increased energy
- Weight loss

Of particular interest to women: I have found that women who eliminate gluten from their diet find it much easier to lose weight and keep it off. Relief from PMS symptoms has been reported by my clients as well.

GLUTEN-FREE FOOD TAGS

You are going to start to see "gluten-free" tag's on many products in the supermarket, especially Whole Foods type markets. It's like a buzzword right now. This is not a bad thing. Remember, what I have found with people is that if they can cut gluten out of their diet it is much easier for them to obtain a desirable body weight. In other words, you will lose weight and keep it off with less effort. It takes a little time to learn which foods do and do not have gluten in them. But once you do, it becomes second nature, and it is not a problem at all. It is definitely worth the effort.

Grains that do not contain gluten:

- Corn
- Rice
- Arrowroot
- Buckwheat
- Millet
- Amaranth
- Quinoa

GMO'S IN PACKAGED FOODS?

Fruits and vegetables are not the only place that you can find GMO's (genetically modified organisms). In fact, you are more likely to find genetically modified substances in your meat, dairy, and packaged food products.

You are probably saying to yourself: How do genetic modifications end up in meat and dairy products? Well, most of the genetically modified corn and soy grown in America ends up in animal feed. They eat GMO grains and you eat them. Simple, huh?

HOW DO GMO'S END UP IN PACKAGED FOODS?

As I just mentioned, most of the corn, soy, canola, and cotton grown in the United States are genetically modified. Corn syrup and high fructose corn syrup is used as a sweetener in most processed foods. Corn, soy, canola, and cottonseed oils are used in almost every type of processed food. Other foods that are genetically modified are rice, wheat, and flax, along with about 50 other forms of produce.

It is estimated that at least 7 out of 10 processed foods are genetically modified. Let me say this another way: **7 out of 10 of the processed and packaged foods that you place in your shopping basket contain genetic modifications**. Here is a short list of some of the more popular products that contain GMO's:

- Coca-Cola & Sprite
- Pepsi
- Hershey's bars
- M&M's
- Campbell's soups
- Progresso soups
- Kellogg's, Post, Quaker, and General Mills cereals
- And the list goes on and on

— Source: Green Living, by the editors of *E*/The Environmental Magazine (Penguin Group)

Go to **www.truefoodnow.org/shoppersguide** for a more comprehensive and printable list of foods that contain genetic modifications. As ingredients change in products all the time, the best thing is to check the ingredients list of the products you buy often. Keep a look out for:

- Corn: corn oil, corn syrup, high fructose corn syrup, corn starch, corn meal
- Soy: soy protein, soy lecithin, soy oil, soy sauce, soy isolates
- Canola: canola oil
- Cotton: cottonseed oil

What I find most interesting is the fact that our federal government does not require food manufacturers to label genetically engineered substances on their ingredients list.

The opposite is true in Europe and other parts of the world. Many countries will not accept food that comes from the United States because they do not want genetically modified substances in their food supply.

This is why you need to make the most informed decisions that you possibly can when shopping for yourself and your loved ones. And this is why I created this course.

REMEMBER

- Stay away from packaged foods whenever possible.
- Processed grains, sugars, and oils are your worst enemy.
- Stay away from gluten.
- Most processed foods contain genetic modifications.
- Make the best choice for the situation you are in.
- If you do eat a packaged food, make sure it's organic.

Which leads us to...

22

DO YOU KNOW ABOUT
ORGANIC LABELS?

ORGANIC = BIG MONEY

It is reported that the organic industry is growing at a rate of nearly 20 percent per year. Because of this it seems that every food manufacturer wants to get its piece of the pie.

This was most apparent at the Natural Products Expo West in the spring of 2007. It seemed that almost every booth carried organic products. Seven years ago, organics accounted for roughly 10 percent of the entire show. What a difference! This obviously equates to big money. Where there is big money there are big corporations. And where there are big corporations there is usually corruption.

SHAME ON WAL- MART

In 2007, it was reported that Wal-Mart was caught mislabeling packaged foods "organic" when they were not organic. Also, the organic farms that Wal Mart claimed to have gotten their products from were from far away places, such as China & India. There is no way to regulate whether or not these products are grown organically when they come from such far away places.

By the way, one of the main reasons for buying organic is to support local farmers.

SO, WHAT DO THE LABELS REALLY MEAN?

You may have noticed that some organic labels have different wording than others.

- 100% Organic
- Organic
- Made With Organic

What does all of this mean? Well, let me explain.

100% Organic: These products are produced using organic methods and contain 100% organic ingredients.

Organic: At least 95% of the ingredients by weight, excluding water, have been organically produced. The remaining ingredients must be recommended by the National Organics Standard Board. Also, the product cannot use both the organic and non-organic versions of an ingredient that is listed on the label as organic.

Made With Organic: Products that contain 70% to 95% organic ingredients may put "Made With Organic" on the front of the label.

All three of these categories prohibit the inclusion of any ingredients which have been genetically modified, irradiated, or produced using sewage or sludge. And yes, commercial produce is subjected to sewage and sludge.

23

PACKAGED FOODS

PASTA

Pasta is just like bread, it is an extremely condensed grain or flour. As we learned in the grains and flours section of this course, 6 cups of a whole grain will make 1 cup of flour and all of the calories from those 6 cups of the whole grain will be in that 1 cup of flour. So it is very calorie dense. Also, most of the pastas on the shelves of markets today are denatured and devitalized. These highly processed pastas will wreak havoc on your body.

Some people love pasta and they have to have it. If you are one of these people and you would like to eat pasta from time to time, make the best choice for the situation you are in.

WHAT IS YOUR BEST CHOICE?

My suggestion is that you stay away from wheat based pasta because it contains gluten.

The form of pasta that I recommend to my clients is organic gluten-free brown rice pasta. Make sure that it says gluten-free on the box. Eating this type of pasta will be a more beneficial choice. Also, it tastes great. Besides the color, you wouldn't even know the difference. It tastes like regular pasta.

PASTA SAUCE

It is preferable to make pasta sauce from scratch with fresh ingredients. It is always best to know exactly what is going into the food that you are eating.

When buying sauces at the grocery store there are a few things that you want to look for:

- Organic
- No preservatives
- No added sugars
- No artificial sweeteners
- Gluten free

It may sound funny, but some sauces do have gluten in them. The reason for this is the fact that some of these sauces have vinegar in them. Some vinegar is grain-based and contains gluten. So do your best to choose a gluten free sauce.

Always look at the ingredients list. Make sure that the sauce contains whole foods and herbs; nothing else.

RICE

White rice is one of the white devils. You should avoid white rice at all costs. White rice is just like white bread, it has gone through processes which strip the grain of all of its vital nutrients until only the carbohydrate remains. When you eat white rice you force your body to use up its stores of vital nutrients to breakdown and process this denatured substance. These nutrients stores are meant to be used for repair and defense against sickness and disease. Also, white rice will cause a spike in insulin which will cause you to store fat. White rice is like a poison to your body.

If you are going to eat rice, it is suggested that you eat the organic whole grain or long grain form. Examples include organic brown rice, organic jasmine rice and organic basmati rice. Look for color. Rice that has a darker color is usually more nutritious.

You will literally be able to taste the nutrition contained in long grain rice; your body quickly becomes accustomed to its taste. After this happens, white rice will taste like cardboard to you.

BEANS AND LEGUMES

Beans and legumes are among the oldest cultivated plants. There are many varieties of beans and legumes; they are an excellent source of protein, minerals, and dietary fiber, as well as a terrific source of antioxidants. Also, the high fiber content in beans prevents blood sugar levels from rising too rapidly by slowing their absorption into your blood stream.

Beans and legumes should be organic if possible. It is best to prepare your own, as opposed to buying them in a can. When preparing them it is best to soak them for a minimum of eight hours. Doing so will deactivate the enzyme inhibitors which they contain. Remember to thoroughly rinse the legumes prior to cooking them. Also, it is best to cook them under low heat or in a crock pot.

SOY SAUCE

Most of us do not give much thought to soy sauce, but we should. Remember that soy is one of the most genetically modified substances on the planet. Here's the problem, most of us eat soy sauce when we are out at restaurants. If this is the case, ask the restaurant server and manager if they carry organic soy sauce. If they don't, request that they start carrying it. It may take some time, but they will eventually catch on. Another alternative when eating out at restaurants is to bring your own sauce.

When purchasing soy sauce for your home, it is best to buy organic. However, your best bet would be to buy Bragg's Liquid Aminos. Bragg's Liquid Aminos taste just like soy sauce, but it is a much healthier choice. It is a high quality vegetable protein from soy. Organic, no genetic modifications, no preservatives, and gluten free, it has all the pluses.

Note: Soy sauce contains gluten unless it is stated gluten free on its label. Bragg's Liquid Aminos are always gluten free.

BRAGG'S HEALTH PRODUCTS

Bragg's Health Products is a family run business operated by Patricia Bragg N.D., P.H.D. I had the opportunity to speak with Patricia Bragg in March 2007. She is a vibrant wonderful person who is truly a health crusader. She definitely practices what she preaches and it shows.

Her company, started by her father Paul C. Bragg N.D., P.H.D., has a wonderful array of high quality health products. Bragg's products are highly respected and highly regarded in the nutrition industry.

Bragg's products which I recommend:

- Bragg's Organic Apple Cider Vinegar
- Bragg's Healthy Organic Vinaigrette
- Bragg's Liquid Aminos

DRESSING

As I previously mentioned, there is a Bragg's Healthy Organic Vinaigrette. It not only tastes great, but it is very healthy for you and it doesn't require refrigeration. It contains organic extra virgin first cold pressed olive oil, organic apple cider vinegar, Bragg's liquid aminos, raw honey, fresh ginger; all of these ingredients are Non-GMO and of the highest quality. It's going to be your best choice as far as the dressings that are available in your grocery store. And it has apple cider vinegar as opposed to the other grain based vinegars that have gluten in them, so this dressing is gluten free as well.

Most dressings, such as ranch and bleu cheese, are obviously not good for you. However, some of the dressings that appear to be good for you actually are not. Slick marketing and misleading labels try to fool you.

For example, some will say, organic natural balsamic vinaigrette and you say to yourself: "Oh wow, it's natural and it's organic... it must be good for me." But you look at the label and it has canola oil, xanthan gum, and sugar. These are not good for you. As with all packaged foods, read the label and look for whole food ingredients that you are familiar with.

Of course, it's always best to make your own fresh salad dressing from wholesome nutritious ingredients.

NUT BUTTERS

While nut butters are not your best source of nutrition, they do come in handy with today's hectic lifestyle. That being said, it is my job to help you make the best decision possible for the situation you are in. There are a wide variety of nut butters on the market today. As with most of the other packaged foods, there are a few that are definitely better than the others.

You definitely want to stay away from commercial nut butters, such as peanut butter that is solid at room temperature. When a nut butter is solid at room temperature it has gone through a process where it has been injected with hydrogen. While doing so makes the peanut butter easier to handle, this process turns the fats in the peanut butter into trans-fats. Trans-fats have no benefit to your body and can only be stored as body fat. It is best to avoid trans-fats at all possible cost since they are thought to be detrimental to your health and the health of your loved ones.

Never choose nut butters that say low fat or reduced fat. These types of foods usually have harmful chemical preservatives added to them. Also, these products always contain hidden fats, usually in the form of monoglycerides and diglycerides.

When selecting nut butters, it is best to first look at the ingredient list. Peanut butter should contain peanuts. Almond butter should contain almonds. There should not be a long list of ingredients on the label. Many commercial nut butters, especially reduced fat nut butters, will have a long list of ingredients; most of which are detrimental to your health.

Next, choose a nut butter that has a layer of oil on top of it. This will tell you that it has not been hydrogenated. If you are worried about the fat in the oil you can simply pour off some of the excess.

My favorite nut butter is raw almond butter. Not only does it taste great, but, since it is raw, it has more beneficial nutrients in it than its roasted counterparts. Raw almond butter tastes great on celery sticks, which is a great snack for children.

JELLIES & FRUIT SPREADS

While I don't recommend the use of jams and jellies I do realize that, in today's world, we lead very hectic lives and there are going to be times when you simply have to prepare a quick and easy meal. That being said, a sandwich on sprouted grain bread with raw almond butter and an organic fruit spread is going to be a much better choice for yourself and your loved ones than any of the prepackaged meals, such as Lunchables, or the highly processed, high fat, highly toxic meats, such as hot dogs or commercial deli meats, available on the market today. As with any of the other food choices you want to make the absolute best choice for the situation you are in.

Because of the vulnerable nature of the fruits found in jams and jellies you definitely want to choose organic as opposed to the pesticide laced commercial brands that are available. Also, 100% organic fruit spreads are preferable over jellies and jams which contain sugar and preservatives.

Things to look for in fruit spreads:

* 100% Organic
* No preservatives
* No added sugar

Simply read the ingredients list to discover exactly what is in the fruit spread you are buying for yourself and your family. Typically, the ingredients should be nothing more than organic fruit and fruit juice concentrate.

CANNED SOUP

I personally do not eat any canned soups. It is always best to make your own fresh soups completely from scratch. However, if you decide to eat canned soups, choose a brand that is organic and has whole food ingredients that you recognize. Stay away from soups that have sugarcane, preservatives, and other chemical additives in their ingredients list.

Remember that Campbell's and Progresso soups contain genetically engineered ingredients.

CANNED TUNA

Because it is a large fish you should limit your intake of tuna. Remember that large fish have a tendency to contain higher levels of mercury than smaller fish. Choose water packed tuna over oil packed tuna. Oil increases the fat content in tuna. Also, the oil that is used to pack tuna in often contains gluten. Water packed tuna is usually gluten free.

LACTO-FERMENTED PRODUCTS

Fermentation is a healthful process commonly used to preserve food. Before the invention of the refrigerator, many foods were commonly fermented.

Types of foods that are commonly fermented include vegetables and raw dairy products:

* Raw Kefir

- Sauerkraut

- Kimchi

- Raw Unfiltered Apple Cider Vinegar

- Olives

- Pickles

- Miso

Lacto-fermentation is a process by which beneficial micro-organisms break down food, prevent the growth of harmful bacteria, and increase nutrient density. Mark McAfee, owner of Organic Pastures, states that his raw milk has 24 kinds of beneficial bacteria (probiotics), while his raw kefir has as many as 65 different kinds of beneficial bacteria.

In other words, the process of fermentation or culturing dramatically increases the nutrient density of an already healthy whole food.

Lacto-fermented foods provide your body with:

- Probiotics: Beneficial bacteria that aid in digestion and enhance your immune system.

- Increased levels of vitamins and minerals.

- Increased production of enzymes.

MAKE YOUR OWN FERMENTED FOODS

I suggest that you learn how to make your own lacto-fermented foods. Doing so will insure that you receive the many health benefits associated with eating these living cultured foods.

Many of the commercially fermented foods that are available on the shelves of our supermarkets do not contain the same health benefits as traditionally fermented foods. Mass production always sacrifices health benefits. Good examples of this are yogurt and pickles, which are subjected to pasteurization. We have already learned that pasteurization kills off the beneficial bacteria contained in our food.

HOW DO YOU MAKE YOUR OWN FERMENTED FOODS?

Luckily, it is relatively easy to make your own fermented foods. Look at the recommended resources section of this manual to find out more information regarding reliable sources for Kefir Starter kits and Culture Starter kits.

My personal favorite lacto-fermented product is raw kefir. It is extremely easy to make and very beneficial.

ARE YOU LACTOSE INTOLERANT?

It is interesting to note that the beneficial probiotic bacteria contained in fermented products, such as kefir, breakdown the lactose contained in it. Because of this, people that are lactose intolerant are able to drink raw kefir (cultured raw milk) without any problems.

FROZEN DINNERS

Most frozen dinners are extremely bad (unhealthy) for you. They contain a variety of harmful ingredients including MSG, chemical preservatives, genetic modifications, processed fats, and sugars.

WHAT ABOUT HEALTHY FROZEN DINNERS?

Many people, especially women, get themselves in trouble eating so called "healthy" frozen dinners. Deceptive marketing leads them to believe that they are eating nutritious meals that are low in calories.

Let's take a look at one of these "healthy" meals:

Healthy Choice
Chicken Parmigiana

Back of box deceptive marketing:

Satisfy Your Appetite... to eat right

"We at Healthy Choice prepare meals that meet the highest quality and nutritional standards. This recipe offers a complete meal and a delicious dessert, so you'll enjoy what you're eating and feel good about it too."

Partial Ingredients List:

Yellow corn flour, corn starch, soybean oil, dextrose, sugar, salt, sodium acid pyrophosphate, monocalcium phosphate, modified food starch, maltodextrin, disodium inosinate, disodium guanylate, natural flavors (MSG), sodium tripolyphosphate, BHT (harmful preservative), artificial flavors (MSG), high fructose corn syrup, corn syrup, honey, brown sugar, molasses, modified corn starch, sodium caseinate, sodium aluminosilicate, ethyl alcohol, polysorbate 80, and the list goes on and on.

Isn't this a shame? By now you understand that these ingredients are extremely detrimental to your health and well being. It is amazing to me that the manufactures of this frozen concoction advertise it as a healthy meal.

GENETIC MODIFICATIONS IN FROZEN DINNERS

According to www.TrueFoodNow.org the following brands of frozen dinners have been shown to contain genetically engineered ingredients:

- Banquet
- Budget Gourmet
- Green Giant
- Healthy Choice
- Lean Cuisine
- Marie Callenders
- Weight Watchers

REMEMBER

When buying packaged foods there are a few things you should look for:

- Organic
- No Genetic Modifications
- No Preservatives
- No Added Sugars
- No Artificial Sweeteners
- Gluten Free

24

CEREALS

As I mentioned earlier, it is best to eliminate or severely limit the amount of grains in your diet, so I do not recommend the use of breakfast cereals. It is much better for you to eat fruit or a homemade breakfast smoothie in the morning to start the day; these choices are much more nutritious and easier for you to digest.

However, those of you who have children will sometimes feel the need to feed them breakfast cereals. Here are some guidelines:

- Stay away from commercial brands such as Honey Nut Cheerios, Frosted Flakes, etc... They are high in sugar and usually contain GMOs.

- Look for organic, 100% whole grain cereals from companies who specialize in these types of cereals such as Nature's Path.

Make sure to read the labels to make sure that there are no addded preservatives or other chemicals in the cereal. You should be able to recognize every ingredient on the box... if you don't, then don't buy it.

Remember that cereal is a packaged convenience food. It does nothing for you in your quest towards a tighter more toned body. Most cereals are processed denatured garbage. Also, they are a very condensed form of carbohydrate, just like the flour in a processed loaf of bread.

WHAT ABOUT KID'S CEREAL?

Cereal marketed to kids is horrible. Most are the breakfast equivalent of cookies, candies, and doughnuts. Slick marketers know exactly how to market foods directly to our children. I believe that this practice should be illegal. I have never seen a kid's cereal that has any benefit for a child.

If you must buy a kid's cereal, buy one that is organic. Organic kid's cereals are still loaded with sugar, but they are not filled with pesticides, harmful chemical preservatives, or genetically engineered substances.

Which leads us to...

FOOD FOR THOUGHT

I will give you a simple rule of thumb for purchasing packaged foods: If the label says that the food is fortified, don't buy it. The term fortified is a key indicator that a food has been processed to the point that all of its nutritional value has been stripped from it. Food manufacturers will add small amounts of vitamins and minerals to the food, so they will be able to list some nutrients on the nutrient content portion of the label.

ALWAYS BUY ORGANIC

When it comes to cereal, always buy organic. Wheat products are similar to corn and soy, whereas they are highly genetically modified and they are subjected to a large amount of pesticides.

Even when you buy organic cereal, you have to be very careful. Look at the ingredients list, **the second ingredient is usually organic cane juice or evaporated cane juice**. This is sugar, it doesn't matter if it's organic or not, it is still a form of table sugar, which is not good for you.

Ezekiel has a sprouted grain cereal. It tastes very good and it is a better choice when it comes to packaged cereals. **Ezekiel cereal is made from organic sprouted grains and contains no sugar or flour.**

OATMEAL IS YOUR BEST BET

Organic Oatmeal is preferred over the other types of prepackaged cereals. However, there are a few guidelines that you need to follow.

- 100% Organic

- Whole oat

- No individual packages

- No microwaves

You must cook oatmeal on a stove not in a microwave. **Individual packets are not acceptable**, since they usually contain added sugar and other substances that are not beneficial to your goals. The ingredients list should say 100% whole oats or rolled oats. I know that oatmeal is very bland, but do not use table sugar or artificial sweeteners to enhance the flavor. Add fresh fruit such as sliced bananas, berries, or sliced apples to enhance the flavor naturally. You may also use a small amount of raw agave nectar if no fruit is available.

REMEMBER

- Avoid all processed cereals including fortified cereals and kid's cereals.

- Organic oatmeal and Ezekiel sprouted grain cereal are your best choices.

25

SNACKS

CHIPS

The more I research chips the more I tell people to stay away from them, especially potato chips. Organic or not, it doesn't matter. If you think about it, the oil used to make the chips cannot be good for you if it is heated over and over again. Also, the chips soak up this harmful denatured oil and you eat it.

> **There is nothing healthy about chips; they are purely a pleasure food. I suggest that you stay away from chips at all costs.**

COOKIES

Cookies are another pleasure food. If you eat a cookie, know that you are eating something that is bad for you. Don't fool yourself by eating vegan or organic cookies. These *are* better choices, but they're still bad for you. Cookies are something that my clients save for their "cheat day" when following one of my holistic fitness programs such as the *16 Week Total Body Makeover.*

POPCORN

Pre-packaged popcorn found on the shelves of supermarkets and convenience stores are very bad for you. Look at the ingredients list and you will find a wide array of chemical additives and preservatives.

Believe me when I tell you that you do not want to feed this unhealthy snack to your family, especially if it is microwave popcorn. Microwaves themselves are especially detrimental to your health.

WARNING!
BUTTER FLAVORING IS
HAZARDOUS TO YOUR HEALTH!

Diacetyl, a chemical component of artificial butter, is known to make factory workers who come in contact with it very sick. According to the Center for Disease Control (CDC), Diacetyl is known to cause irritations in the skin, eyes, and lungs. Factory workers who breathe in its vapors have contracted serious lung problems. The problem is so common that it has been nick-named *popcorn workers lung.* The CDC advises workers who come in contact with this dangerous substance to use tightly sealed containers, wear skin and eye protection, and use respiratory protection.

However, Diacetyl has been deemed safe for human consumption. It is no wonder that so many children and adults in America have lung problems, which are usually diagnosed as asthma. The amount of inhalers prescribed to children in America is devastating.

Diacetyl is used for its buttery aroma and taste in popcorn, bakery products, candy, and frozen foods. Stay away from this poisonous chemical at all costs.

THE HEALTHIER POPCORN ALTERNATIVE

It is possible to make popcorn that is relatively healthy. Follow these guidelines for a healthier snack:

- Use Organic Popping Corn (Remember, corn is the most genetically modified substance on the planet).
- Pop The Corn Yourself.
- Use A Hot Air Popper.
- Season With A Dash Of Himalayan Salt.

Following the above guidelines is an easy to follow, healthy alternative to the dangerous pre-packaged popcorn available on supermarket shelves.

CRACKERS

There's not a whole lot of killer, these are healthy for you, crackers. Treat them like their bread counterparts, try to make the best choice for the situation you are in and keep them to a minimum. Look for 100% whole-grain as opposed to regular wheat flour. Read the labels to make sure there are no preservatives or added sugars in them.

I can go on and on with snacks; cakes, pies, doughnuts, scones, Ding Dongs, and Twinkies. You get the picture. These are all unhealthy. They cause weight gain and contribute to chronic disease.

Here's the deal. When you think of snacks you need to think of something healthy. Remember, food is fuel for your body.

You always want to supply your body with the most quality fuel available, whether you're eating a meal or a snack.

- Raw vegetables.
- Raw fruit.
- Raw nuts or seeds mixed with goji berries.
- Celery sticks with raw almond butter.

These raw snacks are a much healthier choice than the highly processed snacks mentioned above.

REMEMBER

- Most packaged snack foods will sabotage your weight loss efforts. Do your best to avoid them.
- When you think of snacks think of something healthy.

26

CHOCOLATE

Every woman that I have ever met craves chocolate. Reason being, beneficial sources of chocolate contain minerals and polyphenols that women can become deficient in at certain times of the month. There are a lot of studies being done that confirm these claims. **However, as with all other foods, all chocolate is not created equal**. Things to consider when choosing your chocolate:

- Always Buy Organic
- Choose Raw Cacao Beans
- No Processed Sugar or Preservatives

Always Buy Organic: Chocolate and coffee are typically grown outside of the United States. These foreign crops may be subjected to higher levels of pesticide spraying than that allowed in the U.S. I will say it again: Always buy organic.

Choose Raw Cacao Beans: Raw cacao beans have nutritional qualities that are killed or removed when chocolate is cooked and processed. Raw cacao contains enzymes, polyphenols, antioxidants, and a whole host of other beneficial nutrients that are not present in a typical store bought candy bar.

No Processed Sugar or Preservatives: Most dark chocolate candy bars are processed at high heats and contain sugar and preservatives. These candy bars are not good for you and I do not recommend them.

IS THERE A GOOD SOURCE OF DARK CHOCOLATE?

I am often asked this question by the women that I instruct. This is what I tell them: I suggest that you eat raw cacao beans when you crave chocolate. Raw food chef Jenny Ross suggests that you eat a handful of raw cacao mixed with goji berries to satisfy your cravings. A favorite snack of one of my clients is **raw cacao mixed with goji berries and raw pecans; this wonderful combination increases serotonin production in your brain. Serotonin is also known as the *feel good* hormone.**

There *are* some raw food companies who are now making raw chocolate bars. These bars are made from organic raw cacao beans and organic raw agave; nothing else. The best one that I have tasted is made by Ultimate Raw Foods and it is called Ultimate Raw Chocolate. It is touted as chocolate that is good for you.

Ultimate Raw Chocolate Stats:

- Tastes great.
- Made from organic raw cacao and raw agave; that's it.
- No additives or preservatives.
- Contains naturally occurring vitamins, minerals, and polyphenols.

27

CONDIMENTS

Condiments can be a lovely addition to your meals. However, there are a few key points you should consider...

SALT

Salt is probably the most misunderstood condiment of them all. The kind of salt that we are accustomed to is processed and refined table salt. Regular table salt is very bad for you. It is one of the *white devils*. Stay away from it. Table salt has been stripped of all of its beneficial properties until only the sodium chloride (NaCl) remains. Often times, a small percentage of harmful chemicals are added to the salt. Table salt robs your body of its vital nutrient stores in order to process through it. Basically, refined table salt wreaks havoc on your body.

WHAT KIND OF SALT SHOULD YOU USE?

Salt in its natural form contains a variety of minerals which are beneficial to your body. There are two varieties of salts that can be beneficial for you:

1. Sea Salt

2. Himalayan Salt

Sea Salt contains a variety of beneficial nutrients. The amount and type of the nutrients contained in sea salt is dependent on its source of origin. As with all other foods, the process through which sea salt is harvested will determine its nutritional benefit. The salt must be solar dried in order to keep its nutrient value intact. If it is subjected to high heats, such as in an oven, the delicate nutrients will be destroyed.

MY FAVORITE TYPE OF SALT

Himalayan Salt is my favorite type of salt. It has many benefits which are extremely beneficial for you:

* Himalayan Salt contains 84 of the nutritional elements we need. The highest elemental content of any salt.
* Himalayan Salt balances the pH in your body.
* Himalayan Salt contains no environmental pollutants.
* Himalayan Salt helps to regulate blood pressure.

I have listed just a few of the many benefits of Himalayan Salt. It is a bit more expensive than other salts, but it is well worth it. Basically, Himalayan Salt has beneficial nutrients that will be added to your body with nothing taken away.

HERBS & SPICES

Herbs and spices are generally good for you. Do your best to buy organic whenever possible. You can also start your own herb garden. Doing so will insure that you have the highest quality freshest herbs available.

GARLIC

Garlic is a wonderful addition to your diet; it is known as one of the great blood cleansers. Some of the other benefits of garlic include:

* Has antibacterial, antiviral, and antifungal properties.
* Kills intestinal parasites.
* Enhances immune system.
* Helps relieve infections of all types.

KETCHUP

Ketchup used to be very popular, but it has lost some of its loyal followers in recent years. Ketchup is not the best thing for you, but if you are going to eat it, choose one that is organic, preservative free, and does not contain high fructose corn syrup.

SALSA

Salsa has become very popular in recent years, surpassing ketchup in popularity. It is always best to make your own salsa. Most of the salsa found on the shelves of grocery stores contain harmful preservatives. Store bought salsa should be **organic** and **preservative free**.

MAYONNAISE

Stay away from mayonnaise at all costs; especially if you are overweight. It is bad for you. Mayonnaise is not your friend. Hopefully you get the point.

WHAT ABOUT LOW-FAT OR "HEALTHY" MAYONNAISE?

Low-fat mayonnaise, light mayonnaise, vegannaise... they are all unhealthy. In fact, these types of mayonnaise are usually worse than regular mayonnaise. Despite what the commercials say I have never seen a mayonnaise that has any healthy properties in it.

MUSTARD

Mustard is a much better choice than ketchup or mayonnaise. However, make sure to check the ingredients. Mustard should contain mustard seed and water as the only ingredients. Maybe some herbs and spices as well.

> **Note:** Some brands of mustard contain grain vinegar, which contains gluten.

REMEMBER

- Choose Himalayan salt or sea salt.
- Herbs and spices should be organic and free of preservatives, including MSG.
- Ketchup and salsa should be organic and preservative free.
- Stay away from all mayonnaise.
- Mustard is the better choice.
- Garlic is a great addition to any diet.

28

BABY FOOD

You may not have a baby, but you most likely have a relative or friend that does. Do them a favor and pass this little bit of information on to them.

WHAT SHOULD YOU FEED YOUR BABY?

It's always best to feed your baby breast fed mother's milk. As the saying goes, breast is best. In the event that you are not able to breast feed your baby, a Mother's Milk Bank may be an option for you. There are 7 distributing milk banks in North America. To find the locations of Mother's Milk Banks in North America, go to www.BreastFeeding.com and type "Banking on Breastmilk" into its search engine.

A baby needs mother's milk from a beneficial source in order to inoculate his/her gut with beneficial bacteria as well as provide a whole myriad of beneficial properties that cannot be replicated in baby formula.

According to BreastFeeding.com, "...for some babies, receiving breastmilk isn't just a good nutrition and mothering choice, it may be a question of life or death."

> **Note:** I checked all of the baby formulas available at my local grocery store and they were all unhealthy for your baby. All of the baby formulas contained processed sugars, denatured proteins, and harmful preservatives.

FOOD FOR THOUGHT

It is imperative that all pregnant and lactating women eat a diet of exclusively organic food. Organic vegetables, organic fruits, and grass fed organic meat and dairy products (unless you are a vegetarian).

Studies have shown that meat and dairy (milk) products from non-organic sources contain higher levels of pesticide contamination than commercial fruits and vegetables. Well, the same thing goes for human mother's milk. Yes, you read that right, human mother's milk has been found to be contaminated with high levels of pesticides. These pesticides are then transferred to your baby.

If you gain nothing else from this manual, please promise me one thing... Promise Me That You Will Do Everything That You Can To Eat Organic Whole Foods! It's good for you and it's good for your loved ones.

According to Mark McAfee of Organic Pastures, there are infant formulas allowed in the United States that the World Health Organization does not allow in third world countries.

Whatever you do, never feed your baby soy based infant formula. Many studies have shown that soy formulas are bad for baby's health. I will discuss the dangers of soy in detail throughout this section.

> **Note:** Never use a microwave to warm up your baby's food. Microwaves destroy the chemical structures of the delicate nutrients contained in your food.

WHAT ABOUT BABY FOOD?

When your baby is ready to be fed baby food it is best to make it yourself. If you don't have a food processor, buy one. You can put your own organic vegetables and fruits in the processor knowing that you are feeding your baby fresh wholesome ingredients. Babies deserve the most vital, nutritious, life giving, enzyme rich foods that you can possibly give them.

> **It amazes me to see women feeding their children the most convenient easy food that they can find without regards to its nutritional content. You have already learned through this manual that the big corporations do not have your best interests at heart. Well, the same thing goes for your children. Do not depend on corporate America to provide you with the proper food to feed your baby. If you expect your children to develop properly, both physically and mentally, you have to provide them with the proper nutrition. Doing this may take a little extra work, but your children are more than worth it.**

HOMEMADE BABY FOOD RECIPES

Wholesome homemade baby food recipes can be found at WholesomeBabyFood.com. It is a great website containing tons of information, great wholesome recipes, and, best of all, it's free.

WHAT ABOUT PACKAGED BABY FOOD?

Packaged baby food is just like any other packaged food; some will contain healthy ingredients, but most contain tons of preservatives and other chemical additives that are extremely bad for your child.

Also, many of the same principles that apply to bottled whole vegetable and fruit juices apply to baby food. Mainly, the nutrient density of the packaged baby food is greatly diminished until just the carbohydrates remain.

If you find yourself in a situation where you have to buy pre-packaged baby food, follow these guidelines:

- **Organic Whole Food Ingredients:** It is easy to find organic baby food on supermarket shelves these days. At the very least, buy organic.

- **No Preservatives or Chemical Additives:** Read the ingredient list. The list should be small and you should recognize every ingredient. If you don't recognize an ingredient you should immediately put the jar back on the shelf and look for something else. Read every label. If you are buying a jar of pureed carrots, the only ingredient should be organic carrots.

- **Stay Away From Soy:** Soy is not good for your baby. You will see a lot of baby food on the shelves of supermarkets which contain soy. Soy has estrogen like properties, called phytoestrogens, that you do not want to eat and you certainly do not want your baby to eat, especially if it is a boy. Phytoestrogens in soy disrupt the hormonal development in a baby. I read an article recently which stated that babies that are fed a diet of soy products can ingest the estrogen equivalent of two birth-control pills in one day.

REMEMBER

- Babies need mother's milk for proper development.
- Make your own fresh organic baby food.
- Do not feed your baby soy products.

WHAT'S THE DEAL WITH SOY?

Soy is one of the foods that manufacturers are trying to put into everything and baby food is no exception.

Soy is being touted as a miracle health food, but it's not. There is much debate about this, but research that I have done has shown that soy has a myriad of detrimental components in it that are not beneficial for human consumption. Also, soy along with corn are the most genetically modified substances on the planet.

You may be asking: What about the Asian cultures that eat tons of soy?

Well, historically these large Asian cultures did not eat the soy that is available on supermarket shelves today. The type of soy that Asians have historically eaten is fermented soy, such as tempeh or miso. The fermentation process destroys the anti-nutrients in the soy which increases its bioavailability.

The soy available in most of the world today is the highly processed genetically modified soy that is grown and manufactured in the United States and Canada. This unnatural soy is having a dramatic impact on the world as a whole. More than 75% of all of the soy grown in America is genetically modified.

China is getting fat. As American corporations such as McDonald's, Starbucks, and Wal-Mart experience exponential growth in China, so does the Chinese waistline. It is interesting to note that there are more Starbucks in China than in the United States.

It is reported that there are 250 million overweight Chinese. Childhood obesity is also on the rise. A recent USA Today article reports: "Today, 8% of 10 to 12 year-olds in China's cities are considered obese and an additional 15% are overweight, according to Education Ministry data."

As the world becomes more "Americanized" it is also getting fatter. Countries such as France and Brazil who used to laugh at the "fat Americans" are now experiencing a rapid increase in overweight and obesity.

CHILDHOOD OBESITY
RUNNING OUT OF CONTROL

It's true. The incidence of overweight and obesity in children has risen at an alarming rate since 1982. Take a look at the following statistics released by the National Institute of Health.

- 4% of children overweight in 1982
- 16% of children overweight in 1994
- 25% of all white children overweight in 2001
- 33% African American & Hispanic children overweight in 2001

Because of this, diabetes, hypertension (high blood pressure), and other obesity related chronic diseases that are prevalent among adults have now become increasingly common in our children.

Type II diabetes is no longer called adult onset diabetes, due to the fact that a large portion of those contracting the disease are now children. In fact, children account for 45% of all new reported cases of Type II diabetes. Poor dietary habits and inactivity are the major contributing factors to the increase of obesity in youth. It has been reported that this is the first generation in the history of the modern world that will not outlive their parents. I hope that you understand just how imperative it is that you put to use the principles outlined in this course. The health and future of your children depend on it.

29

INTRODUCTION TO BEVERAGES

The Beverage industry is another huge multi-billion dollar industry that, for the most part, does not have your best interest at heart. You need to make the most informed decisions that you possibly can when selecting beverages for yourself and your loved ones. I see people who make painstaking efforts to choose the best foods that they possibly can, but totally blow it when it comes to the drinks that they choose.

In this section we will discuss your best choices for:

- Water
- Vegetable & Fruit Juices
- Coffee & Tea

30

WATER

Your body consists of 70% water and your brain consists of 85% water. It only makes sense that you need to drink plenty of good clean water on a daily basis to remain vibrant and healthy.

Proper hydration is a key element in obtaining a tight and toned body. You cannot look great and feel great without proper hydration. Key functions of water include:

- Proper delivery of nutrients to our cells.

- Proper brain function.

- Elimination of waste products from our cells.

- Help in maintaining a healthy environment in our intestines.

- Proper digestion of food.

- Frequent healthy bowel movements.

FIT FACT

Water is truly the most essential element of life. We can live more than a month without food (I have seen people do this), but we cannot survive more than a few days without water.

As you can see, every function in the body, in one way or another, requires water. Which leads us to...

Benefits of drinking adequate amounts of water:

* Maintain Optimal Health.
* Accelerate Weight Loss.
* Increase Energy.
* Think Clearly.
* Prevent and Heal Disease.

Many of us are dehydrated and don't even realize it. Dehydration can cause a myriad of problems from headaches to high blood pressure. Simply put, a lack of water will cause you to store toxic waste adding unnatural stress on your liver and kidneys.

HOW MUCH WATER SHOULD YOU DRINK IN ONE DAY?

This is one of the questions that I am most often asked. However, there is no standard answer that can be given for this question. You have probably heard many people say that you should drink 8 glasses of water a day or half your body weight in ounces per day or something similar. The problem is this: some people will listen to a statement like the one just mentioned and drink all eight glasses of water in the morning and think they are good for the day. This is faulty thinking.

It has been my experience that water needs will vary from individual to individual. For instance, a carpenter working all day in the sun will require much more water than an office worker sitting behind a desk in an air conditioned office.

A better question would be: How often should I drink water throughout the day?

You should do your best to consume some water every one or two hours. It is more beneficial for you to concern yourself with drinking water consistently throughout the day, rather than focusing on a predetermined amount. Making this one change in your daily regimen will make a positive impact on your weight loss and fitness success.

WHAT KIND OF WATER SHOULD YOU DRINK?

Just like the food that you eat, you need to make the most informed decision possible when choosing the water that you drink. Let's take a look at a few different sources of water and discuss the most beneficial options for each.

TAP WATER

You definitely do not want to drink straight tap water. Tap water contains chlorine, fluoride, and a whole myriad of other contaminants that are detrimental to your health.

Whole House Filtration System: In order to drink tap water you must first filter out all of its harmful contaminants. If you live in a house I suggest that you install a whole house filtration system. Investing in a home filtration system is the most economical route that you can take in regards to your

---

FOOD FOR THOUGHT

Vegetables and fruits contain large amounts of water. Therefore, eating plenty of fruits and vegetables will aid in hydrating you body. This is one more reason for you to eat your fruits and veggies.

---

drinking water. These systems have the added benefit of providing you with purified water to cook your food in.

Reverse Osmosis: A reverse osmosis system is great because it filters out all harmful contaminants including fluoride. The best reverse osmosis systems will contain a second filter that remineralizes the water.

Carbon Filters: Carbon filters are generally the most economical. However, it is best to choose a multistage carbon filter to insure the removal of the greatest amount of contaminants.

As I mentioned, there are multi-stage filters available for your tap water. These filters remove harmful pollutants and add beneficial minerals which increase the alkalinity of the water.

THINK GREEN

Also, it takes considerable resources to bottle water and ship it half way around the world. So, from a Green perspective, a home filtration system that remineralizes your water will have the most positive impact on planet earth.

FIT FACT

Your skin is your largest organ. Because of this, your body can soak up more contaminants in a 10 minute shower than during a whole day of drinking water. A whole house filtration system will prevent the absorption of heavy metals and other contaminants from all of the faucets in your house. If you are not able to install a whole house filtration system, you should consider a shower filter.

BOTTLED WATER

Bottled water is another area where you need to be extremely careful. The National Resources Defense Council (NRDC) estimates that 25 percent or more of bottled water is really just tap water in a bottle.

For Example: Dasani (Coca-Cola) and AquaFina (Pepsi-Cola) bottled waters are purified tap water in a bottle. Using a home filtration system is better for you and our environment.

Also, many people like to buy bottled water because they think it's better for them, but they buy the cheapest water that they can possibly find. If you buy bottled water, do some research, so you will choose the most beneficial water for yourself and your loved ones.

Sometimes you will see bottled water that is steam distilled. Steam distilled water goes through a process which turns water into steam and then back into water. This process takes out every property that the water contains except for the hydrogen and oxygen. All of the impurities are removed, but all of the beneficial minerals are removed as well. This type of water can be beneficial during certain times, such as during a *cleanse*, but on a daily basis you do not want to drink distilled water.

Naturally sourced spring water is your best bet when it comes to bottled water. Often times these waters contain naturally occurring minerals that make them slightly alkaline. Remember that your blood has a slightly alkaline pH between 7.35 and 7.45. Some bottled waters including *Fiji* and *Icelandic Glacial* have a similar alkaline pH. These waters will help your body maintain its healthy alkaline environment.

Read the label of your bottled water to insure that it is from a beneficial source.

> # FIT FACT
>
> An alkaline rich environment has been shown to carry as much as 20% more oxygen in your blood cells. Cancer cells cannot live in an oxygen rich environment. There is much debate over this, but I have found that when people eat foods and drink water that promotes alkalinity in their body they are much healthier. They look healthier, they have more energy, they appear more vibrant, and they do not get sick easily, if at all. People whose bodies are more alkaline tend to have that special glow. I personally do everything I can to keep myself slightly alkaline and I do not get sick. Anything you can do to maintain an alkaline pH in your body is highly advisable.

ALL PLASTIC IS NOT CREATED EQUAL

Another concern with bottled water is the container that it's in. The plastic should always be clear. It should never be cloudy. A good example of cloudy plastics is the 2 1/2 gallon jugs that you find in Arrowhead or Sparklets drinking water. These types of plastics have properties in them that are not beneficial for you, and will leech very easily into the water. Stay away from these cloudy plastic containers. Again, when buying bottled water, make sure that the container that it is in is clear.

However, do not use these plastic bottles more than once. They are disposable bottles that are made to break down very easily. If used more than once, they will start to break down and leach harmful substances into your water.

WHERE CAN YOU LEARN MORE ABOUT DRINKING WATER?

AllAboutWater.org is an excellent website with valuable information including:

- Water Filtration Alternatives.
- The Truth About Bottled Water.
- 10 Benefits of Using a Drinking Water Filter.

VITAMIN WATER & FRUIT WATER

I have never found any benefit to drinking vitamin water, fruit water, or any other type of enhanced water. Take a look at the ingredient list of these enhanced waters; they will usually contain artificial sweeteners, preservatives, and other chemical additives that do not need to be there and are definitely unhealthy. Also, these enhanced waters are usually fortified with man-made vitamins and minerals that may not be bioavailable; in other words, your body may not be able to absorb and utilize them.

REMEMBER

Plain water is always going to be your best bet. Naturally sourced alkaline water which contains naturally occurring bioavailable minerals is not only good for you, but it will also taste delicious. **Nothing can replace the positive effects of drinking good clean water.**

31

VEGETABLE & FRUIT JUICES

There are three basic types of whole fruit juices. One of them is beneficial for you. The other two are disguised "healthy" drinks that do more harm than good.

- Freshly juiced vegetables and fruits.
- Packaged juiced vegetables and fruits.
- Made with real fruit juice.

MY FIT LIFE

When I first started eating fruits and vegetables I ate them almost exclusively from a juicer. Nowadays, I do not use my juicer at all unless I am doing a cleanse. I currently make vegetable and fruit smoothies every morning in a blender and eat whole raw vegetables and some fruits throughout the rest of the day.

FRESHLY JUICED VEGETABLES & FRUITS

Juicing your own fresh organic produce is a great way for you to eat a variety of fruits and vegetables. There are a couple of key benefits to fresh juicing:

- Fresh vegetable and fruit juice is a nutrient dense enzyme rich beverage, power packed with bioavailable amino acids, carbohydrates, vitamins, minerals, phytonutrients, and life giving enzymes; these beneficial juices are like nature's medicine.

- Eat a greater variety of vegetables and fruits than you normally would. Many people, especially when first starting out with their new healthy lifestyle, often times have difficulty eating a wide variety of raw fruits and vegetables. However, juicing affords you a way to quickly and easily ingest fruits and vegetables that you might otherwise never take the time to try.

- You will soon discover that raw fruits and vegetables taste great. Also, your body will become accustomed to the flavor and great nutritional value of these healthy juices. It may sound strange right now, but you will actually begin to crave these healthy fruits and vegetables. Those of you who are already juicing know what I am talking about.

- Once you become accustomed to juicing, you will find yourself eating more raw vegetables and fruits with each of your meals.

Note: People that juice do so because of the enzyme activity. Enzymes are our fountain of youth; they are the reason we eat raw foods, go on *cleanses*, and drink fresh vegetable and fruit juice. Enzymes give you that *glow* to your skin and help you fight off sickness and disease. Enzymes are the key to life.

PACKAGED JUICED WHOLE FRUITS & VEGETABLES

Packaged juiced whole fruits and vegetables, such as Naked Juice and Odwalla, may seem like a great idea, but they actually do more harm than good. This is another example of slick marketing leading you down the wrong path.

You should stay away from these types of juices for these reasons:

- **Pasteurization**: In order to have a shelf life these juices are pasteurized. You have already learned in the dairy section that when you pasteurize food you kill all of the beneficial nutrients including the life giving enzymes.

- **Half-life**: Juiced vegetables and fruits have a half life, which means that the nutrient density of the juice goes down as time goes on. Experts say that after 18 hours most of the nutritional benefits are gone and all that you are left with are the carbohydrates.

- **Dense Carbohydrates**: If you eat one orange its calories will release into your blood stream at a slow rate because of the fiber and other nutrients found in the whole fruit. However, one pint of orange juice may contain the juice from eight or nine oranges and all of the calories from those eight or nine oranges. Since there is no fiber or other nutrients to slow the absorption of this calorie dense juice into your system you will get a spike in your insulin. You will be able to store a small amount of these carbohydrates as glycogen and the rest will be stored as fat, just like the flour from the breads over in the bread section.

- **Pesticide Contamination**: Most of the produce used to manufacture juices are not organic, which means that they will have high levels of pesticide contamination as well as GMO's (genetic modifications).

- **Rotten Produce**: Keep in mind that packaged juices are produced on a large scale. If you have ever juiced vegetables and fruits yourself you know how messy conditions get... very quickly. Just imagine what condition the commercial juicing plants must be in.

    Also, it is impossible for the employees of these large companies to inspect each and every piece of fruit. They are processing hundreds or thousands of pounds of produce at a time. It is highly likely that some of the vegetables or fruits that are being juiced will be rotten. This is one of the reasons that these companies pasteurize their juices. In the latter part of 2006 one of the major whole juice companies had to recall a tainted batch of carrot juice for this very reason. It's just not worth the risk.

MADE WITH REAL FRUIT JUICE

The real fruit juices found on the shelves of your local supermarket are much worse than the pasteurized whole fruit juices. These juices have very little, if any, real fruit juice. They often contain table sugar, high fructose corn syrup, or some other form of processed sugar. These calorie dense juices will spike your insulin levels and cause you to store body fat. **These types of juices are never good for you.**

REMEMBER

- Drink plenty of good clean water.
- Make your own fresh organic vegetable and fruit juices. Doing so will insure that your juice is full of life giving nutrition.
- Stay away from store bought packaged juices; they will cause you to store body fat.

32

COFFEE & TEA

Coffee and tea are two of the most widely consumed beverages in the world. Because of this, coffee and tea are a huge multi-billion dollar industry. This translates into deception, corruption and exploitation on a global scale. Hopefully you understand that you have to be aware of what is going on in the world in regards to your food and beverage.

The type of coffee and tea that you choose to drink can have a huge impact not only on your own personal health, but also on the well being of small farmer's throughout the world. But first...

IS COFFEE & TEA GOOD FOR YOU?

Let's first take a look at coffee. It is estimated that more than 50% of Americans drink coffee. And yes, I am included in this statistic. However, I do not drink coffee for health reasons; I drink coffee because I like the way it tastes.

There is conflicting research when it comes to coffee. Coffee advocates state that it has a whole myriad of beneficial properties including antioxidants. Opponents of coffee state that it is a harmful and addictive substance.

MY PERSONAL OPINION

It is best to keep your coffee consumption to a minimum.

There are two main reasons for the above statement:

1. Coffee is acid forming in your body. If you have listened to this course, you know that I suggest staying away from acid forming foods. Remember, you should do everything that you can to keep your body in an alkaline state.

2. Coffee is a diuretic. It will leech water from your body at a rapid rate if you consume too much of it. If this happens you will become dehydrated.

   So, a little is okay, but large amounts of coffee will be detrimental to your health.

Now, let's take a look at tea. There are many different types of tea:

- Black Tea
- Green Tea
- White Tea
- Red Tea
- Herbal Tea
- Naturally Caffeinated
- Naturally Decaffeinated
- Etc.

I will not discuss all of the attributes of each different type of tea. However, tea is used in many countries for its therapeutic effects. This practice dates back through many centuries. I have found that people tend to drink tea in moderation compared to coffee. For this reason, I am a strong advocate of drinking tea. I personally enjoy chamomile tea and rooibos, which is a red African tea.

COFFEE ALTERNATIVES

There are two coffee alternatives worth mentioning:

- Yerba Mate
- Teeccino

Yerba Mate is usually found in the tea section of your supermarket. It is widely used throughout South America. I have found that it tastes good and it feels good. Millions of people drink it on a daily basis. It's not acid forming like coffee, but it has an uplifting feel to it. Yerba Mate contains an ingredient known as matteine, which is similar to caffeine. However, Yerba Mate will not make you jittery.

Teeccino is marketed as a healthy alternative to coffee. I drink Teeccino on occasion. Teeccino tastes similar to coffee, but is naturally caffeine free. The difference with Teeccino is the fact that it is a mixture of cacao, nuts, chikory, and some other ingredients. It is alkaline forming in your body and is touted as having antioxidants. In other words it is a coffee substitute that is supposed to be good for you.

The best thing to do is drink plenty of good clean water and keep your consumption of coffee and tea to a minimum.

As with all of the other food and beverage in this course, my job is to help you make the most informed decision for the situation you are in.

WHAT TO LOOK FOR

There are a couple of things to look for when selecting coffee, tea, or yerba mate:

- Shade Grown
- Organic
- Fair trade

Coffee is grown in tropical climates; most of it is grown on small farms. Historically, these small coffee farmers have been treated unfairly:

Shade Grown: Coffee farmers have been forced to cut back the trees on their farms in order to increase their yields. These trees are more commonly called rain forest. As you probably know, the destruction of rain forest is a hot topic today.

In other words, **shade grown coffee helps preserve tropical rainforests, which in turn helps to protect our delicate ecosystem and reduce global warming**.

Organic: What you may not know is the fact that coffee grown in direct sunlight requires large amounts of pesticides. As you know, pesticides and herbicides are harmful to you. Also, since countries outside of the United States are not regulated by the FDA, they will typically use a larger amount of pesticides. These high levels of pesticides soak into the coffee beans which in turn get transferred into your body.

Fair Trade: Here's the problem: 70% of the coffee grown in the world is produced by small rural farmers. Their farms are typically five acres or less. Rural farmers in other parts of the world do not realize the dramatic effect commercially grown coffee, tea, and cacao has on consumers and the environment.

Many of these farmers and their workers have been kept in poverty by large corporations. Fair Trade certification was established in order to stop the exploitation of these farmers, workers, and the environment.

Fair Trade is much more than a fair price! Fair Trade principles include:

- *Fair price:* Democratically organized farmer groups receive a guaranteed minimum floor price and an additional premium for certified organic products. Farmer organizations are also eligible for pre-harvest credit.

- *Fair labor conditions:* Workers on Fair Trade farms enjoy freedom of association, safe working conditions, and living wages. Forced child labor is strictly prohibited.

- *Direct trade:* With Fair Trade, importers purchase from Fair Trade producer groups as directly as possible, eliminating unnecessary middlemen and empowering farmers to develop the business capacity necessary to compete in the global marketplace.

- *Democratic and transparent organizations:* Fair Trade farmers and farm workers decide democratically how to invest Fair Trade revenues.

- *Community development:* Fair Trade farmers and farm workers invest Fair Trade premiums in social and business development projects like scholarship programs, quality improvement trainings, and organic certification.

- ***Environmental sustainability*:** Harmful agrichemicals and GMO's are strictly prohibited in favor of environmentally sustainable farming methods that protect farmers' health and preserve valuable ecosystems for future generations.

— Source: www.TransFairUSA.org

Fair Trade Certification has been available since 1999, but it's just now beginning to gain public awareness. I consider it a moral obligation to support the Fair Trade initiative. Fair Trade Certification offers a simple way for conscious consumers to know that their products were produced in a socially, environmentally, and economically responsible manner.

With Fair Trade *you* can make a difference. Look for the Fair Trade Certified label the next time you buy coffee, tea, or cacao.

For more information go to www.transfairusa.org.

REMEMBER

- Drink coffee and tea in moderation.
- Yerba Mate and Teeccino are good coffee alternatives.
- Look for coffee and tea that is organic, Fair Trade, and shade grown.

33

SPORT NUTRITION DRINKS

The sport nutrition drink business is a huge multi-billion dollar business. Yes, you read that right; a multi-billion dollar business. As you can see, there is a lot of money being made off of this processed and packaged food business. And yes, most sport nutrition bars and drinks are nothing more than processed and packaged foods.

Furthermore, most sport nutrition drinks are full of processed sugars, artificial sweeteners, and chemical additives that are detrimental to your weight loss and fitness goals. These drinks are of no benefit to you; you do not need them.

There are three basic types of sport nutrition drinks available on the market today.

1. Energy Drinks and Fat Burning Drinks.
2. Meal Replacement Drinks.
3. Electrolyte Replacement Drinks.

Let's take a look at each type individually...

ENERGY DRINKS & FAT BURNING DRINKS

Energy and fat burning drinks are basically the same thing. These drinks are stimulants that make two basic claims:

1. They give you more energy.
2. They create a thermic fat-burning effect in your body.

First off, the stimulant effect from the substances inside of energy drinks, will give you a false sense of energy followed by an inevitable "crash" which will create a craving for more energy drinks.

Secondly, the supposed thermic fat-burning effect of these drinks gives you a false sense of hope. These drinks do not make you burn fat. If they did, obesity would not be at the all time high that it is today.

The only way for you to efficiently burn body fat is to release it into your muscle cells to be burned as energy.

Furthermore, the stimulant effect from energy drinks causes an unnatural increase in your heart rate. This increase in heart rate is the mechanism which gives you a false sense of increased energy. This is very dangerous. In fact, many people, including young athletes, have died as a direct result of energy drinks and pills. Avoid these dangerous substances at all costs.

In addition to the above mentioned statements, keep in mind that most energy drinks contain sweeteners and chemical additives that are not beneficial to your weight loss goals.

IF YOU WANT ENERGY, YOU NEED TO EAT FOOD

Food is your body's only source of usable energy. Quality food gives your body the necessary calories and nutrients that will make it run at optimal levels. Notice that I mentioned quality food.

Here's the deal, in order to have sustainable energy throughout the day, without the highs and lows, you need to fuel your body with nutrient dense quality food. It is incredible how good you can feel by simply eating healthy whole foods. There is nothing like it.

IF YOU WANT TO BURN FAT, YOU NEED TO BUILD MUSCLE

Muscle is your fat burning furnace. The only way for you to burn fat is to release it into your muscle cells to be burned as energy. Therefore, the more muscle that you have, the more fat you can burn. It only makes sense.

So, if you want to become an energized fat burning machine you have to follow three basic principles:

1. Eat the right foods.
2. Eat when your body is hungry and not for emotional reasons.
3. Follow a proper exercise routine.

Better Living With Whole Foods empowers you with the knowledge necessary to make the most healthful food choices for yourself and your loved ones.

This course, along with an effective exercise routine, such as the *16 Week Total Body Makeover*, are all that you need to take control of your life and achieve your weight loss and fitness goals.

MEAL REPLACEMENT DRINKS AND POWDERS

There are a lot of meal replacement drinks and powders available on the market today, most of which are processed and denatured:

- Slimfast
- Ensure
- Atkins Advantage
- Special-K Protein Water
- Boost
- Myoplex
- Met-Rx

I found all of the above mentioned drinks in my local grocery store. Unfortunately, they are of no benefit to you or me.

It is interesting to note that most of these meal replacement drinks contain both refined sugar and sucralose, a harmful artificial sweetener.

If you can believe this, MSG is contained in almost every one of these drinks. Remember that MSG is a harmful chemical additive that has no place in the foods that you eat or the beverages that you drink. Also, the protein contained in these drinks is highly processed and denatured; your body cannot effectively utilize it. There is no real benefit to drinking these meal replacements. They not only give you a false sense of hope, but also sabotage your fitness and weight loss efforts.

WHAT SHOULD YOU DO?

It is always best to eat whole foods whenever possible. Make the time to prepare meals and bring healthy snacks with you when you know you are going to be away from your home or office for extended periods of time.

That being said, I understand that the world is a very busy place these days, especially for working moms. It is during these times that we tend to opt for the convenience of the nearest drive-thru window. Do not give into this temptation.

If you find yourself frequently in a situation where you do not have access to healthy whole foods, arm yourself with a healthy food bar or healthy whole food meal replacement.

As mentioned earlier, most meal replacement drinks and powders are processed and denatured; they do more harm than good. However, there are some meal replacements that are made from freeze dried whole foods. They do not contain the same nutritional value of fresh whole foods, but they are much better than commercial meal replacements or fast food meals and snacks.

I personally do not use any type of meal replacement powders or drinks. I have figured out a simple system to supply myself with healthy whole foods throughout the day, which I will discuss in the **Putting It All Together** section of this manual.

ELECTROLYTE REPLACEMENT DRINKS

Electrolyte replacement drinks are basically sugar water. They will spike your insulin levels causing you to store body fat. Also, these enhanced drinks usually contain harmful chemical additives including dyes which give them their unique colors.

LET'S TAKE A LOOK AT GATORADE

Gatorade is the most highly marketed and widely used of all sport nutrition drinks. There is an onslaught of advertising dollars forced down our throats from every form of media imaginable.

Gatorade marketing is very slick. They use top athletes, Gatorade University, and official looking chemists and doctors to push their products. In reality, Gatorade is one of those products that are all smoke and mirrors. There is no benefit to drinking it.

Gatorade Ingredients:

- Water
- Glucose-Fructose Syrup
- Natural and Artificial flavors
- Sodium Citrate
- Ester Gum
- Red 40
- Sucrose Syrup
- Citric Acid
- Salt
- Monopotassium Phosphate
- Sucrose Acetate Isobutyrate
- Blue 1

Sucrose syrup and glucose-fructose syrup are highly refined sugars that spike insulin and cause storage of body fat. Remember, a 32 oz. bottle of Gatorade contains 14 teaspoons (56 grams) of processed sugars.

Sucrose acetate isobutyrate is a laboratory made sweetener. I could not find much information on this substance, but it is most likely very unhealthy, as are all man made sweeteners.

Natural flavors are MSG. Remember, MSG has been called edible nicotine because of its harmful addictive properties.

Red 40 and Blue 1 are harmful dyes that give Gatorade its color. Studies have shown that Red 40 causes hyperactivity in children. There are a wide variety of dyes used depending on the color of a particular flavor. It is important to stay away from these harmful substances.

Ester gum is an emulsifier used to suspend oil in water.

DO TOP ATHLETES REALLY DRINK GATORADE?

It's common to see big jugs of Gatorade on the sidelines of professional and college football games. These big jugs are commonly used to pour over the coach's head when a team wins a big game or championship. If you'll notice, the liquid inside of those jugs is not colored, it's clear. In other words, the jugs contain water, not Gatorade. Those big jugs are on the sidelines for marketing purposes. Coaches and trainers know that Gatorade is not good for their athletes.

REMEMBER

* Stay away form sport nutrition drinks, including energy drinks, meal replacements, and electrolyte replacement drinks.

* If you want energy you need to fuel your body with nutrient dense quality food.

* You need to build muscle to burn fat.

* Choose healthy snacks over commercial meal replacements

* Drink plenty of water and eat whole fruits and vegetables in order to replace and maintain fluid and electrolyte levels.

34

SPORT NUTRITION BARS

Two key principles you will learn in this section:

1. You should avoid most sport nutrition bars
2. There is a better alternative

Sport nutrition bars include:

- Meal Replacement Bars
- Protein Bars
- Energy bars

Most of the sport nutrition bars available on the shelves of supermarkets and health food stores are processed denatured junk that contains high levels of refined sugar, artificial sweeteners, hidden fats, hidden carbs, artificial ingredients, and a ton of preservatives.

These supposed *Nutrition Bars* are nothing more than over-glorified candy bars. These include Atkins Bars, South Beach

Diet Bars, Power Bars, Myoplex Bars, Met-Rx Bars, Kashi Go-Lean Bars, and Special-K Bars just to name a few. I would say that 95 – 99% of the nutrition bars available on the market today are junk. Do not eat these convenience foods. They will make you gain weight; especially in your waist, hips, butt, and thighs.

LET'S TAKE A LOOK AT A TYPICAL SPORT NUTRITION BAR

Headline:

Special K Protein Meal Bar

"The Meal Replacement Bar That Helps You Stay On Track"

10 grams of protein

Sounds good doesn't it?

NOW, LET'S LOOK AT THE INGREDIENT LIST

- Sugar
- Corn Syrup
- Fructose
- High Fructose Corn Syrup
- Dextrose
- Rice Starch
- Partially Hydrogenated Palm Kernel Oil
- Soy Lecithin
- Mono- and Diglycerides
- Sorbitan Monostearate
- Polysorbate 60
- BHT (preservative)
- Artificial Flavor
- Wheat Gluten

- Wheat Flour
- Peanut flour

What? I thought this was supposed to be a healthy meal replacement bar.

Let me break this down just for clarification:

Sugar, Corn Syrup, High Fructose Corn Syrup, Dextrose, Rice Starch: These are highly processed sugars that will cause you to store fat.

Partially Hydrogenated Palm Kernel Oil: This is a trans-fat. However, because of an FDA loophole, food manufacturers are not required to label this dangerous fat as a trans-fat.

Soy Lecithin: A highly processed hidden fat which is used as an emulsifier.

Mon- and Diglycerides: Highly processed hidden fats

> **Note:** For more information regarding soy lecithin, monoglycerides, and diglycerides, refer to page 28 of this manual.

Sorbitan Monostearate: An emulsifying agent also known as a synthetic wax. Used in baked goods, cake mixes, imitation whipped cream and **hemorrhoid cream. Yuck!!**

Polysorbate 60: An emulsifier.

> **Note:** An emulsion is a mixture of oil and water. Emulsifiers enable emulsions to form and hold. Sports bars would not hold together without the use of emulsifiers.

BHT (preservative): According to a post on www.drweil.com, BHT has been banned in some European countries and in Japan.

It is thought to cause liver damage, kidney damage, and abnormal behavior patterns.

Wheat Gluten, Wheat Flour, And Peanut Flour: These are all highly processed flours that will cause you to store body fat and may cause allergies and contribute to inflammatory disorders.

Isn't this a shame? Why does the FDA allow these dead non-food bars to be marketed and sold as a healthy meal replacement? They are obviously very bad (unhealthy) for you.

Women and men alike eat these types of bars on a regular basis. In fact, I personally know women that will not give up their nutrition bars. These same women do not lose weight; and they wonder why! You must learn to read labels in order to protect yourself from these harmful foods.

IS THERE A BETTER ALTERNATIVE?

As mentioned previously, most of us have very busy lives. Because of this there will be times when we are hungry, but have no time to eat a whole meal. During these times it would be great if there was a healthy nutrition bar available. Luckily, there are a few companies who actually "get it". These companies offer a better alternative to the processed and denatured sport nutrition bars available on the shelves of your local supermarket.

I do not promote the use of these bars on a daily basis, but they are definitely a better alternative to the denatured sports bars that most people eat. Remember, whole foods will always be your best bet.

A BETTER CHOICE

One of the bars that I recommend is made by Organic Food Bar Inc. Their bars are promoted as the only line of Organic

Food Bars consisting of alkaline forming, enzyme active organic whole foods, sprouted superfoods and antioxidants that provide optimal nutrition for your body.

These whole food nutrition bars are:

- Cold Processed
- High Energy
- 100% Organic
- 100% Vegetarian
- Gluten Free
- GMO Free (no genetic modifications)
- Up to 100% Raw
- No Preservatives, No Additives, No Salt, No Coatings, No Refined Sugar, No Soy, No Peanuts, No Dairy
- Certified Kosher

My favorite is their Omega-3 Flax Bar, it is 100% raw.

I like these bars because they are organic, they taste good, and they are sold all over the United States and in many parts of the world. You can find Organic Food Bars in Whole Foods, Mother's Market, Henry's Market, and Trader Joe's.

REMEMBER

- Stay away from the commercial sport nutrition bars found on the shelves of your local supermarket.
- Eating whole foods will always be your best bet.
- Organic Food Bars are a better alternative.

35

SUPPLEMENTS

There are two main goals to this section:

1. To help you understand what supplements are.
2. To help you understand the need for a healthy diet.

The supplement industry is a huge multi-billion dollar industry that makes most of its money on false promises and deception. We are offered "magic bullets" on a daily basis. Take this pill and you'll be full of energy. Take this drink and you'll fight cancer and heart disease... You know the story. People are led to believe that they can live a life full of indiscretion and remain healthy by taking one or a combination of magic potions. This type of thinking is very harmful.

Look, it's only natural to get caught up in this whirlwind of deceptive marketing. Every health & fitness magazine is filled with page after page of advertisements pushing the latest and greatest supplements. In fact, some of these magazines are nothing more than supplement catalogs with an occasional article.

I am not saying that all supplements are worthless, but most of them are. That being said, quality supplements, used in the correct manner, can be a wonderful contribution to your healthy lifestyle.

WHAT ARE SUPPLEMENTS?

Supplements are exactly what their name implies, an addition to an already healthy eating regimen and wellness lifestyle. Supplements all by themselves will not give you lasting health and weight loss success.

Before taking supplements you must...

FIRST, EAT HEALTHY, THEN ADD SUPPLEMENTS

One of the questions that I am most often asked: "What supplements should I be taking?"

I always answer this question with another question: "What types of foods are you currently eating?"

Most people take supplements because they think they are lacking a specific nutrient. Most times what is lacking is a healthy diet. There is no single ingredient or nutrient that will magically prevent disease or improve health. Vibrant health is accomplished by eating a combination of nutrients found in healthy whole foods, especially raw vegetables and fruits.

There is one other area of concern when talking of supplements...

ALL SUPPLEMENTS ARE NOT CREATED EQUAL

The quality of your supplements is determined by the quality and type of their ingredients as well as the processes by which the ingredients are extracted and formulated. Just like the food that you eat, the quality of your supplements will determine what benefit, if any, they will provide you. Supplements should be derived from natural whole food sources. Synthetic man made supplements should be avoided at all costs; they will do you more harm than good.

RECOMMENDED SUPPLEMENTS

There are a couple of supplements that are worth mentioning:

* MSM
* Multi-Mineral Solution
* Omega-3 Fatty Acid Supplement
* Lacto Fermented Products

MSM: I have been taking MSM since 1992. MSM is the only supplement that I currently take. MSM is the third most abundant substance in your body. It has been called one of the five elements of life. I will discuss MSM in greater detail in a few moments, but first...

Multi-Mineral Solution: According to Dr. Jacob Swilling, a quality mineral solution will make you feel energetic and vibrant. The best form of minerals is a crystalloid solution. A crystalloid solution is the smallest molecule form which allows for almost instant absorption.

Omega-3 Fatty Acids: As I previously mentioned, the Standard American Diet (SAD) contains too many omega-6 fatty acids and not enough beneficial omega-3 fatty acids. Because of this, it could be beneficial for you to include a good omega-3 supplement in your diet, such as cod liver oil.

Lacto-Fermented Products: Lacto fermented products are not supplements; they are actually whole food products with an amazing amount of quality nutrients. Lacto-fermented products are worth mentioning here because they are a fantastic source of added nutrition. These quality foods are packed with life giving enzymes, beneficial bacteria, and a whole host of other nutrients.

REMEMBER

- Eat healthy whole foods, including plenty of raw vegetables and fruits.
- Supplements are an addition to an already healthy lifestyle.
- Supplements should be derived from organic whole foods.

36

MSM AND YOUR HEALTH

MSM, or methylsulfonylmethane, is a natural sulfur compound found in all living things. It is actually one of the most prominent compounds in our bodies, just behind water and sodium. A 160 pound man has approximately 4 pounds of sulfur as body weight.

WHY IS MSM IMPORTANT?

MSM has been called 1 of the 5 elements of life. It originates in the ocean and reaches the human food chain through rainfall. It is the prime source of bio-available sulfur, which is lost from our food by soil depletion, processing, drying, cooking and preserving. MSM is an important nutrient (not a drug or medicine) and is a component of over 150 compounds. It is needed by the body for healthy connective tissues and joint function, proper enzyme activity and hormone balance, along with the proper function of the immune system.

Because it plays such a major role in these healthy body functions and others, it has been found that supplementation with MSM improves many health problems such as: body aches, arthritis, allergies, asthma, emphysema, lung dysfunction, headaches, skin problems, stomach and digestive tract problems, circulation, cell osmosis and absorption.

WHY IS IT LACKING IN OUR DIET?

MSM is lacking in our diet because processing, heating, storage, and preparation of foods destroys essential MSM. Without sufficient MSM in the body, unnecessary illness of varying types may result.

Beth M. Ley, in her book, *MSM: Our Way Back to Health With Sulfur*, lists common signs of sulfur deficiency, including slow wound healing, scar tissue, brittle hair or nails, gastrointestinal problems, arthritis, acne, depression, and more. "The body is in a constant state of repair, but if we do not have all the necessary 'parts'", says Ley, the body will "produce weak, dysfunctional cells."

HOW DOES MSM WORK?

I have found that MSM works for two basic reasons:

1. MSM makes your body a better filter. On a cellular level it makes cell walls more permeable, allowing water and nutrients to freely flow into cells and waste products and toxins to properly flow out. In other words, you are able to absorb nutrients better and remove toxins better. This enables your body to build healthy vibrant cells, free of pain, sickness, and disease.

2. MSM is the component which forms the disulfide bonds that link amino acids together to form proteins in the body. Proteins are not only the major constituents of muscle tissue and

connective tissue; they are the major components of enzymes. Remember that enzymes are our key to life. Every reaction in our body is first activated through enzymes.

In other words, MSM helps your body to function at optimal levels. When your body is functioning at optimal levels, it is free of pain, sickness, and disease.

TREAT THE CAUSE NOT THE SYMPTOM

MSM can be a natural remedy for osteoarthritis, rheumatoid arthritis, fibromyalgia, tendonitis and bursitis, muscular soreness and athletic injuries, carpal tunnel syndrome, post-traumatic inflammation and pain, heartburn and hyperacidity, headaches and back pain, and allergies. People taking MSM may notice other benefits, including softer skin, stronger nails, thicker hair, and softening of scar tissue.

If you'll notice, the above symptoms are caused by hardening of tissues, inflammation of tissues, or both. These symptoms are caused by your body's inability to remove toxins. MSM allows for the removal of these toxins.

This concept is very important. What this means to you is that MSM removes pain and inflammation by alleviating the root cause of the problem; no matter where it may occur in your body. This is in direct contrast to medications, both over the counter and prescription, which merely mask symptoms while increasing levels of toxicity in your body.

There are two main points that you need to take from this:

1. Your body has the ability to heal itself

2. MSM works

Many people, including myself, have reported miraculous success stories directly attributed to MSM.

DOSAGE:

Currently there is no Recommended Daily Allowance for MSM.

I have personally researched MSM for over 15 years. I have found that most people will get the beneficial/ healing effects of MSM by taking 3000mg to 6000mg per day. In order to optimize the effects of MSM you should take it with equal amounts of Vitamin C.

ALL MSM IS NOT CREATED EQUAL

As with everything else in the food and supplement industry, all MSM is not created equal. There is only one type of MSM that I recommend. It is the MSM that I have personally been taking since 1992. Cardinal MSM is the gold standard of all MSM. Cardinal MSM is manufactured in the United States. It is the only form of MSM that I trust for quality, purity, and effectiveness.

MSM is available in capsules, tablets, and powders. I have found that capsules work best. The powder works well, but it is very bitter.

37

THIS INFO IS GREAT AL, BUT WHAT DO YOU DO?

This is definitely the question that I am most often asked by family, friends, and clients; which makes perfect sense to me. I would much rather learn by example than be told what to do. This is by far the most effective way to achieve lasting success.

The principles that I follow are basic yet effective. Reason being, if something is too complex, you will not stick to it for any length of time. The goal here is to adopt a beneficial way of eating that you can follow for the rest of your life.

YOU ARE ON A PERSONAL JOURNEY

One of the things that I found to be most discouraging when I adopted a healthy lifestyle was the negative attitude some people gave me. You will most likely encounter this same experience. It is interesting to note that the negativity will come from both sides of the fence; those that follow an unhealthy eating regimen and those that follow an extremely healthy eating regimen.

People who eat a lot of processed and refined foods like to make fun of those of us who choose to eat healthy. There are many reasons for this. However, I have found that the main underlying reason for their behavior is the fact that they lack what it takes to chart their own course. These people will usually tell you that you are depriving yourself of the really good food that is available. Decadent meals that taste delicious.

These people don't understand that, by eating the way that they do, *they* are depriving *themselves* of the vital nutrients that their bodies need to look better, feel better, and live better than they could ever possibly imagine.

I never defend myself when I am confronted with these situations. I have found that it is best to simply reply by saying: "I actually enjoy eating the way that I do, it brings me a lot of pleasure and satisfaction." This response is simple, effective, and it's the truth.

On the other side of the coin, no matter how healthy you are, no matter how well you eat, there is always going to be someone who is a little more hardcore than you. Just when you think you are doing great, along comes someone to try and burst your bubble. Believe me when I tell you that I encounter these people all the time.

For example: I was discussing my eating regimen with a leading expert in the Raw Food community. I mentioned that every morning I drink a blended smoothie which consists of spinach, banana, and water. I also add some cucumber, beets, or whatever else I feel like adding. This smoothie is very pleasing to me and I feel great when I drink it. However, this "expert" proceeded to tell me that blending produce denatures it to the point that it becomes a processed food. He was actually telling me that there is no nutritional value in my morning beverage. Do you believe that?

I didn't argue the point. I simply told this well meaning individual that I am happy with the results that I am getting from my efforts. I don't know if he was trying to put me down or help me out. It doesn't really matter. All that matters is the fact that I'm happy with the place that I'm in right now.

Here's the point: Follow the guidelines outlined in this course as best you can. That is all that you can do. You should be extremely proud of yourself for making the effort to better your life. In fact, I applaud you for finishing this course. You definitely have what it takes to achieve your goals and take control of your life. **You are very special!**

2 KEY POINTS THAT LEAD TO HAPPINESS & SUCCESS:

1. If you aren't happy with your current eating regimen, just think of how you ate last week and try to eat a little better this week. Before you know it, you'll be living a healthy vibrant life.

2. Don't worry about how someone else is eating. Some of us catch on to the principles of *Better Living With Whole Foods* faster than others and this is okay. Remember, this is not a race, it is merely a journey.

   Let's support each other's efforts by leading by example and striving to be our best.

Which leads us to...

WHERE DO I SHOP?

When shopping for food, I do my best to buy from local sources. Therefore, I get most of my produce at Farmer's Markets or

CSA's (Community Supported Agriculture). Next, I go to a health food market such as Whole Foods Market or Mother's Market to purchase food that is not available at the Farmer's Market. Whole foods markets purchase their produce from local farmers as much as they possibly can. Remember to support your local farmers. The only reason that I ever go to a large commercial supermarket is to buy cleaning supplies, toilet paper, and other non-food essentials.

> **Note:** I never go to Wal-Mart or Sam's Club (Sam's Club is owned by Wal-Mart). Costco or Target is a much better choice. Wal-Mart is not good for our environment or our local economy. Remember, every time that you make a purchase, you are voting with your dollars.

WHAT KIND OF FOOD DO I BUY?

I want to stop right here and remind you that this is a synopsis of the way that I currently eat. I am not suggesting that you eat exactly the same types and amounts of foods that I do. This is merely an example of how I have incorporated the whole foods lifestyle into my life. There are plenty of healthy foods available for you to customize an eating regimen specific to your particular needs.

What I *am* doing is giving you a reference point. It is always beneficial to see how someone else, who is actually living this lifestyle, is doing it. My hope is that, by seeing the way that I actually do things, your life will be made a little easier.

PRODUCE:

Most of the food that I buy is produce; vegetables, fruits, and some raw nuts.

My main staples are:

- Spinach   4 lbs. per week
- Bananas   15 per week
- Lacinto Kale   2 bunches per week
- Carrots   2 bunches per week
- Tomatoes   5 per week
- Persian cucumber   5 per week
- Broccoli   1 lb. per week
- Hot Peppers   1 lb. per week
  (Jalapeno, Serrano,or Fresno chilies)
- Avocados   7 per week
- Celery   1 bunch per week
- Goji Berries   2 lbs. per month
- Raw Almonds   1 lb. per month
- Raw Pecans   2 lbs. per month

I will also eat other vegetables and fruits depending on what is in season during that particular time of the year. With the exception of bananas and goji berries, I usually do not buy produce that is grown on the other side of the country or in different parts of the world. Remember, local is the new organic.

During the summer I eat more fruits than during winter because more fruit is available during this time of the year.

MEAT

I'm a vegetarian, so I don't eat meat. Follow the guidelines in *Better Living With Whole Foods* to choose the healthiest meats to eat if you are a meat eater. Also, be sure to eat meat in moderation.

DAIRY

My dairy consumption fluctuates up and down. In the past I ate raw cheese and raw milk with great results. Right now, I don't eat any cheese; maybe once a month. Currently, I drink about a half gallon of raw milk per week.

EGGS

Currently, I cook a mixed vegetable and egg breakfast approximately once per week.

BREADS & TORTILLAS

Sprouted grain bread: I buy one loaf of flourless sprouted grain bread every other month on average. I will usually eat it with avocados or raw almond butter and organic fruit spread (no added sugar). Note: There are times when I don't eat any bread at all for months at a time.

Also, I eat organic oatmeal with fruit about 2 times per month.

BEANS & LEGUMES

I love to make beans from scratch; mainly pinto beans and black beans. They taste great with vegetables and avocados.

BEVERAGES

I drink my blended vegetable and banana smoothie on a daily basis. Other than that, I drink water, coffee, and tea.

HOW DO I EAT AT HOME?

Basically, I eat all of the foods mentioned above at home. Most of the foods that I eat are raw vegetables and fruits, as well as a small amount of raw nuts.

I do my best to drink my spinach and banana smoothie on a daily basis. I know that it sounds gross, but it tastes awesome and it's an extremely quick, nutrient dense meal. This drink is a much healthier alternative to all of the meal replacement drinks and powders available in supermarkets and health food stores. There is no comparison.

Note: If you try this drink and it is not sweet enough for you, try adding a small amount of raw agave nectar. This usually does the trick for most people.

Other than that, I eat raw veggies and some fruit on a plate. Remember, I keep things very simple. I am not opposed to eating more elaborate healthy meals, but I prefer it if someone other than myself prepares them.

As I mentioned above, I also eat:

* Organic oatmeal approximately 2 times per month.
* Organic eggs with mixed vegetables once per week

One dish that I love to make is black bean soup. I make it from scratch about 2 times per month. It is the best black beans I have ever tasted if I do say so myself ☺.

HOW DO I EAT ON THE ROAD?

This is the area of greatest concern for most of my clientele. At one time or another they will always tell me the same thing: "I am eating well at home, but everything goes out the window when I leave the house. There is just no way for me to eat healthy when I am at work/school." Well, I used to go back and forth with this issue myself, so I know exactly what this is like.

This is what I do: I bring a medium sized ice chest to work. The ice chest is filled with reusable plastic containers that contain healthy foods. I usually bring a ton of veggies including; baby spinach, carrots, tomato, celery, a piece fruit, and whatever else I have at home. Sometimes, I will bring a sprouted grain sandwich made with either avocado or organic raw almond butter and organic blackberry fruit spread.

You can use blue ice to keep everything cold while you are working. I went to my local sporting goods store and bought 2 blocks of blue ice. Keep 1 in your freezer and 1 in your ice chest. Switch them out on a daily basis. Some people try to get away with buying only 1 block of blue ice, thinking that they will freeze it at night and use it during the day. This method will work on most days, but the time will come when you forget to freeze your blue ice and you will be very thankful that you have a spare. Do yourself a favor and buy 2 blocks of blue ice.

> **Warning:** Eating healthy at work is an open invitation for naysayers to make comments about your newfound lifestyle. Don't worry; just keep doing what you are doing. The more you continue to eat healthy, the more impressed your coworkers will become. You may even get some people to join you. It is interesting to note that my coworkers still make fun of the way that I eat... and I work in a health club!

WHAT DO I ORDER AT RESTAURANTS?

Restaurant meals are usually reserved for my cheat day, which I will describe below. However, when trying to eat healthy at a restaurant, do the best you can for the situation you are in.

For example:

On occasion I eat vegetarian chili or black bean chili at Rutabegorz, which is a healthy restaurant that serves both meat and vegetarian dishes. The chili itself is healthy, but the toppings and sides aren't, so I order it without cheese or bread.

Another favorite of mine are the vegetarian tacos at the Durango Grill. I order them without cheese or sour cream and ask them to add avocado. My vegetarian tacos contain a corn tortilla, black beans, pico de gallo (chopped tomato and onions), and avocado.

Here are some other tricks of the trade:

- If you want to eat a hamburger, order it lettuce wrapped, no cheese, with mustard instead of dressing. No french fries.
- Salads and other items should have the dressing on the side, not on top.
- Have pasta sauce served over a bed of spinach instead of pasta.
- When your meal comes, automatically place half of it in a to-go container. Restaurants serve too much food to eat at one sitting.
- Order items a la carte.
- Find restaurants that have healthy items on their menu.
- Customize your own meal.

WHAT DO I EAT AS A QUICK SNACK?

- My special smoothie.
- Raw vegetable or a piece of fruit.
- Raw Organic Food Bar. Usually the Omega-3 Flax Bar.

WHAT ABOUT MY CHEAT DAY?

I don't like to buy cheat foods for the house because I don't want to be tempted during the week. I usually eat my cheat meals at a restaurant. I eat vegetable curry from a Thai restaurant approximately 3 times per month and I eat vegetarian tacos approximately once per month.

I have gotten to the point in my journey that I do not crave sweets very much. However, I usually eat something sweet during the Christmas season. Maybe a piece of pie or a cookie.

EAT GOOD MOST DAYS OF THE WEEK

According to Robin Jones, owner of the Living Temple in Huntington Beach, CA, if you want to do the best for your body and Planet Earth, you should divide your foods into 3 sections:

- **Optimal Foods**, which should make up the bulk of your diet: Raw fruits, greens, nuts, and seeds.
- **OK Foods**, which should be consumed sparingly: Legumes, grains, raw dairy, eggs, and pasture raised meat.
- **Non Foods**, which should be avoided completely; processed and refined foods, such as sodas, doughnuts, white bread, fast food, T.V. dinners, commercial candy bars, and packaged snacks.

Which leads us to...

WHAT IS A "CHEAT DAY" AND WHY DO YOU NEED ONE?

The principles of the cheat day are simple; eat good most days of the week and reserve one day as a cheat day. The cheat day is not a gorge yourself day, but it is a day that you can eat foods that are not so, shall we say, beneficial.

The benefits of the cheat day are two fold:

1. It gives you peace of mind.
2. It gives you an excuse to eat well on the other 6 days of the week.

Let me explain...

Knowing that you have a cheat will give you peace of mind, knowing that you are not on a life sentence of deprivation. Here's my reasoning: Most people in today's world have an all or nothing attitude. Let me know if this sounds familiar. You wake up Monday morning and declare: "This is the day that I am starting my new life! I am going to eat perfect from this day forward and finally fit into my favorite pair of jeans again." Well, if you've gone through this scenario before, you are not alone. The only problem with this is the fact that nobody is perfect, not me, not you, or anybody else. You may last one day, one week, or one month, but the day will come when you give into your cravings and eat something that "isn't on your diet". When this happens you feel like a failure, like you don't have what it takes to lose weight.

Well, the cheat day takes the pressure off of you and gives you permission to splurge 1 day out of the week. Imagine that. You don't have to put yourself on that life sentence of depravity. Doing this will definitely give you peace of mind.

On the flip side of this equation, knowing that you have a cheat day gives you an excuse to eat well on the other six days of the week. For example, it's Tuesday and you feel like drinking a chocolate shake. Instead of giving in to your urges, you make a note of this craving and say to yourself, "I will eat well today and drink a chocolate shake on my cheat day." Isn't that totally awesome? You have an excuse to eat well most days because you know you will have a cheat day coming up in a few days. And not just 1 cheat day, but 1 cheat day every week. That's 52 cheat days per year! What more could you ask for?

I'll let you in on a little secret. As time goes on, the cheat day becomes less and less important. The cheat day eventually turns into a cheat meal. Some weeks, you may not utilize your cheat day, but you will still have the peace of mind knowing that you could use it if you wanted to.

From professional athletes to stay at home moms, understanding and correctly utilizing this one concept has changed the lives of more people than you could ever imagine, including myself!

38

THE ACTION PLAN

Congratulations on sticking with this material to the very end. You now have more than 20 years of my own professional and personal experience. By now you understand that *Better Living With Whole Foods* is not a diet; it is a way of life. **You will look better, feel better, and live better by simply following the principles described in this course.**

We have covered a lot of information together and I realize that it may be a bit overwhelming. This section will help you pull it all together and develop a plan of action that you can incorporate into your everyday life.

8 SIMPLE PRINCIPLES THAT LEAD TO SUCCESS

1. Keep plenty of good quality whole foods in your house, especially plenty of vegetables and fruits.
2. Make a shopping list prior to going to the market. Be sure to utilize the **Foods To Eat** outline and **Beneficial Foods Lists** in the appendix.

3. Eat before you go shopping for food; don't shop hungry.

4. Do most of your shopping at Farmer's Markets and Whole Foods type markets.

5. Be prepared. Take plenty of good quality food with you to work or school.

6. Review the examples of how I incorporate whole foods living into my everyday life.

7. Read this manual often. Doing so will help you keep the principles of *Better Living With Whole Foods* fresh in your mind.

8. Visit www.BetterLivingCommunity.com and join the Better Living Community. It is important to keep yourself involved with people who have similar aspirations.

The Better Living Community will:

- Keep you updated with happenings and events.
- Supply you with approved Better Living recipes from chefs and fellow community members.
- Provide you with valuable tips for equipping your kitchen for healthy eating
- Provide you the opportunity to interact with other members who are on a similar journey.
- Provide you access to webcasts, teleseminars, and Q&A sessions.
- Keep you excited and motivated!

REMEMBER

This is your personal journey. Do the best that you can and be proud of yourself for making the effort to better your life. Do not try to be perfect from day 1. The best thing to do is to think of how you ate last week and eat a little better this week. Always strive for constant improvement, but don't worry about perfection.

"Inch by inch and life's a cinch.
Yard by yard and life is hard."

— Anonymous

I wish you the absolute best in everything you do. If you have any questions or concerns, simply send an email to: info@BetterLivingWithWholeFoods.com; I'd be delighted to hear from you.

Yours in health,

Alexander Morentin, C.E.S.
My Fit Life
PO Box 1462
Brea, CA 92822
www.BetterLivingWithWholeFoods.com
info@betterlivingwithwholefoods.com

AFTERWORD

EXERCISE & WEIGHT MANAGEMENT

Eating well is one component of the health and wellness equation, effective exercise is the other. If you are not already doing so, it is highly recommended that you begin a comprehensive exercise program; one that includes resistance training.

It's true, a proper exercise program will get you dramatic results with less effort and in the shortest amount of time possible. However, the fitness and weight loss industries are just as deceptive as the commercial food industry. This is the reason I have dedicated my life to professing the TRUTH in fitness and nutrition.

If you are in doubt about how to structure an effective exercise routine on your own, it is highly recommended that you implement my most successful Fitness and Fat Loss Program and see how great you can look and feel.

A Fitness Solution Guaranteed to Melt Body Fat!

THE 16 WEEK TOTAL BODY MAKEOVER

The most comprehensive fitness and weight management program available on the market today.

Are You Ready To:

- **Melt Body Fat & Drop Clothing Sizes**
- Lose Your Belly Bulge
- **Firm & Tone Your Entire Body**
- Enjoy Wearing Shorts & Sleeveless Tops Again
- **Gain Confidence & Self-Esteem**
- Rediscover a Passion for Life

The 16 Week Total Body Makeover is a simple, complete, highly effective fitness and weight management program that will get you the results you want in the shortest amount of time possible. Guaranteed! The 16 Week Total Body Makeover utilizes a holistic approach to health and wellness through fitness, nutrition, and beneficial lifestyle change.

For more information go to:

www.16WeekTotalBodyMakeover.com.

Appendix A

FOODS TO EAT

This is a concise outline of approved Better Living foods to eat that are discussed in detail throughout this course.

PRODUCE

Your produce should be fresh, organic, and locally grown. CSA's (community supported agriculture) and Farmer's Markets are your best bet for finding the freshest produce that is in season. Eat a variety of organic vegetables, fruits, and sprouts.

NUTS & SEEDS

- Raw
- Organic
- Sprouted

NUT MILKS

- **Almond Milk:** Freshly made almond milk from sprouted almonds. It's best to make the almond milk yourself.

- **Soy Milk:** I don't recommend soy milk, but if you decide to drink it, it should be organic and contain only two ingredients; filtered water and organic soybeans, nothing else.

SPROUTED GRAIN BREADS

It is best to stay away from breads and flours altogether; especially if your goal is weight loss. If you must eat bread, choose an option that is organic, sprouted grain, and flourless.

TORTILLAS

- **Corn Tortillas:** Corn tortillas should only contain three ingredients; stone ground corn, water, and lime. Buy organic when available.
- **Sprouted Grain Tortillas**

DAIRY

- **Raw Milk:** Organic raw milk from grass fed free range cows that are free of antibiotics, hormones, and pesticides. Full fat raw milk (no low fat or non fat milk).
- **Butter:** Raw butter (best choice) or organic butter (okay choice).
- **Organic Yogurt:** Organic yogurt is pasteurized, but it has a few of the beneficial bacteria added to it. Plain is best. Stay away from sweetened yogurts. Raw kefir is a much better choice.
- **Raw Kefir:** Preferably homemade.

EGGS

Organic, pasture raised or free range, omega-3 eggs obtained from chickens that are free of antibiotics, hormones, and pesticides.

> **Note:** It is preferable if your beef, chicken, dairy, and eggs are obtained from local farmers whenever possible.

MEATS

All meats should be free of antibiotics, hormones, and pesticides.

- **Beef:** Organic free range grass fed beef.
- **Chicken:** Organic pasture raised or cage free chickens.
- **Fish:** Coldwater fish caught in the wild; preferably smaller fish such as Wild Pacific Salmon and Tilapia.
- **Pork:** None
- **Deli Meats:** Not recommended: If you absolutely have to eat them, buy freshly sliced deli meats that are prepared in your supermarket; not prepackaged.

BEANS & LEGUMES

Organic whole beans. It is best to prepare your own.

RICE

Organic whole grain or long grain rice; the darker the color, the better.

OILS

- **Olive Oil:** Organic, extra virgin, first cold pressed olive oil.
- **Coconut Oil:** Raw, unrefined, organic, extra virgin , cold pressed coconut oil.

CEREAL

My two recommendations are:

- Organic oatmeal
- Ezekiel sprouted grain cereal.

PASTA

Gluten-free brown rice pasta.

PASTA SAUCE

It is preferable to make it yourself. Store bought pasta sauce should be organic and contain no preservatives, no added sugars, and be gluten-free.

SOY SAUCE

- Organic
- Gluten-free
- **Healthy Alternative = Bragg's Liquid Aminos.**

SALAD DRESSING

It is best to make your own salad dressing from beneficial ingredients. The best store bought salad dressing is **Bragg's Organic Vinaigrette.**

NUT BUTTERS

Raw organic almond butter.

JELLIES & FRUIT SPREADS

Organic fruit spreads that contain no preservatives and no added sugar.

CANNED TUNA

Water packed tuna.

BABY FOOD

- Mother's milk
- Homemade baby food
- Organic preservative free baby food

SALT

- Himalayan Salt
- Sea Salt

PEPPER

Fresh ground peppercorns.

HERBS AND SPICES

Most herbs and spices are okay. Make sure they are organic. Grow your own from organic seeds if possible.

MUSTARD

Should contain two ingredients; mustard seed and water.

GARLIC

Raw garlic cloves.

WATER

- **Tap Water**: Use a home filtration system.
- **Bottled Water**: Naturally sourced spring water.

FRUIT JUICES

Freshly juiced or freshly squeezed vegetable and fruit juices.

COFFEE & TEA

Look for coffee and tea that is organic, Fair Trade, and shade grown.

Appendix B

FOODS TO AVOID

This is a concise outline of the foods to avoid that are discussed in detail throughout this course.

PROCESSED & REFINED FOODS

Avoid processed and refined foods at all costs. Including the white devils: white bread, white sugar, white flour, iodized salt, and white rice.

FOOD ADDITIVES

Stay away from foods which contain mono-glycerides, di-glycerides, soy lecithin, soybean oil, artificial flavors, natural flavors, chemical preservatives, and dyes. If you do not recognize an ingredient, don't eat it.

BREADS

White breads and whole wheat processed breads. All breads which contain processed flour. Always read the labels.

Remember, if your goal is weight loss, you should avoid bread, flour, and foods which contain gluten.

TORTILLAS

* White flour tortillas
* Whole wheat tortillas: They are as bad as or worse than white flour tortillas.
* Corn flour tortillas

MEATS

Avoid all meats that are subjected to antibiotics, hormones, or pesticides. Most of the beef, chicken, fish, and pork available to consumers are raised in deplorable conditions and fed an unnatural diet that results in very unhealthy meat.

* **Beef:** Avoid grain fed beef; especially those that are raised on commercial feed lots.
* **Poultry:** Commercial chickens raised in crowded factory warehouses.
* **Fish:** Farm raised fish. Do not eat farm raised fish.
* **Pork:** Avoid pork and all pork products.
* **Deli Meats:** Avoid all prepackaged deli meats. Also, stay away from deli meats that contain preservatives, dyes, MSG, and other additives.

DAIRY

* **Pasteurized Milk:** Stay away from all forms of pasteurized milk; they are harmful to you.

- **Organic Pasteurized Milk:** Stay away from all forms of organic pasteurized milk; they are harmful as well.
- **Butter:** You guessed it: stay away from commercial pasteurized butter.
- **Yogurt:** Avoid commercial pasteurized yogurt. Also, stay away from all yogurts that are sweetened with sugar, cane juice, or artificial sweeteners.
- **Margarine:** Avoid margarine like the plague. Margarine is extremely harmful to you.

EGGS

Commercial eggs; they are just as bad as the factory raised commercial chickens that lay them.

PRODUCE

Commercial produce: May have been sprayed with pesticides, irradiated, or genetically modified. Also, stay away from canned fruits and vegetables.

NUTS & SEEDS

Stay away from roasted nuts and seeds. Nuts and seeds that have been subjected to high heat, such as roasting or cooking, are not good for you.

NUT MILKS

- **Soy Milk:** Avoid soy milk, especially if it contains ingredients other than organic soybeans and water. Always read the label. Most soymilk contains harmful preservatives and sweeteners.

- **Almond Milk:** Never buy store bought almond milk. I have never seen almond milk sold in stores that I can recommend.
- **Rice Milk:** Stay away from rice milk.

OILS

Stay away from processed and refined oils including hydrogenated oils. These include canola oil, safflower oil, corn oil, sunflower oil, soybean oil, and cottonseed oil.

CEREALS

Avoid all processed cereals including fortified cereals and kid's cereals.

PASTA

Avoid pasta, especially wheat pasta.

PASTA SAUCE

Avoid sauces that are not organic and contain any of the following: preservatives, sugar, artificial sweetener, canola oil, and gluten.

RICE

Stay away from all forms of white rice. White rice is one of the white devils.

BEANS & LEGUMES

Avoid canned beans that contain harmful chemical preservatives.

SOY SAUCE

Don't use soy sauce unless it is organic and gluten free.

SALAD DRESSING

Most salad dressings found in your supermarket are not good for you. In fact, there is only one that I recommend.

NUT BUTTERS

You definitely want to stay away from commercial nut butters, such as peanut butter that is solid at room temperature. Never choose nut butters that say low fat or reduced fat.

JELLIES & FRUIT SPREADS

Stay away from jellies, jams, and preserves.

BABY FOOD

Stay away from:

- All baby formula
- All soy based baby food
- Commercial baby food containing chemical preservatives

SALT

Refined table salt as well as all iodized salts, including iodized sea salt.

MAYONNAISE

Avoid mayonnaise like the plague.

WATER

- Tap Water: Stay away from plain unfiltered tap water
- Bottled Water: Do not buy bottled water that is filtered tap water, such as Dasani or Aquafina.
- Enhanced Water: Stay away from enhanced waters such as vitamin waters and fruit waters.

FRUIT JUICES

Stay away from all packaged store bought fruit juices including whole fruit juices.

COFFEE & TEA

Stay away from commercially grown coffee and tea.

Appendix C

FOOD LISTS:

ORGANIC VEGETABLES

Alfalfa Sprouts	Mustard Greens
Asparagus	Olives
Beets	Onions
Beet Greens	Parsley
Broccoli	Peppers
Cabbage	Romaine Lettuce
Carrots	Sea Vegetables
Cauliflower	Spinach
Celery	Squash
Chard	Sweet Potatoes
Collard Greens	Swiss Chard
Cucumbers	Tomato
Green Beans	Turnip Greens
Kale	Yams
Mushrooms	Zucchini

ORGANIC FRUITS

Apples	Orange
Apricots	Peaches
Avocados	Pineapple
Banana	Plums
Blackberries	Pomegranate
Blueberries	Prunes
Cantaloupe	Raisins
Figs	Raspberries
Grapefruit	Strawberries
Grapes (with seeds)	Watermelon (with seeds)
Kiwi	Lemon
Lime	

Note:

- Make sure to eat whole fruits as opposed to packaged fruit juices. Packaged fruit juice is loaded with simple sugars; they spike your insulin levels, which results in the conversion to and storage of body fat.

- Solid fruits have fiber and other nutrients, which slow the release of their carbohydrates into the blood stream.

- Freshly juiced vegetables and fruits are okay in moderation.

COMPLEX CARBOHYDRATES

GRAINS

Amaranth Arrowroot Buckwheat

Millet Quinoa

BREADS / CEREALS / PASTA

Sprouted Grain Flourless Bread
Organic Oatmeal (slow cooked – no packets)
Sprouted Grain Cereal
Brown Rice Pasta

RICE

Whole Grain or Long Grain Rice Brown Rice

Basmati Rice Jasmine Rice

BEANS / LEGUMES

Black Beans Garbanzo Beans

Kidney Beans Lentils

Miso Pinto Beans

Tempeh

MEAT & DAIRY

Note: All meats should be free of hormones (Growth Hormone and Steroids), antibiotics, dyes, radiation, virus injections, and pesticides. Preferably grass fed.

BEEF GROUP (3OZ. – 6OZ.)

Organic

Grass Fed

Pasture Raised

POULTRY GROUP (3OZ. – 6OZ.)

Chicken

Turkey

Pasture Raised

Organic

FISH GROUP (3OZ. – 6OZ.)

Fish Caught in the Wild

Wild Pacific Salmon

Tilapia

Croaker

Sardines

Haddock

Summer Flounder

DAIRY GROUP

Raw Milk

Raw Cheese

Raw Butter

Raw Kephir

Raw Colostrum

Eggs

Organic

Pasture Raised

Omega 3

ESSENTIAL FATS

Polyunsaturated fats include fish, raw walnuts, raw pecans, raw almonds, flax.

Monounsaturated fats include avocados, raw cashews, natural peanut butter, olives, cold pressed extra virgin olive oil.

Saturated fats include raw coconut oil.

Omega 6 – Linoleic Acid (We already get too much of these in our modern diet)

Omega 3 – Alpha Linolenic Acid (from plant sources such as flax seeds)

Omega 3 – EPA & DHA (from fish, eggs, and grass fed beef)

If you like nut butters, try raw almond butter, it tastes great.

Do not eat peanut butter if it is solid. This means that it is hydrogenated.

Note: The two oils that I recommend are:

1. First cold pressed extra virgin olive oil in your salads and other non cooked items...
2. Use raw coconut oil when cooking. It can handle heat without denaturing. Olive oil denatures quickly when exposed to heat.

Both of these oils have essential fatty acids that are beneficial to your health.

CONDIMENTS

Himalayan Salt	Celtic Sea Salt
Olive Oil	Balsamic Vinaigrette
Apple Cider Vinegar	Fresh Ground Pepper
Fresh Garlic	Lemon Juice
Oregano	Chili Powder
Cloves	Mustard
Organic Ketchup	Herbs
Ginger	Onion
Raw Agave	Raw Cacao
Cinnamon	

Appendix D

RECOMMENDED RESOURCES

MARKETS & STORES

Whole foods type markets are excellent. While some things do cost more than at a traditional farmer's market or neighborhood supermarket, the key advantage is convenience. You will find everything you need to live a healthy vibrant life all under one roof. Most of the produce is organic and locally grown. Also, you will be able to find specialty items, such as organic raw milk, fermented foods, and fair trade coffee and tea.

- **Whole Foods Market** — www.WholeFoods.com With more than 200 stores, Whole Foods Market is the big daddy in the organic whole foods movement. They are largely responsible for bringing awareness to organic foods and sustainable green living into the mainstream of our society. Whole Foods has recently opened a store in Tustin, California. With over 60,000 square feet, the store is absolutely breathtaking.

- **Mother's Market & Kitchen**
  — www.MothersMarket.com
  Mother's is a wonderful vegetarian organic whole foods market with 4 locations throughout Orange County, California. Mother's also has a tasty vegetarian restaurant in each of its locations.

- **Sprouts — www.sprouts.com**
  Sprouts is a whole foods market with locations in Arizona, California, and Texas.

- **The Living Temple — www.thelivingtemple.com**
  7561 Center Ave, #40
  Huntington Beach, CA 92647
  (714) 891-5117
  The Living Temple carries specialty products including raw foods, books, and dvd's.

FARMER'S MARKETS & COMMUNITY SUPPORTED AGRICULTURE (CSA)

- **Local Harvest — www.localharvest.com**
  The Best Organic Food is What's Grown Closest to You

  This is a wonderful website for organic food and local produce. It maintains a public nationwide directory of small farms, farmers markets, CSAs, and other local food sources. It has an internal search engine which provides sources of local sustainably grown food and allows direct contact with local farmers in your area.

- **AMS at USDA**
  —www.lams.usda.gov/farmersmarkets/map.htm

Farmer's Markets Listed by State

Includes locations, times, and contacts for farmer's markets in every state. All documents are listed in PDF format

- **Jaime Farms — www.jaimefarms.com**

  909.395.7818

  Jaime Farms are the farmers that I personally buy most of my produce from at farmer's markets. They grow all of their produce using 100% sustainable farming methods. Very tasty and very nutritious.

FITNESS & WEIGHT MANAGEMENT PROGRAMS

- **16 Week Total Body Makeover**

  www.16WeekTotalBodyMakeover.com

RAW FOOD RESTAURANTS

- **118 Degrees**

  2981 Bristol St. Ste. B-5

  Costa Mesa, CA 92626

  714.754.0718

  www.shop118degrees.com/

  118 Degrees is located at the Camp in Costa Mesa

  Chef: Jenny Ross

- **Au-Lac**

  16563 Brookhurst Street

  Fountain Valley, CA 92649

  714.418.0658

  www.aulac.com

  Chef: Ito

- **Terra Bella Restaurant**
  1408 Pacific Coast Hwy.
  Redondo Beach, CA 90277
  (310) 316-8708
  www.terrabellacafe.com
- **Cru Raw Food Restaurant**
  1521 Griffith Park Blvd.
  Los Angeles, CA 90026
  323.667.1551
  www.crusilverlake.com
- **Nationwide Directory of Raw Food Restaurants**
  www.rawfoodinfo.com/directories/dir_rawrests.html
  This is the most comprehensive nationwide directory of raw food restaurants that I could find. I highly recommend this site to anyone in search of raw food restaurants.

RAW DAIRY PRODUCTS

- **Organic Pastures Dairy Company**
  7221 South Jameson Avenue
  Fresno, California 93706
  Phone: (559)846-9732
  www.organicpastures.com
  www.realmilk.com

MEAT

- **Local Harvest**
  www.localharvest.org
  This is a wonderful resource for grass-fed meats, organic food, and local produce. It maintains a public nationwide

directory of small farms, farmers markets, CSAs, and other local food sources. It has an internal search engine which provides sources of local sustainably grown food and allows direct contact with local farmers in your area.

- **Eat Wild**

  www.eatwild.com

  An excellent information site for grass-fed pasture raised meats. Supplies a list of pastured farms in your area.

- **Grass Fed Beef**
  Frank Fitzpatrick
  Trabuco Canyon, CA
  714.749.5717

FISH

- **Audubon Society Pocket Seafood Selector**

  www.audubon.org

  Seafood Wallet Card: A wallet sized printable guide to the best and worst seafood choices.

  Note: The selections outlined in the wallet card are environmentally friendly choices. Remember to eliminate or severely limit your intake of shellfish.

CULTURED VEGETABLES & KEFIR

- **Alive! Super Foods**
  2110 Continental Ave.
  Costa Mesa, CA 92627
  800.909.8333

www.culturedvegetables.com

Alive! Super Foods has a great assortment of delicious raw cultured vegetables, cultured juices, and coconut kefir. They are lovingly prepared by healing foods chef Kristen Krofina. I have personally tasted their products and they are truly amazing.

- **Body Ecology**
  800.511.2660

  www.bodyecology.com

  Body Ecology is a reliable easy to use source for kefir starter and cultured vegetable starter kits. The starter kits are great for those of you who prefer to make your own cultured vegetables and juices. Their website has a ton valuable information and articles.

SPROUTED NUTS & SEEDS
NUT & SEED BUTTERS

- **Maranatha Nut Butters**
  nSpired Natural Foods, Inc.
  1850 Fairway Drive
  San Leandro, CA 94577
  510.686.0116

SPROUTED GRAIN BREADS & CEREALS

- **Food For Life Baking Co.**
  PO Box 1434
  Corona, CA 92878
  800.797.5090

  www.FoodforLife.com

Food for life is the maker of Ezekiel sprouted flourless whole grain breads, tortillas, and cereals. Ezekiel sprouted grain products are available in a variety of stores throughout the United States. If you are going to eat bread, tortillas, or cereal, this is the brand that I recommend.

VINEGARS & SALAD DRESSINGS

- **Bragg Live Foods, Inc.**
  Box 7
  Santa Barbara, CA 93102
  800.446.1990

  www.bragg.com

  Apple Cider Vinegar, Salad Dressing, and Olive Oil.

SWEETENERS & SPECIALTY PRODUCTS

- **Ultimate Raw Foods**
  800.737.0798
  714.888.5770

  www.ultimaterawfoods.com

  Ultimate Raw Foods carries the highest quality products available on the market today. Raw Agave, Himalayan Goji Berries, Raw Chocolate, and Raw Coconut Oil just to name a few.

CONDIMENTS

- **Himalayan Crystal Salt**
  American Blue Green, LLC
  877.224.4872

  www.americanbluegreen.com

- **Real Salt**
  Redmond Trading Company, L.C.
  475 West 910 South
  Heber City, Utah 84032
  800-367-7258

FOOD BARS

- **Organic Food Bar, Inc.**
  215 East Orangethorpe Ave. #284
  Fullerton, CA 92832
  800.246.4685

  www.organicfoodbar.com

  Organic Food Bars are the best tasting most nutritious food bars I have ever tried. I like them because they are either 100% raw or close to it. My favorite is the Omega 3 Flax.

COFFEE & TEA

- **TransFair USA**
  www.transfairusa.org
  Valuable information regarding Fair Trade Certification and the impact it has on farmers, our environment, and our community.

- **Peace Coffee**
  2801 21st Ave S #120
  Minneapolis, MN 55407
  (612) 870-3440
  www.peacecoffee.com

- **Eco Teas**
  Mate Revolution, Inc.
  P.O. Box 1192
  Ashland, OR 97520
  Phone: 800-839-0775

  www.yerbamate.com

  Certified organic yerba mate and rooibos tea.

SUPPLEMENTS

- **Superior Health Products**
  13808 Ventura Boulevard
  Sherman Oaks, California 91423
  818.986.9456

  www.superiorhealthproducts.com

  Superior Health Products is a wonderful resource for quality supplements, as well as juicers, water filters, and other related health appliances.

WATER

- **www.AllAboutWater.org**
  This is a valuable website that explains everything you need to know about water, including water filters, bottled water, and water treatment alternatives.

RECOMMENDED BOOKS, DVD'S & WEBSITES

BOOKS

Better Health Through Natural Healing
Dr. Ross Trattler N.D., D.O. and Dr. Adrian Jones N.D., Hinkler books, 2005

The Detox Solution
Dr. Patricia Fitzgerald, Illumination Press, 2001

Diet for A New America
John Robbins, H.J. Kramer Books, 1987

Dr. Mercola's Total Health Program
Dr. Joseph Mercola, Brian Vaszily, Dr. Kendra Pearsall, & Nancy Bentley, Mercola.com, 2006

Fast Food Nation:
The Dark Side of the All American Meal
Eric Schlosser

Fit For Life: A New Beginning
Harvey Diamond, Twinstreams Health, 2000

Green Living: The E Magazine Handbook For Living Lightly On The Earth
The Editors of E/The Environmental Magazine, Penguin Group, 2005

Grub: ideas for an urban organic kitchen
Anna Lappe & Bryant Terry, Tarcher/Penguin, 2006

Healing With Whole Foods
Paul Pitchford, North Atlantic Books, 1993

How To Eat Move and Be Healthy
Paul Chek, Chek Institute Publications, 2004

The Green Food Bible
David Sandoval, Freedom Press, 2007

The Maker's Diet
Jordan S. Rubin, Berkley Publishing Group, 2004

The Miracle of Fasting
Paul C. Bragg N.D., Ph.D. and Patricia Bragg N.D., Ph.D., Health Science

Seeds of Deception
Jeffrey M. Smith

DVDS

The Future of Food
Lily Films, 2004
Hidden Dangers in Kid's Meals: Genetically Engineered Foods
Yes!Books, 2005

WEBSITES

www.BetterLivingWithWholeFoods.com

www.fitness-for-women.net

www.BetterLiving Community.com

www.Mercola.com

www.SeedsofDeception.com

www.sustainabletable.org

www.takechargeofyourhealth.biz

www.WholesomeBabyFood.com

www.Breastfeeding.com

www.PublicCitizen.org

www.ucusa.org

http://www.truefoodnow.org/shoppersguide/

GLOSSARY OF TERMS

Amino Acids: The building blocks of protein. The body can make some (non-essential); others are needed in the diet (essential).

Bacteria: Single-celled microorganisms which can exist either as independent (free-living) organisms or as parasites (dependent upon another organism for life).

Bioavailability: The level by which a nutrient or drug can be absorbed and utilized by the body.

Cage-Free: Birds that are raised without cages. Here's the problem: Many times these birds are raised in crowded factory warehouses that do not have access to the outdoors. Pasture raised is what you are looking for.

Country of Origin Labeling (COOL): This initiative would require perishable foods, including meats, produce, and nuts, to be labeled with the country in which they were produced. If passed, COOL will make it easier for you to shop for locally grown/raised foods.

Community Supported Agriculture (CSA): A system in which consumers support a local farm by paying in advance for agricultural products. This reduces the financial risks for the farmer because the costs of seeds and planting crops are covered in advance by consumers. Throughout the growing season, CSA members receive a portion of the farm's harvest at predetermined drop off points on a weekly basis. Members share the financial risks and the bounty of the harvest.

Enzymes: Enzymes are protein structures that are the catalyst to every chemical reaction in your body. In other words, they are the spark plug, the energy source needed for every action and reaction that occurs inside of you. Without them life would literally cease to exist.

EPA: Environmental Protection Agency. A part of the US federal government that enforces environmental laws and provides information and guidance to policy makers.

Factory Farm: A large-scale industrial site where many animals (generally chickens, turkeys, cattle, or pigs) are confined and treated with hormones and antibiotics to maximize growth and prevent disease. The animals produce much more waste than the surrounding land can handle. These operations are associated with various environmental hazards as well as cruelty to animals.

Farmer's Market: A public market at which farmers and often other vendors sell produce directly to consumers.

FDA: Food and Drug Administration. This government agency regulates industries and labels food and related items such as medicines and cosmetics. The FDA is controlled by big business; they do not have your best interests at heart.

Feedlots: Buildings, lots, or a combination of buildings and lots in which animals are confined for feeding, breeding, raising, and/or holding. The concentration of hundreds or thousands of animals in a confined feedlot facility drastically reduces the welfare of these animals, creates health risks, promotes the spread of disease, and yields tremendous quantities of animal waste, which pollutes the natural environment and threatens human health.

Free Range: This term refers to animals (usually poultry, and the eggs that they produce) that are not confined, meaning that these animals are able to go outdoors to engage in natural behaviors. It does not necessarily mean that the animals spend the majority of their time outdoors. The use of the term "free range" is only defined by the USDA for poultry production, and need only mean that the bird has had some access to the outdoors each day, which could be a dirty or concrete feedlot. USDA considers five minutes of open-air access each day to be adequate. Claims are defined by USDA, but are not verified by third party inspectors.

Genetic Engineering: The science of changing the DNA of a plant or animal. Genetic engineering is harmful to us as a population and is an area of great concern.

GMO: Genetically Modified Organism. This is a plant or animal that has been genetically engineered.

Grain-fed: The animal was raised on a diet of grain and the grain could be supplemented with animal by-products and other miscellaneous matter such as cement dust and/or euthanized cats and dogs. The grain is usually subjected to high amounts of pesticides, which transfer into the meat of the animals. Grain-fed animals tend to be raised on factory farms and should be avoided.

Grass-fed: Animals graze on pasture and eat grasses. They should not be supplemented with grain, animal by-products, synthetic hormones, or be given antibiotics to promote growth or prevent disease (though they might be given antibiotics to treat disease). This is the same as pastured or pasture raised.

Natural Foods: Foods that do not contain artificial ingredients and are minimally processed. They are usually more nutritious than refined foods. Natural foods do not include ingredients such as refined sugars, refined flours, milled grains, hydrogenated oils, artificial sweeteners, artificial food colors, or artificial flavorings.

Obesity: The state of being well above one's normal weight. Obesity is defined in adults as having body fat as a percentage of body weight greater than 25% for men and 30% for women. A person has traditionally been considered to be obese if they are more than 20 percent over their ideal weight. That ideal weight must take into account the person's height, age, sex, and build.

Organic: Organic foods cannot be grown using pesticides, synthetic fertilizers, chemicals, or sewage sludge, cannot be genetically modified, and cannot be irradiated. Organic meat and poultry must be fed only organically-grown feed (without any animal byproducts) and cannot be treated with hormones or antibiotics.

Pastured or Pasture-Raised: Indicates the animal was raised on a pasture and that it ate grasses and food found in a pasture, rather than being fattened on grain in a feedlot or barn. Pasturing livestock and poultry is a traditional farming technique that allows animals to be raised in a humane, ecologically sustainable manner. This is basically the same as grass-fed.

Protein: Proteins are chains of amino acids bonded together in varying lengths.

Runoff: Water from precipitation or irrigation that flows over the ground and into bodies of water. It can contribute to soil erosion and carry harmful pollutants.

Sustainable: A product can be considered sustainable if its production enables the resources from which it was made to continue to be available for future generations. A sustainable product can thus be created repeatedly without generating negative environmental effects, without causing waste products to accumulate as pollution, and without compromising the wellbeing of workers or communities.

Sustainable agriculture: Farming that provides a secure living for farm families; maintains the natural environment and resources; supports the rural community; and offers respect and fair treatment to all involved, from farm workers to consumers to the animals raised for food.

Whole Foods: Foods that are unprocessed and unrefined.

INDEX

ARE YOU READY FOR MORE?

Please contact My Fit Life for more information on our classes, corporate programs, church programs, books, and teleseminars featuring *Better Living With Whole Foods* and the *16 Week Total Body Makeover*. We offer a variety of programs and products designed to support you in your quest towards vibrant health and happiness.☺

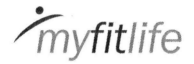

P.O. Box 1462
Brea, CA 92822
Phone: (562) 941-9900
Toll Free (877) 941-9922

www.BetterLivingWithWholeFoods.com

info@BetterLivingWithWholeFoods.com

A Special Gift for You!

Join our FREE healthy newsletter, My Fit Life News You Can Use, and receive a complimentary ebook, *Expert Workout Tips Revealed!* Go to www.BetterLivingWithWholeFoods.com enter your email address, and improve your life... for free!

QUICK ORDER FORM

Yes, I want _____ Copies of *Better Living With Whole Foods* at $21.95 each (California residents please add $1.70 sales tax per book).

Shipping
U.S.: $4.00 for first book and $2.00 for each additional book.
International: $9.00 for first book and $4.00 for each additional book.

Website Orders: www.BetterLivingWithWholeFoods.com

Telephone Orders: Call (877) 941-9922 toll-free. Have your credit card ready.

Email Orders: orders@BetterLivingWithWholeFoods.com

Postal Orders: My Fit Life, P.O. Box 1462, Brea, CA 92822, USA. Telephone: (562) 941-9900

I have enclosed $_____ for my order.

Name: _____

Address: _____

City/State/Zip: _____

Telephone: _____

Email Address: _____

Credit Card # _____Type _____

Exp. Date _____ Signature _____

Call or email for group and corporate quantity discounts.

QUICK ORDER FORM

Yes, I want _____ Copies of *Better Living With Whole Foods* at $21.95 each (California residents please add $1.70 sales tax per book).

Shipping
U.S.: $4.00 for first book and $2.00 for each additional book.
International: $9.00 for first book and $4.00 for each additional book.

Website Orders: www.BetterLivingWithWholeFoods.com

Telephone Orders: Call (877) 941-9922 toll-free. Have your credit card ready.

Email Orders: orders@BetterLivingWithWholeFoods.com

Postal Orders: My Fit Life, P.O. Box 1462, Brea, CA 92822, USA. Telephone: (562) 941-9900

I have enclosed $_____ for my order.

Name: _____

Address: _____

City/State/Zip: _____

Telephone: _____

Email Address: _____

Credit Card # _____Type _____

Exp. Date _____ Signature _____

Call or email for group and corporate quantity discounts.

LES ENFANTS DU FLEUVE

Lisa Wingate

LES ENFANTS
DU FLEUVE

**Traduit de l'anglais (États-Unis)
par Aude Carlier**

LES ESCALES

Titre original : *Before We Were Yours*
© Wingate Media LLC 2017

Les Enfants du fleuve est un roman historique. L'action et les dialogues sont le fruit de l'imagination de l'auteur et ne doivent pas être considérés comme réels. Si certains personnages ont réellement existé, les situations, péripéties et dialogues qui leur sont attribués sont entièrement fictionnels et ne changent pas la nature entièrement fictionnelle de l'œuvre. Pour tous les autres cas, toute ressemblance avec des personnes existantes ou ayant existé est purement fortuite.

Édition française publiée par :
© Éditions Les Escales, un département d'Édi8, 2018
12, avenue d'Italie
75013 Paris – France
Courriel : contact@lesescales.fr
Internet : www.lesescales.fr

ISBN : 978-2-36569-315-8
Dépôt légal : avril 2018
Imprimé en France

Couverture : Hokus Pokus créations
Mise en pages : Nord Compo

Pour les centaines qui ont disparu
et pour les milliers restés parmi nous.
Que vos histoires ne soient jamais oubliées.

Pour ceux qui aident les orphelins d'aujourd'hui
à trouver des foyers durables.
Puissiez-vous connaître la valeur
de votre travail
et de votre amour.

« Saviez-vous, que dans ce pays de la liberté, la terre des braves, existe un grand marché des bébés ? Et les actions qui changent de main... ne sont pas de simples bouts de papier imprimés promettant certains dividendes financiers, mais des bébés bien vivants, de chair et de sang. »

Extrait de l'article
« Le marché des bébés »,
The Saturday Evening Post,
1er février 1930

« Ce sont, comme [Georgia Tann] aimait à le répéter, des ardoises vierges. Ils naissent immaculés et, si vous les adoptez très jeunes, que vous les entourez de beauté et de culture, ils deviendront tout ce que vous voulez qu'ils soient. »

Barbara Bisantz Raymond,
La Voleuse de bébés (The Baby Thief)

Prélude

Le 3 août 1939, Baltimore, Maryland

Mon histoire débute lors d'une nuit d'août caniculaire, en un lieu où mon regard ne se posera jamais. La pièce ne prend vie que dans mon imagination. Je me la figure le plus souvent comme une grande salle. Les murs sont blancs et propres, les draps amidonnés aussi craquants qu'une feuille morte. La suite privée est aménagée avec un raffinement extrême. Dehors, la brise est lasse, et les cigales stridulent dans les grands arbres, cachettes verdoyantes juste sous les portes-fenêtres. Les moustiquaires s'ouvrent vers l'intérieur tandis que le ventilateur tremblote au plafond, brassant un air humide qui n'a aucune envie de se mouvoir.

L'odeur des pins se glisse dans la pièce et les cris de la femme jaillissent tandis que les infirmières la maintiennent de toutes leurs forces sur le lit. Elle est en nage, la sueur ruisselle sur son visage, ses bras et ses jambes. Elle en serait horrifiée si seulement elle en avait conscience.

Elle est jolie. Une âme douce, fragile. Pas du genre à provoquer intentionnellement les événements catastrophiques qui ne font, à cet instant, que commencer. Au cours des longues années de ma vie, j'ai appris que la plupart des gens font de leur mieux pour vivre ensemble. Ils ne cherchent pas à nuire. Si cela arrive, ce n'est souvent qu'un effet secondaire terrible de leur lutte pour leur survie.

Ce n'est pas sa faute, tout ce qui advient après cette dernière poussée impitoyable. Elle met au monde la dernière chose qu'elle aurait pu vouloir. Une chair silencieuse naît – une fille

11

minuscule aux cheveux blonds, jolie comme une poupée, et pourtant bleue et inerte.

La femme n'a sans doute aucun moyen de connaître le sort de son enfant et, dans le cas contraire, les médicaments auront transformé cette connaissance en souvenir flou dès le lendemain. Elle cesse de se démener et se rend au sommeil crépusculaire, bercée par les doses de morphine et de scopolamine qu'on lui a administrées pour l'aider à vaincre la douleur.

Pour l'aider à lâcher prise, ce qu'elle fera.

Une conversation pleine de compassion a lieu tandis que les docteurs recousent et que les infirmières nettoient le reste.

— C'est tellement triste, quand cela finit ainsi. Tellement anormal qu'un être n'ait même pas le temps de respirer une fois dans ce monde...

Un voile est abaissé. Des petits yeux derrière un linceul. Ils ne verront jamais.

La femme entend mais ne comprend pas. Tout glisse sur elle. Comme si elle tentait d'attraper la marée, de la voir s'échapper entre ses doigts, avant de finir par se laisser emporter par elle.

Un homme attend tout près, dans le couloir peut-être, devant la porte. Il est imposant, digne. Bien peu accoutumé à l'impuissance. Il aurait dû devenir grand-père, ce jour-là.

L'exaltation anticipée s'est muée en angoisse déchirante.

— Je suis terriblement navré, monsieur, dit le docteur en s'éclipsant de la pièce. Soyez assuré que nous avons fait tout ce qu'il était humainement possible pour soulager la souffrance de votre fille et sauver le bébé. Je comprends à quel point cela peut être difficile. Je vous prie de transmettre nos condoléances au père de l'enfant lorsque vous parviendrez enfin à le joindre par-delà les mers. Après tant de déceptions, votre famille devait être emplie d'espoir.

— Pourra-t-elle en avoir d'autres ?

— Ce serait malavisé.

— Elle ne s'en remettra pas. Et sa mère non plus, lorsqu'elle l'apprendra. Christine est notre fille unique, voyez-vous. Des rires d'enfants dans la maison... le début d'une nouvelle génération...

— Je comprends, monsieur.

— Quels seraient les risques si elle...

— Sa vie. Et il est très peu probable que votre fille parvienne à mener une nouvelle grossesse à terme. Si elle essayait, les conséquences seraient...

— Je vois.

Dans un élan de réconfort, le médecin pose la main sur l'épaule de l'homme au cœur brisé, du moins est-ce comme cela que je l'imagine. Leurs regards se croisent.

Le docteur jette un coup d'œil par-dessus son épaule pour s'assurer que les infirmières ne peuvent l'entendre.

— Monsieur, puis-je suggérer une chose ? murmure-t-il d'un ton solennel. Je connais une femme, à Memphis...

1

Avery Stafford
De nos jours, à Aiken, en Caroline du Sud

J'inspire un bon coup, glisse au bord de la banquette et défroisse ma veste tandis que la limousine s'arrête sur l'asphalte brûlant. Des camionnettes de journalistes attendent le long du trottoir, soulignant l'importance de notre visite matinale qui aurait pourtant pu sembler anodine.

Dans le déroulement de la journée, rien ne sera laissé au hasard. Ces deux derniers mois passés en Caroline du Sud ont été calibrés pour distiller un message nuancé – esquisser quelques insinuations afin de suggérer un propos, et rien de plus. Aucune déclaration définitive ne doit être faite.

Pour l'instant, du moins.

Et pas avant longtemps, si on m'écoutait.

J'aimerais pouvoir oublier pourquoi je suis revenue dans ma ville natale, mais le simple fait que mon père ne soit pas en train de lire ses notes ou de vérifier le briefing de Leslie – son attachée de presse ultra-efficace – est un rappel indéniable. Pas moyen d'échapper à l'ennemi qui nous accompagne silencieusement dans la voiture. Il est là, sur la banquette arrière, dissimulé derrière le costume gris qui tombe un peu trop lâchement des épaules larges de mon père.

Mon père regarde par la vitre, tête penchée. Il a relégué Leslie et ses assistants à une autre voiture.

— Tu te sens bien ?

Je tends la main vers un long cheveu blond – à moi – pour l'enlever de la banquette afin qu'il ne colle pas à son pantalon lorsqu'il descendra de voiture. Si ma mère était là, elle sortirait une mini-brosse à peluches de son sac, mais elle est à la maison, occupée à préparer le second événement de la journée : une photo de famille de Noël officielle, qui doit être prise quelques mois en avance... juste au cas où le pronostic de mon père s'aggraverait.

Il se redresse un peu, lève la tête. L'électricité statique lui hérisse ses cheveux gris sur le crâne. Même si j'ai bien envie de les remettre en place, je n'en fais rien. Ce serait enfreindre le protocole.

Alors que ma mère s'investit dans le moindre aspect de nos vies – au point de faire la chasse aux peluches sur nos vêtements ou d'organiser une photo de famille de Noël en plein mois de juillet –, mon père est tout le contraire. Il est distant – un îlot de virilité solide dans une maison pleine de femmes. Je sais qu'il tient beaucoup à ma mère, ainsi qu'à mes deux sœurs et moi, mais il ne l'exprime que rarement. Je sais aussi que je suis sa préférée, et celle qui le déroute le plus. Il est le produit d'une époque où les femmes n'allaient à l'université que pour y trouver un mari. Il ne sait pas trop quoi faire de sa fille de trente ans qui est sortie major de promo de la fac de droit de Columbia et qui apprécie vraiment le monde impitoyable des avocats en général et son travail au sein du cabinet d'un procureur fédéral en particulier.

Quelle que soit la raison – et peut-être parce que les rôles de « fille perfectionniste » et « fille attentionnée » étaient déjà pris –, j'ai toujours été la « fille intello ». Comme j'adorais l'école, un accord tacite est vite apparu : il me reviendrait un jour de reprendre le flambeau familial, je serais le fils de remplacement, celle qui succéderait à mon père. Bizarrement, j'avais toujours imaginé que je serais plus âgée quand cela arriverait et que je m'y sentirais prête.

Maintenant, je regarde mon père et je me dis : Comment peux-tu ne pas en avoir envie, Avery ? Voilà ce pour quoi il a travaillé toute sa vie. Ce pour quoi des générations de Stafford ont travaillé depuis la guerre d'Indépendance, bon sang ! Notre famille a toujours eu la fibre du service public. Mon père ne fait pas exception. Depuis qu'il est sorti diplômé de l'académie militaire de West Point et qu'il a servi comme pilote dans l'armée avant ma naissance, il a porté haut le nom de notre famille, avec dignité et détermination.

Bien sûr que tu le veux, me dis-je. Tu l'as toujours voulu. Tu ne t'attendais pas à ce que cela arrive si vite, et encore moins de cette façon. C'est tout.

En mon for intérieur, je m'accroche bec et ongles au meilleur scénario possible. Les ennemis seront vaincus sur les deux fronts – le politique et le médical. Mon père va guérir grâce à l'opération qui l'a fait revenir plus tôt que prévu de la session parlementaire estivale, associée à la pompe à chimio qu'il doit porter attachée à sa jambe une semaine sur trois. Mon retour à Aiken ne sera que temporaire.

Le cancer ne fera bientôt plus partie de nos vies.

La maladie peut être vaincue. D'autres personnes l'ont battue et, s'il y a bien un homme combatif dans ce monde, c'est bien le sénateur Wells Stafford.

Il n'existe pas, où que ce soit, d'homme plus fort ou meilleur que mon père.

— Prête ? me demande-t-il en rajustant son costume.

Je le vois avec soulagement aplatir la crête de coq qui s'était hérissée sur sa tête. Je ne suis pas préparée à franchir la ligne qui sépare la fille de l'aide-soignante.

— Je te suis.

Je ferais n'importe quoi pour lui, mais j'espère qu'il nous reste de longues années avant que nous soyons obligés d'inverser les rôles enfant-adulte. J'ai appris à quel point c'était dur lorsque j'ai vu mon père se débattre avec lui-même quand il a fallu prendre une décision concernant sa propre mère.

Mamie Judy, jadis vive et drôle, n'est plus que l'ombre d'elle-même. Aussi douloureux cela soit, mon père ne peut en parler à personne. Si les médias apprenaient qu'on l'a confiée à une maison de retraite, un établissement très haut de gamme dans une propriété charmante à moins de quinze kilomètres d'ici, ce serait une catastrophe, politiquement parlant. Après le scandale autour d'une série de morts injustifiées et de mauvais traitements dans différentes maisons de retraite privées de notre État, les ennemis politiques de mon père en feraient leurs choux gras, soulignant le fait que seuls les riches peuvent se payer des structures haut de gamme – à moins qu'ils l'accusent d'être un rustre sans cœur ayant mis sa mère au placard car il ne se soucie guère des seniors. Ils prétendraient que mon père est prêt à fermer les yeux sur les besoins des nécessiteux si cela pouvait profiter à ses amis et à ses donateurs de campagne.

En réalité, le choix de placer mamie Judy en maison de retraite n'a rien de politique. Nous sommes comme les autres familles. Toutes les voies possibles sont pavées de culpabilité, bordées de chagrin et grevées de honte. Nous avons pitié d'elle. Nous avons peur pour elle. Imaginer vers où cette cruelle descente dans la démence pourrait la conduire nous rend malades. Avant de la placer là-bas, ma grand-mère a échappé à la surveillance de son infirmière à domicile *et* de ses aides ménagères. Elle a appelé un taxi et a disparu une journée entière avant d'être retrouvée en train d'errer devant des bureaux qui étaient jadis son centre commercial préféré. Comment a-t-elle réussi à arriver là-bas alors qu'elle ne se souvient même pas de nos noms, c'est un grand mystère.

Ce matin, je porte l'un de ses bijoux préférés. Je le sens à peine glisser sur mon poignet lorsque je sors de la limousine. Je fais comme si j'avais choisi mon bracelet libellule en son honneur mais, en vrai, il est là pour me rappeler que, chez les Stafford, les femmes font toujours leur devoir, même lorsqu'elles ne le veulent pas. Le lieu de l'événement de la matinée me met mal à l'aise. Je n'ai jamais aimé les maisons de retraite.

C'est juste une rencontre informelle, me dis-je. La presse est là pour couvrir notre venue, pas pour poser des questions. Nous allons nous serrer la main, visiter le bâtiment, nous joindre aux résidents pour célébrer l'anniversaire d'une pensionnaire qui fête ses cent ans. Son mari en a quatre-vingt-dix-neuf. Il y a bien de quoi sabrer le champagne.

Quand nous ouvrons les portes et que le parfum d'intérieur m'agresse les narines, je me dis que l'odeur n'aurait pas été pire si on avait lâché les triplés de ma sœur dans le couloir avec des bombes de désodorisant. Ça empeste le jasmin, version artificielle. Leslie renifle, hoche la tête, puis nous fait entrer, mon père et moi, ainsi qu'un photographe et plusieurs aides-soignants. Nous sommes venus sans garde du corps. Ils sont sans doute déjà partis pour préparer la rencontre de l'après-midi, à l'hôtel de ville. Au fil des ans, mon père a reçu des menaces de mort de la part de groupes marginaux, de milices privées et de tout un tas de tarés se prétendant tireurs d'élite, bioterroristes ou kidnappeurs. Il prend rarement ces menaces au sérieux, contrairement à son service de sécurité.

Au bout du couloir, nous sommes accueillis par la directrice de la maison de retraite et deux nouvelles équipes de journalistes dotées de caméras. Nous visitons. Ils filment. Mon père sort le grand jeu. Il serre des mains, pose pour les photos, prend le temps de parler avec les gens, se penche vers les chaises roulantes et remercie les infirmières de s'investir chaque jour dans un travail difficile et exigeant.

Je le suis et je l'imite. Un charmant vieillard débonnaire coiffé d'un chapeau melon en tweed flirte avec moi. Avec un accent britannique enchanteur, il me dit que j'ai de beaux yeux.

— Si j'avais cinquante ans de moins, j'userais de mon charme pour que vous acceptiez une invitation à dîner.

— Oh, mais je suis déjà sous le charme, lui réponds-je, et nous rions tous les deux.

L'une des infirmières me prévient que M. McMorris est un Don Juan du troisième âge. Comme pour le prouver, il lui fait un clin d'œil.

Alors que nous suivons le couloir vers la salle où se tient la fête d'anniversaire, je me rends compte que, en fait, je m'amuse bien. Les gens ont l'air contents ici. Si ce n'est pas aussi luxueux que l'établissement de ma grand-mère, on est loin des maisons mal gérées dénoncées par les plaignants lors des derniers procès. D'ailleurs, il y a peu de chance qu'un seul de ces plaignants voie un jour le moindre dollar de dédommagement que la cour leur attribuera. Les financeurs des chaînes de maisons de retraite bénéficient d'un réseau de holdings et de sociétés-écrans qu'ils peuvent mettre en faillite quand ils le souhaitent pour éviter de payer. Voilà pourquoi la découverte d'un lien entre l'une de ces chaînes et l'un des plus vieux amis de mon père – qui est aussi l'un de ses principaux donateurs – est potentiellement dévastatrice. Mon père est un notable vers qui on peut braquer la vindicte populaire et la dénonciation politique.

La haine et l'opprobre sont des armes puissantes. L'opposition le sait bien.

Dans la salle commune, on a installé une petite estrade. Je vais me placer sur le côté, avec les proches de la famille, près des portes-fenêtres qui donnent sur un jardin ombragé où s'épanouit un kaléidoscope floral, malgré la canicule.

Une femme seule se tient sur l'une des allées abritées du jardin. Elle nous tourne le dos, comme si elle ignorait qu'une fête avait lieu derrière elle. Ses mains reposent sur une canne. Elle porte une robe simple en coton couleur crème, ainsi qu'un gilet blanc, en dépit de la chaleur. Son épaisse chevelure grise a été tressée puis enroulée autour de sa tête, ce qui, combiné à sa tenue dépourvue de couleur, lui donne un air fantomatique, une réminiscence d'un passé depuis longtemps oublié. La brise qui caresse la glycine ne semble pas l'effleurer et renforce l'impression qu'elle n'est pas vraiment là.

Je reporte mon attention vers la directrice de l'établissement. Elle salue tout le monde, évoque avec verve les raisons de cette fête – un siècle d'existence, ça ne se croise pas tous les jours, après tout. Avoir été mariée pendant presque toutes ces années et avoir toujours l'être aimé près de soi, c'est encore plus remarquable. Voilà bien un événement digne d'une visite sénatoriale.

Sans compter que ce couple compte parmi les soutiens de mon père depuis ses débuts au sein du gouvernement de la Caroline du Sud. Techniquement, ils le connaissent depuis plus longtemps que moi et ils lui sont presque aussi dévoués. La reine de la fête et son mari lèvent leurs mains frêles bien haut et applaudissent furieusement quand le nom de mon père est prononcé.

La directrice évoque l'histoire des amoureux adorables installés à la table centrale. Lucie est née en France à l'époque où les voitures à cheval encombraient encore les rues. C'est franchement dur à imaginer. Elle a travaillé dans la Résistance pendant la Seconde Guerre mondiale. L'avion de son mari, Frank, un pilote de chasse, s'était fait descendre pendant un combat aérien. Leur histoire semble sortie tout droit d'un film – une romance renversante. Lucie l'a aidé à se déguiser et à quitter le pays, malgré sa blessure. Après la guerre, il est retourné la chercher. Elle habitait toujours dans la ferme familiale avec ses proches, tassés dans la cave, seule pièce épargnée par les bombardements.

Les épreuves que ces deux-là ont traversées m'épatent. Voilà ce qu'il est possible de vivre, quand l'amour est réel et puissant, quand deux personnes sont si dévouées l'une à l'autre, quand on est prêt à tout sacrifier pour être ensemble. Voilà ce que je veux connaître, mais je me demande parfois si c'est possible, pour notre génération moderne. Nous sommes tellement distraits, tellement... occupés.

Je jette un coup d'œil vers ma bague de fiançailles en me disant : Elliot et moi, nous pouvons le faire. Nous nous connaissons tellement bien... Nous avons toujours été proches...

La centenaire se lève doucement de sa chaise pour prendre le bras de son amoureux. Ils se déplacent ensemble, voûtés, tordus, appuyés l'un à l'autre. C'est émouvant, et mon cœur se serre. J'espère que mes parents vivront eux aussi assez longtemps pour connaître cet âge mûr de la vie. J'espère qu'ils profiteront d'une longue retraite... un jour... dans très longtemps, quand mon père aura enfin décidé de lever le pied. Cette maladie ne peut pas l'emporter à cinquante-sept ans. Il est trop jeune. On a trop besoin de lui, à la maison comme à l'extérieur. Il a encore du travail à faire et, après ça, mes parents méritent une retraite où les saisons s'écouleront lentement, où ils auront du temps à passer ensemble.

Dès que je sens l'émotion me serrer ma poitrine, je chasse ces pensées. « Pas de débordement d'émotions en public »– Leslie me le rappelle souvent. « Dans ce domaine, les femmes ne peuvent pas se le permettre. C'est vu comme de l'incompétence, de la faiblesse. »

Comme si je ne le savais pas déjà. Ce n'est pas vraiment différent dans la salle d'audience d'un tribunal. Les avocates y sont toujours jugées, et de plus d'une façon. Nous devons jouer en suivant d'autres règles.

Mon père adresse un salut militaire à Frank lorsqu'ils se retrouvent près de l'estrade. L'homme s'arrête, se redresse et lui retourne son salut avec une précision de soldat. Leurs regards se croisent et cet instant est intense. Très télégénique, même s'il n'est pas destiné aux caméras. Les lèvres de mon père se pincent en une ligne fine. Il se retient de pleurer.

Être si près des larmes, ça ne lui ressemble pas.

Je déglutis car ma gorge se serre de nouveau. Un souffle tremblotant s'échappe de mes lèvres. Je tire mes épaules vers l'arrière, détourne les yeux et me concentre sur la fenêtre pour étudier la femme dans le jardin. Elle n'a pas bougé, les yeux toujours dans le vague. Qui est-elle ? Que cherche-t-elle ?

Le chœur tapageur de « Joyeux anniversaire » doit filtrer à travers la vitre car elle se tourne doucement vers le bâtiment. Je sens moi aussi l'appel de la chanson. Je sais qu'il y a une chance que les caméras glissent vers moi, et que je semblerai distraite à l'écran, mais je n'arrive pas à arracher mon regard de l'allée. Je veux voir le visage de cette femme, au moins. Sera-t-il aussi lisse que le ciel d'été ? Est-ce qu'elle s'est juste égarée, tant mentalement que physiquement, ou bien a-t-elle évité délibérément les festivités ?

Leslie tire d'un coup sec l'arrière de ma veste et me ramène aussitôt à moi comme une écolière surprise en train de parler dans le rang.

— Joyeux anni... Concentre-toi, chante-t-elle tout près de mon oreille.

Je hoche la tête tandis qu'elle s'éloigne, son smartphone en main, pour pouvoir prendre sous un meilleur angle des photos qui iront sur le compte Instagram de mon père. Le sénateur est présent sur tous les réseaux sociaux à la mode, même s'il n'en maîtrise aucun. Son chargé de communication est un petit génie.

La cérémonie se poursuit. Des flashes crépitent. Des parents joyeux essuient quelques larmes et filment tandis que mon père offre une lettre de félicitations encadrée.

Le gâteau est apporté sur une desserte, orné de cent bougies flamboyantes.

Leslie est ravie. La joie et l'émotion envahissent la pièce comme de l'hélium propulsé dans un dirigeable. Encore un peu de bonheur et nous nous envolerons tous.

Tout à coup, quelqu'un me touche la main et le poignet, des doigts m'encerclent si soudainement que je sursaute avant de me reprendre pour ne pas faire une scène. La poigne qui me tient est froide, osseuse, tremblante mais étonnamment forte. En baissant la tête, je reconnais la femme du jardin. Elle redresse son dos courbé et lève vers moi des yeux qui ont la couleur des hortensias qui poussent chez moi, à Drayden Hill – un bleu clair et doux, bordé d'un cercle brumeux plus clair encore. Ses lèvres plissées tremblotent.

Avant que j'aie le temps de réagir, une infirmière vient la chercher en la prenant fermement par les épaules.

— May, dit-elle en me lançant un regard contrit, venez par ici. Vous ne devez pas embêter nos invités.

Plutôt que de me lâcher le poignet, la vieille dame s'accroche un peu plus à moi. Elle semble désespérée, comme si elle avait besoin de quelque chose, mais je ne vois pas du tout ce que cela peut être.

Elle scrute mon visage, sa tête levée vers moi.

— Fern ? murmure-t-elle.

2

May Crandall
De nos jours, Aiken, Caroline du Sud

Parfois, c'est comme si les verrous de mon esprit étaient trop rouillés, usés. Les portes s'ouvrent et se ferment à volonté. Un coup d'œil à l'intérieur par ici. Un trou par là. Un endroit sombre que j'ai peur de contempler.

Je ne sais jamais ce que je vais trouver.

Il n'y a aucun moyen de prédire quand une barrière s'ouvre soudain, ni pourquoi.

Des « moments gâchettes ». Voilà comme les psychologues appellent cela, à la télé. Comme si le choc embrasait la poudre et propulsait un projectile tourbillonnant dans le canon d'un fusil. Une métaphore appropriée.

Le visage de cette femme me fait cet effet.

Une porte s'ouvre vers un passé lointain. Je la franchis en titubant – malgré moi, au début –, en me demandant ce qui peut bien être enfermé dans cette pièce. Dès que je l'appelle Fern, je sais très bien que ce n'est pas vraiment à Fern que je pense. Je suis remontée bien plus loin. C'est Queenie que je vois.

Queenie, notre maman si forte, qui nous a transmis à tous ses jolies boucles dorées. Sauf à cette pauvre Camellia.

Mon esprit, léger comme une plume, glisse sur les cimes, au creux des vallées. Je vole vers une berge basse du Mississippi, où j'ai vu Queenie pour la dernière fois. L'air chaud et doux de cette nuit d'été à Memphis m'enveloppe, mais la nuit est fourbe.

Elle n'est pas douce. Elle ne pardonne pas.

Après cette nuit-là, il n'y aura plus de retour en arrière possible.

Douze ans, encore maigre et noueuse comme un poteau, je balance mes jambes dans le vide, sous le bastingage de l'humble bateau où nous habitons, guettant le reflet ambré de notre lanterne dans les yeux d'un alligator. Les alligators s'aventurent rarement si haut sur le fleuve mais, selon la rumeur, on en aurait aperçu quelques-uns dans le coin récemment. Du coup, les guetter devient une sorte de jeu. Les gamins pauvres de notre genre qui vivent sur des bateaux de fortune s'amusent comme ils le peuvent.

Et, cette nuit-là, nous avons encore plus besoin de nous changer les idées que d'habitude.

Près de moi, Fern grimpe sur la rambarde et scrute les bois à la recherche de lucioles. À presque quatre ans, elle apprend à compter. Elle pointe son doigt dodu et se penche sans se soucier des crocos.

— J'en vois une, Rill ! J'en vois une ! s'écrit-elle.

Je l'attrape par la robe pour la tirer en arrière en râlant :

— Si tu tombes, hors de question que je plonge encore pour te repêcher.

En vérité, cela ne lui ferait sans doute pas de mal. Ça lui donnerait une bonne leçon. Notre bateau est amarré dans une jolie lagune en face de Mud Island. Près de la poupe de l'*Arcadie*, l'eau ne m'arrive qu'aux hanches. Fern pourrait s'y tenir debout sur la pointe des pieds mais, de toute façon, nous nageons comme des têtards tous les cinq, même le petit Gabion qui ne sait pas encore prononcer une phrase entière. Quand on est né sur le fleuve, c'est aussi naturel que de respirer. On connaît ses bruits, ses humeurs et ses petits insectes. Pour une famille de rats d'eau comme nous, le fleuve est notre foyer. Un endroit sûr.

Cependant, ce soir-là, je perçois quelque chose dans l'air... quelque chose d'anormal. La chair de poule hérisse mes bras et picote mes joues. J'ai toujours eu des pressentiments. Je ne l'avouerai jamais à personne, pourtant, c'est vrai. Malgré la touffeur de cette nuit d'été, je suis soudain glacée. Là-haut, le ciel est lourd et les nuages semblent prêts à exploser. Un orage couve, mais je pressens autre chose.

Dans la cabine, les petits gémissements de Queenie s'accélèrent, malgré les avertissements de la sage-femme.

— M'ame Foss, faut arrêter de pousser, là, et tout de suite, dit-elle de sa voix épaisse comme de la mélasse. Ce p'tiot que vous avez là, il vient dans l'mauvais sens, il s'ra pas longtemps de not' monde et vous non plus. C'est tout. Calmez-vous. Tranquille.

Queenie émet un son grave et déchirant, comme un bateau qu'on arrache de la boue du bayou. Alors qu'elle nous a mis au monde, tous les cinq, en poussant à peine un grognement, cette fois, ça prend beaucoup plus de temps. Je frotte mes bras pour en chasser les sueurs froides et je sens soudain une présence dans les bois. Une présence mauvaise. Elle regarde vers nous. Que fait-elle là ? Est-ce qu'elle vient pour Queenie ?

J'ai envie de dévaler la passerelle et de courir sur la rive en criant : « Va-t'en ! Dégage d'ici ! Tu peux pas prendre ma maman ! »

Je le ferais vraiment. Si je n'avais pas peur des alligators. Au lieu de quoi, je reste assise, aussi immobile qu'un pluvier dans un nid. J'écoute les mots de la sage-femme. Elle parle tellement fort que je l'entends aussi bien que si j'étais à l'intérieur.

— Oh, grand Dieu ! Oh, misère ! Y en a pas qu'un, là-dedans. Je vous assure !

Mon père marmonne quelque chose. Le bruit de ses bottes parcourt le plancher dans un sens, hésite, puis repart dans l'autre.

La sage-femme reprend :

— M'sieur Foss, j'peux plus rien pour vous. Si vous amenez pas votre femme vite fait au docteur, ces bébés verront pas la lumière du jour, et leur mère y restera aussi.

Briny, mon père, ne répond pas tout de suite. Il cogne ses deux poings contre le mur, si fort que les cadres de Queenie tremblent. Quelque chose se décroche, j'entends le claquement du métal contre le bois et je devine ce qui est tombé, et où. Dans ma tête, je vois la croix de fer avec l'homme triste pardessus, et je veux me précipiter à l'intérieur, l'attraper, m'agenouiller près du lit et murmurer des mots polonais mystérieux, comme le fait Queenie par les nuits d'orage, lorsque Briny est loin du bateau, que la pluie s'infiltre dans le plafond et que des vagues martèlent la coque.

Mais je ne connais pas la langue étrange et dure que Queenie a apprise dans la famille qu'elle a abandonnée pour s'enfuir jusqu'au fleuve avec Briny. Les quelques mots de polonais que je connais ne voudraient rien dire si j'essayais d'en faire une phrase. Et pourtant, si je pouvais serrer la croix de Queenie dans ma main, je les dirais à l'homme de métal que Queenie embrasse lorsque l'orage gronde.

Je serais prête à tout essayer pour que l'accouchement finisse enfin et que Queenie retrouve le sourire.

De l'autre côté de la porte, les bottes de Briny raclent le plancher et j'entends la croix ricocher sur le sol. Briny regarde par la fenêtre sale, prise à la maison qu'il a démontée pour construire ce bateau-maison avant même ma naissance. Comme la mère de Briny était sur son lit de mort et que, cette année-là encore, les récoltes avaient été détruites par les inondations, le banquier aurait pris la maison, de toute façon. Briny s'est dit que le fleuve les sauverait. Il avait raison. Lorsque la Dépression a frappé, Queenie et lui vivaient déjà très bien sur l'eau. « Même la Dépression ne peut affamer le fleuve, dit-il chaque fois qu'il raconte cette histoire. Le fleuve a sa propre magie. Il prend soin de son peuple. Et pour toujours. »

Cette nuit, pourtant, cette magie tourne mal.

— M'sieur ! Vous entendez que je vous cause ?

La sage-femme devient méchante.

— Moi, j'veux pas leur sang sur mes mains. Vous emmenez vot' femme à l'hôpital. Tout de suite.

Derrière la vitre, le visage de Briny se referme. Comme ses yeux. Il se frappe le front, laisse retomber son poing contre le mur.

— L'orage...

— Je me fous d'savoir si le diable lui-même vient danser par ici, m'sieur Foss. Y a rien que je puisse faire pour cette pauvresse. Rien du tout. Je veux pas avoir ça sur les mains, non, monsieur.

— Elle n'avait... jamais eu de mal... avec les autres. Elle...

Queenie pousse un cri strident, et le bruit résonne dans la nuit comme le feulement d'un chat sauvage.

— Écoutez, vous avez oublié de me dire que'que chose : avant, elle avait jamais eu deux bébés d'un coup non plus.

Je me relève et j'emmène Fern de l'autre côté, sur le pont avant, avec Gabion, qui a deux ans, et Lark, qui en a six. Camellia, le nez à la fenêtre de la cabine pour regarder à l'intérieur, jette un coup d'œil vers moi. Je ferme le portillon menant à la passerelle pour les piéger tous sur le pont et dis à Camellia de ne pas laisser les petits passer par-dessus. Elle me répond par un froncement de sourcils. À dix ans, elle a le sale caractère de Briny, et aussi ses cheveux et ses yeux sombres. Elle n'aime pas qu'on lui dise ce qu'elle doit faire. Elle est aussi têtue qu'une mule et deux fois plus bête, parfois. Si les petits font des bêtises, on sera encore plus dans le pétrin qu'on ne l'est déjà.

— Ça va aller, leur promets-je en tapotant leurs têtes blondes comme on cajolerait des chiots. Queenie passe un mauvais moment, c'est tout. Elle a pas besoin qu'on vienne l'embêter en plus. Vous restez sages. Le vieux rougarou, il rôde dans les parages la nuit, j'ai entendu son souffle il y a un instant. C'est dangereux de sortir.

Maintenant que j'ai douze ans, je ne crois plus au rougarou, au croque-mitaine ni à Jack le Fou, le capitaine des pirates du fleuve. Enfin, presque plus. Je me demande si Camellia a un jour cru aux folles histoires de Briny.

Elle tend la main vers la poignée de la porte.

— Ne fais pas ça, je lui souffle. J'y vais.

On nous a dit de rester dehors, ce que Briny ne nous demande que lorsqu'il est très sérieux. Mais, là, Briny n'a pas l'air de savoir ce qu'il faut faire, et je m'inquiète pour Queenie et pour mon nouveau frère ou ma nouvelle sœur. Nous tous, nous étions tellement impatients de savoir ce que ce serait... Le bébé n'était pas censé arriver maintenant, par contre. Ça fait tôt – plus tôt même que Gabion, qui était minuscule et qui s'est glissé dans le monde avant même que Briny ait le temps d'arrimer le bateau et de trouver une femme pour les aider pendant l'accouchement.

Ce nouveau bébé-là ne semble pas décidé à nous faciliter autant les choses. Il ressemblera peut-être à Camellia, quand il sera né, il sera peut-être tout aussi têtu.

Ces nouveaux bébés, je me souviens soudain. Je me rappelle qu'il y en a plus d'un, comme une portée de chiots, et ce n'est pas normal. Trois vies gisent à demi dissimulées par le rideau que Queenie a cousu à partir de sacs de farine Golden Heart. Trois vies qui essaient de s'arracher les unes aux autres, mais qui n'y arrivent pas.

J'ouvre la porte, et la sage-femme se jette sur moi avant que je me sois décidée à entrer. Sa main se referme autour de mon bras. J'ai l'impression que ses doigts en font deux fois le tour. Je baisse les yeux et je vois le cercle de peau sombre contre ma peau pâle. Elle pourrait me briser en deux si l'envie lui en prenait. Pourquoi ne peut-elle pas sauver mon petit frère ou ma petite sœur ? Pourquoi ne peut-elle pas le tirer du corps de ma mère pour le mettre au monde ?

Queenie s'accroche au rideau, elle hurle, elle crie, arc-boutée dans le lit. Une demi-douzaine de crochets en fil de fer s'arrachent. Je vois le visage de ma mère, ses longs cheveux blonds comme les blés collés à sa peau, ses yeux bleus, ses yeux bleus si doux, si beaux, qui nous ont été transmis à tous sauf à Camellia, exorbités. La peau de ses joues est tellement étirée qu'elle est parcourue de fines veines comme des ailes de libellule.

— Pa' ?

Mon murmure arrive au terme du cri de Queenie, mais il semble encore vibrer dans l'air. Je n'appelle jamais Briny « pa' » et Queenie « 'man », sauf en cas d'extrême urgence. Ils étaient si jeunes lorsqu'ils m'ont eue, je crois qu'ils n'ont pas pensé à m'apprendre les mots « maman » et « papa ». J'ai toujours eu l'impression que nous étions des amis du même âge. Mais, de temps en temps, j'ai besoin qu'ils soient un père ou une mère. La dernière fois, c'était il y a des semaines, lorsque nous avons vu le pendu dans l'arbre, mort, le corps boursouflé.

Est-ce que Queenie ressemblera à ça si elle meurt ? Est-ce qu'elle partira en premier, et ensuite les bébés ? Ou est-ce que ce sera l'inverse ?

Mon estomac est tellement noué que je ne sens plus la grosse main autour de mon bras. Je suis peut-être même contente qu'elle soit là, pour me garder debout, m'ancrer sur place. J'ai peur de m'approcher plus près de Queenie.

— Dis-lui, toi ! me lance la sage-femme.

Elle me secoue comme une poupée de chiffon, elle me fait mal. À la lumière de la lanterne, ses dents brillent d'un blanc éclatant.

Le tonnerre gronde non loin, une bourrasque frappe la cloison de la cabine à tribord, la sage-femme trébuche en m'entraînant vers l'avant. Le regard de Queenie croise le mien. Elle me dévisage comme le ferait une petite fille, comme si je pouvais l'aider, et qu'elle m'implorait de le faire.

Je déglutis péniblement pour retrouver ma voix. Je balbutie de nouveau :

— P-pa' ?

Il continue de fixer droit devant lui. Pétrifié comme un lapin sentant le danger approcher.

Par la fenêtre, je vois Camellia, le nez écrasé contre la vitre. Les petits ont grimpé sur le banc pour regarder à l'intérieur. De grosses larmes roulent sur les joues rebondies de Lark. Elle ne supporte pas de voir le moindre être vivant souffrir. Dès qu'elle en a l'occasion, elle rejette à la rivière les petits poissons qui servent d'appâts. Dès que Briny part chasser des opossums, des canards, des écureuils, ou des daims, elle fait une scène comme si son meilleur ami avait été abattu juste sous ses yeux.

Elle compte sur moi pour sauver Queenie. Les autres aussi.

Un éclair frappe au loin. La lumière jaunâtre de la lampe à huile tremble avant de s'éteindre. J'essaie de compter les secondes jusqu'au coup de tonnerre, pour savoir à quelle distance se trouve l'orage, mais je suis trop secouée.

Si Briny n'emmène pas Queenie très vite au docteur, ce sera trop tard. Comme toujours, nous sommes amarrés sur la rive sauvage. Memphis se trouve de l'autre côté des eaux sombres et vastes du Mississippi.

Je tousse pour me dénouer la gorge et raidis mon cou pour qu'elle ne se serre plus.

— Briny, tu dois l'emmener de l'autre côté.

Il pivote vers moi, doucement. Son visage est toujours terne, pourtant on dirait qu'il attendait cela – que quelqu'un, à part la sage-femme, lui dise que faire.

— Briny, tu dois la porter jusqu'à la barque, avant que l'orage soit sur nous.

Bouger notre bateau prendrait trop de temps, je le sais. Briny le saurait aussi s'il pouvait encore réfléchir.

— Dis-lui ! me presse encore la sage-femme.

Elle s'élance vers Briny en me poussant devant elle.

— Si vous sortez pas cette femme de ce rafiot, elle s'ra morte avant l'aube !

3

Avery Stafford
De nos jours, à Aiken, en Caroline du Sud

— Avery ! On a besoin de toi en bas !

Rien ne peut nous faire passer plus vite de trente à treize ans que la voix d'une mère rebondissant dans l'escalier comme une balle de tennis après un coup droit slicé.

— J'arrive ! Une seconde.

Elliot ricane, au téléphone. C'est un bruit à la fois familier et réconfortant. Il évoque une série de souvenirs qui remontent jusqu'à notre enfance. Entre la mère d'Elliot et la mienne qui ne nous quittaient pas des yeux, nous n'avons jamais ne serait-ce qu'envisagé de sortir du rang, et encore moins de faire les actes indicibles auxquels se livraient les autres adolescents en espérant nous en tirer à bon compte. Nous étions plus ou moins condamnés à bien nous conduire. Ensemble.

— On a besoin de toi, on dirait, ma chérie.

— Oui, pour la photo de Noël.

Je me penche vers le miroir pour écarter de mon visage mes boucles blondes, qui retombent aussitôt. Ma balade rapide jusqu'à l'écurie après la visite de la maison de retraite a fait ressortir les anglaises de mamie Judy. Je m'y attendais, mais une jument a mis bas pendant la nuit et je ne peux pas résister à l'appel d'un poulain nouveau-né. Maintenant, j'en paie le prix. Aucun lisseur professionnel de la création n'est de taille à lutter contre la brise humide du fleuve Edisto.

— Une photo de Noël en juillet ? glousse Elliot, ce qui me rappelle à quel point il me manque.

Vivre si loin l'un de l'autre est vraiment difficile, et cela ne fait que deux mois.

— Elle s'inquiète pour la chimio. Même si on lui a dit que mon père ne perdrait pas ses cheveux avec celle-là, elle redoute quand même que cela arrive.

Il n'y a vraiment aucun docteur sur Terre capable de rassurer ma mère quant au cancer du côlon de mon père. Elle a toujours tout dirigé à la maison et elle est bien décidée à ne pas abdiquer maintenant. Si elle dit que la chevelure de mon père va perdre en épaisseur, cela sera sans doute le cas.

— Cela ne m'étonne pas d'elle, s'esclaffe Elliot encore une fois.

Il est bien placé pour le savoir. Sa propre mère, Bitsy, et la mienne sortent du même moule.

— Elle est juste morte de peur à l'idée de perdre mon père.

Ma gorge se serre. Ces derniers mois nous ont rongés de l'intérieur, exposant chacun de nous à une hémorragie interne silencieuse.

— C'est normal, répond Elliot avant de se taire pendant un moment qui me paraît une éternité.

J'entends les touches du clavier de son ordinateur cliqueter. Ça me rappelle qu'il a une société de courtage balbutiante à diriger et son succès représente tout pour lui. Il n'a pas besoin que sa fiancée l'appelle au beau milieu de sa journée de travail sans raison particulière.

— Heureusement que tu es là-bas, Avy.

— J'espère que ça les aide un peu. Parfois, je me dis que je leur ajoute du stress au lieu de les soulager.

— Tu dois être auprès d'eux. Tu dois passer cette année en Caroline du Sud pour y établir ta résidence... au cas où.

Elliot me le rappelle chaque fois que nous avons cette conversation – chaque fois que je dois lutter contre l'envie de prendre un vol pour le Maryland, pour retrouver mon ancien bureau au cabinet du procureur fédéral, où je n'avais pas de raison de m'inquiéter de traitements contre le cancer, de photo de Noël en avance, d'électeurs, de gens comme cette femme à l'air désespéré qui m'a agrippée par le poignet dans la maison de retraite.

— Hé, Avy, attends deux secondes. Désolé. C'est la folie ce matin.

Elliot me met en attente pour prendre un autre appel, et mes pensées refilent aussitôt vers les événements de la matinée. Je revois cette femme – May – dans le jardin, avec son gilet blanc. Puis elle est près de moi, son visage à peine au niveau de mon épaule, ses mains osseuses resserrées autour de mon poignet, la canne qui pend à son bras. Son regard me hante, à cet instant encore. Elle semble tellement sûre de me reconnaître. Elle est certaine de savoir qui je suis.

— Fern ?

— Pardon ?

— Fernie, c'est moi. (Les larmes lui montent aux yeux.) Oh, ma chérie, tu m'as tellement manqué. Ils m'ont dit que tu étais partie. Je savais que tu ne pourrais jamais briser notre pacte.

Pendant une fraction de seconde, je veux être cette Fern, pour qu'elle soit heureuse – pour qu'elle puisse cesser un instant de fixer la glycine, toute seule. Elle semblait tellement isolée, là-bas. Perdue.

On m'épargne de devoir lui dire que je ne suis pas celle qu'elle cherche. L'aide-soignante arrive, rouge et visiblement secouée.

— Je m'excuse, me murmure-t-elle. Mme Crandall est nouvelle.

Elle passe son bras fermement autour des épaules de la vieille dame et l'oblige à desserrer sa main de mon poignet. Cette Mme Crandall a une force surprenante. Elle cède centimètre par centimètre, et l'aide-soignante chuchote doucement :

— Allez, May. Je vais vous raccompagner à votre chambre.

Je la regarde partir avec l'impression que je devrais faire quelque chose pour elle, mais je ne sais pas quoi.

Elliot revient en ligne et je suis de retour dans le présent.

— Bref, dit-il, reste flegmatique. Tu peux le faire. Je t'ai vue affronter les meilleurs avocats des grandes villes. Aiken ne devrait pas te poser trop de problèmes.

— Je sais... Je suis désolée de t'embêter. C'est juste que... j'avais besoin d'entendre ta voix, j'imagine.

Je sens le rouge me monter au cou. Je ne suis pas si dépendante, d'habitude. C'est peut-être une conséquence de la maladie de mon père et de la situation de mamie Judy, toujours est-il qu'une conscience aiguë et douloureuse de la mortalité de tout être me colle à la peau. Comme un brouillard épais et persistant sur le fleuve. Je suis obligée d'avancer à tâtons, sans voir le danger.

J'ai vécu une vie enchantée. Je ne l'avais peut-être pas compris avant cet instant.

— Ne sois pas si dure envers toi-même, reprend Elliot avec tendresse. Tu as beaucoup à gérer. Donne-toi du temps. Tu ne régleras rien en te tracassant pour l'avenir.

— Tu as raison. Je le sais bien.

— Tu peux me l'écrire, s'il te plaît ?

La blague d'Elliot me fait rire.

— Jamais de la vie.

J'attrape mon sac à main sur le bureau, à la recherche de quelque chose pour m'attacher les cheveux. En renversant tout sur le lit, je trouve deux épingles à cheveux argentées. Ça fera l'affaire. Je me dégagerai le visage et laisserai mes cheveux onduler pour la photo. Ça plaira à mamie Judy lorsqu'elle la verra. Ce sont *ses* boucles que j'essaie de dompter, après tout, et elle les portait toujours de cette façon.

— Ah, ça te ressemble déjà plus, Avy.

Elliot salue quelqu'un qui vient d'entrer dans son bureau et nous nous disons rapidement au revoir pendant que je me coiffe, puis je jette un dernier coup d'œil vers le miroir en défroissant la robe droite verte que j'ai enfilée pour la photo. J'espère que la styliste de ma mère ne vérifiera pas la marque. Je l'ai achetée dans une grande surface en passant. Mes cheveux ont l'air corrects, par contre. Même la styliste approuvera... si elle est là... ce dont je ne doute guère. Leslie et elle sont tombées d'accord sur mon apparence : il y a du travail, comme elles disent.

On frappe doucement à ma porte. Je lance une mise en garde :

— N'entre pas. Il y a une pieuvre dans le placard !

Courtney, ma nièce de dix ans, passe sa tête ornée de boucles blondes dans l'embrasure de la porte. Elle aussi tient de mamie Judy.

— La dernière fois, tu m'as dit qu'il y avait un grizzly, là-dedans, râle-t-elle, les yeux au ciel, pour me faire comprendre que, si cette petite blague l'amusait peut-être encore quand elle avait neuf ans, elle est devenue nulle depuis qu'elle a officiellement atteint un âge à deux chiffres.

— Un grizzly mutant métamorphe, je te ferais dire, réponds-je en taclant au passage le jeu vidéo qui l'obsède un peu trop ces derniers temps.

Avec une fournée surprise de triplés dans la maison, Courtney se retrouve souvent livrée à elle-même. Elle ne semble pas se plaindre de cette nouvelle liberté, mais je m'inquiète pour elle.

La main sur la hanche, elle me lance avec arrogance :

— Si tu ne descends pas tout de suite, tu auras bien besoin de ton grizzly, parce que Pomme d'amour va lâcher les chiens sur toi.

Pomme d'amour, c'est le petit nom que mon père a donné à ma mère.

— Ooooh, je tremble de peur !

Ici, à Drayden Hill, les terriers écossais sont tellement chou-choutés qu'ils accueilleraient sans doute un cambrioleur en levant la patte, persuadés qu'il leur apporte des friandises de luxe venant de la boulangerie canine.

Je sors de ma chambre en ébouriffant ma nièce au passage et je m'élance dans l'escalier en criant :

— Allison ! À cause de ta fille, la photo de famille prend du retard !

Courtney pousse un cri indigné et nous faisons la course dans l'escalier. Elle gagne parce qu'elle est petite et agile, et que je porte des talons hauts. Je n'ai pas besoin de paraître plus grande mais ma mère ne serait pas contente si j'arrivais en chaussures plates pour la photo de Noël.

Dans la salle de réception, le photographe et son équipe ne rigolent pas. Ils ont une mission. S'ensuit une séance où rien n'est laissé au hasard. Le temps qu'on en finisse, les ados de ma sœur aînée sont au bord de la crise de nerfs et, moi, je suis prête pour une bonne sieste. Au lieu de quoi, j'attrape un des triplés et je me lance dans une guerre de guili sur le canapé. Les deux autres rejoignent bientôt la bagarre.

— Avery, pour l'amour du ciel ! proteste ma mère. Regarde dans quel état tu te mets ! Tu es censée partir avec ton père dans vingt minutes, je te rappelle.

Leslie jette un coup d'œil vers moi, prouvant sa capacité à regarder dans deux directions à la fois, tel un iguane. Elle agite un doigt vers ma robe verte.

— C'est trop formel pour la rencontre à l'hôtel de ville, et ta tenue de ce matin ne l'est pas assez. Mets le tailleur-pantalon bleu avec les guipures le long de l'ourlet. Très sénatorial sans être trop solennel. Tu vois duquel je parle ?

— Oui.

Je préférerais continuer à me chamailler avec les triplés ou discuter avec les enfants de Missy, ma sœur aînée, qui veulent partir comme animateurs en colonie de vacances, mais personne ne me demande mon avis.

J'embrasse mes nièces et mes neveux et je file me changer à l'étage. Dans peu de temps, je dois repartir en limousine avec mon père.

Dès que nous sommes installés, il sort son téléphone portable et fait défiler les fichiers jusqu'au briefing vocal concernant la rencontre de l'après-midi. Entre Leslie, ses différents assistants et autres secrétaires, tant ici qu'à Washington, et les journaux, il est toujours très bien informé. Il n'a pas le choix. Dans le climat politique actuel, il y a un risque réel de changement dans l'équilibre sénatorial si son combat contre le cancer le forçait à se retirer. Mon père préférerait rejoindre la tombe plutôt que de laisser cela se produire. La longue période durant laquelle il a ignoré ses symptômes pour rester à Washington en est la preuve, tout comme le fait que j'aie été rappelée à la maison afin que j'y établisse ma résidence principale et qu'on me prépare au poste, juste au cas où, comme le dirait Elliot.

En Caroline du Sud, le nom de Stafford a toujours dépassé les partitions politiques, mais la mauvaise presse autour des scandales des maisons de retraite nous a tous fait transpirer comme des touristes à Charleston en plein été. De nouveaux rebondissements paraissent chaque semaine – des pensionnaires décédés pour des escarres non traitées, des établissements au personnel non diplômé, des endroits bien loin de répondre aux normes fédérales exigeant au moins une heure vingt de soins par jour et par patient, et qui recevaient tout de même des financements publics. Des familles dévastées qui avaient cru leurs proches entre de bonnes mains. C'est horrible et déchirant – et l'infime lien établi avec mon père a fourni à nos ennemis politiques une réserve inépuisable d'armes très chargées émotionnellement. Ils veulent faire croire à tous que, en échange de donations monstrueuses, mon père serait prêt à user de son influence pour aider un ami à profiter de la souffrance humaine sans qu'il soit poursuivi pour cela.

Quiconque connaît mon père ne peut être dupe. Il n'est pas en position de demander à ses soutiens et à ses donateurs de montrer leurs bilans comptables et, même si c'était le cas, la vérité serait enfouie sous des couches et des couches de corporations semblant en règle au premier coup d'œil.

— On ferait mieux de se briefer un peu, déclare-t-il en démarrant le mémo vocal.

Il tient son téléphone entre nous en se penchant vers moi et, soudain, j'ai de nouveau sept ans. Je ressens une espèce d'effusion, la même que lorsque ma mère m'emmenait dans les couloirs sacrés du Capitole, s'arrêtait devant les quartiers de mon père et me permettait d'y entrer seule. Sans un bruit, je m'approchais d'un pas solennel du bureau de la secrétaire et j'annonçais que j'avais rendez-vous avec le sénateur.

— Ah bon ? Voyons ça, répondait Mme Dennison à chaque fois, un sourcil haussé, réprimant un sourire, tandis qu'elle appuyait sur le bouton de l'interphone. Sénateur, une certaine... Mlle Stafford est là pour vous. Est-ce que je la fais entrer ?

Après avoir réussi à me faire admettre à l'intérieur, je rejoignais mon père qui m'accueillait avec une poignée de main en disant :

— Bonjour, mademoiselle Stafford. Je me réjouis que vous ayez pu venir. Êtes-vous prête à aller à la rencontre des électeurs, aujourd'hui ?

— Oui, monsieur !

Ses yeux pétillaient toujours fièrement lorsque je tournoyais pour lui montrer que je m'étais bien habillée pour l'occasion. L'une des meilleures choses qu'un père puisse offrir à sa fille, c'est de lui faire comprendre qu'elle est à la hauteur de ses attentes. Mon père a fait ça pour moi et, malgré tous mes efforts, je ne pourrai jamais vraiment payer la dette que j'ai envers lui. Je ferais n'importe quoi pour lui et pour ma mère aussi.

Nous sommes assis épaule contre épaule, à écouter les détails des activités de cette fin de journée, les sujets qui devraient être abordés et les problèmes qui doivent être évités. On nous donne des réponses soigneusement préparées aux questions concernant les mauvais traitements en maisons de retraite, les procès avortés, les sociétés-écrans qui font faillite comme par magie avant que les dommages et intérêts puissent être payés. Que compte faire mon père pour régler tout cela ? A-t-il fait pression sur certaines personnes pour protéger des donateurs et de vieux amis du bras de la justice ? Se servira-t-il maintenant de son influence pour aider les milliers de seniors qui luttent pour trouver des soins de qualité ? Et pour ceux qui vivent encore chez eux, qui sont confrontés aux dégâts commis par les récentes inondations records, qui sont forcés de choisir entre faire les réparations, manger, payer leur facture d'électricité ou renouveler leurs traitements médicaux ? À son avis, que faut-il faire pour les aider ?

Les questions se suivent inlassablement. Chacune est accompagnée d'au moins une réponse bien argumentée. Beaucoup comportent plusieurs options, que nous pouvons choisir selon le contexte ou d'éventuelles réfutations. La réunion de cet après-midi sera une opération de communication soigneusement encadrée, mais il y a toujours un risque, même mineur, qu'une personne mal intentionnée obtienne le micro. Le ton pourrait monter.

On nous explique même comment répondre si jamais quelqu'un révélait où nous avons placé mamie Judy. Pourquoi payons-nous un établissement aux tarifs journaliers sept fois plus élevés que le montant remboursé aux seniors à faibles revenus ?

Pourquoi ? Parce que le docteur de mamie Judy nous a recommandé Magnolia Manor comme étant le meilleur choix et qu'elle connaissait déjà l'endroit. L'une de ses amies d'enfance habitait dans cette propriété avant qu'elle soit réaménagée, si bien qu'elle a l'impression d'être chez elle. Si nous pensons avant tout à son bien-être, nous sommes aussi inquiets pour sa sécurité. Comme beaucoup de familles, nous nous trouvons confrontés à un problème complexe pour lequel il n'existe aucune réponse simple.

Problème complexe… pas de réponse simple…

J'enregistre ça tel quel dans un coin de ma tête, au cas où je serais interrogée. Il vaut mieux que je n'improvise pas lorsque des sujets si personnels sont abordés.

— C'était parfait pour ton image, la visite de ce matin, Wells, déclare Leslie en se glissant dans notre voiture pendant une pause-café à quelques pâtés de maisons de l'hôtel de ville. Nous sommes bien partis pour tuer cette affaire dans l'œuf.

Elle est encore plus déterminée que d'habitude.

— Cal Fortner et son équipe peuvent bien essayer de profiter de cette histoire de maisons de retraite. Ils ne font que tendre le bâton avec lequel ils se feront battre.

— Le bâton ? À ce niveau-là, c'est tout un fagot.

La blague de mon père tombe à plat. Il y a un plan bien élaboré dans l'opposition, une stratégie globale visant à faire passer mon père pour un élitiste coupé de la réalité, un habitué de Washington qui, après des dizaines d'années passées au Capitole, ne voit plus les besoins des habitants de son État d'élection.

— Nous retournerons toutes leurs attaques à notre avantage, déclare Leslie avec confiance. Écoutez, il y a un petit changement de programme. Nous allons entrer dans le bâtiment par l'arrière. Il y a une manifestation dans la rue, juste en face de l'entrée.

Elle se tourne vers moi avant de reprendre :

— Avery, nous allons te faire monter sur scène, cette fois-ci. Pendant la conférence, le sénateur sera assis en face de l'intervenant, pour créer une ambiance détendue. Tu seras à côté de ton père, sur le canapé, à sa droite – la fille inquiète revenue à la maison pour veiller sur sa santé et s'occuper des affaires familiales. Tu es la seule célibataire, libre parce que tu n'as pas d'enfants à élever ; tu as aussi un mariage à organiser ici, à Aiken, etc. Tu connais la chanson. Rien de trop politique, mais n'aie pas peur de montrer tes connaissances des dossiers et leurs ramifications juridiques. Le ton de la rencontre doit être détendu, naturel, si bien qu'une question plus personnelle pourrait t'être adressée. Il n'y aura que des journaux locaux dans la salle, ce qui peut être l'occasion idéale pour toi de te montrer au public sans trop de pression.

— Bien sûr.

J'ai passé les cinq dernières années avec des jurés qui guettaient mes moindres faits et gestes et des avocats de la défense qui me surveillaient de près. Les participants à une conférence méticuleusement préparée ne me font pas peur.

C'est du moins ce que je me dis. Pour une raison qui m'échappe, mon pouls s'emballe et ma gorge est soudain sèche et rêche.

— Montre-leur ton visage de pro, ma puce, me lance mon père avec ce que nous appelons parfois « son clin d'œil à un million de dollars ».

Son œillade pleine de confiance en soi, comme du miel chaud, épais et irrésistible.

Si seulement j'avais ne serait-ce que la moitié de son charisme...

Leslie continue à nous briefer. Elle parle encore lorsque nous arrivons à l'hôtel de ville. Contrairement à notre visite à la maison de retraite, il y a un service de sécurité, cette fois-ci, dont des agents de la police d'État. J'entends le vacarme de la foule à l'avant du bâtiment et une voiture de police est stationnée à l'entrée de la ruelle.

Lorsqu'on nous fait sortir de la limousine dans la cohue, Leslie a l'air prête à frapper quelqu'un. Sous mon tailleur bleu marine très sobre, je transpire nerveusement.

— Honore ton père et ta mère ! hurle un manifestant par-dessus le brouhaha.

J'ai une folle envie de tourner les talons, de remonter le trottoir et de leur dire ce que je pense. Comment osent-ils ?

— Pas de camps de concentration pour les seniors ! entendons-nous alors que nous entrons dans le bâtiment.

— C'est quoi, leur problème ? Ils sont débiles ou quoi ? marmonné-je.

Leslie m'adresse un regard de mise en garde avant de hausser discrètement les épaules vers les policiers. Elle me fait comprendre que, en public, je dois garder mes opinions pour moi, sauf si elles ont été soumises à approbation. Seulement, moi, je suis prête à me battre... ce qui est peut-être une bonne chose. Mon pouls ralentit résolument et je sens mon visage de pro se mettre en place.

Dès que la porte se referme, les choses se calment. Nous sommes accueillis par Andrew Moore, le coordinateur du programme de la conférence organisée par l'Association de défense des droits des seniors, un organisme très influent. Andrew semble étonnamment jeune pour un tel poste. Il ne peut pas avoir plus de vingt-cinq ans. Avec son costume gris impeccable, sa cravate un peu de travers et son col de chemise qui bouffe n'importe comment, on dirait un petit garçon à qui on a préparé ses affaires mais qu'on a laissé s'habiller tout seul. Il nous explique qu'il a été élevé par ses grands-parents, qui ont dû faire d'énormes sacrifices pour lui. Son investissement au sein de l'ADDS est sa façon à lui de leur rendre la pareille. Lorsque quelqu'un mentionne le fait que je suis avocate, il me dévisage et laisse entendre que son organisme aurait bien besoin de recruter un avocat digne de ce nom. Je réponds par une plaisanterie :

— Je note, on ne sait jamais.

En attendant le début du débat, nous discutons de tout et de rien. Il paraît aimable, honnête, énergique et engagé. Je suis soudain plus optimiste : nous aurons peut-être un débat équitable.

On nous présente rapidement d'autres personnes. Dont le journaliste local qui officiera comme modérateur. Nous glissons les micros sous nos vestes, les fixons à nos revers avant d'accrocher les boîtiers de transmission à nos ceintures.

Nous attendons dans les coulisses pendant que le journaliste s'adresse au public. Il remercie les organisateurs, rappelle à tout le monde le format de la conférence avant de finir par nous présenter. La foule applaudit et nous montons sur scène en saluant joyeusement l'assistance. Tout le monde reste courtois même si, en scrutant la salle, je remarque quelques mines inquiètes, sceptiques ou hostiles. D'autres dévisagent le sénateur d'un air qui ne peut être interprété que comme de l'admiration béate.

Mon père parvient sans mal à répondre aux questions simples et à esquiver les quelques sujets qui ne peuvent être traités par une brève déclaration. Il n'y a pas de solutions toutes faites au problème du financement des années de retraite – beaucoup plus nombreuses que pour les générations précédentes –, à celui des familles recomposées ni au basculement culturel qui fait que nous nous tournons vers une prise en charge professionnelle des seniors plutôt qu'une prise en charge à la maison par des proches.

Malgré ses réponses bien tournées, je devine qu'il est un peu décontenancé. Il tarde à réagir lorsqu'un jeune homme lui demande :

— Monsieur, j'aimerais savoir ce que vous avez à répondre à l'accusation de Cal Fortner, affirmant que l'objectif des chaînes de maisons de retraite privées est de parquer les personnes âgées à moindre coût afin d'augmenter leurs profits, et que votre acceptation des multiples donations de L. R. Lawton et de ses partenaires financiers indique que vous soutenez ce modèle pour lequel les profits sont plus importants que les conditions de vie des gens. Reconnaissez-vous que, dans ces établissements, les seniors reçoivent des soins – quand ils en reçoivent – par un personnel peu ou pas qualifié et payé au salaire minimum ? Votre détracteur demande que la législation fédérale reconnaisse quiconque tire des bénéfices d'une maison de retraite ou de ses sociétés mères comme personnellement responsable des soins qui y sont pratiqués, et redevable des dommages et intérêts attribués lors d'un procès. Fortner demande aussi qu'on taxe les individus fortunés tels que vous pour financer une augmentation des retraites les plus basses. Au vu des événements récents, soutiendrez-vous de telles propositions au Sénat ? Et, si oui ou non, pour quelles raisons ?

J'entends presque Leslie grincer des dents derrière le rideau. Ces questions n'étaient nulle part dans le programme et je suis certaine qu'elles ne sont pas non plus sur la fiche que tient ce jeune homme.

Mon père hésite, comme frappé de stupeur. *Allez* – je l'encourage mentalement. Une goutte de sueur dégouline dans mon dos. Mes muscles se crispent et j'agrippe l'accoudoir du canapé pour m'empêcher de gigoter nerveusement.

Le silence qui s'éternise est une vraie torture. J'ai l'impression que des minutes entières s'écoulent. Même si je sais que ce n'est pas si long.

Mon père finit par se lancer dans une longue explication des régulations fédérales existantes concernant les maisons de retraite, et des taxes et autres caisses fédérales qui financent Medicaid, la sécurité sociale pour les plus pauvres. Il semble compétent et imperturbable. De nouveau maître de la situation. Il fait clairement apparaître qu'il n'est pas en position de modifier seul le mode de financement de Medicaid, le code des impôts et l'état actuel de prise en charge des seniors, mais que ces questions auront toute son attention lors de la prochaine session parlementaire.

La conférence se poursuit selon le programme prévu.

Une question finit par m'être adressée et le modérateur me regarde avec indulgence. Je donne la réponse prévue à celui qui voulait savoir si j'étais oui ou non venue pour me préparer à reprendre le siège de mon père au Sénat. Je ne dis pas oui, je ne dis pas non plus jamais de la vie. Je finis par répondre :

— De toute façon, ce serait prématuré... sauf si je voulais me présenter contre lui. Et qui serait assez fou pour faire une chose pareille ?

Des rires parcourent l'assistance et je leur adresse le clin d'œil que j'ai hérité de mon père. Il est tellement content qu'il se redresse et semble avoir pris vingt centimètres lorsqu'il répond aux questions suivantes, et puis la séance prend fin.

Lorsque je rejoins les coulisses, je m'attends à ce que Leslie me félicite par quelques tapes dans le dos. Au lieu de quoi, elle m'attrape par le coude, l'air soucieuse et, tandis que nous sortons, elle se penche vers moi.

— La maison de retraite a appelé. Apparemment, tu as perdu un bracelet, là-bas, c'est vrai ?

— Quoi ? Un bracelet ?

Je me souviens soudain que j'en avais mis un ce matin. Je ne sens rien autour de mon poignet et, après vérification sous ma manche, effectivement, il a disparu.

— On l'a trouvé sur l'une des pensionnaires. La directrice a épluché les photos qu'elle avait prises avec son portable, c'est comme ça qu'elle a su qu'il était à toi.

La vieille dame de la maison de retraite... celle qui m'a prise par le poignet...

Je me souviens maintenant des petites pattes en or des trois libellules me griffant le poignet lorsque May Crandall a été écartée de moi. Elle a dû partir avec.

— Oooh, je crois que je sais ce qui s'est passé.

45

— La directrice s'est excusée profusément. La coupable est une nouvelle pensionnaire, elle a du mal à s'adapter. On l'a trouvée il y a deux semaines dans une maison au bord du fleuve, avec le cadavre de sa sœur et une douzaine de chats.

— C'est terrible !

Mon imagination s'emballe et je vois malgré moi la scène lugubre, épouvantable.

— Je suis certaine que c'était un accident – cette histoire de bracelet, je veux dire. Elle m'a pris la main pendant le discours de mon père. L'aide-soignante a été presque obligée de l'arracher à moi.

— Ça n'aurait jamais dû arriver.

— Ce n'est pas grave, Leslie. Vraiment.

— Je vais envoyer quelqu'un pour le récupérer.

Je repense aux yeux bleus de May Crandall, à la façon dont elle me dévisageait d'un air désespéré. Je l'imagine s'éloignant avec mon bracelet, l'examinant seule dans sa chambre, le passant sur son poignet pour l'admirer avec ravissement.

Si ce n'était pas un bijou de famille, je la laisserais le garder.

— Tu sais quoi ? Je crois que je vais y aller moi-même. Le bracelet appartenait à ma grand-mère.

La suite du programme nous oblige à nous séparer là, mon père et moi. Il va passer un peu de temps à son bureau avant d'aller dîner avec l'un de ses donateurs pendant que ma mère reçoit une réunion des Filles de la Révolution américaine[1] chez nous, à Drayden Hill.

Les yeux de Leslie lancent des éclairs. J'ai peur qu'on en vienne aux mains, alors j'ajoute une excuse imparable.

— Puisque j'ai un petit peu de temps, je comptais de toute façon en profiter pour aller prendre le thé avec mamie Judy.

Après la conférence sur le thème des conditions de vie des seniors, je me sens coupable de ne pas avoir été la voir depuis presque une semaine.

---

1. Filles de la Révolution américaine (FRA) : société réservée aux descendantes des combattants pour l'indépendance des États-Unis.

Leslie hoche la tête en serrant les dents : visiblement, elle trouve ma décision idiote et bien peu professionnelle.

Je n'y peux rien. Je pense encore à May Crandall et à la pléthore d'articles concernant la maltraitance en maison de retraite. Je veux peut-être m'assurer que May n'est pas venue me trouver parce qu'elle avait des ennuis là-bas.

Ou peut-être que son histoire triste et macabre a piqué ma curiosité. On l'a trouvée il y a deux semaines dans une maison au bord du fleuve, avec le cadavre de sa sœur...

Est-ce que sa sœur s'appelait Fern ?

4

Rill Foss
1939, Memphis, Tennessee

Queenie est pâle comme du lait écrémé, son corps crispé et dur lorsque Briny la dépose sur le pont avant du bateau pour aller chercher la barque, qui est accrochée à un tas de bois flotté un peu plus loin. Queenie pleure et hurle à pleins poumons, la joue collée au plancher lisse.

Lark recule dans la nuit, à l'ombre de la cabine, mais les petits, Fern et Gabion, s'approchent, à quatre pattes. Ils n'ont jamais vu d'adultes se comporter de cette façon.

Gabion se penche vers notre mère, comme s'il n'était pas sûr que cette chose dans la robe rose à fleurs de Queenie soit bien elle. Queenie, c'est la lumière, le rire et toutes les vieilles chansons qu'elle chante avec nous quand nous naviguons sur le fleuve d'une ville à l'autre. Cette femme qui montre les dents, qui jure, qui gémit et qui pleure ne peut pas être elle, et pourtant, si.

— Lill, Lill ! lance Gabion car, à tout juste deux ans, il n'arrive pas à dire mon nom, Rill.

Il agrippe l'ourlet de ma jupe et tire dessus tandis que je m'agenouille pour tenir la tête de notre mère.

— Keenie bobo ?

— Taisez-vous ! crache Camellia en tapant sur les mains des petits alors que Fern fait mine de caresser les longues boucles dorées de Queenie.

C'est sa chevelure qui a tapé dans l'œil de Briny et qui l'a charmé. « Tu trouves pas que ta maman ressemble à une prin-cesse de conte de fées ? me demande-t-il parfois. La reine du

48

royaume d'Arcadie, c'est ta maman. Ça veut dire que t'es une princesse aussi, pas vrai ?

Mais ma mère n'est plus du tout jolie, maintenant, avec son visage barbouillé de sueur et sa bouche déformée par la douleur. Les bébés vont la faire éclater. Son ventre se contracte et enfle sous sa robe. Elle m'attrape le poignet et s'y cramponne pendant que, dans la cabine, la sage-femme s'essuie les mains et rassemble ses instruments dans un panier d'herbes tressées.

— Vous devez l'aider ! je hurle. Elle est en train de mourir !

— Vos histoires, moi, j'veux plus m'en mêler, répond la femme, dont le corps lourd fait tanguer le bateau et balancer la lanterne qui crachote. Plus du tout. Vous êtes que des « chie dans l'eau » stupides.

Elle est furieuse comme un chien de bidonville parce que Briny refuse de la payer. Il affirme qu'elle avait promis de mettre un bébé au monde, ce qu'elle n'a pas fait, et qu'elle devrait s'estimer heureuse qu'il la laisse prendre les deux poissons-chats dodus qu'il a tirés des palangres un peu plus tôt, ainsi qu'un peu de charbon pour sa lanterne. Elle pourrait essayer de se venger, mais elle est plus noire que le goudron, et nous sommes blancs, et elle sait ce qui pourrait arriver si elle nous cherchait des ennuis.

On devait manger les poissons-chats au dîner, ce qui ne nous laisse rien qu'un petit pain de maïs à nous diviser en cinq. Une pensée parmi une demi-douzaine d'autres qui tourbillonnent dans ma tête.

Est-ce que je devrais rassembler des habits pour Queenie ? La brosse à cheveux ? Ses chaussures ?

Est-ce que Briny a assez d'argent pour payer un vrai docteur ? Sinon, qu'arrivera-t-il ?

Et s'il se fait arrêter par la police ? C'est arrivé une fois, quand on faisait le tour des salles de billard des villes de la côte. Mon père gagne sa vie en jouant au billard. Personne ne peut le battre, et il est assez doué au piano pour que, dans les salles de billard, des gens le paient pour ça aussi mais, depuis la crise, l'argent liquide se faire rare. Maintenant, la plupart du temps, il joue au billard ou du piano en échange d'objets qu'on peut ensuite troquer contre ce dont nous avons besoin.

Est-ce qu'on a une réserve secrète d'argent ? Est-ce que je devrais poser la question à Briny à son retour ? Lui rappeler qu'il en aura peut-être besoin ?

Comment va-t-il réussir à traverser le fleuve dans le noir alors que l'orage provoque déjà des vagues ?

La sage-femme se tourne sur le côté pour passer la porte, et son panier rebondit sur ses fesses. Quelque chose de rouge en dépasse, et je le reconnais tout de suite, même dans la pénombre – le joli chapeau de Queenie avec les plumes, celui que Briny a gagné dans un petit endroit crasseux nommé Boggyfield.

— Remettez ça où vous l'avez pris ! crié-je. C'est le chapeau de ma mère !

La femme plisse ses yeux sombres et pointe son menton vers moi.

— Moi, j'ai perdu ma journée ici, mam'zelle, et vos deux poissons, vous pouvez vous les garder. Du poisson, j'en ai assez. Je prends ce chapeau.

Elle cherche Briny du regard avant de se diriger vers la passerelle, sur le côté du pont.

Je voudrais l'arrêter, mais je ne peux pas. Sur mes genoux, Queenie hurle en s'agitant dans tous les sens. Sa tête tombe sur le pont dans un bruit creux, comme une pastèque. Je l'attrape avec mes deux mains.

Camellia bondit pour passer devant la femme et lui barrer le passage, les bras tendus d'un côté du bastingage à l'autre.

— J'vous laisserai pas emporter le chapeau de ma mère !

La femme fait un pas de plus mais, si elle connaissait Camellia, elle y réfléchirait à deux fois. Ma sœur n'a peut-être que dix ans, mais elle n'a pas hérité que de la chevelure noire et épaisse de Briny ; elle a son caractère, aussi. Lorsque Briny se met en rogne, il est « aveuglé par la colère », comme le dit le vieux Zede. « Et être aveuglé par la colère, sur le fleuve, ça peut nous faire tuer. » Zede a mis mon père en garde plus d'une fois quand nos bateaux se sont retrouvés amarrés côte à côte, c'est-à-dire très souvent. Zede est l'ami de mon père depuis qu'il est venu vivre sur le fleuve. C'est lui qui a appris à Briny à se débrouiller ici.

— T'as la langue bien pendue, toi ! Quel culot !

Une grande main sombre se referme sur le bras de Camellia et, quand la femme essaie de la soulever, ma sœur s'accroche si fort au bastingage que j'ai peur que son épaule se déboîte.

Il ne faut pas deux secondes à Camellia pour se tourner et mordre à belles dents. La femme crie, recule d'un pas trébuchant qui fait tanguer le bateau.

Queenie hurle.

Le tonnerre gronde au loin.

Des éclairs surgissent, la nuit se transforme en jour avant de remettre son voile noir.

Où est Briny ? Pourquoi met-il autant de temps ?

Je pense au pire. Et si la barque s'était détachée et que Briny n'arrivait pas à la retrouver ? Et s'il était parti en emprunter une autre à quelqu'un ? Pour une fois, je regrette que Briny soit si obstinément solitaire. Il ne va jamais sympathiser avec les autres familles qui vivent comme nous sur des bateaux, et ceux qui connaissent l'*Arcadie* savent qu'ils ne doivent pas passer nous voir sans y être invités. Pour Briny, sur le fleuve, il y a des gens bien et d'autres indignes de confiance, et il vaut mieux garder ses distances avant de savoir qui appartient à quel groupe.

À force de donner des coups de pied, Queenie fait tomber Gabion, qui se cogne le bras en poussant une longue plainte suraiguë. Lark file se cacher dans la cabine maintenant que la sage-femme n'y est plus. Queenie est en train de mourir dans mes bras. J'en suis sûre.

Camellia reste campée devant la passerelle. Son regard de chien de garde semble mettre la femme au défi de réessayer de passer. Camellia se bat toujours pour un rien. Elle est capable d'attraper des serpents à mains nues et de se bagarrer avec les garçons du fleuve sans se poser de questions.

— Laissez le chapeau de ma mère ! hurle-t-elle si fort qu'elle couvre les plaintes de Gabion. Et le poisson aussi. Dégagez de notre bateau avant qu'on aille dire à la police qu'une dame de couleur a essayé de nous tuer notre maman et de nous voler en plus ! Ils vous pendront dans un arbre, voilà !

Elle laisse sa tête rouler sur le côté et tire la langue, et mon estomac se soulève. Deux semaines plus tôt, un mercredi, on a vu un homme pendu dans un arbre plus bas, sur le fleuve. Un grand Noir en salopette. Il n'y a pas de maison à des kilomètres alentour, il était là depuis assez longtemps pour que les buses s'en soient déjà prises à lui.

Seule Camellia est capable de se servir de ça pour arriver à ses fins. Ça me rend malade, rien que d'y penser.

C'est peut-être pour ça que Queenie est si mal en point, me murmure une voix. Parce que Briny ne s'est pas arrêté pour détacher cet homme, retrouver sa famille afin qu'il soit enterré convenablement. C'est peut-être lui qui nous scrute depuis les bois, maintenant.

Queenie avait supplié Briny de gagner la rive pour s'occuper du corps, mais il avait refusé. « Il faut penser aux enfants, Queenie, avait-il dit. On sait pas c'est qui qui lui a fait ça, ni qui pourrait le surveiller. Vaut mieux continuer tout droit sur le fleuve. »

La sage-femme arrache le chapeau de Queenie de son panier, le jette par terre, marche dessus d'un pas si lourd que le bateau tangue de nouveau, avant de descendre la passerelle et de ramasser la lanterne qu'elle avait laissée sur la berge. Pour finir, elle prend l'enfiloir avec les deux poissons-chats. Puis elle s'éloigne en nous couvrant de jurons.

— Va au diable toi-même ! lui renvoie Camellia, penchée au-dessus du bastingage. C'est ce qui arrive aux voleurs !

Elle se retient de répéter tous les gros mots proférés par la femme. Au cours de ses dix années d'existence, Camellia a mangé plus de savon que de vraie nourriture, en tout cas suffisamment pour nettoyer l'intérieur d'une baleine. C'est un miracle que des bulles ne lui sortent pas des oreilles.

— Quelqu'un arrive. Tais-toi, Gabion.

Elle attrape Gabby, lui plaque la main sur la bouche et écoute les bruits de la nuit. Moi aussi, j'entends le grondement d'un moteur. Je lance à Fern :

— Va voir si c'est Briny.

Quand elle se lève d'un bond pour obéir, Camellia pousse Gabby vers elle.

— Fais-le taire, lui ordonne-t-elle avant de traverser le pont pour se pencher par-dessus le garde-fou côté fleuve et, pour la première fois de la soirée, j'entends une once d'espoir dans sa voix lorsqu'elle annonce :

— On dirait qu'il a trouvé Zede.

Le soulagement m'enveloppe comme une couverture chaude. Si quelqu'un est capable d'arranger les choses, c'est bien le vieux Zede. Je ne savais même pas qu'il était dans les environs de Mud Island, mais Briny, lui, était sans doute au courant. Ils arrivent toujours à savoir où est l'autre, sur le fleuve. La dernière fois que j'avais entendu parler de lui, Zede était dans les terres pour s'occuper d'une sœur qui avait dû entrer au sanatorium à cause de la tuberculose.

Je murmure à l'oreille de Queenie :

— Zede est là.

Elle semble m'entendre, se calmer un peu, peut-être. Zede saura quoi faire. Il va apaiser la violence de Briny, chasser les nuages des yeux de mon père et le faire réfléchir.

— Zede est là, Queenie. Ça va s'arranger. Ça va s'arranger...

Je me répète ça jusqu'à ce qu'ils lancent la corde de la barque à Camellia et qu'ils grimpent sur la passerelle.

Briny traverse le pont en deux pas, tombe à genoux près de Queenie et la prend dans ses bras, la tête tout près de celle de ma mère. Je sens son poids me quitter, sa chaleur disparaître de ma peau. La rosée du soir se met à tomber et, tout à coup, j'ai froid. Je me lève, augmente la flamme de la lanterne et croise les bras fermement pour me réchauffer.

Zede s'accroupit tout près, regarde Queenie dans les yeux, déplie un peu le drap, et il y a du sang partout. Il pose une main sur son ventre, là où une tache rouge progresse sur sa robe.

— Mademoiselle Floss ? fait-il d'une voix calme et claire. Mademoiselle Floss ? Vous m'entendez ?

Elle émet ce qui pourrait être un « oui », mais le son meurt entre ses dents serrées et elle enfouit son visage dans la poitrine de Briny.

La bouche de Zede forme une ligne sinistre dans son épaisse barbe grise. Ses yeux rougis semblent pendouiller dans leurs orbites. Il inspire par ses larges narines poilues et expire entre ses lèvres pincées. Il sent fort le whisky et le tabac, des odeurs réconfortantes. C'est la seule chose qui soit normale, dans cette soirée.

Il croise le regard de Briny et secoue un peu la tête.

— Queenie, ma fille, on va te descendre du bateau, tu m'entends ? On doit t'emmener à l'hôpital dans ma *Jenny*. Ça va remuer, la traversée. Tu dois être courageuse, d'accord ? Tu peux faire ça pour moi ?

Il aide Briny à la soulever et ses hurlements déchirent la nuit comme les femmes déchirent leur voile funéraire à La Nouvelle-Orléans. Elle s'avachit, inerte, dans les bras de Briny, avant même d'arriver au canot.

— Tiens-la, dit Zede à Briny, avant de me regarder et de tendre vers moi son doigt tordu, cassé pendant la guerre hispano-américaine. Tu fais rentrer tous les petits dans la cabine et tu les mets au lit, grande sœur. Restez à l'intérieur. Je reviendrai vite, avant l'aube, si l'orage vient pas par là. Sinon, la *Lizzy Mae* est attachée un peu plus bas. Votre barque est là-bas. J'ai un p'tit jeune avec moi, sur la *Lizzy*. Il est pas trop beau à voir, en ce moment – il a essayé d'embarquer en douce dans un train et il s'est fait ramasser par les contrôleurs. Mais il vous fera pas de mal. Je lui ai dit de prendre la barque et de venir vous voir demain matin si je donnais pas de nouvelles.

Il tourne la manivelle, le moteur Waterwitch se met à ronronner, et je regarde l'eau bouillonner à la lueur de la lanterne.

Je ne veux pas voir les yeux fermés de Queenie ni sa bouche qui pendouille comme ça.

Camellia leur lance la corde, qui atterrit pile sur la proue de la barque.

Zede tend ensuite l'index vers Camellia.

— Toi, t'écoutes ta sœur, m'dame butée. Tu fais rien sans demander d'abord à Rill. C'est compris ?

Camellia fronce tellement le nez que ses taches de rousseur se rejoignent sur ses joues.

— C'est compris ? répète Zede.

Il sait laquelle de nous deux est la plus susceptible de partir en vadrouille et de s'attirer des ennuis.

— Mellia ! braille Briny, qui retrouve un instant ses esprits.

— Oui, m'sieur, lâche-t-elle à contrecœur.

Quand Briny se tourne vers moi, on dirait qu'il m'implore plus qu'il me parle.

— Surveille les petits, Rill. Prends soin de tout le monde, jusqu'à ce qu'on revienne. Queenie et moi.

— On sera sages. Promis. Je veillerai sur eux. On n'ira nulle part.

Zede tourne la barre, met les gaz et le Waterwitch emporte ma maman dans les ténèbres. Tous les cinq, nous nous précipitons contre la rambarde, où nous restons côte à côte pour suivre la *Jenny* du regard jusqu'à ce que l'obscurité l'avale tout entière. Nous écoutons la coque claquer contre les vagues, montant et tombant, le moteur grondant, se taisant, grondant encore. Sa voix se fait un peu plus lointaine à chaque fois. Au loin, les remorqueurs font sonner leurs cornes de brume. Un maître d'équipage siffle des consignes. Un chien jappe.

Puis la nuit sombre dans le silence.

Fern s'enroule autour de ma jambe comme un singe et Gabby va rejoindre Lark dans la cabine car c'est sa sœur préférée. Pour finir, nous n'avons plus rien à faire à part rentrer à notre tour et nous débrouiller pour le dîner. Il ne nous reste que le pain de maïs et des poires que Briny a troquées à Wilson, dans l'Arkansas, où nous sommes restés trois mois et où on a même été à l'école jusqu'aux vacances d'été. À ce moment-là, Briny a eu de nouveau la bougeotte. Il était prêt à repartir sur l'eau.

En temps normal, il n'arrête jamais le bateau près d'une grande ville comme Memphis, mais Queenie se plaignait de crampes depuis avant-hier. Même si c'était plus tôt que ce qu'elle avait prévu, après cinq bébés, elle savait qu'il valait mieux amarrer le bateau et rester tranquilles.

À l'intérieur de l'*Arcadie*, on gémit, on s'inquiète, on a chaud, on râle. Camellia se plaint parce que j'ai fermé la porte au lieu de tirer juste la moustiquaire, et on se croirait dans un four malgré les fenêtres ouvertes.

— Taisez-vous, dis-je en préparant le dîner.

Nous nous asseyons par terre en cercle, tous les cinq, parce qu'il nous semble déplacé de nous installer à table en laissant deux places vides au bout.

— 'ai faim, se plaint Gabion, les lèvres boudeuses, dès qu'il a fini sa part.

Il mange plus vite qu'un chat errant.

Je découpe un bout de ma tranche de pain de maïs et le fais tournoyer vers lui.

— Tu as gobé ta part trop vite.

Il ouvre la bouche comme un oisillon son bec chaque fois que je m'approche, et je finis par jeter le morceau de pain à l'intérieur.

— Mmm, fait-il en se frottant le ventre.

Fern reprend le jeu, et puis Lark aussi. Pour finir, c'est Gabby qui mange presque tout le pain. Sauf la part de Camellia, parce qu'elle a dévoré tout son morceau.

— J'irai tirer les lignes demain matin, dit-elle comme si cela compensait sa tendance égoïste.

— Zede nous a dit de ne pas bouger, lui rappelé-je.

— Quand Zede reviendra. Ou quand le garçon se montrera. J'irai à ce moment-là.

Elle ne peut pas manœuvrer les lignes toute seule, elle le sait.

— La barque n'est même pas ici. Briny l'a prise pour rejoindre le bateau de Zede.

— Elle sera là demain.

— Briny aussi, il sera là demain. Avec Queenie et les bébés.

Nous échangeons un regard – juste Camellia et moi. Je sens que Lark et Fern nous observent, mais nous sommes les deux seules à comprendre suffisamment la situation pour partager notre inquiétude. Camellia tourne la tête vers la porte et moi aussi. Nous savons toutes les deux que personne n'entrera par là ce soir. Nous ne sommes jamais restés seuls la nuit. Queenie était toujours là, même lorsque Briny partait chasser ou jouer au billard ou pêcher des grenouilles.

Gabion s'écroule sur le tapis tressé de Queenie, les yeux fermés, ses longs cils couleur sable chatouillant ses joues. Je dois encore lui mettre un lange pour la nuit – j'attendrai qu'il dorme profondément, comme le fait Queenie. Maintenant qu'il va sur le pot dans la journée, il pique une crise dès qu'on s'approche de lui avec un lange.

Dehors, le tonnerre gronde, les éclairs fusent et le ciel se met à cracher de la brume. Est-ce que Zede et Briny ont réussi à traverser avec notre maman ? Est-ce qu'elle est dans un endroit où les docteurs peuvent la soigner, comme ils l'ont fait quand Camellia a eu une appendicite ?

— Ferme les fenêtres qui donnent sur le fleuve. Ce serait idiot de laisser la pluie entrer, conseillé-je à Camellia, qui ne proteste même pas.

Pour la première fois de sa vie, elle est perdue. Elle ne sait pas ce qu'il vaut mieux. Le problème, c'est que je ne le sais pas non plus.

La bouche de Gabion s'ouvre toute seule et il se met à ronfler. C'est au moins un des petits qui ne fera pas de scène ce soir. Avec Lark et Fern, ce sera une autre paire de manches. Les grands yeux bleus de Lark s'emplissent de larmes et elle murmure :

— Ze ve-e-eux Queenie. Z'ai peur.

Moi aussi, je veux Queenie, mais je ne peux pas le lui dire.

— Tais-toi, voyons. Tu as six ans. Tu n'es plus un bébé. Ferme les fenêtres avant que le vent ne se lève et mets ta chemise de nuit. On va changer les draps du grand lit et on y dormira tous ensemble. Comme quand Briny n'est pas là.

Si mon corps est fourbu et las, mon esprit tournicote comme un fou. Il n'arrive pas à penser clairement. Il ne réussit qu'à faire tournoyer des mots qui n'ont pas de sens, comme le Waterwitch brasse les eaux peu profondes en remuant des feuilles, des brindilles, des appâts et de la vase.

Et ça continue tellement que j'entends à peine les gémissements, les plaintes, les hoquets et les reniflements, que Camellia aggrave en traitant Fern de chochotte, Lark de bébé et en utilisant un gros mot qu'elle n'est même pas censée connaître.

Pour finir, quand nous sommes tous dans le grand lit et que j'éteins les lanternes, je ramasse l'homme de métal tombé au sol et je le raccroche au mur, à sa place. Briny n'a pas besoin de lui, mais Queenie, si et, ce soir, c'est le seul qui est là pour veiller sur nous.

Avant d'aller au lit, je m'agenouille et je murmure tous les mots polonais que je connais.

5

Avery

— Ça ne me prendra pas longtemps, dis-je à Ian.

Le stagiaire de Leslie vient de se garer sous le portique de la maison de retraite.

— Oh... fait-il alors qu'il est déjà à moitié sorti de voiture. D'accord. Je vais rester là pour m'occuper de mes e-mails.

Il semble déçu que je n'aie pas besoin d'une escorte. Je sens son regard curieux me suivre tandis que je descends de voiture et que j'entre dans le hall d'accueil.

La directrice m'attend dans son bureau. Le bracelet de mamie Judy est posé devant elle. Les yeux en pierres précieuses des libellules scintillent lorsque je glisse le trésor perdu à mon poignet.

Nous discutons un peu de la fête du matin avant qu'elle ne s'excuse de m'avoir dérangée.

— Mme Crandall nous donne du souci, admet-elle. La pauvre, la plupart du temps, elle ne parle à personne. Elle se contente de... traîner dans les couloirs et dans le parc jusqu'à ce qu'on ferme les portes pour la nuit. Puis elle reste dans sa chambre, sauf si des bénévoles viennent jouer du piano. Elle semble adorer la musique, mais même pendant la chorale, elle refuse de parler aux autres résidents. Le chagrin et le déracinement, c'est parfois trop pour l'esprit et le corps.

J'imagine aussitôt quelqu'un disant la même chose de mamie Judy. Mon cœur se serre pour cette pauvre femme, May.

— J'espère qu'elle n'est pas contrariée. Je suis certaine qu'elle n'a pas fait exprès de prendre ce bracelet. J'aurais bien voulu le lui laisser, mais c'est un bijou qui est depuis longtemps dans notre famille.

— Oh, grand Dieu, non. Il vaut mieux qu'elle le rende. Une chose que nos pensionnaires ont parfois du mal à accepter, c'est qu'une grande partie de leurs possessions n'ait pas été transférée ici avec eux. Ils ont tendance à repérer de petits objets dans l'établissement et pensent qu'on les leur a dérobés en douce. Nous rendons souvent à leurs propriétaires des biens volés. Mme Crandall est encore en période d'adaptation, après avoir quitté sa maison.

— Je sais que c'est une transition difficile.

La maison de ma propre grand-mère sur Lagniappe Street est fermée, avec tout ce qu'elle contient. Nous ne sommes pas encore prêts à décider de ce qu'il faut faire d'une vie de souvenirs, d'innombrables trésors de famille. La maison sera transmise à la génération suivante, comme c'est toujours le cas. Avec un peu de chance, l'une de mes sœurs y emménagera et la plupart des meubles anciens pourra y rester.

— Est-ce que Mme Crandall reçoit de la visite de sa famille ?

J'évite soigneusement de parler de la sœur décédée. Je me sens suffisamment coupable de parler de cette femme comme si c'était... une étude de cas. C'est une personne, comme mamie Judy.

La directrice secoue la tête, les sourcils froncés.

— Elle n'a pas de proches dans le coin. Son fils unique est décédé il y a des années. Elle a des petits-enfants, mais c'est une famille recomposée, et aucun d'eux ne vit dans les parages, ce qui complique la situation. Ils font de leur mieux et, pour être honnête, Mme Crandall n'a pas facilité les choses. Elle avait d'abord été admise dans un établissement plus près de chez elle, puis elle a essayé de s'enfuir. La famille l'a fait transférer ici en pensant qu'un peu de distance pourrait faciliter son adaptation. Elle a cherché à s'échapper trois fois en deux semaines. Bien sûr, il n'est pas inhabituel que les nouveaux résidents soient désorientés et posent quelques difficultés. Nous espérons que son comportement s'améliorera une fois qu'elle se sera un peu habituée. Je m'en voudrais d'être obligée de la transférer dans l'unité Alzheimer, mais…

Elle interrompt sa phrase en pinçant les lèvres, comprenant sans doute qu'elle n'est pas censée me dire tout cela.

— Je suis désolée, dis-je en ayant l'impression de n'avoir fait qu'aggraver une situation déjà difficile. Est-ce que je pourrais la voir… pour la remercier de m'avoir rendu le bracelet ?

— Elle ne l'a pas rendu… à proprement parler. L'infirmière l'a trouvé sur elle.

— J'aimerais au moins lui dire que je suis contente de l'avoir récupéré.

En fait, je suis surtout inquiète de l'approche très… clinique de la directrice. Et si j'avais attiré des ennuis à May ?

— Ce bracelet était l'un des bijoux favoris de ma grand-mère.

Je baisse les yeux vers les libellules dorées ciselées, avec leurs yeux en pierres précieuses et leurs dos multicolores.

— Nous n'interdisons pas les visites, ici, mais il vaudrait mieux que vous vous absteniez. Mme Crandall refusera sans doute de vous parler, de toute façon. Nous l'informerons que le bracelet a été remis à sa propriétaire et tout ira bien.

Nous terminons la discussion en évoquant aimablement la fête d'anniversaire, puis nous nous séparons à la porte de son bureau. Alors que je me dirige vers la sortie, je passe devant un panneau indiquant les noms et les numéros des chambres, arrangés proprement sur des porte-étiquettes en métal.

MAY CRANDALL, 107. Je tourne dans le couloir.

La chambre 107 se trouve tout au fond. La porte est ouverte. Le lit dans la première moitié de la chambre est vide. Le rideau de séparation est tiré. J'entre et murmure :

— Il y a quelqu'un ? Madame Crandall ?

Ça sent le renfermé et la lumière est éteinte mais j'entends une respiration rauque.

— Madame Crandall ?

Encore un pas, et je vois des pieds qui sortent des couvertures de l'autre lit, derrière le rideau. Les orteils sont rabougris et recourbés. Comme s'ils n'avaient pas touché le sol depuis longtemps. Ça ne doit pas être elle.

J'étudie la partie de la chambre occupée par Mme Crandall. L'endroit est exigu, impersonnel, déprimant. Alors que le nouveau mini-appartement de mamie Judy est équipé d'un canapé, d'un fauteuil, d'un guéridon pour jouer aux cartes, et décoré avec autant de ses photos préférées que possible, cette pièce semble dire que son occupant n'a pas l'intention d'y rester. Le seul objet personnel repose sur la table de nuit – une photo dont le cadre est doté d'un pied en velours poussiéreux à l'arrière.

Même si je sais que je ne devrais pas faire ma curieuse, je revois encore May lever vers moi ses yeux bleu couleur œuf de rouge-gorge, comme si elle avait besoin de quelque chose. Désespérément. Et si elle avait essayé de fuir cet endroit parce que quelqu'un la maltraite ? Dans un cabinet de procureur fédéral, on croise forcément des cas horribles de maltraitance de seniors. Lorsque des crimes sont commis dans notre État et qu'ils incluent du télémarketing frauduleux, du vol d'identité ou des détournements de pensions de retraite, cela tombe sous notre juridiction. Il arrive bien trop souvent que des jeunes attendent juste de faire main basse sur l'argent de leurs grands-parents. Mme Crandall a peut-être des petits-enfants merveilleux, mais j'ai du mal à imaginer pourquoi ils la laissent toute seule ici au lieu de la faire transférer plus près d'eux, où ils pourraient s'assurer qu'elle est bien traitée.

Je veux juste être sûre que tout va bien, me dis-je. J'ai, chevillé au corps, le sens du devoir des Stafford. Il me pousse à me sentir responsable du bien-être d'inconnus, surtout s'ils sont vulnérables et marginalisés. Les œuvres de bienfaisance, c'est le deuxième boulot à plein temps, non officiel, de ma mère.

Le cadre élaboré est tourné vers le mur, malheureusement. Il a été moulé dans le genre de celluloïd ivoire nacré qui aurait été assorti aux poudriers des dames, aux brosses, aux peignes et aux tire-boutons dans les années trente et quarante. Même en me penchant en avant, je ne vois pas la photo.

Pour finir, je n'y tiens plus. Je tourne le cadre. Sépia, blanchie sur les côtés, la photo présente un jeune couple sur le bord d'un lac ou d'un étang. L'homme porte un chapeau en feutre élimé et tient une canne à pêche. Son visage est difficile à distinguer – yeux et cheveux sombres. Il est bel homme et sa posture, un pied sur une bûche, les épaules étroites rejetées en arrière, évoque la confiance en soi, l'arrogance, presque. Comme s'il mettait au défi le photographe.

La femme est enceinte. Le vent fait bouffer sa robe fleurie, soulignant un ventre qui semble trop gros pour être porté par ses longues jambes fines. Les anglaises de sa chevelure blonde épaisse descendent presque jusqu'à sa taille. Elle est coiffée comme une petite fille, avec un ruban au nœud défait qui empêche ses cheveux de lui tomber dans les yeux. C'est le plus saisissant, chez elle : on dirait une adolescente déguisée pour une pièce de théâtre. *Les Raisins de la colère*, peut-être.

Ce qui me frappe ensuite, c'est à quel point elle me rappelle ma grand-mère. Je cligne des yeux, me penche plus près, repense aux photos que nous avons accrochées avec soin il n'y a pas longtemps dans la chambre de mamie Judy. Il y en a une en particulier – un cliché de son voyage post-bac. Elle est assise sur une jetée, à Coney Island, et sourit à l'appareil.

Cette ressemblance n'est sans doute que le fruit de mon imagination. À en juger par les habits qu'ils portent, cette photo est trop ancienne pour être celle de mamie Judy. Ma grand-mère, toujours au dernier chic, ne se serait jamais habillée comme ça, mais, malgré tout, en scrutant à travers le cadre en verre, je ne pense qu'à une chose : ce pourrait être elle. Je lui trouve aussi une ressemblance avec ma nièce, Courtney, et, bien sûr, avec moi.

Je sors mon portable pour prendre une photo et j'essaie de faire la mise au point malgré la pénombre.

La mise au point patine. J'appuie quand même. La photo est floue. Je me rapproche du lit pour recommencer. Je ne sais pas pourquoi, mais j'aurais l'impression de passer les bornes en allumant la lumière et, en me servant du flash, il y aura un reflet sur le verre du cadre. Pourtant, je veux une photo. Mon père pourra peut-être me dire s'il reconnaît ces personnes... à moins que, une fois chez moi, en regardant de nouveau ce cliché, je me rende compte que j'ai exagéré cette ressemblance. La photographie est ancienne et pas très nette.

— Il faut être bien mal élevé pour entrer chez les gens sans y avoir été invitée.

Je sursaute avant d'appuyer sur le bouton « prise de vue ». Puis mon téléphone m'échappe des mains. Il tourbillonne dans l'air et je suis comme un personnage de dessin animé, à bouger au ralenti, mes doigts n'agrippant que de l'air.

May Crandall entre dans la chambre alors que je récupère mon téléphone sous son lit.

— Je suis désolée. Je voulais juste...

Il n'y a aucune bonne excuse pour mon intrusion. Aucune.

— Qu'est-ce que vous vouliez, précisément ?

Quand je me tourne, elle recule d'un pas, surprise. Son menton rentre dans son cou avant d'en ressortir tout doucement.

— Vous êtes revenue.

Son regard s'arrête sur le cadre, et je comprends qu'elle sait qu'il a été bougé.

— Vous êtes l'une d'*eux* ?

— Eux ?

— Ces gens.

Sa main volette dans l'air, indiquant le personnel de la maison de retraite.

— Ils me retiennent prisonnière ici.

Je repense à l'histoire que Leslie m'a racontée – la maison, le cadavre de la sœur. Dans cette histoire, il n'y a peut-être pas que du chagrin et de la désorientation. Je ne connais vraiment rien sur cette femme.

— Je vois que vous avez mon bracelet, reprend-elle, le doigt pointé vers mon poignet.

Les mots de la directrice me reviennent en tête. « La plupart du temps, elle ne parle à personne. Elle se contente de... traîner dans les couloirs et dans le parc... »

Pourtant, elle me parle, à moi.

Je me surprends à approcher le bracelet, une main par-dessus, et le mettre tout contre ma poitrine.

— Je suis désolée. Ce bracelet est à moi. Il a dû glisser lorsque vous m'avez prise par le poignet, tout à l'heure... ce matin... au repas d'anniversaire.

Elle me regarde en clignant des yeux, comme si elle ne voyait pas du tout de quoi je lui parle. A-t-elle déjà oublié la fête ?

— Vous avez eu le même ?

— Le même repas d'anniversaire ? Bien sûr que non.

Sa contrariété bouillonnante affleure à la surface de sa peau, puissante et corrosive.

La directrice a peut-être sous-estimé les problèmes de cette femme ? J'ai entendu dire que la démence et la maladie d'Alzheimer pouvaient se manifester par de la paranoïa et des signes d'agitation. Moi, je n'en ai jamais été témoin. Mamie Judy a les idées confuses et elle s'énerve contre elle-même, mais elle est aussi douce et gentille que d'habitude.

— En fait, je voulais parler du bracelet. Vous en avez eu un identique ?

— Eh bien, oui... jusqu'à ce qu'ils vous le donnent.

— Non. Je le portais déjà quand je suis arrivée ici ce matin. C'est un cadeau de ma grand-mère. C'était l'un de ses bijoux favoris. Autrement, j'aurais...

Je me retiens de poursuivre. *J'aurais pu vous le laisser.* Elle pourrait le prendre comme un manque de respect, comme si je la traitais comme une enfant.

Elle me regarde longuement. Tout à coup, elle semble tout à fait lucide, perspicace, même.

— Je pourrais peut-être rencontrer votre grand-mère, pour que nous tirions cela au clair. Elle habite dans les environs ?

Il y a un changement brutal d'atmosphère dans la pièce. Je le sens et cela n'a rien à voir avec la climatisation qui se met en route au-dessus de nos têtes. Elle attend quelque chose de moi.

— J'ai peur que cela soit impossible. Je le regrette, mais je n'y peux rien.

En vérité, je n'exposerais jamais ma douce grand-mère à cette femme étrange et amère. Plus elle parle, plus il m'est facile de l'imaginer terrée chez elle avec le cadavre de sa sœur.

— Elle n'est plus de ce monde, alors ?

— Si. Elle a déménagé pour s'installer dans une maison de retraite.

— Récemment ?

— Il y a un mois environ.

— Oh... oh, quel dommage. Est-ce qu'elle est heureuse, au moins, là-bas ?

S'ensuit un regard implorant, désespéré, et je suis soudain prise de pitié pour elle. Quel genre de vie a-t-elle vécu ? Où sont les amis, les voisins, les collègues... les gens qui devraient lui rendre visite maintenant, par devoir à défaut d'envie ? Mamie Judy reçoit de la visite au moins une fois par jour, parfois deux ou trois.

— Je le pense. En vérité, elle se sentait seule, chez elle. Maintenant qu'elle est dans cet établissement, elle a des gens à qui parler, il y a des journées jeux et des fêtes auxquelles elle peut assister. Ils font des activités manuelles et il y a une bibliothèque remplie de livres.

Je ne doute pas qu'ils proposent le même genre de divertissements ici. Je peux peut-être profiter de cette conversation pour encourager May Crandall à laisser une chance à sa nouvelle vie et arrêter de donner du fil à retordre au personnel. Le tour que prend notre conversation me laisse penser qu'elle n'est pas aussi perturbée qu'elle le prétend.

Elle ignore habilement mes sous-entendus et change de sujet.

— Je crois que je l'ai connue, votre grand-mère. On devait aller au même club de bridge, précise-t-elle avant de tendre vers moi le bout de son index courbé et noué. Vous lui ressemblez beaucoup.

— C'est ce qu'on dit. Oui. J'ai hérité de ses cheveux. Mes sœurs, non, mais moi, oui.

— Et de ses yeux.

La conversation prend une tournure intime. Elle me scrute, comme si elle voyait jusqu'à la moelle de mes os.

Qu'est-ce qui se passe ?

— Je... je lui parlerai de vous quand je la reverrai. Enfin, elle ne se souviendra peut-être pas de vous. Elle a des bons et des mauvais jours.

— Comme nous tous, non ?

Les commissures des lèvres de May se soulèvent un peu et je me surprends à rire nerveusement.

En changeant de position, je cogne la lampe de chevet avec mon coude, la rattrape et renverse cette fois-ci le cadre. Je le récupère de justesse et m'y cramponne en résistant à l'envie de le regarder de plus près.

— Elles le font toujours tomber. Les filles qui travaillent ici.

— Je pourrais le poser sur la commode.

— Non, je veux le garder près de moi.

— Oh... d'accord.

J'aimerais tellement prendre une nouvelle photo... À cet angle, il n'y a pas de reflet et le visage ressemble encore plus à celui de ma grand-mère. Est-ce que cela pourrait être elle, déguisée pour un spectacle, peut-être ? Je sais qu'elle était présidente du club de théâtre, au lycée.

— Je m'interrogeais justement à propos de cette photo, quand vous êtes entrée.

Maintenant que nous sommes en meilleurs termes, il ne semble plus déplacé de l'interroger.

— La femme sur cette photo me rappelle ma grand-mère, un peu.

Mon téléphone vibre – je l'ai mis en mode silencieux depuis la rencontre à l'hôtel de ville. Ça me rappelle qu'Ian m'attend depuis longtemps dans la voiture. Mais le message vient de ma mère, pas de lui. Elle veut que je la rappelle.

— Les mêmes cheveux, reconnaît May Crandall d'un ton neutre. Enfin, ce n'est pas si rare.

— Oui, j'imagine que vous avez raison.

Elle ne m'offre aucune information supplémentaire. À contre-cœur, je repose le cadre sur la table de nuit.

May fixe mon téléphone qui vibre de nouveau, encore un texto de ma mère exigeant une réponse. Je sais que je ferais mieux de ne pas l'ignorer.

— J'étais ravie de vous rencontrer, dis-je pour prendre congé.

— Vous devez partir tout de suite ?

— J'en ai bien peur. Mais je demanderai à ma grand-mère si votre nom lui dit quelque chose.

Elle s'humecte les lèvres et fait un petit bruit avec sa bouche.

— Vous reviendrez et, ce jour-là, je vous raconterai l'histoire de cette photo.

Elle pivote avec une agilité étonnante sans se servir de sa canne et se dirige vers la porte.

— Enfin, peut-être, ajoute-t-elle.

Elle est partie sans me laisser le temps de répondre. J'en profite pour prendre une meilleure photo du cliché encadré, puis je file à mon tour.

Dans le hall d'entrée, Ian fixe son téléphone. Apparemment, il en avait assez d'attendre dans la voiture.

— Désolée d'avoir été si longue, dis-je.

— Oh, c'est rien. Ça m'a donné l'occasion de faire du tri dans mes messages.

La directrice nous passe devant, sourcils froncés, en se demandant sans doute pourquoi je suis encore là. Si je n'étais pas une Stafford, elle viendrait à coup sûr m'interroger. Au lieu de quoi, elle tourne délibérément la tête et s'éloigne. Même au bout de deux mois passés en Caroline du Sud, je ne m'habitue pas à être traitée comme une rock star juste à cause de mon nom de famille. Dans le Maryland, il m'est arrivé de côtoyer des gens pendant des mois avant qu'ils se rendent compte que mon père est sénateur. J'ai apprécié cette opportunité de faire mes preuves par moi-même.

Ian et moi nous dirigeons vers la voiture. Comme nous nous retrouvons rapidement coincés dans un bouchon pour cause de travaux sur la voie, j'en profite pour appeler ma mère. Je sais que je ne pourrai pas l'interroger à la maison, avec sa réunion des FRA. Ensuite, elle sera trop occupée à s'assurer que toutes les assiettes en porcelaine et les verres à punch ont retrouvé leur place d'origine. C'est Pomme d'amour. Une maniaque du rangement.

Par ailleurs, elle n'oublie jamais un nom.

Après qu'elle m'a demandé de « passer en vitesse » à sa réunion des FRA pour serrer quelques mains et marquer quelques points auprès de « femmes de » importantes, je l'interroge :

— Est-ce qu'on connaît une certaine May Crandall ?

« Convainquez les femmes, et vous aurez les votes, disait toujours mon père. Il faut être idiot pour sous-estimer leur pouvoir. »

— Je ne crois pas... répond ma mère d'un ton songeur. Crandall... Crandall...

— May Crandall. Elle doit avoir l'âge de mamie Judy. Elles ont peut-être joué au bridge ensemble ?

— Oh, certainement pas. Mamie Judy ne jouait au bridge qu'avec ses amies.

Par « amies », elle entend de vieilles connaissances de la famille, dont les liens avec nous remontent à plusieurs générations, pour la plupart. Des gens de notre cercle social.

— Lois Heartstein, Dot Greeley, Mini Clarkson... Tu les connais déjà toutes.

— D'accord.

Après tout, May Crandall n'est peut-être qu'une vieille dame perturbée, la tête pleine de souvenirs confus qui n'ont qu'une vague ressemblance avec la réalité. Mais ça n'explique pas la photo sur la table de nuit.

— Pourquoi ?

— Oh, rien. Je l'ai rencontrée aujourd'hui à la maison de retraite.

— Comme c'est charmant. Tu as été bien gentille de discuter avec elle. Ces personnes peuvent vraiment souffrir de la solitude. Elle nous connaît sans doute de nom, Avery. Comme beaucoup.

Je grimace en espérant que Ian n'entend pas la fin de la phrase de ma mère. C'est très gênant.

La question de la photo continue à me titiller.

— Qui va voir mamie Judy, ce soir ?

— Je comptais y aller. Après la réunion des FRA, si ce n'est pas trop tard, soupira ma mère. Ton père ne pourra pas.

Pomme d'amour endosse fidèlement les responsabilités familiales lorsque le travail de mon père le retient.

— Et si tu restais à la maison pour te reposer, ce soir ? J'irai, moi.

— Mais tu viens d'abord à la réunion ? insiste ma mère. Bitsy est rentrée de son voyage au lac Tahoe. Elle meurt d'envie de te voir.

Tout à coup, j'éprouve la sensation horrible, désespérée, qu'un animal sauvage doit ressentir lorsque les portes d'une cage se referment sur lui. Pas étonnant que ma mère veuille tellement que je vienne à sa réunion. Bitsy est de retour. Connaissant les autres invitées, je peux compter sur un interrogatoire à feux croisés visant à savoir si Elliot et moi avons décidé de la date du mariage, choisi notre service et l'argenterie, discuté du lieu et de la saison – intérieur, extérieur, hiver, printemps.

Nous ne sommes pas pressés. Nous sommes tous les deux très occupés, ces derniers temps. Nous attendons juste le bon moment... Tout ça, ce n'est pas la réponse que Bitsy veut entendre. Une fois que les FRA et elle m'auront acculée dans un coin, elles ne me lâcheront pas avant de m'avoir extorqué les réponses qu'elles attendent.

Le cœur serré, je comprends alors que je n'aurai peut-être pas le temps de passer à Magnolia Manor ce soir pour interroger mamie Judy à propos de la photographie.

6

Rill

Dans mon rêve, nous sommes libres sur le fleuve. Le moteur de Ford T que Briny a installé à l'arrière du bateau nous entraîne facilement à contre-courant, à croire que nous ne pesons rien du tout. Queenie est assise sur le toit de la cabine, comme si elle chevauchait un éléphant. Sa tête est rejetée en arrière, ses longs cheveux cascadent de sous son chapeau à plume rouge. Elle chante une chanson qu'elle a apprise d'un vieil Irlandais croisé dans un campement de bateaux.

— Elle est belle comme une reine, pas vrai, ta maman ? demande Briny.

Le soleil chauffe, les bruants chanteurs gazouillent, les notes de basse jaillissent du fleuve. Une nuée de pélicans en forme de grosse flèche pointant au nord nous survole, ce qui veut dire que nous avons encore tout l'été devant nous. Il n'y a pas un seul bateau à aubes, pas une seule péniche, pas un seul remorqueur ni une barque à l'horizon. Le fleuve est à nous.

Juste à nous.

— Et, du coup, tu es quoi, toi ? me demande Briny dans mon rêve.

— La princesse Rill du royaume d'Arcadie ! crié-je.

Briny me coiffe d'une couronne de chèvrefeuille et répète mon titre, comme les rois dans les livres de contes.

Le matin, quand je me réveille, je sens encore un goût sucré sur ma langue. Il dure jusqu'à ce que j'ouvre les yeux et que je me demande pourquoi nous sommes tous les cinq dans le lit de Queenie et Briny, alignés sur le matelas comme les prises d'un pêcheur, tout glissants de sueur.

Queenie n'est pas là. J'ai à peine le temps de me formuler cette idée avant de comprendre ce qui m'a tirée de mon rêve.

Quelqu'un frappe à la porte.

Mon cœur fait un bond dans ma poitrine, je saute moi aussi pour descendre du lit et je passe un châle de Queenie autour de ma chemise de nuit. C'est Zede, de l'autre côté de la porte et, même à travers la vitre, je vois que son visage à barbe blanche est triste, long comme un jour sans pain. Mon estomac se noue.

Dehors, l'orage s'en est allé. Une belle journée s'annonce. L'air matinal est déjà chaud et humide mais, dès que j'ouvre la porte pour sortir, je sens le vent froid à travers la vieille chemise de nuit que Queenie a dû rallonger parce que j'avais tellement grandi... Elle disait qu'une jeune fille de mon âge ne devrait pas montrer autant ses jambes.

Je resserre un peu plus le châle sur ma poitrine, pas à cause de Zede, ni parce que j'ai des formes à cacher – Queenie dit que ça arrivera quand le temps sera venu, pas tout de suite –, mais parce qu'il y a un garçon dans le bateau à moteur de Zede. Il est maigre comme un clou et grand. Sa peau est sombre, comme celle d'un Cajun ou d'un Indien. Pas encore un homme, je pense, mais plus vieux que moi. Quinze ans et quelques. Zede a toujours quelqu'un sous son aile. C'est le grand-papy de tout le fleuve.

Le garçon se cache le visage sous une casquette de vendeur de journaux miteuse, les yeux baissés vers le fond du bateau, pas levés vers moi. Zede saute les présentations.

Je sais ce que ça signifie, même si j'aurais préféré l'ignorer.

La main de Zede est lourde sur mon épaule. Elle est censée me réconforter, pourtant je voudrais la fuir en courant, détaler quelque part sur la rive, mes pieds volant si vite qu'ils laisseraient à peine des traces dans le sable rejeté là par le courant.

J'ai la gorge si serrée... je ravale mes larmes. Le visage de Fern s'écrase contre la fenêtre, derrière moi. J'imagine qu'elle s'est réveillée et qu'elle m'a suivie. Elle ne me laisse jamais m'éloigner.

— Les bébés de Queenie n'ont pas survécu.

Zede n'est pas du genre à tourner autour du pot.

Quelque chose meurt en moi – un petit frère ou une petite sœur que je comptais bercer comme une poupée de porcelaine toute neuve.

— Ni l'un ni l'autre ?

— C'est ce qu'a dit le docteur. Qu'il a pas pu les sauver. Que ça n'aurait rien changé si Briny avait amené ta maman plus tôt à l'hôpital. Les bébés n'étaient pas faits pour être de ce monde, c'est tout.

Je secoue la tête très fort, à croire que j'essaie d'extirper ces mots de mes oreilles comme de l'eau après une baignade. Ça ne peut pas être vrai. Pas dans le royaume d'Arcadie. Le fleuve est notre magie. Briny nous a toujours promis qu'il prendrait soin de nous.

— Briny, qu'est-ce qu'il a dit ?

— Il est dévasté. Je l'ai laissé là-bas avec ta maman. Ils devaient signer des papiers à l'hôpital et je ne sais quoi. Ils ne lui avaient pas encore dit, pour les bébés. J'imagine que Briny le fera quand elle sera bien réveillée. Elle s'en remettra, a dit le toubib.

Mais je connais Queenie. Non, elle ne s'en remettra pas. Rien ne la rend plus heureuse qu'un tout nouveau bébé tout doux à cajoler.

Zede m'annonce qu'il ferait mieux de retourner à l'hôpital. Briny n'allait pas bien, ce matin.

— Je suis passé au campement, en bas, sur le fleuve, pour voir si y avait pas une femme qui pourrait s'occuper de vous, surtout des petits, mais y avait pas grand monde. Y a eu du grabuge avec la police et la plupart des gens sont partis sur le fleuve. J'ai amené Silas pour qu'il vous surveille le temps que je puisse ramener votre père à la maison.

Il pointe le garçon dans le bateau, qui lève la tête, surpris. Il ne savait pas que Zede comptait le laisser là, j'imagine.

— On n'a besoin de personne.

En fait, je veux juste que Queenie et Briny rentrent à la maison et nous emmènent sur le fleuve. Je le veux tellement, ça me transperce le nœud que j'ai dans le ventre.

— On a rien à lui faire à manger, déclare Camellia, à la porte, pour donner son avis.

— Eh, bien le bonjour à toi aussi, mam'zelle Rayon de soleil.

Zede l'appelle toujours comme ça, parce qu'elle en est l'exact opposé.

— J'allais pêcher des grenouilles, annonce-t-elle comme si on l'avait nommée capitaine de l'*Arcadie*.

— Hors de question, abois-je. On n'a pas le droit de quitter le bateau. Aucun de nous.

Zede pointe ma sœur du doigt.

— Vous tous, vous restez à l'intérieur.

Les yeux plissés, il tourne la tête vers le fleuve.

— Je sais pas ce qu'a fait fuir les gens du campement de Mud Island. Heureusement que vous êtes tous par ici, tout seuls, dans ce lagon. Ne faites pas de bruit. Et n'attirez pas l'attention sur vous, ni rien.

Un poids nouveau s'écrase sur ma poitrine. Très lourd. L'angoisse se pose en moi et s'y fait un nid. Je ne veux pas que Zede s'en aille.

Fern se glisse vers nous pour s'accrocher à ma jambe. Je la prends dans mes bras et cale ses folles boucles blondes sous mon menton. Ça me réconforte.

Quand Gabion sort à son tour, je le prends aussi et leur poids cloue mes pieds au sol. Le châle de Queenie, trop serré autour de mes épaules, m'entaille la peau.

Zede me confie de nouveau mon frère et mes sœurs puis fait monter Silas, le garçon, sur l'*Arcadie*. Une fois déplié, Silas est plus grand que je le pensais. Il est maigre comme un coucou mais il serait beau s'il n'avait pas la lèvre éclatée et un œil au beurre noir. S'il s'est fait prendre en embarquant en douce dans un train, comme l'a dit Zede, il a eu de la chance que les contrôleurs ne lui fassent rien de pire.

Il prend appui sur le bastingage et, d'un saut, s'y assied, comme s'il comptait rester là.

— Tu veilles sur eux, maintenant, lui ordonne Zede.

Silas hoche la tête, même si ça lui déplaît visiblement. Un épervier passe devant nous, à l'affût d'une proie, et Silas l'observe avant de braquer son regard vers Memphis.

Zede nous laisse de la nourriture – un sac de farine de maïs, une botte de carottes, dix œufs et du poisson salé.

Silas suit du regard Zede qui grimpe dans son bateau et disparaît.

— T'as faim ?

Silas se tourne vers moi et je me souviens à cet instant que je suis encore en chemise de nuit. Je sens l'air moite sur ma gorge, là où le col est tiré vers le bas à cause des enfants sur mes hanches.

Il se détourne, comme s'il l'avait remarqué.

— J'imagine, dit-il.

Ses yeux sont noirs comme minuit sur l'eau. Ils reflètent tout ce qu'il regarde – un héron pêchant tout près, les branches tombantes d'un arbre à moitié brisé, le ciel matinal avec ses nuages d'écume blanche... moi.

— Tu sais cuisiner ?

À son ton, je devine qu'il m'en croit déjà incapable.

Je relève le menton, redresse les épaules. Le châle de Queenie me scie un peu plus la peau. Je crois que je n'aime pas trop Silas.

— Oui. Je sais cuisiner.

— Pff ! crache Camellia.

— Toi, tais-toi, dis-je en posant les petits pour les pousser vers elle. Et surveille-les. Où est Lark ?

— Encore au lit.

— Surveille-la aussi.

Lark est capable de filer en douce sans que personne ne le remarque. Un jour, elle s'est égarée dans une petite clairière près d'une crique et s'y est endormie, et il nous a fallu une journée et la moitié d'une nuit avant qu'on la retrouve. Queenie était folle d'inquiétude.

— J'imagine que je dois te surveiller pour que tu mettes pas le feu à la cabine, grommelle Silas.

Ça y est, c'est décidé : je ne l'aime pas du tout, ce garçon.

Malgré tout, lorsque nous franchissons la porte, il me regarde et sa lèvre fendue se soulève d'un côté, et je me dis qu'il n'est peut-être pas si odieux que ça.

Nous allumons un feu dans le poêle et nous cuisinons du mieux possible. Lui et moi, nous n'y connaissons pas grand-chose. Le poêle, c'est le territoire de Queenie et je ne m'y suis jamais intéressée. Je préfère rester dehors, à regarder le fleuve et les animaux, à écouter Briny inventer des histoires de chevaliers, de châteaux d'Indiens venus de l'Ouest, d'endroits très lointains. Briny est allé dans le monde entier, j'ai l'impression.

Silas en a vu pas mal aussi. Pendant que nous préparons à manger et que nous nous mettons à table, il nous raconte ses histoires de passager clandestin dans les trains, sa traversée de cinq États en faisant du stop, grattant un peu de nourriture ici et là, dans les camps de travailleurs itinérants, vivant de la terre comme un Indien sauvage.

— Pourquoi t'as pas de maman ? demande Camellia en finissant la galette de maïs qui est à peine brûlée sur le bord.

Lark hoche la tête, elle aussi, elle veut savoir mais elle est trop timide pour demander.

Silas agite une fourchette classieuse en argent que Briny a trouvée dans le sable près de l'épave d'un vieux bateau à aubes.

— J'en avais une. Je l'aimais bien, jusqu'à mes neuf ans. Ensuite, je suis parti et je l'ai plus revue.

— Et pourquoi ? demandé-je en l'observant pour voir s'il nous taquine.

Queenie me manque déjà tellement que je ne m'imagine pas qu'on puisse rester loin de sa mère exprès.

— Elle s'est mariée à un gars qu'aimait boire du whisky et donner des baffes. J'ai supporté ça un an avant de comprendre que je serais mieux tout seul.

Son regard cesse un instant de pétiller et il ne reste plus que de l'obscurité dans ses yeux. Mais ça ne dure pas, il hausse les épaules, sourit, et ses petites fossettes reviennent creuser ses joues.

— Je suis parti avec une équipe de moissonneurs qui passaient par chez nous. J'ai été jusqu'au Canada, pour cueillir des pommes et faucher le blé. Après, je suis redescendu vers le sud en trouvant du travail en chemin.

— Et t'avais que dix ans ? s'étonne Camellia en faisant claquer ses lèvres pour lui faire comprendre qu'elle n'en croit pas un mot. T'as vraiment fait tout ça ? Mon œil !

Souple comme un chat, il se tourne sur sa chaise, relève le bas de sa chemise délavée et nous montre les cicatrices qui barrent son dos. Tous les cinq, nous nous écartons d'un bond de la table. Même Camellia ne trouve rien d'intelligent à répondre.

— Estimez-vous heureux d'avoir une maman et un papa gentils, reprend Silas en regardant durement ma sœur. Ne vous mettez jamais dans la tête de partir, s'ils sont bons envers vous. C'est pas le cas de tous les parents, je vous le dis.

Nous restons silencieux un instant et Lark a les larmes aux yeux. Silas sauce le jaune d'œuf dans son assiette et prend une gorgée d'eau. Il nous regarde par-dessus le bord de sa tasse en fer-blanc et fronce les sourcils comme s'il ne comprenait pas pourquoi nous faisons la tête.

— Dis-moi, Petit Bout, dit-il en pinçant doucement le nez de Lark, et ses cils battent comme les ailes d'un papillon, je t'ai déjà parlé de la nuit où j'ai rencontré Banjo Bill et Henry, son chien danseur ?

Aussitôt, il part dans une autre histoire, puis une autre encore. Le temps file pendant que nous terminons notre repas et que nous nettoyons la pièce.

— Tu cuisines pas si mal, déclare Silas en se léchant les babines après qu'on a fini de laver les assiettes dans le seau, sur le porche.

Là, on se rend compte que Fern a mis sa robe à l'envers, parce qu'elle s'est habillée toute seule, et Gabion court partout à moitié nu, à la recherche de quelqu'un pour le nettoyer car il est allé en douce dans les cabinets extérieurs à l'arrière du bateau. Heureusement qu'il n'est pas tombé dans le trou, jusqu'au fleuve. Il n'y a pas de fond aux toilettes d'un bateau-maison comme le nôtre, juste de l'eau.

Je dis à Camellia de l'emmener sur le porche et de lui tremper les fesses dans l'eau avant de le sécher. Ce sera le plus simple.

Les narines de Camellia se dilatent. La seule chose qui lui fait peur, dans la vie, c'est le caca. Et c'est précisément pour ça que je la force à nettoyer Gabby. Elle le mérite. Elle n'a pas levé le petit doigt pour nous aider pendant toute la matinée.

— Mellia ! Mellia ! piaille notre frère tandis que ses petites jambes dodues l'emmènent d'un pas chancelant vers la porte, les fesses à l'air. Gabby cracra !

Ma sœur me fait une grimace, ouvre la porte à la volée et traîne Gabion dehors en le tirant par le bras au point qu'il avance sur la pointe de ses petits orteils.

— Je vais le faire, murmure Lark pour mettre fin à la dispute.

— Tu laisses Camellia s'en occuper. Tu es trop petite.

Silas et moi échangeons un regard et il esquisse un sourire.

— Tu vas pas t'habiller de la journée ?

Je baisse les yeux et je me rends compte que je ne me suis toujours pas changée, que je n'y ai même pas pensé, tellement j'étais captivée par les histoires de Silas.

— Je ferais mieux de m'y mettre, dis-je en riant de moi-même avant de décrocher ma robe du portemanteau. Mais tu dois sortir. Et essaie pas de m'espionner.

J'avais une drôle d'idée en tête pendant que Silas et moi on préparait à manger et on s'occupait des petits. Je m'imaginais qu'on était le papa et la maman, que ça, c'était notre maison. Ça m'aidait à ne pas penser à Queenie et Briny, qui n'étaient toujours pas là.

Mais hors de question que je me déshabille devant lui, ni devant quiconque. J'ai grandi tellement cette année que je m'habille derrière le rideau, comme Queenie. Je ne laisserais personne me voir toute nue, comme je ne laisserais personne me fouetter le dos jusqu'à y laisser des cicatrices.

— Tu parles, lâche Silas, les yeux au ciel. Pourquoi je t'espionnerais ? Tu n'es qu'une gamine.

Je me sens bouillir de la tête aux pieds et j'ai les joues en feu. Dehors, Camellia s'esclaffe.

Je rougis encore plus. Si je le pouvais, je les ferais tomber tous les deux à l'eau, Silas et elle. À défaut, je lance :

— Et emmène les petits. Une femme a besoin d'intimité.

— Qu'est-ce que t'en sais ? T'es pas une femme. T'es rien qu'une petite poupée avec des bouclettes, me taquine Silas, ce que je ne trouve pas drôle, surtout quand Camellia peut l'entendre.

Fern, Lark et elle se sont mis en rang sur le pont pour profiter du spectacle.

Tous mes muscles se crispent. Je ne me mets pas facilement en colère mais, quand je m'y mets, c'est comme un brasier en moi.

— Eh bien, toi, tu n'es qu'un... qu'une brindille ! Une brindille sur pattes, voilà ! T'es tellement maigre que tu risques de t'envoler au moindre coup de vent !

Je lève la tête vers lui, le menton en avant, les poings sur les hanches.

— Au moins, moi, mes cheveux ressemblent pas à une serpillière.

Il prend son chapeau sur le crochet et sort d'un pas lourd. Il doit être sur la passerelle lorsqu'il lance :

— Tu ferais bien de rentrer dans un cirque. Tu y serais à ta place. Tu pourrais faire le clown !

Je me regarde dans le miroir mural et je vois des boucles blondes dans tous les sens, et un visage rouge comme la tête d'un pic-vert. Avant même de me rendre compte de mon allure, je me précipite à la porte et je hurle :

— C'est ça, va-t'en, Silas... Silas... je sais même pas ton nom de famille, si seulement t'en as un. On n'a pas besoin de toi de toute façon et...

Sur la rive, il s'accroupit soudain et agite la main vers moi. Sous le chapeau, je ne vois pas son visage mais il est évident qu'il y a un problème. Il a vu quelque chose dans les bois.

Je n'ai soudain plus chaud du tout.

— C'est ça, dégage ! renchérit Camellia en se mêlant à la dispute. Et remets pas les pieds sur notre bateau, brindille à pattes !

Silas nous jette un coup d'œil en agitant encore la main. Il se glisse dans les sous-bois et les branches se referment sur lui.

— T'es même pas caché ! Je te vois encore !

— Chut, Camellia !

J'ouvre la porte à la volée et je pousse Fern et Lark à l'intérieur.

Camellia me dévisage, sourcils froncés. Elle est penchée par-dessus la rambarde, où elle tient Gabion par les bras. Ses fesses trempent dans l'eau pendant qu'il donne des coups de pied en gloussant. Camellia fait semblant de le lâcher puis le rattrape, et il pousse un cri avant que je les rejoigne.

— Rentrez tout de suite.

Je me penche pour attraper mon frère par le bras mais Camellia me donne une tape sur la main et laisse Gabby pendre par un seul bras.

— Il s'amuse et il fait chaud à l'intérieur.

Son épaisse chevelure brune tombe en avant et ses pointes qui trempent dans l'eau dessinent des arabesques d'encre.

— Tu veux aller nager ? demande-t-elle à Gabby, et, l'espace d'un instant, je crois qu'elle va le rejoindre dans l'eau.

Sur la rive, Silas sort la tête des buissons, un doigt sur la bouche, pour tenter de nous faire taire.

— Quelque chose ne va pas, dis-je en attrapant Gabion par la main, si brusquement que le bras de ma sœur suit le mouvement.

— Aïe ! fait-elle quand son coude se cogne dans la rambarde.

Plus loin sur la berge, les feuilles frémissent et je vois une tache noire – le chapeau d'un homme, peut-être.

— Rentrez vite ! Il y a quelqu'un, là-bas !

— Tu dis ça juste parce que tu veux que le garçon revienne, renifle Camellia, qui ne peut pas voir Silas alors qu'il doit être à trente centimètres de l'endroit où une branche craque soudain en poussant une corneille à s'envoler.

— Là. Tu vois ?

Elle voit la tache noire. Quelqu'un arrive, c'est sûr mais, au lieu de rentrer dans la cabine, Camellia contourne le bateau.

— Je vais descendre par l'arrière pour voir qui c'est.

— Non !

Je m'énerve mais, en vérité, je ne sais pas quoi faire.

J'ai envie de larguer les amarres et pousser l'*Arcadie* hors du banc de sable pour partir sur le fleuve. Comme l'eau est calme, ce matin, nous n'aurions pas de mal à mettre le bateau à flot, sauf que je n'oserai jamais. Avec juste Camellia, moi et peut-être Silas pour empêcher l'*Arcadie* de percuter un banc de sable ou de se faire pulvériser par une barge ou un bateau à aubes, on ne sait pas ce qui pourrait nous arriver sur le fleuve.

— Rentrons, dis-je. Il croira peut-être que le bateau est vide et passera son chemin.

Mais qui viendrait là par hasard, dans ce petit lagon isolé de tout ?

— C'est peut-être juste quelqu'un qui chasse les écureuils, suggère Camellia, pleine d'espoir. Si ça se trouve, il nous en donnera pour le dîner si on demande gentiment.

Elle sait se montrer polie quand elle veut, quand quelqu'un a des friandises à distribuer ou des beignets à partager autour d'un feu de camp.

— Zede nous a dit de rester discrets. Et Briny nous flanquerait une sacrée raclée s'il le découvrait.

Briny n'a jamais levé la main sur nous mais il nous menace parfois de le faire. Cette idée inquiète suffisamment Camellia pour qu'elle traverse le pont en vitesse avec moi jusqu'à la cabine.

Nous barrons la porte, nous grimpons dans le grand lit, nous tirons le rideau et nous tendons l'oreille. Il me semble entendre les pas d'un homme sur le rivage. Et puis j'ai l'impression qu'il est parti. Ce n'était peut-être qu'un chasseur ou un vagabond...

— Ohé, du bateau !

— Chut !

Ma voix tremblote. Des yeux écarquillés, inquiets, se tournent vers moi. Quand on grandit sur le fleuve, on sait qu'on doit se méfier des inconnus. Parfois, le fleuve, c'est là où vont des hommes qui fuient le mal qu'ils ont fait ailleurs.

Camellia se penche vers moi.

— C'est pas Zede.

Son souffle effleure le duvet de ma nuque.

Le bateau tangue un peu. Quelqu'un pose un pied sur la passerelle.

Lark se blottit contre moi et Fern grimpe sur mes genoux, sa joue tout contre mon cœur.

L'*Arcadie* glisse vers le rivage, déséquilibré par le poids entier de l'homme. Il est costaud. Qui qu'il soit, Silas n'est pas de taille.

Je plaque un doigt sur mes lèvres. Nous nous figeons tous les cinq comme des faons quand la biche s'en va chercher à manger.

L'homme est sur le pont, maintenant.

— Ohé, du bateau ! crie-t-il encore.

Allez-vous-en... Il n'y a personne.

Il essaie d'ouvrir la porte, la poignée tourne doucement.

— Y a quelqu'un là-dedans ?

La porte heurte la barre et ne va pas plus loin.

Une ombre plane devant le carré de lumière que la fenêtre projette sur le plancher. La tête d'un homme, le contour d'un chapeau. Il a un bâton ou une batte dans la main. Il s'en sert pour taper contre la vitre.

Un policier ? J'en ai bien peur. Les policiers font des descentes dans les campements de bateaux quand l'envie leur prend. Ils cassent tout, maltraitent les gens du fleuve, prennent ce qu'ils veulent et nous chassent de là. C'est une des raisons pour lesquelles on amarre toujours notre bateau dans notre coin, sauf si Briny, exceptionnellement, a besoin d'un coup de main.

— Je peux vous aider, m'sieur l'agent ?

La voix de Silas arrête l'inconnu qui se dirigeait vers l'autre fenêtre pour voir à l'intérieur. Leurs ombres s'étirent longuement sur le sol, l'une dépassant l'autre d'une tête.

— Tu vis là, fiston ?

— Nan. J'suis juste venu chasser. Mon père est par là-bas.

— Y a des enfants qui vivent ici ?

La voix n'est pas haineuse, mais elle est intéressée. Et si Silas se faisait arrêter pour avoir menti ?

— J'en sais rien du tout. Je viens juste d'arriver là.

— Ah ouais ? Je crois que tu me racontes des salades, espèce de chie dans l'eau. Je t'ai entendu parler à quelqu'un, sur ce bateau.

— Non, m'sieur, répond Silas, sans se démonter. J'ai vu des gens partir dans une barque… oh… y a bien deux heures. C'est quelqu'un du camp que vous avez dû entendre. Les voix portent loin, sur le fleuve.

L'homme s'approche brusquement de Silas.

— T'avise pas de me donner de leçon sur le fleuve, fiston. C'est mon fleuve, et j'ai passé la moitié de la matinée à chercher ces gamins. Tu les fais sortir, pour que je puisse les emmener en ville voir leur maman et leur papa.

Comme Silas ne répond pas, le policier se penche vers lui, leurs ombres se joignent au niveau du visage.

— Fiston, ça me ferait vraiment de la peine que t'aies des problèmes avec la justice. Et comment que t'as récolté cet œil au beurre noir, d'abord ? T'as fourré le nez dans quelque chose que t'aurais pas dû ? T'as des parents pour s'occuper de toi ou t'es un vagabond ?

— Mon oncle Zede. C'est lui qui s'occupe de moi.

— Je croyais que tu chassais là avec ton paternel ?

— Oui, lui aussi.

— Si tu mens à un policier, tu vas te retrouver en cabane, raclure de fleuve.

— Je mens pas.

J'entends d'autres voix tout près, maintenant. Des hommes qui crient dans les fourrés et un chien qui aboie.

— Dis aux gamins de sortir. Leurs parents nous ont envoyés les chercher.

— Et comment il s'appelle, leur père ?

Camellia et moi, nous échangeons un coup d'œil. Ses yeux sont grands comme des soucoupes. Elle secoue la tête. Elle pense comme moi. Briny n'enverrait jamais la police ici et, si jamais il l'avait fait, cet homme aurait su dès le début où trouver le bateau.

Qu'est-ce qu'il peut bien nous vouloir ?

Nous regardons par le trou dans le rideau la grande ombre soulever la petite par le col de chemise. Silas tousse et suffoque.

— Ne joue pas au plus malin avec moi, fiston. Je suis pas venu pour toi mais, si tu me causes encore du souci, on va t'emmener aussi. Tu verras où finissent les gosses des rues maigrelets comme toi, dans cette ville.

J'ai sauté du lit avant que Camellia ait le temps de m'en empêcher.

— Non, Rill, non !

Elle m'attrape par la chemise de nuit, le tissu lui glisse entre les doigts.

Quand j'ouvre la porte, la première chose que je vois, ce sont les pieds de Silas qui pendouillent à quinze centimètres du sol. Son visage est violet. Quand il essaie de donner un coup de poing, l'agent se contente de rigoler.

— Tu veux te battre contre moi, gamin ? Et si on te mettait la tête sous l'eau une minute ou deux, pour te refroidir ?

— Non ! Arrêtez ! crié-je alors que d'autres hommes arrivent.

Il y en a sur le rivage et, à tribord, un bateau à moteur approche en grondant. Je ne sais pas ce que nous avons fait de mal – à part être des vagabonds du fleuve – mais nous sommes faits comme des rats. Cela n'arrangerait rien si Silas était tué ou embarqué avec nous.

L'agent le relâche aussitôt et Silas se cogne la tête contre la paroi de la cabine.

— Va-t'en, Silas, dis-je d'une voix si tremblante que les mots sont à peine audibles. Rentre chez toi maintenant. Tu n'es même pas censé être là. Nous voulons aller voir nos parents.

Je me dis que ça ira mieux si nous coopérons. Toute seule, j'aurais pu sauter du pont sur la rive et m'enfuir dans les bois avant que les hommes aient le temps de m'attraper, mais avec mes petites sœurs et Gabion, c'est impossible. Si je sais une chose de Briny, c'est qu'il voudrait qu'on reste ensemble, quoi qu'il arrive.

Je me redresse pour regarder l'agent de police et j'essaie de toutes mes forces d'avoir l'air d'une adulte.

Il sourit.

— Voilà une bonne fille.

— Mon père va bien ?

— Bien sûr.

— Et ma mère ?

— On ne peut mieux. Elle a demandé à ce que vous alliez la voir.

Je n'ai pas besoin de scruter son regard pour savoir qu'il ment. Impossible que Queenie aille « on ne peut mieux », en ce moment. Où qu'elle soit, elle a le cœur brisé, pour les bébés.

Je ravale la boule qui me noue la gorge et la sens descendre en moi, aussi acérée qu'un éclat de glace tout juste taillé hors du bloc.

— Je vais chercher les autres enfants.

L'agent s'approche, m'attrape le bras comme pour me retenir.

— T'es une jolie ratounette, toi, non ?

Sa langue glisse sur ses dents et, pour la première fois, il est assez près pour que je voie son visage sous le bord de son chapeau brillant. Ses yeux sont gris et méchants, mais pas froids comme je m'y attendais. Ils sont intéressés, même si je ne sais pas pourquoi. Son regard glisse sur ma figure, mon cou, jusqu'à l'épaule qui dépasse de la chemise de nuit à ce moment-là.

— Quelqu'un devrait te remplumer un peu.

Derrière lui, Silas se relève tant bien que mal, cligne des yeux, chancelle. Il pose une main sur la hache posée près du tas de bois.

« Non », j'essaie de lui dire mentalement. N'entend-il pas les hommes sur le rivage et le bateau à moteur qui se rapproche ?

De la cabine me parvient un petit couinement, juste assez sonore pour que je le reconnaisse. La porte des cabinets extérieurs. Camellia essaie de s'enfuir par l'arrière.

Fais quelque chose.

— M-mon petit frère vient d'aller sur le pot. Je dois le nettoyer avant qu'on s'en aille, sinon il y aura du caca partout. À moins que v-vous vouliez le faire.

C'est ma seule idée. Les hommes n'aiment pas les bébés sales. Briny refuse de les toucher, à part pour les plonger dans le fleuve si Queenie, Camellia ou moi ne sommes pas là pour le faire.

L'agent fronce le nez, me lâche et tourne la tête vers les bruits qui viennent de derrière lui. Silas ôte sa main en vitesse de la hache et se relève, les poings serrés au bout de ses bras tout maigres.

— Vous feriez mieux de vous dépêcher, répond le policier dans un sourire tout sauf amical. Votre maman attend.

— Tu peux t'en aller, Silas. Allez.

Je m'arrête sur le seuil pour le foudroyer du regard en pensant : Va-t'en. Cours !

Les yeux du policier glissent de moi à Silas. Il tend la main vers sa ceinture, son pistolet, sa matraque, ses menottes de métal noires. Que compte-t-il faire ?

— Allez, va-t'en ! hurlé-je en poussant Silas. Briny et Zede ne voudraient pas que tu restes ici !

Nos regards se croisent. Il secoue un peu la tête, je hoche la mienne. Il ferme tout doucement les yeux avant de les rouvrir, de pivoter et de dévaler la passerelle.

— Il y en a une dans l'eau ! hurle un autre policier sur la berge.

Les hommes dans le bateau beuglent et le moteur gronde.

Camellia ! Je me tourne brusquement pour courir dans la cabine mais les pas lourds du policier me suivent. Il m'écarte et je percute le poêle pendant qu'il se précipite à l'arrière où la porte est grande ouverte. Fern, Lark et Gabion sont blottis contre la rambarde. L'homme les pousse à l'intérieur, brutalement, et ils tombent les uns sur les autres en criant et en pleurant.

— Mellia ! Mellia ! gémit Gabion, le doigt pointé vers les cabinets extérieurs, où notre sœur a réussi à se glisser par le trou des toilettes jusqu'au fleuve.

Elle sort péniblement de l'eau pour gagner le rivage, sa chemise de nuit trempée collée à ses longues jambes bronzées. Un policier lui court après pendant que le bateau les suit de loin.

Elle escalade un tas de bois flotté, aussi rapide et agile qu'une biche.

Gabion pousse un cri suraigu.

Le policier à l'arrière du bateau tire son pistolet de son holster.

— Non !

J'essaie de me précipiter vers lui mais Fern s'est accrochée à mes jambes. Nous tombons toutes les deux sur le sol, fauchant Lark au passage. Elle hurle et, la dernière chose que je vois avant qu'une caisse en bois me cache la vue, c'est le policier sur la rive qui saute par-dessus une branche, tend le bras et attrape Camellia par ses longs cheveux bruns.

Quand je me relève, elle est en train de se débattre comme une folle, donnant des coups de pied en hurlant et en grognant. Ses bras et ses jambes s'agitent dans tous les sens lorsque le policier l'écarte de lui.

Les hommes dans le bateau renversent la tête en arrière et éclatent de rire comme des ivrognes devant une bagarre de salle de billard.

Ils doivent se mettre à trois pour faire monter ma sœur dans le bateau et à deux pour la maîtriser à bord. Lorsqu'ils s'arrêtent près de l'*Arcadie,* ils l'ont carrément clouée au sol. Ils sont pleins de boue et furieux parce qu'elle sent comme le fond des cabinets et qu'elle a collé sa puanteur sur tout le monde.

L'agent sur l'*Arcadie* se plante sur le seuil, les bras croisés, l'épaule contre le chambranle de la porte comme s'il était installé confortablement.

— Vous allez vous changer gentiment, maintenant... dehors, là où je peux vous voir. On n'a pas envie qu'un autre d'entre vous se fasse la malle.

Hors de question que je m'habille devant lui. Du coup, je m'occupe d'abord de Gabion, Lark et Fern. Ensuite, je me contente d'enfiler ma robe par-dessus ma chemise de nuit, même s'il fait bien trop chaud pour que ce soit supportable.

L'agent de police s'esclaffe.

— Très bien, si c'est ce que tu veux. Maintenant, soyez bien gentils et bien calmes, et nous vous emmènerons voir votre papa et votre maman.

Je fais ce qu'il dit, je le suis hors de la cabine en refermant la porte derrière nous. Je ne peux plus avaler ma salive, ni respirer ni même penser.

— Heureusement que les quatre autres n'étaient pas aussi difficiles, déclare un agent qui tient Camellia contre le fond du bateau à moteur, les bras croisés dans son dos. Celle-là est une vraie tigresse.

— Je dirais plutôt un sanglier, vu l'odeur, plaisante l'autre policier présent dans le bateau.

Il nous aide à monter à bord, soulève Gabion, puis Fern et Lark en leur disant de s'asseoir par terre. Camellia me foudroie du regard quand je les imite.

Elle pense que tout est ma faute, que j'aurais dû résister, empêcher tout ça.

Elle a peut-être raison.

— Elle va les adorer, ceux-là, beugle l'un d'eux alors que le moteur vrombit et nous éloigne de l'*Arcadie*.

Il pose sa grosse main sur les cheveux de Lark, qui baisse aussitôt la tête pour venir à quatre pattes se blottir contre moi. Fern l'imite. Seul Gabion ne se rend pas compte et n'a pas peur.

— Elle aime les blondinets, pas vrai ? s'esclaffe celui qui était monté à bord de l'*Arcadie*. Par contre, je ne sais pas ce qu'elle va faire de cette petite mouffette.

Du menton, il désigne Camellia. Elle renifle grassement et lui crache dessus. Il lève la main, comme pour la gifler, puis éclate de rire et se contente d'essuyer le crachat sur son pantalon.

— À l'entrepôt Dawson, encore ? demande celui qui est à la barre.

— C'est ce que j'ai entendu.

Je ne sais pas combien de temps nous restons sur l'eau. Nous traversons le fleuve, puis nous empruntons le canal où la rivière Wolf se jette dans le Mississippi. Quand nous contournons Mud Island, Memphis nous apparaît entièrement. Les grands bâtiments se dressent vers le ciel comme des monstres attendant de nous avaler tout rond. J'envisage de me jeter à l'eau. D'essayer de m'enfuir. De me battre. Je regarde les bateaux qui passent devant nous – des remorqueurs, des bateaux à aubes, des bateaux de pêche et des barges. Même un bateau-maison. Je pense à crier en agitant les bras pour appeler au secours.

Mais qui nous aiderait ?

Nous sommes avec la police.

Est-ce qu'ils nous emmènent en prison ?

Une main se pose sur mon épaule, comme si quelqu'un avait lu dans mes pensées. Elle reste là jusqu'à ce que nous accostions. En haut de la colline, je vois encore des immeubles.

— Maintenant, tu vas être bien sage et tu vas empêcher ton frère et tes sœurs de s'attirer des ennuis, me murmure celui qui était monté à bord de l'*Arcadie*.

Puis il dit aux autres de tenir la tigresse encore un peu, le temps qu'elle nous voie tous les quatre.

Nous avançons sur le caillebotis à la queue leu leu, moi avec Gabion sur la hanche. Le martèlement des machines et la puanteur du goudron chaud m'agressent et je perds l'odeur du fleuve. Nous traversons une rue, où j'entends une femme chanter, un homme hurler, un marteau frapper du métal. Des brins de coton échappés des balles flottent dans l'air comme des flocons de neige.

Dans un buisson rabougri au bord d'un parking, un cardinal rouge pousse sa chanson claire : Fuis, fuis, fuis.

Il y a une voiture, tout près. Une grosse voiture. Un homme en uniforme en descend, contourne l'automobile pour aller ouvrir la portière arrière afin qu'une femme puisse s'extraire de la banquette. Elle nous regarde de haut, les yeux plissés à cause du soleil. Elle n'est ni jeune ni vieille, entre les deux. Elle est lourde et corpulente, et ses bourrelets pointent sous sa robe fleurie marron. Ses cheveux, mi-gris mi-châtains, sont coupés court.

Son visage me rappelle un héron. Elle nous observe pendant que les policiers nous mettent en rang. Son regard glisse sur nous, rapide et saccadé, pour évaluer la situation.

— Ils devraient être cinq, dit-elle.

— L'autre arrive, mademoiselle Tann, répond l'agent. Elle a fait un peu plus de difficultés. En tentant de s'échapper par le fleuve.

Elle fait claquer sa langue trois fois contre ses dents, tuit, tuit, tuit.

— Toi, tu ne ferais pas une chose pareille, n'est-ce pas ? demande-t-elle.

Elle prend le menton de Fern dans sa main et se penche tant qu'elles sont presque nez à nez.

— Tu ne ferais pas la vilaine fille, n'est-ce pas ?

Les yeux bleus de Fern s'écarquillent, elle secoue la tête.

— Quel joli lot, ces petites trouvailles, dit la femme – Mlle Tann. Cinq précieux enfants aux boucles blondes. C'est parfait.

Elle tape des mains et les replie sous son menton. Les coins de ses yeux se plissent et sa bouche se pince, en une ligne si fine qu'elle a beau sourire, ses lèvres ont disparu.

— Juste quatre, rectifie l'agent.

D'un signe de tête, il lui montre Camellia, qui arrive du fleuve escortée par un policier qui la tient par la peau du cou. Je ne sais pas ce qu'ils lui ont dit, mais elle ne se débat plus.

Mlle Tann fronce les sourcils.

— Eh bien... celle-ci n'a pas hérité des beaux traits de sa famille, n'est-ce pas ? Elle est plutôt banale. J'imagine qu'on trouvera tout de même preneur pour elle. Nous y parvenons presque toujours.

Elle recule soudain d'un pas, la main plaquée sur le nez.

— Dieu du ciel ! Quelle est donc cette pestilence ?

Mlle Tann n'a pas l'air contente lorsqu'elle voit dans quel état est ma sœur. Elle ordonne aux officiers d'installer Camellia sur le plancher de la voiture et nous autres sur la banquette. Il y a déjà deux autres enfants par terre – une fillette blonde de l'âge de Lark et un garçon un peu plus grand que Gabion. Ils me regardent tous deux avec leurs grands yeux bruns épouvantés. Ils ne disent pas un mot, ne bougent pas d'un poil.

Mlle Tann essaie de me prendre Gabion des bras avant que je monte en voiture. Elle fronce les sourcils lorsque je me cramponne à lui.

— Un peu de tenue ! crache-t-elle, et je lâche.

Une fois que nous sommes tous en voiture, elle tient Gabion sur ses genoux, le met debout pour qu'il puisse voir par la vitre. Il sautille, montre du doigt et babille, tout excité. Il n'était jamais monté dans une auto.

— Eh bien, regardez-moi ces bouclettes !

Elle fait glisser ses doigts sur la tête de mon petit frère pour relever ses cheveux blonds comme les blés, si bien qu'ils moutonnent comme ceux des petits baigneurs qu'on reçoit en lot à la foire.

Gabion pointe le doigt vers la vitre, ravie.

— Dada ! Dada !

Il a remarqué une petite fille qui est en train de se faire photographier, assise sur un poney pie noir et blanc, devant une grande maison.

— Il va falloir qu'on te lave pour te débarrasser de la puanteur du fleuve, n'est-ce pas ? Ensuite, tu seras un petit garçon adorable.

Mlle Tann fronce le nez. Je me demande ce qu'elle veut dire par là. Qui va nous laver et pourquoi ?

L'hôpital ne nous laissera peut-être pas entrer dans cet état. Nous devons peut-être d'abord nous laver... pour voir Queenie ?

— Il s'appelle Gabion, dis-je pour qu'elle sache comment l'appeler. Gabby, pour faire plus court.

Sa tête pivote aussitôt vers moi, comme celle d'un chat qui a vu une souris dans le garde-manger. Elle me fixe comme si elle avait oublié que j'étais dans la voiture.

— Retiens-toi de parler, à moins qu'on t'interroge.

Son bras s'élance comme un serpent, pâle et dodu, s'enroule autour de Lark pour l'écarter de moi.

Je baisse les yeux vers les deux enfants épouvantés blottis l'un contre l'autre sur le plancher, puis vers Camellia. Le regard de ma sœur me dit qu'elle a compris ce que je sais déjà, même si je ne veux pas y croire.

Nous ne nous dirigeons pas vers l'hôpital pour voir nos parents.

7

Avery

La maison de retraite baigne dans la douce lumière du soleil matinal. Même si un parking tout neuf remplace la vaste pelouse d'antan, Magnolia Manor évoque une époque révolue – des réunions d'après-midi raffinées autour d'une tasse de thé, des bals des débutantes chatoyants et des dîners formels autour de la longue table en acajou qui trône toujours dans la salle à manger. On s'imagine facilement Scarlett O'Hara s'éventant sous les chênes drapés de mousse qui ombragent la galerie et ses colonnes blanches.

Je me souviens de la vie antérieure de cet endroit, ne serait-ce qu'un petit peu. Ma mère m'y avait emmenée pour une *baby shower* lorsque j'avais neuf ou dix ans. En cours de route, elle m'avait raconté qu'elle y avait assisté à un cocktail très important pour son cousin, qui se présentait au poste de gouverneur de la Caroline du Sud. Étudiante, à l'époque, la politique était bien la dernière chose qui l'intéressait. Elle n'était arrivée que depuis trente minutes à Magnolia Manor lorsqu'elle avait remarqué mon père à l'autre bout de la pièce. Elle s'était ensuite arrangée pour découvrir qui il était. En apprenant qu'il était un membre de la famille Stafford, elle avait mis le cap sur lui.

Vous connaissez la suite. Un mariage entre deux dynasties politiques. Le grand-père de ma mère avait été député de la Caroline du Nord avant de prendre sa retraite, et son père occupait le poste au moment du mariage.

Cette histoire me fait sourire tandis que je grimpe les marches de marbre et que je tape le code sur le clavier étrangement moderne fiché dans le mur à côté de la porte. Des gens importants vivent encore ici. Tout le monde n'a pas le droit d'entrer. Tristement, tout le monde n'a pas le droit de sortir non plus. Derrière le manoir, le vaste domaine a été précautionneusement entouré de grilles de fer forgé décoratives, trop hautes pour être enjambées. Le portail est fermé à clef. Le lac et les fontaines peuvent être admirés, mais pas approchés... impossible d'y tomber.

La plupart des résidents doivent être protégés d'eux-mêmes. C'est la triste vérité. Au fur à mesure qu'ils déclinent, ils sont déplacés d'une aile à l'autre, montant progressivement vers de plus hauts niveaux de soins, qu'on leur prodigue avec douceur. On ne peut nier que Magnolia Manor est un établissement plus haut de gamme que celui où vit May Crandall, mais ils doivent tous les deux relever le même défi : apporter dignité, soins et confort lorsque la vie prend une tournure difficile.

Je me faufile jusqu'à l'unité de soins de la mémoire – ici, personne ne penserait à l'appeler grossièrement l'unité Alzheimer. Je passe par une autre porte verrouillée pour entrer dans un salon, où la télévision passe une rediffusion de *Police des plaines* à plein volume.

Une femme assise près de la fenêtre me lance un regard vide. Derrière la vitre, j'aperçois les fleurs fuchsia couvertes de rosée du rosier grimpant, fraîches et pleines de vie.

Celles qui montent devant la fenêtre de mamie Judy arborent un jaune joyeux. Lorsque j'entre dans sa chambre, elle s'est assise dans son fauteuil à oreilles pour les admirer. Je m'arrête sur le seuil pour me blinder avant de lui signaler ma présence.

Je me prépare à la voir m'adresser le même regard vide que la femme dans le salon – sans le moindre signe de reconnaissance.

J'espère que ce ne sera pas le cas. C'est imprévisible.

— Bonjour, mamie Judy !

J'ai parlé fort et d'un ton gai. Pourtant, mes paroles mettent un moment à provoquer une réaction.

Elle se tourne lentement, feuillette les pages éparpillées de son esprit puis me répond tout aussi gentiment qu'à l'habitude :

— Bonjour, ma chérie. Comment vas-tu, par ce bel après-midi ?

En fait, c'est le matin. Comme prévu, la réunion des FRA s'est terminée tard la veille au soir et, malgré tous mes efforts, je n'ai pas pu échapper à l'interrogatoire concernant le mariage. J'étais comme une sauterelle sans défense qu'on aurait lâchée dans un poulailler. Maintenant, j'ai la tête fourrée de suggestions, de dates que je ne devrais pas choisir car quelqu'un d'important ne sera pas en ville, et de propositions de prêt d'assiettes de porcelaine, d'argenterie, de verres en cristal et de linge de table.

— Je vais très bien, merci.

Je traverse la pièce pour aller la serrer dans mes bras, espérant que cet instant intime ravivera ses souvenirs.

Pendant une fraction de seconde, j'y crois. Elle me regarde profondément dans les yeux, soupire puis me dit :

— Tu es vraiment jolie. Quels beaux cheveux tu as !

Elle effleure mes boucles en souriant.

La tristesse me gonfle le cœur. Je suis venue dans l'espoir d'obtenir des réponses à propos de May Crandall et de la vieille photographie sur sa table de nuit. Cela semble mal parti.

— « Il était une fois, une petite fille avec une boucle sur le front », récite ma grand-mère en me souriant.

Des doigts froids, à la peau fine comme du papier à cigarette, me caressent la joue.

— « Et quand elle était gentille, elle était vraiment adorable », poursuis-je.

Mamie m'accueillait toujours avec ce poème lorsque j'allais lui rendre visite dans sa maison de Lagniappe Street, quand j'étais enfant.

— « Mais quand elle était méchante, elle était exécrable », conclut-elle.

Elle me fait un grand sourire et m'envoie un clin d'œil, et nous rions ensemble. Comme au bon vieux temps.

Je m'assieds dans le fauteuil de l'autre côté de la petite table ronde.

— J'ai toujours aimé que tu me taquines avec cette comptine.

Dans la maison de Pomme d'amour, on n'attendait surtout pas des petites filles qu'elles soient méchantes ou exécrables, mais mamie Judy a toujours été connue pour son culot, qui confinait parfois à l'inconvenance. Elle avait pris position sur des sujets tels que les droits civiques et l'éducation des femmes bien avant que cela soit acceptable pour une femme d'avoir des opinions.

Elle me demande si j'ai vu Welly-Boy, le surnom qu'elle donne à mon père, Wells.

Je lui raconte la visite médiatique du matin à la maison de retraite puis la rencontre à l'hôtel de ville et enfin la très, très, très longue réunion des FRA à Drayden Hill. Je lui épargne le bavardage autour du mariage, bien sûr.

Pendant que je parle, mamie Judy hoche la tête d'un air approbateur, plisse un œil et fait des commentaires perspicaces.

— Wells ne doit pas laisser ces gens se déchaîner contre lui. Ils adoreraient traîner un Stafford dans la boue, mais ça n'arrivera pas.

— Bien sûr que non. Il s'en est tiré à merveille, comme d'habitude.

Je ne précise pas à quel point il avait l'air fatigué, je n'évoque pas non plus sa courte absence pendant l'échange.

— C'est bien mon fils ! Très comme il faut. Je me demande comment il a pu élever une fille capable d'être exécrable.

— Pff ! Mamie !

Je pose ma main sur la sienne et lui serre les doigts. La voilà qui plaisante et m'offre un moment de complicité. C'est vraiment un bon jour.

— Je crois que ça a sauté une génération.

Je m'attends à une repartie immédiate. Au lieu de quoi, elle se contente de dire :

— Oh, comme bien des choses.

Elle se laisse aller en arrière dans son fauteuil, sa main quittant la mienne. Je sens qu'un moment précieux est en train de s'achever.

— Mamie, je voulais te demander quelque chose.

— Ah bon ?

— J'ai fait la connaissance d'une dame, hier. Elle m'a dit qu'elle te connaissait. May Crandall. Ce nom te dit quelque chose ?

Elle se souvient toujours des noms des vieux amis et des anciennes connaissances. Comme si le livre de ses souvenirs s'était ouvert en tombant et qu'un vent persistant arrachait d'abord les pages les plus récentes. Plus les souvenirs sont anciens, plus ils ont de chance de rester intacts.

— May Crandall...

Quand elle répète ce nom, je vois tout de suite qu'elle le reconnaît. Je tends déjà la main vers mon téléphone pour lui montrer la photo lorsqu'elle reprend :

— Non, ça ne me dit rien.

Je lève les yeux de mon sac à main. Elle me regarde d'une façon très directe, ses cils fins et blancs pointant au-dessus de ses yeux couleur océan qui semblent soudain étrangement perçants. J'ai peur que nous nous retrouvions dans un de ces moments où elle s'arrête au milieu d'une conversation et, sans crier gare, recommence depuis le début avec une phrase du genre : « Je ne savais pas que tu viendrais aujourd'hui. Comment vas-tu ? » Au lieu de quoi, elle me demande :

— Pourquoi me poser cette question ?

— Je l'ai rencontrée hier... à la maison de retraite.

— Oui, tu me l'as dit. Mais beaucoup de gens ont entendu parler des Stafford, ma chérie. Nous devons toujours être prudents. Les gens cherchent toujours à faire des scandales.

— Des scandales ?

Ce mot me fait bondir.

— Bien sûr.

Le téléphone me semble soudain glacial entre mes doigts.

— Je ne savais pas que nous avions des squelettes dans nos placards.

— Grand Dieu, non. Bien sûr que non.

Je cherche la photo sur mon téléphone et regarde le visage de la jeune femme qui me rappelle encore plus ma grand-mère maintenant que je suis en face d'elle.

— Elle avait cette photo. Tu connais ces gens ?

Ce sont peut-être des cousins issus d'une branche illégitime de la famille ? Et que ma grand-mère ne veut pas reconnaître comme faisant partie de l'arbre généalogique ? Tous les clans doivent en avoir quelque part. Peut-être une cousine qui s'est enfuie avec un homme peu recommandable et est tombée enceinte ?

Je tourne l'écran vers elle, guettant sa réaction.

— Queen... murmure-t-elle en tendant la main pour rapprocher le téléphone de son visage. Oh...

Les larmes lui montent aux yeux. Perlent et débordent, laissant de longs sillons sur ses joues.

— Mamie ?

Elle est partie à des millions de kilomètres.

Non, pas des millions de kilomètres, des millions d'années. Elle se souvient de quelque chose. Elle sait qui est sur la photo. Queen. Qu'est-ce que ça veut dire ?

— Mamie ?

— Queenie, dit-elle en caressant l'écran du bout du doigt.

Puis elle se tourne vers moi avec une intensité qui me cloue sur mon fauteuil.

— Nous ne devons laisser personne le découvrir... dit-elle à voix basse.

Elle jette un coup d'œil vers la porte, se penche vers moi avant d'ajouter en chuchotant :

— Ils ne doivent jamais savoir, pour l'*Arcadie.*

Il me faut un instant avant de pouvoir répondre. Mon esprit tourbillonne. *Est-ce que je l'ai déjà entendue utiliser ce mot ?*

— Quoi ? Mamie, c'est quoi... cette Arcadie ?

— Chut ! fait-elle si brusquement qu'elle postillonne sur la table. Si jamais ils le découvrent...

— Ils ? Qui ça, ils ?

La poignée de la porte tourne, et ma grand-mère s'adosse à son fauteuil, les mains pliées sagement l'une sur l'autre. Un coup d'œil rapide m'enjoint à faire de même.

J'ai beau faire semblant de me détendre, trop de possibilités tourbillonnent dans ma tête – tout, depuis une affaire étouffée à la Watergate impliquant mon grand-père jusqu'à une société secrète de femmes politiques agissant en tant qu'espionnes de la guerre froide. Dans quoi ma grand-mère a-t-elle trempé ?

Une employée aimable entre avec du café et des biscuits. À Magnolia Manor, les résidents ont non seulement des repas, mais aussi des en-cas et des boissons chaudes.

Ma grand-mère agite le dos de sa main discrètement vers mon téléphone, la tête tournée vers la jeune femme.

— Qu'est-ce que vous voulez ?

Cette dernière n'est pas troublée par cet accueil inhabituellement sec.

— C'est le café du matin, madame Stafford.

— Oui, bien sûr, répond ma grand-mère en me faisant de nouveau signe, discrètement, que je devrais ranger mon téléphone. Nous prendrons une tasse avec plaisir.

D'un coup d'œil, je regarde l'heure sur mon téléphone. Il est plus tard que je ne le pensais. Je suis censée rejoindre mon père pour le déjeuner avant de l'accompagner à une inauguration à Columbia. « Une occasion en or d'être vue en action dans la capitale de mon État natal », comme l'a formulé Leslie. La presse sera là, ainsi que le gouverneur de Caroline du Sud. Après les remous récents dénonçant les parachutés de Washington et autres politiciens carriéristes, ce genre d'événement local est important. Je le sais mais, ce que j'ai vraiment envie de faire, c'est de rester avec ma grand-mère suffisamment longtemps pour pouvoir clarifier cette histoire autour de May Crandall et découvrir ce que l'Arcadie vient faire là-dedans.

Elle parle peut-être d'un endroit ? Arcadie, la ville de Californie ? Ou celle de Floride ?

— Je dois vraiment y aller, mamie. On m'a demandé d'accompagner papa à une inauguration.

— Grand Dieu, je ne dois pas te retenir, alors.

La jeune femme apporte des tasses de café malgré tout.

— Juste au cas où, dit-elle.

— Tu peux l'emporter, plaisante ma grand-mère, vu que la tasse est en porcelaine.

— Je n'ai pas besoin d'une nouvelle dose de caféine ce matin. Je risquerais de rebondir partout. J'étais juste passée t'interroger sur May...

— Tsss ! siffle-t-elle, le doigt en l'air, pour m'empêcher de finir le nom.

Elle me foudroie du regard, comme si je venais de jurer dans une église.

L'employée sent qu'il est temps de repartir avec son chariot.

— Fais attention, Rill, me murmure ma grand-mère.

— Qu-quoi ?

Son intensité me surprend de nouveau. Que se passe-t-il, dans son esprit ? Rill. Est-ce que c'est un nom ?

— Les murs ont des oreilles, ajoute-t-elle, les doigts tendus vers ses tempes.

Son humeur change aussitôt. Elle soupire, penche le pichet de lait en porcelaine et en verse un nuage dans son café.

— Tu en veux ? me demande-t-elle.

— Je dois y aller.

— Oh, quel dommage. J'aurais tellement voulu que tu puisses rester bavarder. C'était gentil à toi de passer me voir.

Depuis mon arrivée, cela fait au moins une demi-heure que nous discutons. Elle a déjà oublié. L'*Arcadie*, quoi que ce soit, a déjà disparu dans les brumes.

Elle m'offre un sourire aussi franc qu'impersonnel. Complètement sincère. Elle ne sait plus trop qui je suis, mais elle essaie d'être polie.

— Reviens me voir quand tu seras moins pressée.

— Je n'y manquerai pas.

Je dépose une bise sur sa joue et sors de la pièce sans réponse, et avec plus de questions encore.

Je ne peux pas laisser tomber cette histoire maintenant. Je dois découvrir de quoi il retourne. Il faudra que je déterre d'autres sources d'information, et je sais où commencer à creuser.

8

Rill

L'ombre de la grande maison blanche glisse sur la voiture et l'engloutit tout entière. De hauts magnolias feuillus bordent la propriété, créant un mur de verdure qui me rappelle le château de la Belle au bois dormant. Il nous cache de la rue, où les enfants jouent dans des parcs et où des mamans poussent des landaus le long du trottoir. Il y a une poussette devant cette maison. Elle est vieille et il lui manque une roue, si bien qu'elle penche. Si on y mettait un bébé, il tomberait aussitôt.

Un petit garçon est perché comme un singe dans l'un des magnolias. Il est grand comme Lark, à peu près – il doit avoir cinq ou six ans. Il nous regarde entrer à bord de la voiture, il ne sourit pas, il n'agite pas la main, il ne bouge pas. Lorsque la voiture s'arrête, il disparaît dans les feuilles.

Une seconde plus tard, je le vois s'éloigner de l'arbre à quatre pattes et se glisser sous le haut grillage qui entoure le jardin à l'arrière de la maison et la propriété voisine. Le petit bâtiment d'à côté a pu être jadis une école ou une salle paroissiale. Là-bas, des enfants jouent sur des bascules et des balançoires, mais les portes et les fenêtres sont condamnées avec des planches et il n'y a presque plus de peinture sur la façade en bois. Des ronces poussent sur la galerie à l'avant, ce qui me fait de nouveau penser à la Belle au bois dormant.

Toujours assise par terre, Camellia tend le cou pour voir dehors.

— C'est l'hôpital ? lance-t-elle à Mlle Tann, avec un regard qui lui laisse comprendre qu'elle ne le croira pas une seule seconde.

Ma sœur, qui s'est reposée pendant le trajet, est prête à repartir à la charge.

Mlle Tann se tourne vers elle et change Gabion de place – il dort profondément sur ses genoux. Ses petits bras pendouillent, ses doigts dodus s'ouvrent et se referment. Ses lèvres bougent comme s'il envoyait des baisers à quelqu'un dans son rêve.

— Vous ne pouvez pas vous rendre à l'hôpital dans cet état, n'est-ce pas ? Imprégnés de la puanteur du fleuve et infestés de vermine. Mme Murphy prendra soin de vous et, si vous êtes très très sages, alors nous reparlerons de l'hôpital.

Une lueur d'espoir, telle la flamme d'une bougie, tente de s'allumer en moi, mais je ne trouve rien pour l'alimenter. Elle s'éteint dès que Mlle Tann me regarde.

Fern me grimpe dessus et se presse contre moi, les genoux dans mon ventre.

— Je veux Briny, murmure-t-elle en geignant.

— On descend. C'est l'heure de rentrer. Vous serez très bien ici, nous assure Mlle Tann. Si vous êtes sages. Me suis-je bien fait comprendre ?

— Oui, m'dame.

J'essaie de répondre au nom de tous mais Camellia refuse d'abandonner si facilement.

— Où est Briny ?

Elle est très contrariée par toute cette histoire et une colère noire couve en elle. Je le sens comme un orage à l'approche.

— Chut, Camellia ! Fais ce qu'elle dit.

— Très bien, répond Mlle Tann dans un sourire. Vous voyez ? Tout peut très bien se passer. Mme Murphy prendra soin de vous.

Elle attend que le chauffeur vienne ouvrir la portière. Puis elle descend en premier, mon petit frère sur un bras, tirant Lark par la main. Lark me dévisage, les yeux écarquillés mais, comme toujours, elle ne proteste pas. Elle est aussi calme qu'un chaton dans le foin.

— À ton tour, me dit-elle.

Je me dépêche de sortir et mes genoux cognent au passage le garçon et la fille aux yeux bruns qui étaient installés par terre. Fern me serre si fort par le cou que je ne peux presque plus respirer.

— Vous deux, maintenant.

Les deux enfants inconnus sortent dans l'allée.

— Et maintenant, à toi.

La voix de Mlle Tann se fait plus grave lorsqu'elle regarde Camellia. Elle m'envoie Gabion et Lark, et se place juste devant la portière, les jambes écartées, son corps bouchant le passage. Ce n'est pas une petite femme. Elle fait une tête de plus que moi et semble robuste.

— Allez, Camellia.

Je l'implore d'être sage, et elle sait ce que je lui demande. Jusque-là, elle n'a pas bougé d'un poil. Elle a une main cachée dans son dos et j'ai peur qu'elle tente de sortir par l'autre portière. À quoi ça nous avancerait ? Nous ne savons pas où nous sommes ni quelle direction prendre pour retrouver le fleuve ou l'hôpital. Notre seul espoir, c'est que, si nous sommes sages comme nous le demande Mlle Tann, nous pourrons voir Briny et Queenie.

Ou bien que Silas leur dise ce qui nous est arrivé et que nos parents viennent nous chercher.

L'épaule de Camellia se soulève un peu et j'entends le cliquetis de la poignée. La portière ne bouge pas et je vois les narines de Camellia se dilater. Quand elle se tourne pour pousser de toutes ses forces, Mlle Tann soupire et se penche à l'intérieur.

Lorsqu'elle en ressort, elle tire Camellia par ses vêtements.

— Ça suffit comme ça ! Tu vas te calmer et te tenir correctement.

— Camellia, arrête ! crié-je.

— Mellia, non, non ! ajoute Fern, comme en écho.

Gabion rejette la tête en arrière et hurle si fort que son cri rebondit sur la maison et part vers les arbres.

Mlle Tann tourne le poignet pour avoir une bonne prise sur Camellia.

— Est-ce qu'on se comprend, toutes les deux ? demanda Mlle Tann, les joues rouges et trempées de sueur, ses yeux gris exorbités derrière ses lunettes.

Lorsque Camellia pince les lèvres, je m'attends à ce que Mlle Tann la gifle pour lui faire passer son air de rébellion, mais elle n'en fait rien. Au lieu de quoi, elle murmure quelque chose près de l'oreille de ma sœur avant de se dresser au-dessus d'elle.

— Tout ira bien, maintenant, n'est-ce pas ?

Camellia a toujours l'air d'avoir avalé un citron.

L'instant est en équilibre, comme une bouteille au bord du pont de l'*Arcadie,* attendant de basculer et d'être emportée par le fleuve.

— N'est-ce pas ? répète la femme.

Même si les yeux sombres de Camellia lancent des éclairs, elle hoche la tête.

— Très bien.

Mlle Tann nous met en rang et Camellia grimpe les marches avec nous. Derrière la grille, des garçons et des filles de toutes les tailles nous observent. Aucun d'eux ne sourit.

À l'intérieur de la grande maison, ça sent mauvais. Comme les rideaux sont tirés dans toutes les pièces, il fait sombre. Un grand escalier se dresse dans l'entrée. Deux garçons sont assis sur les marches. L'un d'eux me rappelle Silas, mais en plus grand, sauf que ses cheveux sont aussi roux que de la fourrure de renard. Ces garçons ne ressemblent pas du tout aux autres enfants dans le jardin ou à celui dans l'arbre. Ils ne peuvent pas tous être frères et sœurs.

Qui sont-ils ? Combien sont-ils ? Est-ce qu'ils vivent tous ici ? Est-ce qu'ils sont tous là pour se débarbouiller avant d'aller voir leurs papas et leurs mamans à l'hôpital ?

Qu'est-ce que c'est que cet endroit ?

On nous emmène dans une pièce où une femme attend derrière un bureau. Elle est petite, comparée à Mlle Tann, et ses bras sont si maigres qu'on voit ses os et ses veines. Son nez pointe sous ses lunettes, crochu comme le bec d'une chouette. Il se fronce lorsqu'elle nous regarde. Puis elle sourit, se lève et salue Mlle Tann.

— Comment allez-vous aujourd'hui, Georgia ?

— Très bien, merci, madame Murphy. La matinée a été plutôt productive, si j'ose dire.

— Je le vois, en effet.

Mme Murphy s'approche de nous et laisse courir ses doigts sur le bureau en traçant des sillons dans la poussière. Un coin de ses lèvres se soulève et une canine apparaît.

— Dieu du ciel. Où avez-vous débusqué ces petits bouts ?

Les enfants se blottissent contre moi, même ceux que je ne connais pas. Je m'accroche à Fern, perchée sur une de mes hanches, et Gabion, calé sur l'autre. Je commence à ne plus sentir mes bras, mais je ne les lâcherai pas.

— Ils font tous pitié, non ? demande Mlle Tann. Je crois que nous les avons tirés de là juste à temps. Avez-vous de la place pour eux tous ? Ce serait le plus simple. Je pense en déplacer certains très rapidement.

— Regardez-moi ces cheveux… s'extasie Mme Murphy en s'approchant de plus près, suivie par Mlle Tann.

Le corps de cette dernière bascule d'un côté puis de l'autre lorsqu'elle marche. Je remarque seulement qu'elle a une patte folle.

— Oui, c'est quelque chose, n'est-ce pas ? Quatre blondinets bouclés de la même famille et… celle-ci.

Elle renifle en jetant un coup d'œil vers Camellia.

— Oh, elle ne peut pas venir de la même fournée, s'étonne Mme Murphy avant de se tourner vers moi. C'est ta sœur ?

— O-oui, m'dame.

— Et elle s'appelle… ?

— C-Camellia.

— Quel nom distingué pour une petite chose aussi banale. Sans parler de ces taches de rousseur ridicules. On dirait que la cigogne t'a lâchée dans le mauvais nid.

— Elle n'est pas du genre à coopérer, la met en garde Mlle Tann. Elle nous a déjà causé du souci. Un vrai petit mouton noir, et c'est rien de le dire.

Mme Murphy plisse les yeux.

— Allons bon. Eh bien, j'attends vraiment de bonnes manières dans cette maison. Ceux qui échouent à répondre à mes attentes n'auront pas le droit de rejoindre les autres enfants à l'étage.

Elle fait glisser sa langue sur ses dents.

J'ai soudain très froid. Fern et Gabion me serrent le cou un peu plus fort. Ce que veut dire Mme Murphy est assez clair. Si Camellia la met en colère, ils l'emmèneront et la mettront... ailleurs.

Camellia hoche la tête mais je devine qu'elle n'en pense pas moins.

— Ces deux autres aux cheveux blond filasse ont... été trouvés en cours de route.

Mlle Tann réunit le garçon et la fille qui ont voyagé par terre avec Camellia. Ils ont tous les deux de longs cheveux blond cendré et de grands yeux marron. À voir comment le petit garçon s'accroche à la fille, je suis sûre qu'elle est sa grande sœur.

— Encore des rats du fleuve, évidemment, même si le camp, là-bas, était presque désert. Ils ont dû avoir vent de notre venue, d'une façon ou d'une autre.

— Quels visages adorables...

— Oui, vraiment. Ceux-là, avec leurs boucles, sont vraiment angéliques. On va se les arracher, je le prédis.

Mme Murphy s'éloigne.

— Mais Dieu du ciel ! Ils empestent comme le fleuve. Je ne peux pas tolérer cela dans ma maison, pour sûr. Ils devront rester dehors jusqu'à l'heure du bain.

— Ne les laissez pas sortir avant que vous soyez certaine qu'ils ont pleinement compris les règles qui s'appliquent ici.

Mlle Tann pose la main sur l'épaule de Camellia et la tête de Camellia tremble tellement que je devine que les doigts de la femme la serrent fort.

— Celle-ci est une fuyarde. Elle a essayé de s'échapper de la voiture, entre autres. Ces génisses du fleuve savent se reproduire, mais quand il s'agit d'éduquer leur marmaille, il n'y a plus personne. Cette fournée va demander du travail.

— Bien sûr. Comme toujours, non ? répond Mme Murphy avant de fixer de nouveau son attention sur moi. Et toi, comment t'appelles-tu ?

— Rill. Rill Foss.

Je ne comprends rien à ce qu'elles disent et mon cœur bat la chamade. Si mes genoux tremblent sous le poids de mon petit frère et de ma petite sœur, ce n'est pas la seule raison. Je suis morte de peur. Mlle Tann compte nous laisser ici ? Pour combien de temps ?

— Quand pourrons-nous aller voir nos parents ? demandé-je malgré moi. Ils sont à l'hôpital. Maman a eu un bébé et...

— Chut, me coupe Mme Murphy. Chaque chose en son temps. Tu vas d'abord emmener les enfants dans le couloir et les faire asseoir contre le mur de la cage d'escalier, du plus petit au plus grand. Attendez là et je ne veux entendre aucun bruit ni aucune chamaillerie. Compris ?

— Mais...

Cette fois-ci, Mlle Tann pose la main sur mon épaule. Ses doigts se resserrent autour de mon os.

— Je compte sur toi pour ne pas faire de difficultés. Tu es sans doute plus intelligente que ta sœur.

Une douleur lancinante descend dans mon bras et je sens Gabion glisser.

— O-oui, m'm. Oui, m'dame.

Elle me relâche. Je remonte Gabby sur ma hanche. Je voudrais me masser l'épaule mais je m'abstiens.

— Et... Rill. Qu'est-ce que c'est que ce nom ?

— Ça vient du fleuve. C'est mon papa qui l'a choisi. Il dit que c'est aussi joli qu'une chanson.

— On va te trouver un prénom correct. Un vrai nom pour une vraie jeune fille. May, ça fera l'affaire. May Weathers.

— Mais je m'app...

— May.

Elle me pousse vers la porte, et les enfants me suivent d'un pas traînant. Elles mettent de nouveau Camellia en garde, elle doit rester assise en silence dans l'entrée.

Les petits geignent et gémissent comme des chiots lorsque j'essaie de les arracher de mes bras pour les installer par terre. Les deux garçons sont partis en haut de l'escalier. Dehors, d'autres enfants jouent à la déli-délo. J'ai appris ce jeu dans les écoles qu'on a fréquentées. Tous les ans avant la rentrée, Queenie et Briny essaient d'amarrer le bateau près d'une ville fluviale pour que Camellia et moi – et Lark, maintenant – puissions y aller. Le reste du temps, nous lisons des livres et Briny nous apprend l'arithmétique. Il est imbattable en mathématiques. Camellia est très douée pour le calcul. Et même Fern connaît déjà son alphabet, alors qu'elle est trop petite pour aller à l'école. À la rentrée prochaine, Lark entrera au cours préparatoire...

Lark lève vers moi ses grands yeux de souris et un mauvais pressentiment monte en moi, comme un tourbillon dans une rivière aux eaux noires. Il n'a nulle part où aller. Il peut juste tourner, tourner, tourner en rond.

— Est-ce qu'ils nous emmènent en prison ? murmure la petite fille dont je ne connais même pas le nom.

— Non, bien sûr que non. On met pas de petits enfants en prison.

N'est-ce pas ?

Camellia glisse un regard en coin vers la porte d'entrée. Elle se demande si elle a une chance de filer d'ici sans se faire prendre.

— Ne fais pas ça, dis-je dans un murmure.

Mme Murphy nous a dit ne pas faire de bruit. Plus nous serons sages, plus nous aurons de chance qu'ils nous emmènent où nous voulons.

— Nous devons rester ensemble. Briny viendra nous chercher dès qu'il apprendra qu'on n'est plus à bord de l'*Arcadie.* Bientôt, Silas lui dira ce qui s'est passé. Nous devons tous être au même endroit quand il arrivera. Tu m'entends ?

Je parle comme Queenie l'hiver, quand il y a des blocs de glace sur le fleuve et qu'elle refuse que nous nous penchions sur la rambarde de peur qu'un bloc nous percute et nous fasse tomber dans l'eau. Dans ces moments-là, quand c'est non, c'est non, et elle fait tout pour que ce soit clair. Elle ne se met pas souvent dans cet état.

Tout le monde hoche la tête sauf Camellia. Même l'autre petite fille et son frère.

— Mellia ?

— Mmmmm, cède-t-elle.

Elle remonte ses jambes contre sa poitrine, enroule ses bras autour, et baisse la tête en laissant cogner son front contre ses genoux pour bien nous faire comprendre qu'elle n'est pas contente.

Quand je demande aux deux autres enfants comment ils s'appellent, ils ne veulent pas répondre. De grosses larmes coulent sur les joues du garçon et sa sœur le tient fort contre elle.

Un oiseau vient percuter la porte vitrée, et le bruit nous fait tous sursauter. Je tends le cou pour voir s'il s'est relevé pour s'envoler. C'est un joli petit cardinal. C'est peut-être celui qu'on a entendu près du fleuve, qui nous aurait suivis. Là, il sautille en chancelant, et ses plumes brillent d'un rouge éclatant sous les rayons longs et paresseux du soleil de l'après-midi. J'aimerais pouvoir le prendre au creux de mes mains avant qu'un chat l'attrape – on en a vu au moins trois dans les buissons en arrivant ici – mais j'ai trop peur. Mlle Tann croirait que j'essaie de m'enfuir.

Lark se met à genoux pour mieux voir, la lèvre tremblante. Je chuchote :

— Il va bien. Assieds-toi. Sois sage.

Elle obéit.

L'oiseau sautille vers les marches si bien que je dois m'écarter un peu du mur pour le suivre des yeux. Envole-toi. Dépêche-toi. Envole-toi avant qu'ils t'attrapent.

Mais il reste là, le bec ouvert, tout son corps haletant.

Envole-toi. Rentre chez toi.

Je le surveille. Si un chat approche, je pourrais peut-être lui faire peur à travers la fenêtre.

Des voix se glissent soudain sous la porte du bureau. Je me lève tout doucement et m'approche sur la pointe des pieds.

Je comprends quelques phrases de Mlle Tann et Mme Murphy, mais ça ne veut rien dire :

— ... rempli les papiers aussitôt à l'hôpital pour les cinq frères et sœurs. Simple et rapide. Le meilleur moyen de briser des liens. À vrai dire, le plus difficile a été de déterminer l'endroit exact où se situait leur coque de noix. Leur bateau est amarré à l'écart, face à Mud Island, m'a dit la police. La petite aux taches de rousseur a tenté de s'enfuir par le trou des toilettes. Il n'y a pas que l'odeur du fleuve, que vous avez sentie.

Elle caquette de rire, un rire sec comme le cri d'une corneille.

— Et les deux autres ?

— On les a trouvés en train de cueillir des fleurs près d'un de ces nids de rats de rivière. Leurs papiers seront bientôt en ordre. Cela ne posera sans doute pas de problème. Ils semblent aussi d'un tempérament doux. Hmmm... Sherry et Stevie. Voilà des noms qui conviendront. Mieux vaut commencer tout de suite à les habituer. Ils sont adorables, n'est-ce pas ? Et jeunes. Ils ne resteront peut-être pas longtemps. Nous avons prévu une petite présentation le mois prochain. Je compte sur vous pour qu'ils soient prêts.

— Oh, ils le seront.

— May, Iris, Bonnie... Beth... et Robby pour les cinq autres, je pense. Quant à leur nom de famille, Weathers fera l'affaire. May Weathers, Iris Weathers, Bonnie Weathers... Cela sonne joliment.

Un nouveau rire. Si fort et puissant qu'il m'éloigne de la porte.

Les derniers mots que j'entends sont ceux de Mme Murphy.

— J'y veillerai. Ils seront préparés comme il se doit, n'en doutez pas.

Le temps qu'elles sortent, j'ai déjà filé à ma place et vérifié que tout le monde est bien aligné contre le mur. Même Camellia relève la tête et s'assied en tailleur, comme à l'école.

Nous attendons, immobiles comme des statues, pendant que Mme Murphy raccompagne Mlle Tann à la porte. Seuls nos yeux se tournent pour les regarder discuter sur le seuil.

Le petit cardinal a sautillé sur les marches, mais il reste là, sans défense. Aucune des deux femmes ne le remarque.

Envole-toi.

Je pense au chapeau rouge de Queenie. Envole-toi jusqu'à Queenie et dis-lui où nous trouver.

Envole-toi.

Mlle Tann descend quelques marches en boitant et bute presque dans l'oiseau. Je retiens mon souffle et Lark hoquette. Puis Mlle Tann s'arrête pour ajouter une chose.

Quand elle se remet en route, le cardinal s'envole enfin.

Il dira à Briny où nous sommes.

Mme Murphy rentre dans le bâtiment, elle ne sourit pas. Elle retourne dans son bureau, face à nous, et ferme la porte.

Nous restons assis, là, à attendre. Camellia replonge la tête dans ses genoux.

Fern s'appuie contre mon épaule. La petite fille – Sherry, selon Mlle Tann – tient la main de son petit frère.

— A faim, murmure-t-il.

— Moi aussi, répond Gabion, bien trop fort.

— Chut, fais-je en passant ma main sur ses doux cheveux. Il ne faut pas faire de bruit. Comme à cache-cache. Comme dans un jeu.

Il plaque ses mains sur sa bouche et fait de son mieux. À juste deux ans, il se retrouvait toujours à l'écart de nos jeux d'imagination à bord de l'*Arcadie*, si bien qu'il est content d'être inclus, pour une fois.

J'aimerais que ce ne soit qu'un grand jeu. Que j'en connaisse les règles et que je sache ce qu'on obtient si on gagne.

Pour l'instant, tout ce que nous pouvons faire, c'est rester assis par terre et attendre ce qui va nous arriver ensuite.

Et on attend, on attend, on attend.

Et il nous semble qu'une éternité s'est passée quand Mme Murphy ressort. J'ai faim, moi aussi, mais je vois à son visage que nous ferions mieux de ne rien demander.

Elle se dresse devant nous, les poings sur ses hanches qui saillent sous sa robe noire fleurie.

— Sept de plus... dit-elle, sourcils froncés, en regardant l'escalier.

Elle souffle vers nous, et c'est comme un brouillard glacial. Qui sent mauvais.

— Eh bien, ce n'est pas comme si on avait le choix, puisque vos parents sont incapables de s'occuper de vous.

— Où est Briny ? Où est Queenie ? braille soudain Camellia.

— Tais-toi !

Mme Murphy vacille sur ses jambes tandis qu'elle nous passe en revue, et maintenant je reconnais l'odeur que j'ai sentie lorsqu'elle est revenue dans l'entrée. Celle du whisky. J'ai fréquenté suffisamment les salles de billard pour le savoir.

Mme Murphy pointe Camellia du doigt.

— C'est à cause de toi si tout le monde doit rester assis là au lieu de jouer dehors.

Elle s'éloigne d'un pas lourd et zigzaguant.

Nous restons assis. Les petits se sont enfin endormis, Gabion étalé à même le sol. Quelques autres enfants passent devant nous – plus jeunes ou plus âgés, garçons et filles. La plupart portent des vêtements trop grands ou trop petits. Pas un d'entre eux ne regarde vers nous. Ils passent comme s'ils ne remarquaient pas notre présence. Des femmes en robe blanche et en tablier blanc traversent l'entrée en vitesse, dans un sens puis dans l'autre. Elles non plus, elles ne nous voient pas.

J'enroule mes doigts autour de mes chevilles et serre fort pour m'assurer que je suis toujours là. J'ai presque l'impression de m'être transformée en Homme invisible, comme dans le livre de M. H. G. Wells. Briny adore cette histoire. Il nous l'a lue des tas de fois, et Camellia et moi, nous la rejouons avec d'autres enfants des campements de bateaux, sur les rives. Personne ne peut voir l'Homme invisible.

Je ferme les yeux et je joue un moment à être cet Homme invisible.

Fern a soudain envie d'aller aux toilettes mais, avant que j'aie le temps de décider ce qu'on doit faire, elle fait sous elle. Une femme brune en uniforme blanc nous passe devant et remarque l'urine qui coule sur le sol. Elle attrape Fern par le bras.

— Pas de ça ici ! Tu dois utiliser les toilettes comme il se doit.

Elle sort un lange de son tablier et le jette sur la flaque.

— Nettoie-moi ça, m'ordonne-t-elle. Mme Murphy va avoir une attaque.

Elle emmène Fern et j'obéis. Quand ma petite sœur revient, sa robe et ses sous-vêtements ont été rincés, et elle les porte mouillés. La dame nous dit que nous pouvons nous aussi aller aux toilettes mais que nous devons nous dépêcher et retourner ensuite près de l'escalier.

Nous venons à peine de nous rasseoir lorsqu'un coup de sifflet retentit dehors. J'entends des enfants courir dans tous les sens. Des tas d'enfants. S'ils ne parlent pas, leurs pas résonnent si fort que le vacarme se glisse sous la porte qui donne à l'arrière de la maison, au bout du hall. Ils y restent un moment, puis on entend un tapage épouvantable, comme s'ils se dépêchaient de monter un autre escalier.

À l'étage, les planches craquent et grincent comme le plat-bord et le pont de l'*Arcadie*. Ce sont des bruits réconfortants – je ferme les yeux et fais comme si je pouvais, d'un vœu, nous ramener tous à bord de notre petit bateau où nous étions en sécurité.

Mon vœu est de courte durée. Une femme en blanc s'arrête devant nous et nous ordonne :

— Venez par là.

Nous nous mettons debout pour la suivre. Camellia passe en premier, moi en dernier, pour garder les petits entre nous, y compris Sherry et Stevie.

La dame nous fait passer par la porte au fond du hall et tout est différent, par là. Les murs sont vieux et laids. Des lambeaux de papier peint et de toile de jute pendouillent des murs. Il y a une cuisine sur le côté. Deux femmes de couleur s'affairent au-dessus d'une marmite posée sur le poêle. J'espère que nous mangerons bientôt. J'ai l'impression que mon estomac a rétréci à la taille d'une cacahuète.

Cette simple pensée me donne envie de manger des cacahuètes.

Un grand escalier s'élève à l'autre bout de la cuisine. Les marches n'ont presque plus de peinture, comme s'il avait été beaucoup emprunté. La moitié des barreaux manquent à la rambarde. Deux ou trois dépassent, comme les quelques dents qu'il reste au vieux Zede quand il sourit.

La femme en blanc nous emmène à l'étage et nous aligne contre le mur d'un couloir. D'autres enfants forment d'autres files près de nous, et j'entends de l'eau couler dans une baignoire.

— On ne parle pas, nous prévient la femme. Vous attendrez ici en silence jusqu'à ce que ce soit votre tour d'aller au bain. Vous enlèverez vos vêtements que vous plierez soigneusement à vos pieds. Tous vos vêtements.

J'en ai des sueurs froides et, lorsque je regarde autour de nous, je me rends compte que les autres enfants, grands et petits, sont déjà en train d'obtempérer.

9

Avery

— May Crandall. Tu es sûre que ça ne te dit rien, maman ?

Je suis assise dans la limousine avec mon père et ma mère, en route vers l'inauguration à Columbia.

— C'est elle qui a trouvé mon bracelet à la maison de retraite, hier.

Je dis « trouvé », ça sonne mieux que « l'a volé à même mon poignet ».

— Le modèle Greer avec les libellules en grenat – celui que mamie Judy m'avait donné. Je crois que cette femme l'a reconnu.

— Ta grand-mère le portait souvent, répond ma mère. N'importe qui la connaissant de vue pourrait s'en souvenir. Il est assez particulier.

Elle consulte sa banque de données mentale en pressant ses lèvres aux contours parfaits.

— Non, ce nom ne me dit rien. Elle fait peut-être partie des Crandall d'Asheville ? Je suis sorti avec un garçon de cette famille quand j'étais jeune – avant ton père, évidemment. Tu lui as demandé de quelle famille elle est ?

Pour Pomme d'amour, comme pour toutes les femmes du Sud bien nées de sa génération, c'est une question naturelle qu'on pose lorsqu'on rencontre quelqu'un. « Ravie de vous connaître. Il fait beau aujourd'hui, n'est-ce pas ? Maintenant, dites-moi, de quelle famille êtes-vous ? »

— Je n'ai pas pensé à lui demander.

— Franchement, Avery ! Qu'est-ce qu'on va faire de toi ?

116

— M'envoyer en maison de correction ?

Mon père ricane et lève les yeux de sa mallette pleine de documents.

— Allons, Pomme d'amour, je ne lui ai pas laissé une minute pour souffler. Et personne ne pourrait archiver aussi bien que toi ce genre de détails.

— Oh, tais-toi donc, glousse-t-elle en lui donnant une petite tape.

Il lui prend la main et lui baise les doigts, alors que je suis coincée entre eux. J'ai l'impression d'avoir treize ans.

— Eeeerk. Y a des enfants dans la salle, dites donc.

Depuis que je suis rentrée chez moi, j'ai réadopté des mots comme « dites donc », que j'avais expurgés de mon vocabulaire à force de vivre dans un État du Nord. J'ai décidé depuis que c'était des mots tout à fait acceptables. Comme notre bon vieux plat typique de la Caroline du Sud – les cacahuètes bouillies –, ils remplissent parfaitement leur rôle dans bien des situations.

— Tu te souviens d'une May Crandall, Wells ? Une amie de ta mère ?

— Je ne crois pas.

Mon père lève le bras pour se gratter la tête, avant de se rappeler qu'on l'a arrosé de laque. Des déplacements en plein air nécessitent une préparation supplémentaire. Il n'y a rien de pire que de finir dans les journaux avec une tête d'épouvantail. Leslie s'est assurée que j'avais attaché les miens. Pomme d'amour et moi, nous sommes assorties, en fait. C'est la journée du chignon banane.

— Arcadie, dis-je soudain pour voir si ce mot les fait réagir. Est-ce que c'était le nom d'un des clubs de mamie ? Ou d'une association de joueurs de bridge ? Ou est-ce qu'elle connaissait quelqu'un qui vivait là-bas ?

Ni mon père ni ma mère ne se comportent bizarrement en l'entendant.

— Arcadie, la ville de Floride, tu veux dire ? demande ma mère.

— Je ne sais pas trop. Elle a évoqué ce nom alors qu'on discutait de ses clubs de bridge.

Je ne leur dis pas que la façon dont elle l'a prononcé m'a mise mal à l'aise.

— Comment est-ce que je pourrais en savoir plus ?

— Toute cette histoire te préoccupe drôlement, on dirait.

J'ai failli sortir mon téléphone pour lui montrer la photo. Failli. Ma main s'arrête à mi-chemin au-dessus de mon sac et je finis par lisser ma jupe, à la place. J'entrevois une nouvelle ridule de contrariété sur le visage de ma mère. Elle n'a pas besoin d'un énième sujet d'inquiétude. Si je lui montre la photo, elle sera certaine qu'il s'agit d'un infâme complot et que May Crandall veut nous extorquer quelque chose. Ma mère est une anxieuse professionnelle.

— Non, ça ne me préoccupe pas, maman. Je suis juste curieuse. Cette femme semble si seule…

— C'est gentil à toi, sauf que mamie Judy ne serait pas de bonne compagnie pour elle de toute façon, même si elles se connaissaient. J'ai dû demander au groupe des filles du lundi d'arrêter d'aller la voir à Magnolia Manor. Mamie Judy est frustrée quand trop de vieilles amies passent la voir. Elle est gênée de ne plus se souvenir de leurs noms et de leurs visages. C'est plus difficile lorsque ce n'est pas la famille. Elle s'inquiète de ce que les gens disent sur elle.

— Je sais.

Je ferais peut-être mieux de laisser tomber mais cette histoire me titille. Comme une voix qui me chuchote sans cesse à l'oreille, qui me hante et me tourmente. Elle ne me lâche pas de l'après-midi. Nous bavardons avec des gens, nous les écoutons ; nous applaudissons lorsque mon père coupe le ruban. Nous passons du temps dans l'espace VIP du country club local, nous côtoyons le gouverneur et nous discutons avec des huiles d'entreprises importantes. J'arrive même à donner gratuitement des conseils juridiques concernant la bataille autour du gaz de schiste et la législation actuelle qui pourrait ouvrir grandes les portes à ce type d'exploitation dans la Caroline du Nord voisine. Économie *versus* environnement – l'éternel combat entre ces poids lourds pour remporter le soutien de l'opinion publique et, bien sûr, de la législation à venir.

Même en discutant des questions de coût et de profit, qui me passionnent vraiment en temps normal, dans un coin de ma tête, je pense à mon téléphone portable, là, dans mon sac à main, à la réaction de ma grand-mère face à cette photo.

Je sais qu'elle a reconnu la femme photographiée. Queen... ou Queenie.

Ce n'est pas une coïncidence. Impossible.

Arcadie. Arcadie... et puis quoi ?

Dans la voiture qui nous ramène au bureau de mon père à Aiken, je glisse quelque excuse innocente à mes parents pour leur échapper un instant – une course à faire. En vérité, je retourne voir May Crandall. Il se passe vraiment quelque chose, et je me porterai mieux en sachant de quoi il s'agit. Ensuite, je pourrai décider de ce qui doit être fait.

Mon père semble sincèrement déçu que nos chemins se séparent. Il a prévu une réunion « stratégie » avec son équipe avant de rentrer pour le dîner. Il espérait que j'y assisterais.

— Oh, grand Dieu, Wells, Avery a tout de même le droit d'avoir une vie privée, intervient ma mère. Elle a un beau fiancé avec qui elle doit rester en contact, tu te rappelles ?

Ses frêles épaules se soulèvent et elle m'offre un sourire de conspiratrice avant d'ajouter :

— Et un mariage à organiser. Ils ne peuvent rien préparer s'ils ne se parlent jamais.

Sa voix est chantante, pleine d'impatience. Elle me tapote le genou et se penche vers moi. Me glisse un regard lourd de sous-entendus. « Il est temps de mettre la machine en route », me dit-il. Elle cherche quelque chose dans son sac, laisse un court silence s'installer, avant de faire mine de changer de sujet.

— Le jardinier a apporté une nouvelle sorte de paillis, l'autre jour... pour les azalées... c'est une recommandation du paysagiste de Bitsy. Ils en ont mis partout à l'automne dernier et leurs azalées sont deux fois plus développées que les nôtres. Au printemps prochain, les jardins de Drayden Hill feront l'envie de... eh bien... tout le monde. Vers la fin du mois de mars. Ce devrait être juste... paradisiaque.

Les mots « parfait pour un mariage » restent suspendus dans l'air. Lorsque nous avons annoncé nos fiançailles, Elliot à fait promettre à Bitsy et Pomme d'amour qu'elles n'interviendraient pas, ne feraient pas un hold-up sur l'organisation du mariage. Ça les tue, vraiment. Elles auraient déjà tout prévu si nous les avions laissées faire, mais nous sommes décidés à attendre le bon moment pour arranger tout ça, et de la façon qui nous conviendra le mieux. Pour l'instant, mon père et Pomme d'amour devraient se concentrer à cent pour cent sur la santé de papa, au lieu de s'inquiéter pour des histoires de tulle et de plan de table.

Mais on ne peut pas dire ça à Pomme d'amour.

Je fais comme si je n'avais pas compris l'allusion.

— Je crois que Jason pourrait faire pousser des roses dans un désert.

Jason s'occupait déjà des jardins de Drayden Hill bien avant que je parte pour l'université. Il sera ravi d'avoir une occasion de montrer ses talents. Mais Elliot n'acceptera jamais une idée venue de nos deux mères. Elliot adore la sienne mais, en tant qu'enfant unique, il est épuisé par ses efforts constants pour diriger sa vie.

Chaque chose en son temps, me dis-je. *Papa, cancer, politique.* Voilà les trois grands axes de ma vie, pour le moment.

La voiture s'arrête devant le bureau. Le conducteur nous ouvre la portière et je me glisse dehors, ravie de me sentir libre.

Une dernière allusion me suit sur le trottoir :

— Dis à Elliot de remercier sa mère, pour le paillis des azalées.

— Promis, lancé-je avant de filer vers ma voiture, où j'appelle bel et bien Elliot.

Il ne décroche pas. Il y a des chances pour qu'il soit en réunion, même s'il est déjà tard. Ses clients financiers sont internationaux, si bien que des demandes peuvent arriver à n'importe quelle heure de la journée.

Je lui laisse un rapide message concernant les azalées. Ça le fera rire et il en a souvent besoin à la fin d'une journée hautement stressante.

Au premier croisement, je reçois un appel de ma sœur, Allison.

— Salut, Allie. Quoi de neuf ?

Allison rit, mais elle semble épuisée. Les triplés chahutent derrière elle.

— Y a-t-il la moindre chance pour que tu puisses aller chercher Courtney à son cours de danse ? Les garçons sont malades et on s'est déjà changés trois fois aujourd'hui et... Oui. On est de nouveau tout nus. Tous les quatre. Courtney doit attendre devant son cours en se demandant où j'ai bien pu passer...

Je fais rapidement demi-tour pour me diriger vers le studio de Mlle Hannah, où j'avais été en mon temps tout aussi pitoyable au cours de danse qu'à celui de théâtre. Heureusement, Courtney a un vrai talent. Lors du spectacle du printemps, elle a été formidable.

— Bien sûr. J'y vais tout de suite. Je ne suis pas très loin, j'y serai dans dix minutes, tout au plus.

Allison pousse un long soupir de soulagement.

— Merci. Tu me sauves la vie. Aujourd'hui, c'est toi, ma sœur préférée.

Savoir qui est la favorite d'Allison est une blague récurrente depuis l'enfance. Comme c'est la sœur du milieu, c'est elle qui choisit. Missy, l'aînée, était plus intéressante mais, comme j'étais plus jeune, j'étais influençable.

— Ça, ça vaut largement un passage supplémentaire à l'autre bout de la ville, ris-je.

— Et, s'il te plaît, ne dis pas à maman que les garçons sont malades. Elle viendrait chez moi, et je ne veux pas risquer qu'elle rapporte je ne sais quel microbe à papa. Dépose Courtney chez Shellie. Je t'envoie son adresse par texto. J'ai déjà appelé ses parents. Ils veulent bien que Courtney passe la nuit chez eux.

— D'accord. Ça marche.

De nous trois, Allison est celle qui ressemble le plus à Pomme d'amour. Elle est aussi rigoureuse comme un général à quatre étoiles mais, depuis la naissance des garçons, elle est débordée par une armée ennemie.

— Je suis presque au studio. Je t'envoie un message dès que j'ai sauvé ta fille.

Nous raccrochons et, quelques minutes plus tard, je m'arrête devant le cours de danse. Courtney attend au pied du bâtiment. Son visage s'éclaircit lorsqu'elle se rend compte qu'elle n'a pas été abandonnée.

— Hé, salut, tata Avy ! lance-t-elle en se glissant dans la voiture.

— Salut, ma grande !

— Maman m'a encore oubliée ?

Elle lève les yeux au ciel et laisse tomber sa tête de côté, un geste qui lui donne beaucoup plus que ses dix ans.

— Non... tu me manquais, c'est tout. Je me disais qu'on pourrait passer un peu de temps ensemble, aller au parc, faire du toboggan, jouer dans le fort en bois, ce genre de chose...

— Bon, et sérieusement, tata ?

Je suis un peu peinée qu'elle rejette si vite cette idée. Elle est trop mûre pour son âge. J'ai l'impression qu'hier encore elle me tirait par le pantalon en me suppliant d'aller grimper avec elle dans les arbres de Drayden Hill.

— D'accord... c'est bien ta mère qui m'a appelée pour que je passe te chercher, mais seulement parce que les garçons sont malades. Je suis censée te déposer chez Shellie.

Son visage s'illumine et elle se redresse à côté de moi.

— Trop cool !

Comme je lui lance un regard en coin outré, elle ajoute.

— Je ne parlais pas de la maladie des triplés, je t'assure.

Je lui propose un arrêt chez le marchand de glaces, notre activité préférée de jadis, mais elle me dit qu'elle n'a pas faim. Elle a hâte d'arriver chez sa copine, du coup, j'allume le GPS et je suis les instructions.

Ma nièce dégaine son téléphone portable pour envoyer un texto à son amie et mes pensées divaguent. Arcadie et May Crandall me font presque oublier le pincement que je ressens à voir Courtney foncer droit vers l'adolescence. Quelle sera la réponse de May lorsque je l'interrogerai sur ce mot, Arcadie ?

J'ai de moins en moins de chance de pouvoir le découvrir aujourd'hui. Le temps que je dépose Courtney, ce sera l'heure du dîner à la maison de retraite. Le personnel sera occupé, et May aussi.

Je sors de la rue principale pour zigzaguer dans des ruelles bordées d'arbres où se dressent des maisons coloniales entourées de pelouses parfaitement entretenues. Nous sommes presque arrivées lorsque je comprends pourquoi le trajet jusqu'à la maison de Shellie me semble si familier. La maison de ma grand-mère, sur Lagniappe Street, est tout près.

— Hé, Court', tu veux venir faire un tour avec moi chez mamie ?

Je n'aime pas l'idée d'y aller seule, mais je viens de me dire que je trouverai peut-être des réponses dans les affaires de ma grand-mère.

Courtney baisse son téléphone et me jette un regard ébahi.

— Ça me ferait un peu bizarre, tata. Il n'y a personne, là-bas, et tous les bibelots de mamie y sont encore.

Sa lèvre inférieure se fait boudeuse. Ses grands yeux bleus me fixent d'un air sérieux. C'est dur pour les enfants d'accepter le déclin rapide de mamie Judy. C'est la première fois qu'ils sont confrontés, même de très loin, à la question de la fin de vie et de la mortalité.

— J'irai avec toi si tu as vraiment besoin de moi.

— Non, c'est bon.

Je passe Lagniappe Street sans tourner. Inutile de mêler Courtney à tout ça. Je reviendrai après l'avoir déposée chez son amie. Elle est visiblement soulagée.

— OK. Merci d'être venue me chercher, tata.

— De rien, ma grande.

Quelques minutes plus tard, elle remonte en trottant l'allée qui mène à la maison de Shellie, et je me mets en route vers Lagniappe Street, prête à un voyage dans le passé.

Une bouffée de chagrin pur me serre la gorge lorsque je m'engage dans l'allée en voiture. Où que je regarde, il y a des souvenirs. Les roses que j'aidais ma grand-mère à entretenir, le saule qui nous servait de cabane, à moi et une petite fille de la rue, la baie vitrée de l'étage en encorbellement digne du château de Cendrillon, la grande terrasse qui servait de décor pour les photos de fin d'année scolaire, les bassins où les carpes Koï multicolores pointaient à la surface pour attraper des miettes de biscuit.

Je sens presque la présence de ma grand-mère sur la galerie en bois qui longe la maison, à la façon des bâtisses coloniales de la ville de Charleston. En grimpant les marches du perron, je m'attends presque à ce qu'elle soit là. Il est dur de se rendre compte que ce n'est pas le cas. Jamais plus elle ne viendra m'accueillir ici.

Je suis la galerie jusqu'à la véranda, à l'arrière, où la porte est ouverte. Elle est défraîchie et sent la poussière. Les odeurs humides, terriennes, ont disparu. Les étagères et les pots de fleurs ont été enlevés. Ma mère les a sans doute donnés à quelqu'un qui en avait l'usage.

La clef de la maison est cachée à sa place habituelle. Elle reflète un rayon de soleil tardif lorsque j'enlève une brique descellée en bas du mur. De là, je me glisse à l'intérieur et j'éteins l'alarme. Ensuite, je reste plantée dans le salon en me demandant : Et maintenant ?

Le parquet grince sous mes pas, ce qui me fait sursauter même si c'est un bruit ancien, familier. Courtney avait raison. La maison paraît vide et lugubre, ce n'est plus le foyer qu'elle a été. À partir de mes treize ans, je venais dormir ici pendant l'année scolaire dès que mes parents étaient à Washington, comme ça je pouvais continuer à aller en classe avec mes copines.

Maintenant, je me fais l'impression d'être une fouineuse, une voleuse.

C'est idiot, de toute façon. Tu ne sais même pas ce que tu cherches.

Des photos, peut-être ? Est-ce que la femme sur la table de nuit de May Crandall se trouve aussi dans l'un des vieux albums ? Ma grand-mère a toujours été l'historienne de la famille, la gardienne de l'héritage des Stafford, celle qui, sans relâche, tape des étiquettes sur sa vieille machine à écrire pour les coller partout. Il n'y a pas un meuble, un tableau, une œuvre d'art ou une photo dans cette maison qui n'ait pas été minutieusement étiqueté avec son origine et le nom de ses propriétaires précédents. Ses effets personnels – tous ceux qui comptent pour elle – sont répertoriés de la même façon. Le bracelet libellule m'a été transmis dans une boîte patinée par le temps avec une étiquette jaune scotchée dessous.

Juillet 1966. Un cadeau. Des pierres de lune pour les premières photographies envoyées cette année de la Lune par la sonde américaine Surveyor. *Des grenats pour l'amour. Des libellules pour l'eau. Des saphirs et des onyx pour la mémoire. Créé par Greer Designs, Damon Greer, joaillier.*

En dessous, elle a ajouté :

Pour Avery,

Parce que tu es celle qui rêve des rêves nouveaux, qui ouvre de nouvelles voies.

Que les libellules t'emmènent dans des lieux qui dépassent ton imagination.

Mamie Judy

Il est étrange, et je ne m'en rends compte que maintenant, qu'elle n'ait pas précisé de qui lui venait ce cadeau. Je me demande si je peux trouver cette information dans ses carnets.

Il ne se passait pas une semaine sans qu'elle documente soigneusement les détails de ses journées, gardant trace de tous ceux qu'elle voyait, ce qu'elle portait, ce qui était servi aux repas. Si May Crandall et elle étaient amies, ou si elles jouaient au bridge dans le même club, son nom s'y trouvera sans doute.

« Un jour, tu liras ces notes et tu connaîtras tous mes secrets », m'avait-elle dit jadis quand je lui avais demandé pourquoi elle notait tout si méticuleusement.

Cette réponse sonne presque comme une permission, à présent, mais, alors que je traverse la maison sombre, je me sens un peu coupable. Ce n'est pas comme si ma grand-mère était décédée. Elle est toujours parmi nous. Ce que je fais, c'est de l'indiscrétion, et pourtant je ne peux pas me sortir de l'idée qu'elle veut que je comprenne quelque chose, que c'est important, aussi étrange que cela puisse paraître, pour nous deux.

Dans son petit bureau à côté de la bibliothèque, son dernier carnet de rendez-vous est toujours sur la table. Il est resté ouvert à la page où elle a disparu pendant huit heures et a fini perdue, et déboussolée, devant l'ancien centre commercial. Un mardi.

L'écriture est à peine lisible. Elle tremblote et penche. Elle ne ressemble pas du tout au joli script arrondi de ma grand-mère. Trent Turner, Edisto, c'est la seule chose notée ce jour-là.

Edisto ? Est-ce que c'est ça, qu'il s'est passé le jour où elle a disparu ? Elle a cru, pour une raison ou pour une autre, qu'elle allait au cottage de l'île d'Edisto pour… rencontrer quelqu'un ? Peut-être en avait-elle rêvé la nuit d'avant et s'était éveillée en pensant que c'était vrai ? À moins qu'elle revive des événements de son passé ?

Qui est ce Trent Turner ?

Je feuillette d'autres pages.

Je ne trouve nulle part de May Crandall parmi les rendez-vous de ma grand-mère au cours des mois passés. Pourtant, May m'a donné l'impression qu'elles s'étaient vues récemment.

Plus je remonte, plus l'écriture se clarifie. Et je retrouve les événements routiniers où je suivais jadis ma grand-mère comme son ombre : des réunions du Club des femmes de la fédération, du comité de la bibliothèque, des FRA, du club de jardinage au printemps. Cela me fait de la peine de voir que, sept mois plus tôt, avant sa dégringolade mentale, elle était encore raisonnablement en forme, à suivre sa vie sociale, même si une amie ou deux avaient glissé à mes parents que Judy avait des absences.

Je continue à feuilleter le carnet en m'interrogeant, en me souvenant, en pensant à cette année charnière. La vie peut changer du jour au lendemain. Ce carnet de notes ne fait que renforcer ma conscience nouvelle de cette vérité. Nous faisons des projets, mais nous ne contrôlons rien.

Les notes du mois de janvier de ma grand-mère commencent avec une seule ligne griffonnée de travers dans la marge, juste avant le jour de l'an. Edisto et Trent Turner, de nouveau. Puis un numéro de téléphone noté en dessous.

Elle était peut-être en relation avec une entreprise pour faire faire des travaux dans le cottage ? Dur à imaginer. L'assistante de mon père s'occupe des affaires de ma grand-mère depuis la mort de mon grand-père, il y a sept ans. S'il y avait eu des arrangements à faire, elle s'en serait occupée.

Il n'y a qu'une façon de le savoir, j'imagine.

J'attrape mon portable et je compose le numéro.

Le téléphone sonne une fois, deux fois.

Je commence à me demander ce que je vais dire si quelqu'un décroche. « Euh... je ne sais pas trop pourquoi j'appelle. J'ai trouvé votre nom dans un vieux carnet chez ma grand-mère, et... Et... quoi ? »

Un répondeur se met en route.

— Agence immobilière Turner. Trent à l'appareil. Nous ne sommes pas là pour le moment mais, si vous laissez un message...

Une agence immobilière ? J'en suis abasourdie. Est-ce que mamie Judy envisageait de vendre la maison d'Edisto ? C'est dur à imaginer. Le cottage appartenait à sa famille avant même qu'elle se marie avec mon grand-père. Elle l'adore.

Mes parents m'auraient prévenue si nous nous séparions de l'endroit. Il doit y avoir une autre explication mais, puisque je n'ai aucun moyen de le savoir, je retourne à mes fouilles.

Je trouve le reste de ses carnets dans une bibliothèque ancienne en bois, là où ils ont toujours été. Ils sont bien rangés par ordre chronologique, depuis l'année où elle a épousé mon grand-père jusqu'à aujourd'hui. Pour le plaisir, je sors le plus ancien. La couverture de cuir d'un blanc laiteux est sèche et parcourue de crevasses marron si bien qu'on dirait un morceau de porcelaine antique. À l'intérieur, l'écriture est pleine de boucles, presque enfantine. Les pages sont remplies de soirées de clubs d'étudiantes, de dates d'examen, d'enterrements de vie de jeune fille, de motifs de services de table et de rendez-vous le soir avec mon grand-père.

Dans l'une des marges, elle s'est entraînée à signer de son futur nom d'épouse, les arabesques des lettres témoignant de l'ivresse du premier amour.

Sur une page, elle a noté :

Visite chez les parents d'Harold à Drayden Hill. Séance d'équitation. Saut de plusieurs obstacles. Harold dit de le cacher à sa mère. Elle nous veut en un seul morceau pour le mariage. J'ai trouvé mon prince charmant. Sans le moindre doute.

L'émotion me noue la gorge. Une émotion douce-amère.

« Sans le moindre doute. »

Est-ce qu'elle le pensait vraiment ? Est-ce qu'elle avait vraiment... senti que mon grand-père était le bon quand elle l'a rencontré ? Est-ce que Elliot et moi, nous aurions dû avoir ce genre de... coup de foudre, plutôt qu'une évolution tranquille passant de nos jeux d'enfants à une amitié entre adultes, puis aux rendez-vous galants et enfin aux fiançailles, parce qu'au bout de six ans on a l'impression que c'est le moment ? Est-ce qu'il y a quelque chose qui cloche, entre nous, parce que ça s'est fait tranquillement, sans précipitation ?

Mon portable sonne et, quand je l'attrape, je prie pour que ce soit lui.

La voix que j'entends est masculine et amicale, mais ce n'est pas celle d'Elliot.

— Bonjour, Trent Turner à l'appareil. J'ai reçu un appel de ce numéro. Désolé de vous avoir raté. Qu'est-ce que je peux faire pour vous ?

— Oh... euh... dis-je, incapable de trouver mieux pour briser la glace avant de balancer : J'ai trouvé votre nom dans l'agenda de ma grand-mère.

J'entends des bruits de papier en arrière-fond.

— Est-ce que nous avions un rendez-vous prévu ici, à Edisto ? Pour chercher un cottage ? Ou une location peut-être ?

— Je ne sais pas trop. En fait, j'espérais que vous pourriez me le dire. Ma grand-mère a des problèmes de santé. J'essaie de comprendre les notes sur son carnet.

— Quel jour avions-nous rendez-vous ?

— Je ne suis pas certaine qu'elle en avait un. Je me disais qu'elle avait peut-être appelé pour vendre un bien. Le cottage Myers.

Dans la région, il n'est pas rare que les propriétés soient connues sous le nom de leurs anciens propriétaires. Les parents de ma grand-mère avaient fait construire la maison d'Edisto pour échapper aux étés trop chauds et moites de l'intérieur des terres.

— C'est au nom de Mme Stafford. Judy Stafford.

Je me prépare au changement de ton qui suit invariablement l'annonce de ce nom. Partout dans l'État, les gens nous adorent ou nous haïssent mais, en tout cas, ils savent qui nous sommes.

— Staff... for... Stafford... marmonne-t-il.

Il n'est peut-être pas d'ici ? Maintenant que j'y pense, son accent ne ressemble pas du tout à celui de Charleston. Ce n'est pas non plus celui de la région de Lowcountry, pourtant, il a un petit côté traînant. Du Texas, peut-être ? J'ai passé une partie de mon enfance à fréquenter des enfants d'ailleurs, ce qui fait que je suis douée pour reconnaître les accents, à la fois américains et étrangers.

Un silence bizarre s'installe. Il reprend d'un ton plus réservé :

— Je ne suis là que depuis neuf mois, mais je peux vous promettre que personne n'a appelé pour vendre ou louer le cottage Myers. Je suis désolé de ne pouvoir rien faire de plus pour vous.

Je sens qu'il essaie soudain de se débarrasser de moi. Pourquoi ?

— Si c'était avant le premier de l'an, mon grand-père, Trent Sr., était sans doute son interlocuteur. Il est décédé il y a six mois.

— Oh. Toutes mes condoléances, dis-je en me sentant aussitôt proche de lui, et pas seulement parce qu'il se trouve dans un lieu qui m'a toujours été cher. Vous avez une idée de la raison pour laquelle ma grand-mère était en contact avec lui ?

Une autre pause gênée, comme s'il pesait soigneusement ses mots.

— Pour être franc, oui. Il avait des papiers pour elle. C'est vraiment tout ce que je peux vous dire.

L'avocate en moi bondit. Je flaire le témoin qui cache des informations.

— Quel genre de papiers ?

— Je suis désolé. J'ai fait une promesse à mon grand-père.

— Quel genre de promesse ?

— Si elle vient ici en personne, je pourrai lui donner l'enveloppe qu'il a laissée pour elle.

Des sonnettes d'alarme retentissent dans ma tête. Qu'est-ce que c'est que cette histoire, bon sang ?

— Elle n'est pas en état de voyager.

— Dans ce cas, je ne peux rien pour vous. Désolé.

Sur ces mots, il raccroche.

10

Rill

Le silence et une odeur d'humidité règnent dans la pièce. J'ouvre les yeux, les referme très vite, les laisse se rouvrir tout doucement. Une brume de sommeil m'enveloppe encore l'esprit si bien que je ne vois pas très bien. Comme le brouillard du fleuve qui se glisse la nuit à travers les vitres de la cabine de notre bateau.

Rien n'est à sa place. Au lieu des portes et des fenêtres de l'*Arcadie* se dressent d'épais murs de pierre. L'air sent comme les compartiments fermés où on conserve les caisses de provisions et de combustible. L'odeur de moisi et de terre humide rampe jusqu'à mon nez et s'y tapit.

J'entends Lark gémir dans son sommeil. Et des grincements de charnières au lieu du doux bruissement des couchettes de Lark et Fern.

Je cligne des yeux, lève la tête et distingue une minuscule fenêtre très haut, près du plafond. La lumière du matin parvient à passer à travers, mais elle est fade et grisâtre.

Un buisson gratte la vitre. Ses branches produisent un petit couinement. Une rose miteuse pendouille, à moitié brisée.

Tout me revient d'un seul coup. Je me rappelle m'être couchée sur le matelas empestant l'humidité, fixant la rose par la fenêtre tandis que le jour déclinait, et que les respirations de mon frère et mes sœurs s'allongeaient, ralentissaient tout autour de moi.

Je me rappelle l'employée en blanc nous conduisant en bas des escaliers, devant la chaudière et les tas de charbon, jusqu'à cette petite pièce.

« Vous dormirez ici jusqu'à ce qu'on sache si vous restez pour de bon. Pas de bruit et pas de chahut. Vous devez rester sages. Et ne pas quitter vos lits. » Elle nous a montré du doigt cinq lits pliants, du genre que les soldats utilisent parfois dans leurs camps d'entraînement le long du fleuve.

Puis elle est partie en fermant la porte derrière elle.

Nous nous sommes blottis en silence sur nos lits, même Camellia. Moi, j'étais surtout contente que nous nous retrouvions de nouveau seuls, tous les cinq. Pas d'employées, pas d'autres enfants nous fixant de leurs regards curieux, inquiets, tristes, méchants, vides, morts et durs.

Tout ce qui s'est passé hier défile dans ma tête comme au cinématographe. Je vois l'*Arcadie*, les policiers, Silas, la voiture de Mlle Tann, la file pour le bain à l'étage. Un frisson me descend de la tête aux pieds. Il m'avale comme un remous d'eau croupie, réchauffée par le soleil de l'été, empoisonnée par tout ce qui est tombé dedans.

Je me sens sale, aussi bien dedans que dehors. Et cela n'a rien à voir avec l'eau du bain trouble, brunie par le sable et le savon de tous les enfants passés avant moi, y compris mes sœurs et Gabion.

Au lieu de quoi, je vois l'employée qui se dresse au-dessus de moi pendant que j'entre dans le bain, lui tournant le dos pour me cacher.

— Lave-toi, dit-elle en pointant le savon et le linge. On a pas le temps de traînasser. Vous, les chie dans l'eau, vous z'êtes pas trop connus pour vot' pudeur, de toute façon, pas vrai ?

Je ne sais pas ce qu'elle veut dire ni ce que je dois répondre. Je ne suis peut-être pas censée répondre.

— Je t'ai dit de te laver ! hurle-t-elle. Tu crois que j'ai toute la journée ?

Je sais déjà que ce n'est pas le cas. Je l'ai entendue beugler la même chose aux autres enfants. J'ai entendu des gémissements, des geignements et des crachotements lorsque des têtes se retrouvaient sous l'eau pour être rincées. Heureusement, aucun de nous, les enfants Foss, ne craignons de mettre la tête sous l'eau. Les petits et même Camellia ont fait la queue sans trop de souci. Je veux faire la même chose, sauf que la femme a l'air de m'avoir dans le nez, peut-être parce que je suis l'aînée.

Je m'accroupis au-dessus de l'eau parce qu'elle est sale et froide.

Elle s'approche pour me regarder de plus près et me fixe d'une façon qui me donne la chair de poule.

— En fait, t'es pas si grande que tu peux pas être avec les petits. Mais ça va pas durer, on devra bientôt te mettre ailleurs.

Je tourne un peu plus l'épaule et me lave aussi vite que possible.

Ce matin, je me sens encore sale après avoir senti quelqu'un me scruter comme ça. J'espère qu'on sera partis d'ici avant le jour du prochain bain.

Je veux que la petite rose dehors se volatilise. Je veux que la fenêtre se transforme, que les murs deviennent du bois, que le sol de ciment change, fonde et disparaisse. Je veux un vieux parquet patiné par nos pieds et le fleuve qui ondule sous nos lits et la douce mélodie que Briny joue à l'harmonica dehors sur le pont.

Je me suis réveillée au moins dix fois pendant la nuit. Au petit jour, Fern se glisse près de moi, la toile du lit s'affaisse et nous rapproche tant l'une de l'autre que c'est un miracle qu'elle puisse respirer, sans parler de dormir.

Chaque fois que je me laisse sombrer, je me retrouve sur l'*Arcadie*. Chaque fois que je me réveille, je me retrouve ici, dans cet endroit, et j'essaie de comprendre.

« Vous dormirez ici jusqu'à ce qu'on sache si vous restez pour de bon... »

Comment ça... pour de bon ? Ils ne vont pas nous emmener voir Briny et Queenie à l'hôpital, maintenant que nous avons passé la nuit ici et que nous nous sommes lavés ? Est-ce que nous irons tous les voir, ou juste certains d'entre nous ? Je ne peux pas laisser les petits ici. Et si ces gens leur faisaient du mal ?

Je dois protéger mon frère et mes sœurs, mais je ne peux même pas me protéger moi-même.

Les larmes poissent ma bouche. Je me suis dit que je ne pleurerai pas. Que ça ne ferait qu'effrayer les petits. Je leur ai promis que tout irait bien et, jusqu'à maintenant, ils m'ont crue, même Camellia.

Je ferme les yeux, m'enroule autour de Fern, laisse les larmes couler et tremper ses cheveux. Les sanglots me soulèvent le ventre et compressent ma poitrine, et je les ravale comme des hoquets. Fern continue de dormir profondément. Peut-être que son rêve lui faire croire que c'est juste le fleuve qui berce son lit.

Ne t'endors pas, me dis-je. Je dois reposer Fern dans son propre lit pliant avant que quelqu'un vienne. Je ne dois pas nous attirer d'ennuis. La dame nous a dit de ne pas quitter nos lits.

Juste une minute ou deux. Juste une minute ou deux, et puis je me lèverai et je m'assurerai que tout le monde est bien là où il doit être.

Je dérive, m'éveille, dérive, m'éveille. Mon cœur cogne fort contre mes côtes lorsque j'entends quelqu'un respirer tout près – pas l'un d'entre nous, quelqu'un de plus grand. Un homme. C'est peut-être Briny.

À peine ai-je cette idée que des odeurs de vieille graisse, d'herbe verte, de poussière de charbon et de sueur se glissent dans la pièce. Ce n'est pas Briny. Lui, il sent l'eau du fleuve et le ciel. La brume du matin l'été et le gel et le feu de bois l'hiver.

Mon esprit s'éclaircit et j'écoute. Des pieds font deux pas sur le seuil, puis s'arrêtent. Ce n'est pas la démarche de Briny.

Je remonte les couvertures sur la tête de Fern, j'espère qu'elle ne se réveillera pas, qu'elle ne bougera pas à cet instant. Il fait encore très sombre, seule une vague lumière entre par la fenêtre. Il ne remarquera peut-être pas que Fern n'est pas dans son lit.

Quand je tourne la tête, je le vois à peine du coin de l'œil. Il est massif, plus grand et plus gros que Briny, et de loin, mais c'est tout ce que je vois. Ce n'est qu'une ombre, qui se dresse là. Il ne bouge pas, ne dit rien. Il reste là, à nous regarder.

Même si j'ai le nez qui coule à force de pleurer, je ne l'essuie pas, je ne renifle pas. Je ne veux pas qu'il sache que je suis réveillée. Qu'est-ce qu'il fait là ?

Camellia se tourne dans son lit.

Non, me dis-je. Chut. Est-ce qu'elle le regarde ? Est-ce qu'il peut voir si ses yeux sont ouverts ?

Il entre dans la pièce. Avance, s'arrête, avance, s'arrête. Il se penche sur le lit de Lark, touche son oreiller. Il trébuche un peu et bute dans le cadre en bois.

Je l'observe par la fente de mes yeux à demi clos. Il s'approche de mon lit, ensuite, et se penche un instant. L'oreiller crisse près de ma tête. Il le frôle deux fois, très légèrement.

Puis, après s'être arrêté aux autres lits, il finit par partir, par fermer la porte.

Je relâche le souffle que je retenais, inspire profondément et reconnais l'odeur de la menthe poivrée. Quand je rabats les couvertures et que je réveille Fern, il y a deux petits bonbons sur l'oreiller. Ils me font aussitôt penser à Briny. Quand Briny rapporte de l'argent des salles de billard ou qu'il travaille sur un bateau-théâtre à quai, il revient toujours à l'*Arcadie* avec un rouleau de bonbons Beech-Nut Luster-Mints dans la poche. Ce sont les meilleurs. Briny nous pose des devinettes et, si nous trouvons la bonne réponse, on gagne un bonbon. « S'il y a deux cardinaux dans un arbre et un au sol, trois merles bleus dans un buisson et quatre au sol, et une grande et vieille corneille sur la clôture et une chouette dans la grange, combien y a-t-il d'oiseaux au sol ? »

Plus on grandit, plus les devinettes deviennent compliquées. Plus les questions sont dures, plus les bonbons Beech-Nut sont bons.

L'odeur de menthe me donne envie de courir jusqu'à la porte et de regarder derrière pour voir si Briny est là. Mais ces bonbons ne sont pas les mêmes. Ils n'impriment pas la bonne forme au creux de ma main quand je les ramasse et que je vais reposer Fern dans son lit.

Près de la porte, Camellia gobe le sien et le croque aussitôt.

J'envisage de laisser les bonbons sur les oreillers des petits mais, à la place, je décide qu'il vaut mieux les ramasser. Si les employées viennent, j'ai peur que ces bonbons nous attirent des ennuis.

— Voleuse !

C'est la première fois que Camellia ouvre la bouche depuis que nous avons fait la queue pour aller au bain, la veille au soir. Elle est assise dans son lit, l'épaule de sa chemise de nuit bien trop grande lui tombant jusqu'au coude. Après le bain, l'une des employées a fouillé dans une pile de linge et nous a trouvé de vieux vêtements de nuit.

— Il nous en a donné un à chacun. Tu ne peux pas les garder tous pour toi. C'est pas juste.

— Chut ! fais-je, parce qu'elle est si bruyante que je m'attends à ce que la porte s'ouvre à la volée et qu'on soit tous punis. Je les garde pour plus tard, pour tout le monde.

— T'es qu'une voleuse.

— Pas du tout.

Évidemment, Camellia est redevenue elle-même, aujourd'hui et, comme tous les matins, elle est de mauvaise humeur. Elle a toujours des réveils difficiles, même avec des bonbons à la menthe. La plupart du temps, je lui rends la monnaie de sa pièce mais, là, je suis trop fatiguée pour ça.

— Je les garde pour plus tard, je t'ai dit. Je veux pas qu'on ait d'ennuis.

Les épaules de ma sœur s'affaissent.

— Des ennuis, on en a déjà, répond-elle, et ses cheveux noirs tombent devant ses yeux, aussi emmêlés que les crins d'un cheval. Qu'est-ce qu'on va faire, Rill ?

— On va être sages, pour que ces gens nous emmènent voir Briny. Tu ne dois plus essayer de t'enfuir, Camellia. Tu ne peux pas te battre contre eux, d'accord ? Si nous les mettons en colère, ils ne nous conduiront pas à l'hôpital.

Elle me fixe durement, ses yeux noisette si plissés qu'elle ressemble aux Chinois qui lavent le linge dans les villes fluviales, sur la rive, dans leurs grandes bassines.

— Tu crois vraiment qu'ils vont nous y emmener ? Aujourd'hui ?

— Si on est sages.

J'espère que ce n'est pas un mensonge, mais je n'en suis pas sûre.

— Pourquoi est-ce qu'il nous ont amenés ici ? demande-t-elle, la gorge nouée. Ils pouvaient pas nous laisser tranquilles ?

Je réfléchis à toute vitesse, j'essaie de comprendre. Je dois trouver une explication, pour moi comme pour Camellia.

— Je pense qu'ils ont fait une erreur. Ils ont dû croire que Briny ne reviendrait pas pour s'occuper de nous. Briny leur dira que si, dès qu'il verra qu'on n'est plus là. Il leur expliquera que quelqu'un a fait une grosse erreur et il nous ramènera à la maison.

— Aujourd'hui, c'est sûr ?

Son menton tremble et elle remonte sa lèvre inférieure, pincée comme quand elle s'apprête à se battre avec un garçon.

— Je te le parie. Je parie qu'il va venir aujourd'hui.

Elle renifle et essuie sa morve sur son bras.

— Hors de question que ces femmes me recollent dans la baignoire, Rill. Je les laisserai plus me toucher.

— Qu'est-ce qu'elles t'ont fait, Camellia ?

— Rien, dit-elle, le menton en avant. Mais je les laisserai pas recommencer, c'est tout.

Elle tend la main vers moi.

— Si tu veux pas distribuer les bonbons aux autres, donne-les-moi. Je meurs de faim.

— On les garde pour plus tard... S'ils nous laissent sortir là où jouaient les autres enfants hier, je les distribuerai.

— Tu as dit que Briny allait venir tout à l'heure.

— Je ne sais pas quand. Je sais juste qu'il va venir.

Elle hausse les sourcils comme si elle n'en croyait pas un mot, puis se tourne vers la porte.

— Peut-être que cet homme peut nous aider à sortir d'ici. Celui qui nous a apporté des bonbons. C'est notre ami.

J'y ai déjà pensé. Mais qui est cet homme ? Pourquoi est-il entré ici ? Est-ce qu'il veut vraiment être notre ami ? C'est le premier à se montrer gentil envers nous, dans la maison de Mme Murphy.

— On va attendre Briny, dis-je. On doit être sages jusque-là, c'est...

La poignée de porte cliquette. Camellia et moi nous laissons tomber sur nos lits au même instant pour faire semblant de dormir. Mon cœur bat à toute vitesse sous la couverture rugueuse. Qui est là ? Notre nouvel ami ou quelqu'un d'autre ? Est-ce qu'il ou elle nous a entendues parler ?

J'ai bientôt la réponse à mes questions. Une femme aux cheveux châtains portant une robe blanche entre dans la chambre. Je l'observe de sous la couverture, par un coin si élimé qu'on voit au travers. Elle est aussi trapue qu'un bûcheron, et sa taille est épaisse. Ce n'est pas l'une de celles qu'on a vues hier.

Sur le seuil, elle fronce les sourcils, regarde nos lits puis les clefs dans sa main.

— Lefez-vous, fous tous !

Elle parle comme la famille de Norvégiens dont le bateau est resté arrimé un peu plus bas que le nôtre pendant un mois l'été dernier. Elle dit « fous » au lieu de « vous », mais je la comprends quand même. Elle n'a pas l'air fâchée, juste très, très fatiguée.

— Tebout ! Et pliez les coufertures !

On se lève tous, sauf Gabion. Je dois le tirer du lit, il trébuche et tombe sur les fesses pendant que je m'occupe de son linge.

— Quelqu'un t'autre est fenu cette nuit, non ?

Elle tient une clef entre deux doigts.

Est-ce qu'on doit lui dire, pour l'homme aux bonbons à la menthe ? Peut-être qu'il n'avait pas le droit d'entrer dans notre chambre ? Peut-être qu'on aura des ennuis s'ils découvrent qu'on n'a rien dit.

— Non, m'dame. Personne d'autre. Juste nous, répond Camellia avant moi.

— Et toi, tu es la fauteuse de troubles, à ce qu'on m'a dit.

Elle braque un regard dur vers Camellia, qui se ratatine un peu.

— Non, m'dame.

— Personne n'est entré, dis-je.

Je suis bien obligée de confirmer. Qu'est-ce que je peux faire d'autre, après le mensonge de ma sœur ?

— Sauf si c'est arrivé pendant qu'on dormait.

La femme tire la cordelette de la lampe au plafond. Elle clignote et nous battons des paupières, aveuglés.

— Cette porte aurait tû être fermée. Elle l'était, n'est-ce pas ?

— On sait pas, répond Camellia. On est restés au lit toute la nuit.

La femme me regarde, je hoche la tête, puis je m'active à ranger la chambre. Je voudrais me débarrasser des bonbons mais j'ai trop peur pour ça, du coup, je les garde serrés dans ma main, ce qui ne m'aide pas à plier les couvertures mais la dame ne remarque rien. En fait, elle est surtout pressée de nous faire sortir de là.

Quand on sort pour de bon, je vois l'homme massif debout, là, dans le sous-sol, appuyé contre un manche à balai, près de la grosse chaudière noire pourvue d'une rangée d'ouvertures qui lui dessinent comme une bouche de citrouille d'Halloween. L'homme nous regarde passer. Camellia lui sourit, et il lui rend son sourire. Ses dents sont vieilles et hideuses, et ses cheveux châtains clairsemés pendouillent devant son visage en queue de rat graisseuse mais, malgré tout, son sourire fait plaisir à voir.

On a peut-être bien un ami dans cet endroit, finalement.

— Monsieur Riggs, si fous n'afez rien à faire, occupez-fous de la branche tombée dans la cour cette nuit avant que les enfants sortent, lui ordonne la femme.

— Bien, madame Pulnik.

S'il esquisse un sourire en agitant un peu le balai tandis que Mme Pulnik commence à monter l'escalier, en vrai, il ne balaie rien du tout.

Camellia le regarde par-dessus son épaule et il lui fait un clin d'œil. Ce clin d'œil me rappelle Briny ; du coup, peut-être que j'aime bien ce M. Riggs un petit peu.

Là-haut, Mme Pulnik nous emmène dans la buanderie et nous donne des vêtements pris sur une pile de linge. Elle appelle ça des tenues de jeu, mais c'est à peine mieux que des haillons. Elle nous dit de nous habiller et d'aller aux toilettes, et nous obéissons, et le petit-déjeuner ressemble drôlement au dîner qu'on a eu hier soir après le bain – une cuillerée de bouillie de maïs. Nous sommes en retard. Les autres enfants sont déjà sortis de table pour aller jouer. Une fois qu'on a raclé nos bols, on nous dit de sortir aussi et de ne pas essayer de quitter le jardin ni la cour, sinon « Gare ! ».

— Et fous ne defez pas fous approcher de la clôture, nous met en garde Mme Pulnik en attrapant Camellia et Lark par le bras avant qu'on atteigne la porte. Un garçon a creusé un tunnel tessous hier. Mme Murphy l'a envoyé dans le placard. Aller dans le placard, c'est très très très mauvais. Dans le placard, il fait noir. Fous comprenez ?

— Oui, m'dame, dis-je d'une voix rauque en prenant Gabby dans mes bras et en tendant la main vers Lark pour qu'elle la lâche.

Ma petite sœur est immobile comme une souche, rien ne bouge chez elle sauf les larmes qui dégoulinent sur ses joues.

— Je m'assurerai qu'ils respectent les règles jusqu'à ce qu'on puisse voir notre maman et notre papa.

Mme Pulnik pince ses lèvres en cul-de-poule.

— Bien, dit-elle. C'est une sache décision. Pour fous tous.

— Oui, m'dame.

Nous sortons aussi vite que possible. Le soleil nous donne l'impression d'être au paradis, et le ciel semble immense, tendu entre les peupliers et les érables, et le sol de terre en bas des marches est frais et tendre. Sûr. Je ferme les yeux et j'écoute les murmures des feuilles et les oiseaux entonner leurs chants du matin. Je reconnais leurs voix, une par une, troglodyte de Caroline, cardinal, passereau. Les mêmes oiseaux qui étaient là hier matin quand je me suis réveillée sur notre petit bateau.

Les petites agrippent ma robe pendant que Gabby gigote dans mes bras pour essayer de descendre, et Camellia se plaint car nous restons plantés là. J'ouvre les yeux et vois qu'elle fixe la haute clôture de fer noire qui entoure la cour. Du chèvrefeuille, du houx et des azalées denses la recouvrent presque entièrement, plus haut que nos têtes. Je ne vois qu'un portail, et il donne sur le terrain de jeux derrière la salle paroissiale délabrée. La grille continue là-bas aussi.

Camellia est bien trop grande pour se glisser en dessous mais elle a l'air de chercher le meilleur endroit pour essayer quand même.

— Allons au moins jusqu'aux balançoires, geint-elle. On pourra surveiller la route, de là-bas... pour quand Briny viendra nous chercher.

Nous avançons dans la cour, moi portant Gabion, mes sœurs blotties les unes contre les autres derrière moi, même Camellia qui, d'habitude, se retrouve prise dans une bagarre dès qu'on arrive dans une nouvelle école. Les autres enfants nous fixent parce que nous sommes nouveaux. Nous faisons comme si de rien n'était. Nous sommes plutôt bons, à ce jeu – ne pas être trop amical avec les autres ; veiller les uns sur les autres ; faire comprendre aux autres que, s'ils s'en prennent à l'un de nous, ils feraient mieux d'être de taille à nous affronter tous en même temps. Mais, cette fois-ci, c'est différent. Nous ne connaissons pas les règles de cet endroit. Il n'y a pas de maîtresse qui surveille la cour. Il n'y a pas un adulte en vue. Rien que des enfants, qui arrêtent tous de sauter à la corde ou de jouer à la déli-délo.

Je ne vois pas la petite fille qui est venue du fleuve hier avec nous. Son petit frère – celui que Mlle Tann a appelé Stevie – est assis par terre avec un camion en fer-blanc qui a perdu toute sa peinture ainsi qu'une roue.

— Où est ta sœur ?

Quand je m'accroupis à côté de lui, le poids de Gabion me déséquilibre si bien que je dois poser une main au sol pour m'empêcher de tomber.

Les épaules de Stevie se lèvent et s'abaissent, et ses grands yeux bruns se remplissent de larmes.

— Tu peux venir avec nous, lui dis-je.

— Celui-là, c'est pas notre problème, grommelle Camellia.

Je lui ordonne de se taire.

Stevie fait la moue, hoche la tête et tends les bras vers moi. Il porte une grosse marque de morsure sur l'un d'eux et je me demande qui lui a fait ça. Je le prends contre moi et me relève. Il est plus âgé que Gabion, mais il pèse autant que lui. Il est maigre comme tout.

Deux filles en train de jouer avec une dînette en fer cabossée regardent vers nous. Elles ont ratissé des feuilles mortes afin de dégager un coin pour jouer à l'ombre de l'abri du puits, comme Camellia et moi le faisons parfois dans les bois.

— Vous voulez jouer ? demande l'une d'elles.

— Fichez-nous la paix, réplique Camellia. On a pas le temps. On va dans la cour d'à côté pour guetter notre papa.

— Vous feriez mieux de pas y aller.

Les filles retournent à leurs jeux et nous continuons à avancer.

Au portillon menant à la cour voisine, un grand garçon roux surgit de derrière les buissons de houx. Là, je vois qu'il y a une cachette dans les fourrés, au bout d'un tunnel. Ils sont quatre ou cinq, là-dedans, à jouer aux cartes. L'un d'eux se taille une lance avec un canif. Il me jette un coup d'œil et teste le bout pointu avec son doigt.

Le grand rouquin se tient devant le portail, les bras croisés.

— Viens par là, m'ordonne-t-il comme s'il était chargé de s'occuper de moi. Eux, ils peuvent aller jouer.

Je comprends bien ce qu'il veut dire. Il veut que j'aille me fourrer dans les buissons avec eux quatre. Sinon, mon frère et mes sœurs ne pourront pas aller aux jeux.

Je pique un fard. Je sens le sang me monter au visage. *Qu'est-ce qu'il a en tête ?*

Camellia dit tout haut ce que je viens de penser.

— On ira nulle part avec vous.

Elle écarte un peu les pieds, tend le menton, qui arrive au niveau du torse du rouquin, et ajoute :

— T'es pas notre chef.

— C'est pas à toi que je parle, mocheté. T'es un vrai laideron. On te l'a jamais dit ? J'parle à ta jolie sœur, là.

Camellia a les yeux exorbités. Elle est folle de rage.

— J'suis moins moche que toi, Poil de carotte. Ta mère a pleuré le jour où t'es né, non ? Je parie que si !

Je passe Gabion à Fern. Le petit Stevie ne veut pas qu'on le lâche. Ses bras restent crochetés à mon cou. Si nous devons nous battre, je n'ai pas besoin d'un mioche pendu à moi. Le rouquin est sans doute trop costaud pour Camellia et moi, et si ses copains sortent de leur trou, on aura vraiment de gros ennuis. Il n'y a toujours aucune employée en vue, et l'un de ces affreux jojos a un couteau.

Le rouquin a les narines qui frémissent et décroise les bras. Voilà, ça vient. Camellia a lancé un défi qu'on ne peut pas relever, cette fois-ci. Ce garçon fait au moins quinze centimètres de plus que moi, et je suis grande.

Mon esprit cavale comme un écureuil par une journée de printemps, sautant de branche en branche. *Réfléchis. Trouve quelque chose.*

« Sers-toi toujours de ta cervelle, Rill, me dit Briny dans ma tête, et tu te tireras des ennuis plus vite que l'éclair. »

— J'ai des bonbons à la menthe, dis-je soudain en plongeant la main dans la poche de ma robe d'emprunt. Je vous donne tout, mais vous devez nous laisser passer.

Le garçon a un mouvement de recul et me demande les yeux plissés :

— Tu les as eus où ?

— Je mens pas, réponds-je avec difficulté car Stevie me serre trop fort. Tu nous laisses passer ou quoi ?

— File-moi les bonbecs.

Les autres bagarreurs s'extirpent déjà de leur planque pour pouvoir attraper leur part.

— Ils sont à nous ! proteste Camellia.

— Tais-toi.

Je sors les bonbons. S'ils sont un peu sales à force d'être restés dans ma main toute la matinée, je doute que ces gars-là s'en soucient.

Le rouquin ouvre la main, et j'y lâche les pastilles. Il lève le tout si près de son visage qu'il louche, il a l'air encore plus bête qu'avant. Un sourire lent, méchant, se dessine sur ses lèvres. Une de ses dents de devant est cassée.

— C'est l'vieux Riggs qui vous les a donnés ?

Je ne veux pas attirer d'ennuis à cet homme. C'est le seul à s'être montré gentil avec nous jusqu'à maintenant.

— C'est pas tes oignons.

— C'est notre ami.

Camellia ne sait pas se taire. Peut-être qu'elle pense effrayer les garçons en leur disant que cet homme costaud nous aime bien.

Mais le rouquin continue à sourire. Il se penche vers mon oreille, si près que je sens son haleine puante et sa chaleur sur ma peau. Il murmure :

— Laisse jamais Riggs te coincer toute seule. C'est pas le genre d'ami que tu veux.

11

Avery

De la mousse espagnole drape les arbres, aussi finement ouvragée qu'un voile de mariée en dentelle. Une aigrette bleue prend son envol au-dessus du marais salant, effrayée par le passage de ma voiture. Elle vole d'abord gauchement, comme s'il lui fallait un moment pour se sentir à l'aise en l'air, pour trouver ses marques. Elle bat vigoureusement des ailes puis flotte au loin, guère pressée de redescendre sur terre.

Je sais ce que c'est. Pendant deux semaines, j'ai essayé de partir en douce pour venir dans l'île d'Edisto. Entre les réunions et les déplacements déjà programmés, puis les complications de santé de mon père, ça s'est avéré impossible.

J'ai passé les six derniers jours dans des cabinets de médecins, tenant la main de ma mère, tandis qu'on tentait de comprendre pourquoi, alors que le cancer et les saignements intestinaux étaient censés avoir été éradiqués par l'opération, mon père était de nouveau anémique et si faible qu'il tenait à peine debout. Après des examens à n'en plus finir, nous pensons avoir trouvé la cause. La solution était simple – chirurgie laparoscopique pour dissoudre des vaisseaux sanguins éclatés dans son système digestif, un problème non lié au cancer. Opération ambulatoire. Vite fait bien fait.

Sauf que rien n'est simple lorsqu'on essaie de se cacher du reste du monde, et mon père insiste pour ne révéler à personne qu'il a subi une nouvelle opération, même mineure. Leslie est complètement d'accord là-dessus. Elle a annoncé à la presse que mon père a souffert d'une grosse intoxication alimentaire ; il reprendra le programme de ses déplacements dans quelques jours.

Missy, ma grande sœur, est venue sauver les apparences en assistant à plusieurs événements de charité qui ne pouvaient être annulés.

— Tu as l'air épuisée, Avy, m'a-t-elle dit. Et si tu partais un peu, puisque Leslie a décalé tous les rendez-vous, de toute façon ? Va voir Elliot. Allison et moi, nous pourrons garder un œil sur la suite des événements à Drayden Hill.

— Merci... mais... tu en es sûre ?

— Vas-y. Parlez de votre mariage. Tu pourras peut-être le convaincre de courber l'échine sous le poids de la pression maternelle.

Je ne lui ai pas dit que, à part quelques conversations rapides, Elliot et moi n'avons même pas commencé à parler de l'organisation du mariage. Nous sommes bien trop occupés pour ça.

— Elliot a dû partir pour Milan pour rencontrer un client, mais je pense que je vais descendre à Edisto, voir notre vieille maison. Est-ce que quelqu'un y a été récemment ?

— Scott et moi y avons emmené les enfants quelques jours... oh... au printemps dernier, je pense. Le service d'entretien s'en occupe très bien. Tout sera prêt à ton arrivée. T'as bien mérité quelques jours de vacances.

J'étais déjà en train de faire ma valise avant même qu'elle ait le temps de me dire de saluer la plage de sa part. En quittant la ville, j'ai décidé de passer à la maison de retraite de May Crandall – ce que j'avais bien trop tardé à faire. Un employé m'a avertie qu'elle avait été hospitalisée suite à une infection pulmonaire. Il n'a pas pu me dire si c'était grave ni quand May devait revenir.

Ce qui signifie que ces mystérieux papiers à Edisto sont ma seule piste, du moins pour le moment. Trent Turner refuse de prendre mes appels. Point. Je n'ai pas le choix, je dois le voir en personne. L'enveloppe qu'il détient a fini par hanter mes pensées toute la journée. Ça m'obsède, j'invente des histoires dans lesquelles il joue des rôles différents. Parfois, c'est un maître chanteur qui a découvert une horrible vérité à propos de ma famille et a vendu ces informations aux opposants de mon père ; voilà pourquoi il refuse de me parler au téléphone. À d'autres moments, c'est l'homme sur la photographie de May Crandall. La femme enceinte qu'il tient contre lui est ma grand-mère, et elle a vécu une espèce de vie cachée avant d'épouser mon grand-père. Une romance d'adolescente. Un scandale étouffé pendant des générations.

Elle a abandonné l'enfant, et il a vécu ailleurs pendant tout ce temps. À présent, notre héritier dépossédé veut sa juste part de l'argent de la famille, sinon « Gare ! ».

Tous mes scénarios semblent dingues, mais ils ne sont pas complètement improbables. J'ai appris des choses en lisant entre les lignes des carnets de ma grand-mère. Mon bracelet libellule a une histoire plus complexe liée à Edisto. « Un présent magnifique pour une journée magnifique à Edisto », peut-on lire. « Juste nous. »

C'est ce « juste nous » qui me tracasse. À la page d'avant, elle a noté qu'elle venait de recevoir une lettre de mon grand-père, parti avec les enfants dans les montagnes pour la semaine.

Juste nous...

Qui donc ? Qui lui offrait des cadeaux à Edisto en 1966 ?

Ma grand-mère y allait souvent seule, au fil du temps, mais elle n'y restait pas seule. Ça, ces carnets le disaient clairement.

Est-il possible qu'elle ait eu une liaison ?

Mon estomac se soulève alors que le pont Dawhoo se dresse devant moi. Je ne peux pas y croire. Malgré la pression d'une vie vécue en public, ma famille a toujours été connue pour ses mariages solides comme le roc. Ma grand-mère aimait profondément mon grand-père. Sans compter que mamie Judy est l'une des personnes les plus droites que je connaisse. C'est un pilier de la communauté et une habituée de l'Église méthodiste. Elle ne cacherait jamais, au grand jamais, un secret au reste de la famille.

Sauf si ce secret pouvait nous nuire.

Et c'est exactement ce qui me terrifie.

C'est aussi pourquoi je ne peux pas laisser une enveloppe se promener dans la nature avec le nom de ma grand-mère dessus et je ne sais quelles informations clandestines à l'intérieur.

— Que tu le veuilles ou non, Trent Turner, j'arrive, dis-je en inhalant l'air iodé. Que voulais-tu donc à ma grand-mère ?

Pour tromper l'attente chez le médecin et dans la voiture au cours de ces dernières semaines, j'ai essayé de faire des recherches sur Trent Turner Sr., Trent Turner Jr., le grand-père et le père du Trent Turner à qui j'ai parlé au téléphone, et qui est donc Trent Turner III. J'ai cherché des liens politiques, des casiers judiciaires ou n'importe quoi qui pourrait expliquer leur rapport avec ma grand-mère. J'ai utilisé tous mes trucs d'avocate favoris. Malheureusement, je n'ai rien trouvé de concluant. Selon une nécrologie datée de sept mois dans le journal de Charleston, Trent Turner Sr., qui a partagé toute sa vie entre Charleston et Edisto, était le propriétaire de l'agence immobilière Turner. Juste un type ordinaire. Banal, quoi. Son fils, Trent Turner Jr., est marié et vit au Texas, où il possède lui aussi une agence immobilière.

Trent Turner III ne semble pas non plus sortir le moins du monde de l'ordinaire. Il a joué au base-ball à l'université de Clemson – et plutôt bien. Jusqu'à récemment, il travaillait dans l'immobilier d'entreprise principalement à New York. Un communiqué de presse local datant de quelques mois annonce qu'il a quitté la ville pour reprendre l'affaire de son grand-père à Edisto.

Je m'interroge malgré moi. Pourquoi un homme qui vendait des gratte-ciel déménagerait-il tout à coup pour un trou paumé comme Edisto où il s'occupe de bungalows côtiers et de locations saisonnières ?

Je le découvrirai bien assez tôt. J'ai cherché l'adresse de son agence. D'une façon ou d'une autre, je compte bien sortir de l'agence immobilière Turner avec l'enveloppe de ma grand-mère et tout son contenu, quoi que ce soit.

Malgré la nervosité qui me noue le ventre, la magie d'Edisto commence à agir sur moi quand je descends le pont vers l'île et que je continue sur la route, devant des petites maisons abîmées par les éléments et quelques commerces blottis parmi les pins et les chênes à feuilles persistantes. Au-dessus de moi, le ciel arbore une nuance de bleu parfaite.

Cet endroit est en grande partie fidèle à mes souvenirs. Il a un air paisible, gracieux, peu visité. Ce n'est pas pour rien si les habitants du coin disent que la vie s'écoule lentement à Edisto. Les vieux chênes se penchent au-dessus de la route, comme pour la protéger du monde extérieur. Les arbres chargés de mousse projettent des ombres denses sur la petite voiture que j'ai empruntée dans la grange de Drayden Hill pour le voyage. Les routes secondaires peuvent être un peu cahoteuses à Edisto et, de plus, venir en BMW ne me semblait pas une bonne idée étant donné mes interrogations sur le contenu de l'enveloppe et une éventuelle affaire de chantage.

L'agence immobilière Turner n'est pas difficile à trouver. Elle est ancienne mais pas nécessairement impressionnante, une villa bleu océan sur Jungle Road, à deux pâtés de maisons de la mer. Maintenant que je suis là, elle me semble vaguement familière mais, quand j'étais enfant, je n'avais aucune raison d'y entrer, évidemment.

Alors que je me gare et que je traverse le parking saupoudré de sable, je suis momentanément jalouse de l'homme que je viens voir. Je pourrais travailler dans un endroit pareil. Je pourrais même y vivre. Se réveiller au paradis, tous les matins. J'entends, tout près, des rires et des bruits venus de la plage. Des cerfs-volants colorés planent au-dessus des arbres, maintenus en l'air par une brise constante.

Deux petites filles tournent au coin de la rue, agitant derrière elles de longs rubans attachés à des bâtons. Trois femmes me passent devant à vélo, en riant. De nouveau, je me sens envieuse, et je me dis : Pourquoi est-ce que je ne viens pas ici plus souvent ? Pourquoi est-ce que je n'appelle jamais mes sœurs ou ma mère pour leur dire : « Hé, et si on lâchait tout pour aller passer quelques jours au soleil ? Passer du temps entre filles nous ferait du bien, non ? » Pourquoi Elliot et moi ne sommes-nous jamais venus ici ?

La réponse est amère, si bien que je m'y attarde pas longtemps. Nos emplois du temps sont toujours remplis par autre chose. Voilà pourquoi.

Et qui les remplit, ces emplois du temps ? Nous, j'imagine.

Enfin, souvent, on a l'impression de ne pas avoir le choix. Si on ne s'emploie pas constamment à consolider la forteresse familiale, le vent et les éléments se glisseront à l'intérieur et éroderont les accomplissements d'une douzaine de générations précédentes. La belle vie demande beaucoup d'entretien.

Je monte les marches du perron de l'agence immobilière Turner en inspirant un bon coup pour me donner du courage. Une pancarte dit : ENTREZ. C'EST OUVERT... J'obéis donc. Une clochette signale mon arrivée mais il n'y a personne derrière le comptoir.

À l'accueil, des chaises en vinyle coloré longent les murs. Un distributeur d'eau fraîche attend avec des verres en carton. Des présentoirs proposent une infinité de brochures. Une machine à pop-corn me rappelle que j'ai sauté le déjeuner. Des photos magnifiques de l'île décorent les lieux. La base du comptoir au fond de la pièce est recouverte de dessins d'enfants et de photos montrant des familles heureuses posant devant leurs nouvelles maisons de plage. Toutes les époques sont représentées. Certains clichés en noir et blanc semblent venir tout droit des années cinquante. Je m'approche pour les examiner, à la recherche de ma grand-mère. En vain.

Puisque personne ne se matérialise en sortant d'un des bureaux, je lance :

— Bonjour ? Il y a quelqu'un ?

Ils sont peut-être sortis un instant ? Un silence de mort règne dans l'agence.

Mon estomac grogne, réclamant du pop-corn.

Je suis sur le point de faire une offensive sur la machine lorsque la porte de l'agence s'ouvre. Je repose le sac à pop-corn et je me retourne.

— Bonjour ! Je ne savais pas qu'il y avait du monde.

Je reconnais Trent Turner III pour l'avoir vu sur le Net, mais c'était une photo prise de loin, de plain-pied, devant l'agence. Il était barbu et coiffé d'une casquette. Ce qui ne le flattait pas. Aujourd'hui, il est rasé de frais. Avec son pantalon en toile, ses mocassins usés portés sans chaussettes et son polo bien coupé, on l'imagine sans mal attablé à une terrasse, quelque part, sous un parasol... ou dans une pub vantant la vie tranquille en bord de mer. Il a les yeux bleus et ses cheveux blond clair juste assez longs semblent suggérer : « Moi, je vis au rythme de la plage. »

Il traverse la pièce en jonglant avec deux-trois sacs de nourriture et une boisson. Je me retiens de dévorer son butin du regard. À l'odeur, je crois reconnaître des crevettes grillées et des chips. Mon estomac offre une nouvelle protestation sonore.

— Désolée, je... il n'y avait personne quand je suis arrivée.

— J'ai fait un saut dehors pour aller me chercher à manger.

Il pose son déjeuner sur le comptoir et cherche des yeux une serviette en papier avant de se résigner à essuyer des gouttes de sauce cocktail vagabondes avec une feuille A4. Notre poignée de main est poisseuse, mais amicale.

— Trent Turner, se présente-t-il, sûr de lui. Qu'est-ce que je peux faire pour vous ?

Son sourire me pousse à le trouver aimable. Le sourire des gens habitués à ce qu'on les apprécie. Il semble... honnête, j'imagine.

— Je vous ai appelé il y a deux semaines.

Pas besoin de lui rappeler tout de suite mon nom.

— Vente ou location ?

— Pardon ?

— Le bien que vous cherchez. Est-ce que c'est pour louer ou pour acheter ?

Il farfouille visiblement dans sa banque de souvenirs. Mais il n'y a pas qu'un intérêt professionnel, chez lui. J'ai l'impression qu'il y a une touche de... quelque chose d'autre.

Je me surprends à lui rendre son sourire.

Je me sens aussitôt coupable. Est-ce qu'une femme fiancée – aussi solitaire soit-elle – devrait réagir ainsi ? C'est peut-être juste parce que Elliot et moi, nous nous sommes à peine parlé en deux semaines. Il est à Milan depuis tout ce temps. Avec le décalage horaire, c'est compliqué. Il est concentré sur son boulot. Moi, sur mes affaires de famille.

Je finis par répondre :

— Ni l'un ni l'autre.

Pas la peine de retarder davantage l'inéluctable. Le fait que ce type est beau et agréable ne change pas la réalité.

— Je vous ai appelé parce que j'ai trouvé votre numéro dans la maison de ma grand-mère.

Mon amitié à peine éclose avec Trent Turner est, sans aucun doute, vouée à être tuée dans l'œuf.

— Je suis Avery Stafford. Vous m'avez dit que vous aviez une enveloppe destinée à ma grand-mère, Judy Stafford, vous vous souvenez ? Je suis venue la récupérer.

Il change aussitôt d'attitude. Ses avant-bras musclés se croisent sur son torse sculpté et le comptoir se transforme aussitôt en table de négociations. Hostiles, les négociations.

Il semble contrarié. Très.

— Je suis désolé que vous ayez perdu votre temps en venant jusqu'ici. Je vous l'ai dit, je ne peux donner ces documents qu'à ceux à qui ils ont été adressés. Pas même aux membres de la famille.

— J'ai une procuration.

Je sors déjà le papier de mon sac à main démesuré. En tant que seule avocate de la famille, et puisque mes parents sont déjà bien occupés avec les problèmes de santé de mon père, c'est moi qui ai les pouvoirs de mamie Judy. Je les déplie et tourne les pages vers lui alors qu'il lève les mains en signe de protestation.

— Elle n'est pas en état de s'occuper de ses propres affaires. J'ai l'autorisation pour…

Il rejette mon recours sans même un regard vers les papiers.

— Ce n'est pas une affaire juridique.

— Si, puisqu'il s'agit de son courrier.

— Ce n'est pas un courrier. Il s'agit plutôt de… remettre en ordre les archives de mon grand-père.

Il détourne les yeux, regarde les palmiers agités par le vent, fuit mon insistance.

— C'est à propos du cottage d'Edisto, alors ?

Il s'agit bel et bien d'une question immobilière, en fait, mais pourquoi faire tant de secrets autour de la question ?

— Non.

Sa réponse est désespérément brève. D'habitude, quand on fait une mauvaise déduction à un témoin, il répond en nous donnant par inadvertance au moins un élément de la bonne réponse.

À l'évidence, Trent Turner n'en est pas à sa première négociation, et de loin. En fait, je sens qu'il a déjà vécu cette même négociation auparavant. Il a parlé de « ces documents » et de « ceux à qui ils étaient adressés », comme si plusieurs personnes étaient concernées. Est-ce que d'autres familles que la mienne sont retenues en otage ?

— Je refuse de partir tant que je n'ai pas découvert la vérité.

— Il y a du pop-corn.

Son trait d'humour ne fait que m'embraser un peu plus.

— Ce n'est pas une blague.

— J'en ai bien conscience.

Pour la première fois, il semble un peu compatir. Ses bras se décroisent. Une main glisse brusquement dans ses cheveux. D'épais cils châtains frôlent sa joue quand il ferme les paupières. Des rides apparaissent au coin de ses yeux, suggérant une vie antérieure sous haute pression.

— Écoutez, j'ai fait une promesse à mon grand-père… sur son lit de mort. Et croyez-moi – c'est mieux comme ça.

Je ne le crois pas. Justement.

— S'il le faut, je vous traînerai en justice pour les avoir.

— Les archives de mon grand-père ? s'esclaffe-t-il dans un rire sardonique qui me dit qu'il n'aime guère les menaces. Bonne chance à vous. Elles étaient à lui. Elles m'appartiennent, à présent. Il faudra vous contenter de ça.

— Pas si ça peut nuire à ma famille.

Son expression me dit que j'ai presque mis dans le mille. Ça me rend malade. Ma famille a vraiment un secret inavouable, enfoui là. Qu'est-ce que c'est ?

Trent soupire longuement.

— C'est juste... C'est mieux comme ça, vraiment. C'est tout ce que je peux vous dire.

Le téléphone sonne et il répond, espérant visiblement que l'interruption me poussera à partir. Son interlocuteur a dix mille questions à lui poser sur les locations de maisons de plage à Edisto et les activités qu'on trouve sur l'île. Trent prend le temps de lui parler de tout, de la pêche au grand tambour jusqu'à la chasse aux fossiles de mastodontes et aux pointes de flèche sur la plage. Il donne à son client une jolie leçon d'histoire sur les familles riches qui résidaient à Edisto avant la guerre de Sécession. Il évoque les crabes violonistes, la vase et la récolte des huîtres.

Il s'envoie quelques crevettes frites dans la bouche et les savoure tout en écoutant son interlocuteur. Il me tourne le dos, s'appuie au comptoir.

Je retourne à la chaise près de la porte et je scrute son dos pendant qu'il offre une litanie de commentaires sur Botany Bay. J'ai l'impression qu'il décrit les deux mille hectares de la réserve naturelle centimètre carré par centimètre carré. Je tape du pied et fais pianoter mes doigts. Il prétend ne rien remarquer mais je le surprends lorsqu'il me jette un coup d'œil en coin.

Je sors mon téléphone pour faire défiler mes e-mails. Dans le pire des cas, je pourrai toujours regarder sur Instagram ou Pinterest les idées que ma mère et Bitsy m'ont conseillées, pour le mariage.

Trent se penche vers un ordinateur, vérifie une information, parle location et créneaux disponibles.

Le client finit par se décider pour la date et le lieu de ses vacances idéales. Trent lui confie que ce n'est pas lui qui s'occupe des réservations. Sa secrétaire est coincée chez elle avec un bébé malade, mais il va lui envoyer un mail et elle prendra soin de confirmer tout ça.

Enfin, après ce qui m'a paru au moins trente minutes de blabla, il se redresse de toute sa hauteur et braque les yeux vers moi. Une bataille de regard s'ensuit. Cet homme est, peut-être bien, aussi entêté que moi. Malheureusement, il pourra sans doute tenir plus longtemps. Il a des vivres.

Il raccroche, se tapote la lèvre avec un doigt replié, secoue la tête et soupire :

— Même si vous campez là, ça ne changera rien.

Son agacement commence à être visible. On progresse. Je l'ai au moins ébranlé.

Je me dirige calmement vers la machine à pop-corn et le distributeur à eau, et je me sers.

Ainsi équipée pour le sit-in, je retourne m'asseoir.

Il tire un fauteuil de bureau en face de l'ordinateur, s'assied et disparaît derrière un casier à quatre tiroirs.

À la première bouchée de pop-corn, mon estomac émet un rugissement retentissant, à défaut d'être gracieux.

La barquette de crevettes apparaît soudain au bord du comptoir. Des doigts d'homme la poussent vers moi, mais il ne dit pas un mot. À cause de ce geste prévenant, je me sens coupable, et plus encore lorsque, dans un claquement résolu, il ajoute une canette de soda neuve à son offrande. Sans l'ombre d'un doute, je suis en train de lui pourrir sa journée parfaite.

Je prends une poignée de crevettes et retourne m'asseoir. En fait, la culpabilité et les crevettes, ça se marie très bien.

Des touches de clavier cliquettent. Un autre soupir monte de derrière le casier. Le temps continue de passer. Le fauteuil de bureau émet un couinement outré, comme si Trent s'était adossé brusquement.

— Chez vous, les Stafford, vous n'avez personne pour faire ce genre de truc à votre place ?

— Parfois. Mais pas dans le cas présent.

— Je suis certain que vous avez l'habitude d'obtenir ce que vous voulez.

Son insinuation est cuisante. Je me suis battue contre ça toute ma vie – l'idée que mes seules qualifications étaient d'avoir une jolie frimousse blonde et un nom de famille prestigieux. Maintenant, avec l'envolée des spéculations concernant mon avenir politique, j'en ai plus que marre de l'entendre. Mon nom de famille ne m'a en rien aidée à sortir major de promo de la fac de droit de Columbia.

— J'ai travaillé pour arriver où je suis, merci.

— Pff !

— Je ne demande aucune faveur. Et je n'en attends aucune.

— Dans ce cas, je peux appeler la police et vous faire évacuer de ma salle d'attente, comme je le ferais si une personne lambda s'incrustait ici et refusait de partir quand je le lui demande ?

Les crevettes et le pop-corn s'agglomèrent en une boule dure juste sous mon sternum. Il n'oserait pas... si ? J'imagine déjà la couverture médiatique. Leslie me pendrait haut et court.

— Ça arrive souvent ?

— Non, sauf quand quelqu'un a bu quelques bières de trop sur la plage. Et c'est plutôt rare, à Edisto. Il n'y a pas beaucoup d'agitation, par ici.

— Oui, je sais. Et j'ai l'impression que c'est l'une des raisons pour lesquelles vous ne voudrez pas mêler la police à tout ça.

— L'une des raisons ?

— J'imagine que vous n'êtes pas sans savoir que certaines personnes n'auraient pas hésité à menacer ma famille de révéler des informations qui pourraient être dévastatrices... si ces informations existaient. Et ce genre de comportement est illégal.

Trent bondit aussitôt de son fauteuil et moi du mien. Nous nous faisons face comme deux généraux ennemis.

— Vous êtes à un cheveu de faire la connaissance de la police d'Edisto.

— Qu'est-ce que votre grand-père voulait à ma grand-mère ?

— Ce n'était pas du chantage, si c'est ce que vous insinuez. Mon grand-père était un honnête homme.

— Pourquoi lui a-t-il laissé une enveloppe ?

— Ils avaient des affaires en cours.

— Quel genre d'affaires ? Pourquoi n'en a-t-elle parlé à personne ?

— Elle pensait peut-être que c'était mieux comme ça.

— Est-ce qu'elle venait ici pour... voir quelqu'un ? Est-ce qu'il l'a découvert ?

Il a un mouvement de recul, ses lèvres s'ourlent pour découvrir ses dents.

— Non !

— Alors dites-moi !

Je suis passée en mode tribunal, concentrée sur une seule chose – découvrir la vérité.

— Donnez-moi cette enveloppe !

Il abat sa main sur le comptoir, ébranle tout ce qui s'y trouve, puis le contourne en quelques pas. Nous nous retrouvons face à face. J'ai beau me dresser de toute ma hauteur, il me domine toujours. Je refuse de me laisser intimider. On va régler cette affaire. Là. Tout de suite.

La clochette de la porte retentit et j'y prête à peine attention. Je suis concentrée sur un regard bleu bordé de blanc, des dents serrées.

— Pffiou ! Qu'est-ce qu'il fait chaud, dehors ! T'as du popcorn, aujourd'hui ?

Je jette un coup d'œil par-dessus mon épaule et vois sur le seuil un homme en uniforme – un employé du parc national ou un garde-chasse, peut-être – dont le regard va et vient entre Trent Turner et moi.

— Oh, je ne savais pas que tu avais de la visite.

— Entre et mets-toi à l'aise, Ed, lance Trent avec un enthousiasme amical qui se volatilise quand il se tourne vers moi. Avery allait partir, de toute façon.

12

Rill

Ce n'est que deux semaines plus tard que j'apprends que les enfants d'ici sont des « pupilles » de la Société des foyers d'accueil du Tennessee. Je ne sais pas ce que « pupille » veut dire quand j'entends Mme Murphy le prononcer la première fois au téléphone. Je ne peux pas demander non plus, puisque je ne suis pas censée l'écouter. J'ai découvert que, si je me glissais sous les azalées qui longent la maison, je pouvais m'approcher suffisamment pour écouter à travers les moustiquaires des fenêtres de son bureau.

— Bien évidemment, tous les enfants sont des pupilles de la Société des foyers d'accueil du Tennessee, Dortha. Je comprends la situation difficile dans laquelle se trouve votre belle-fille. Lorsqu'ils sont malheureux, bien des hommes tombent dans l'alcoolisme et... le badinage. C'est tellement difficile, pour une épouse... Accueillir enfin un enfant à la maison pourrait bien égayer l'atmosphère et régler entièrement le problème. La paternité, cela vous change un homme. Je suis certaine que cela ne serait pas un problème, puisque vous n'aurez pas de difficultés à régler les frais. Oui... oui... rapidement, bien sûr. Une surprise pour leur anniversaire. Comme c'est charmant. J'ai de bien jolis chérubins, en ce moment. Évidemment, c'est Mlle Tann qui prend toutes les décisions. Je ne suis payée que pour loger les enfants.

Grâce à cette conversation, je le comprends tout de suite, le sens de ce nouveau mot. Pupille, cela désigne un enfant qui n'a jamais été récupéré par ses parents. Ici, les enfants disent que, si nos parents ne viennent pas nous chercher, Mlle Tann nous donne à d'autres adultes, qui nous emmènent chez eux. Parfois, ces gens nous gardent et parfois non. J'ai trop peur de poser des questions, car nous n'avons pas le droit d'en parler, mais je sens que c'est pour ça qu'on n'a jamais revu la grande sœur de Stevie depuis le jour de notre arrivée. Mlle Tann l'a donnée à quelqu'un. Sherry était une pupille.

Heureusement, ce n'est pas notre cas. Nous sommes à Briny, et il va venir nous chercher, dès que Queenie ira mieux. Ça prend plus de temps que je ne le pensais, et c'est pour ça que j'ai commencé à écouter sous la fenêtre de Mme Murphy. J'espère entendre des nouvelles de Briny. Quand j'interroge les employées, elles me disent juste d'être sage, sinon je devrais rester ici encore plus longtemps. Comme je ne peux rien imaginer de pire, je fais de mon mieux pour que nous soyons bien sages, tous les cinq.

Je prends un risque, en venant sous cette fenêtre comme ça, et je le sais. Nous n'avons pas le droit de nous approcher des parterres de fleurs de Mme Murphy. Si elle savait que j'épie ses conversations téléphoniques et ses discussions sur la galerie lorsque des gens viennent... j'ai quelques idées sur ce qu'elle m'infligerait.

Elle s'approche de la moustiquaire et, à travers les feuilles de l'azalée, je vois un panache de fumée de cigarette. Il s'attarde dans l'air humide comme un génie sorti de la lampe d'Aladin, et mon nez me chatouille et menace de me faire éternuer. Je me couvre le visage avec la main, une branche bouge. Un coup de marteau cogne contre mes côtes, de l'intérieur.

— Madame Pulnik ! hurle-t-elle. Madame Pulnik !

Je suis prise de sueurs froides. Ne cours pas. Ne cours pas. Des pas précipités résonnent dans le hall, à l'intérieur.

— Qu'y a-t-il, madame Murphy ?

— Dites à Riggs de mettre du poison ce soir sous les azalées. Ces maudits lapins sont revenus dans mon parterre.

— Je fais lui dire tout de suite.

— Et faites en sorte qu'il s'occupe de la cour, à l'avant, et qu'il arrache les mauvaises herbes. Dites-lui qu'il peut demander aux plus grands garçons de l'aider. Mlle Tann vient nous voir demain. L'endroit doit être présentable, sinon « Gare ! ».

— Bien, madame Murphy.

— Que deviennent les petits dans l'infirmerie ? Le jeune garçon aux yeux violets, en particulier. Mlle Tann veut le voir. Elle l'a promis pour une commande à New York.

— Il est léthargique, j'en ai bien peur. Il est très maigre, aussi. Il mange peu de porridge. Je ne crois pas qu'il puisse foyager.

— Voilà qui ne va pas plaire à Mlle Tann. Et ça ne me plaît pas non plus. On pourrait croire que, après avoir grandi au fond des ruelles et dans les caniveaux, ces petits mioches des rues seraient plus résistants.

— C'est frai, oui. L'état de la fille à l'infirmerie se dégrade aussi. Depuis deux jours, elle refuse de manger. Il faudrait peut-être appeler le docteur, oui ?

— Non, bien sûr que non. Au nom du ciel, pourquoi appellerais-je le docteur pour une petite diarrhée ? Les enfants ont toujours la courante. Donnez-lui de la racine de gingembre. Voilà qui devrait faire l'affaire.

— Comme fous foulez.

— Et comment va le petit Stevie ? Il est à peu près de la même taille que le garçon à l'infirmerie. Un peu plus vieux, mais ça peut être changé. De quelle couleur sont ses yeux ?

— Marron. En revanche, il a pris l'habitude de mouiller son lit. Et il refuse de dire le moindre mot. Je ne crois pas qu'un client serait content de lui.

— Cela n'est pas tolérable. Attachez-le dans son lit et laisse-le dedans pendant une journée entière s'il le mouille de nouveau. Une ampoule ou deux, ça lui apprendra. Dans tous les cas, des yeux marron n'iront pas pour cette commande. Bleu, violet ou vert. Cela a été spécifié très clairement. Pas marron.

— Robby ?

Ma gorge se serre. Robby, c'est comme ça qu'elles appellent mon petit frère. Il n'y a pas d'autres Robby dans la maison.

— Non, je le crains. Les cinq ont été réservés pour une présentation particulière.

Je ravale la boule de feu qui me noue la gorge et la fait descendre jusqu'à mon estomac. « Une présentation particulière. » Je crois que je sais ce que ça veut dire. J'ai vu des parents venir ici de temps en temps. Ils attendent sur le perron et les employées leur amènent leurs enfants, bien lavés, bien habillés, bien peignés. Les parents leur donnent des présents et les serrent dans leurs bras et pleurent lorsqu'ils doivent repartir. Ça doit être ça, une présentation.

Briny va bientôt venir nous voir.

Mais ça m'inquiète aussi. La semaine dernière, un homme est venu voir son fils, et Mme Murphy lui a dit qu'il n'était plus là. « Il a été placé. Je suis vraiment navrée. » Voilà ce qu'elle a dit.

— Il est forcément là, a protesté l'homme. Lonnie Kemp. C'est mon petit gars. J'ai pas signé de papiers pour qu'il soit adopté. Le foyer l'accueille juste le temps que je retombe sur mes pieds.

Ça n'a pas ébranlé Mme Murphy, même quand l'homme a fondu en larmes.

— Il n'est plus là, malgré tout. Le juge des affaires familiales a décidé que cela valait mieux pour lui. Il a été accueilli par des parents qui pourront subvenir à tous ses besoins.

— Mais c'est mon fils.

— Ne soyez pas égoïste, monsieur Kemp. Ce qui est fait est fait. Pensez à l'enfant. Il recevra tout ce que vous n'auriez jamais pu lui offrir.

— C'est mon fils…

L'homme est tombé à genoux et a sangloté, là, sur le perron.

Mme Murphy s'est contentée de rentrer et de fermer la porte. Au bout d'un moment, M. Riggs est venu relever l'homme pour le raccompagner à la rue et le remettre au volant de sa fourgonnette. Il est resté assis là toute la journée, à regarder la cour, à la recherche de son fils.

J'ai peur que Briny ait le même problème, lorsqu'il viendra. Sauf que Briny ne restera pas là à pleurer. Il défoncera la porte et il se passera quelque chose d'horrible. M. Riggs est un homme imposant. Mlle Tann connaît la police.

— Prenez le plus grand soin du petit garçon à l'infirmerie, ordonne Mme Murphy. Donnez-lui un bon bain chaud et un peu de crème glacée. Un biscuit au gingembre, peut-être. Dorlotez-le un peu. Je demanderai à Mlle Tann si elle peut reporter la commande d'un jour ou deux. Je veux qu'il soit en état de voyager. Vous comprenez ?

— Oui, madame Murphy.

Mme Pulnik crache sa réponse à travers ses dents serrées, signe qu'il vaudrait mieux pour moi qu'elle ne me surprenne pas sous les azalées aujourd'hui. Quand elle est de cette humeur, on a intérêt à courir vite et à bien se cacher, parce qu'elle cherche quelqu'un pour se passer les nerfs.

La dernière chose que j'entends, c'est Mme Murphy qui traverse la pièce et hurle dans le couloir :

— Et n'oubliez pas qu'il faut empoisonner ces lapins !

Je ramasse une branche brisée et je pousse sans bruit des feuilles sur l'empreinte de mes genoux pour que M. Riggs ne se rende pas compte que j'étais là. Je ne voudrais pas qu'il le dise à Mme Pulnik.

Mais ce n'est pas ce qui me fait le plus peur. Ce qui me fait le plus peur, c'est que M. Riggs sache que quelqu'un est venu ici. Pour arriver jusqu'aux azalées, on doit se glisser devant les portes du sous-sol. Riggs les laisse ouvertes et, s'il peut, il y entraîne des enfants, par tous les moyens possibles. Personne ne raconte ce qui se passe en bas, même les plus grands garçons. « Si quelqu'un en parle, disent-ils, Riggs l'attrape, lui brise la nuque et dit qu'il est tombé d'un arbre ou qu'il a trébuché sur les marches du perron. Ensuite, il transporte son corps dans une brouette jusqu'aux marais et le donne à manger aux crocos, et personne n'entend plus jamais parler de lui ou d'elle. »

James, le grand rouquin, est là depuis suffisamment longtemps, il l'a vu arriver pour de vrai. On lui donne des bonbons à la menthe, et il nous dit ce que nous devons savoir pour vivre ici, chez Mme Murphy. Nous ne sommes pas amis mais, avec des bonbons, on achète plein de choses, ici. Tous les matins, à notre réveil, il y a un petit tas de bonbons glissés sous la porte de notre chambre. La nuit, j'entends M. Riggs rôder. Il essaie de tourner la poignée, sauf qu'elle est fermée à clef, et les employées emportent toujours le trousseau lorsqu'elles nous couchent le soir. Et tant mieux. Parfois, j'entends M. Riggs monter à l'étage après être passé devant notre porte. Je ne sais pas où il va, mais je suis contente que nous soyons en bas, au sous-sol. Il fait froid, les lits de camp grattent et sentent mauvais, et nous devons utiliser un pot de chambre la nuit mais, au moins, personne ne peut nous attraper dans notre sommeil.

J'espère que Briny viendra avant que des lits se libèrent en nombre suffisant pour qu'on nous fasse monter à l'étage.

Riggs est justement sur le seuil de la porte du sous-sol lorsque j'arrive au bout du buisson d'azalées. Je le vois juste à temps pour reculer d'un pas et laisser les branches se refermer sur moi.

Même s'il regarde dans ma direction avant de descendre les marches, il ne peut pas me voir. Je suis de nouveau comme l'Homme invisible. La Fille invisible. Voilà qui je suis.

J'attends jusqu'à ce que je sois sûre qu'il est parti, puis je sors de ma cachette en rampant, aussi discrète qu'un petit lynx. Les lynx sont trop forts, car ils peuvent être à cinquante centimètres de nous sans qu'on les remarque. J'inspire un bon coup, je passe en courant devant la porte du sous-sol et je contourne le figuier. Après le figuier, on est en sécurité. Riggs sait que les employées regardent souvent par les fenêtres. Il ne fera rien si quelqu'un peut le voir.

Camellia m'attend de l'autre côté de la petite colline, derrière la cour de la salle paroissiale. Lark et Fern sont assises de chaque côté d'une bascule, avec Gabion au milieu. Stevie est assis par terre, à côté de Camellia. Il me grimpe sur les genoux dès que je m'assieds.

— Tant mieux, râle Camellia. Il va enfin me lâcher. Il pue la pisse.

— C'est pas sa faute.

Stevie me passe les bras autour du cou et se blottit contre moi. Il est poisseux et sent mauvais. Quand je lui frotte la tête, il gémit et s'écarte. Il y a un œuf de pigeon sous ses cheveux. Ici, les employées aiment taper les enfants sur la tête, là où ça ne se voit pas.

— Si, c'est sa faute, rétorque Camellia. Il pourrait parler aussi, s'il voulait. Il s'attire des ennuis avec les dames de service, en plus. Je lui ai dit qu'il ferait mieux d'arrêter, sinon gare à lui.

Camellia a un sacré culot de dire ça. Si l'un d'entre nous se retrouve au placard pendant notre séjour ici, ce sera elle. Je ne sais toujours pas ce qui arrive, dans ce placard, mais ça doit être horrible. Il y a tout juste deux jours, Mme Murphy s'est dressée devant la table du petit-déjeuner et nous a dit : « Quand on aura attrapé le voleur de nourriture, il ira au placard, et pas que pour un jour. »

Depuis, plus rien n'a disparu du garde-manger.

— Stevie a peur, c'est tout. Sa sœu...

Je me retiens de finir ma phrase. Il sera encore plus triste si je parle de sa sœur. Parfois, j'oublie que, même s'il ne parle plus, il comprend toujours tout ce qu'on dit.

— Qu'est-ce que t'as entendu, à la fenêtre ?

Camellia déteste le fait que je n'autorise personne d'autre à aller sous les azalées. Elle me scrute et me renifle chaque fois que je reviens, pour savoir si j'ai trouvé des bonbons à la menthe pendant que j'y étais. Elle croit que les garçons mentent, pour M. Riggs. Si je ne la surveille pas, elle essaiera d'y aller en douce pendant que nous jouons dehors. Je ne peux pas lui tourner le dos cinq secondes, sauf si je lui confie la garde des petits pour m'éloigner.

— Elle n'a rien dit sur Briny.

J'essaie toujours de comprendre ce que j'ai entendu sous la fenêtre de Mme Murphy. Je ne sais pas ce que je dois répéter ou non à Camellia.

— Il viendra pas. Il s'est retrouvé en taule ou j'sais pas quoi et il peut plus sortir. Queenie est morte.

Je me relève aussitôt, sans lâcher Stevie.

— C'est pas vrai ! Ne dis pas des trucs comme ça, Mellia !
Je te l'interdis !

Dans la cour, la bascule s'arrête et des pieds raclent le sol
pour immobiliser les balançoires. Les enfants se sont tournés
vers nous. Ils ont l'habitude de voir les grands se bagarrer,
rouler au sol en donnant des coups de pied et de poing. Ça
n'arrive que rarement chez les filles.

— Si, c'est vrai !

Camellia se lève d'un bond, le menton en avant, ses longs
bras maigres repliés, ses poings sur les hanches. Elle plisse
tellement les yeux qu'on ne les voit presque plus derrière ses
taches de rousseur et son nez se retrousse. On dirait un cochon
moucheté.

— Non, c'est faux !

— Si, c'est vrai !

Stevie gémit et se tortille pour s'échapper. J'imagine que je
ferais mieux de le lâcher. Il file vers la bascule, où Lark le
prend dans les bras.

Camellia brandit son poing. Ce ne sera pas la première fois
qu'on se bagarrera en s'échangeant des coups, en se crachant
dessus et en se tirant les cheveux.

— Hé, oh ! Arrêtez ça !

Avant que je m'en aperçoive, James bondit de la cachette
des grands et se dirige vers nous.

Camellia hésite juste assez longtemps pour qu'il la rejoigne.
Ses grandes mains l'attrapent par le col de sa robe et la fichent
par terre, violemment.

— Et reste couchée, gronde-t-il, le doigt en l'air.

Elle n'obéit pas, évidemment. Elle se relève d'un saut, plus
furieuse qu'une abeille qu'on essaie de chasser. Il la refait tomber.

— Hé ! crié-je. Arrête ça !

Je défends ma sœur, même si elle s'apprêtait à m'assommer.

James regarde vers moi en souriant, et sa langue pointe derrière sa dent cassée.

— Vraiment ? fait-il.

Quand Camellia essaie de lui donner un coup de poing, il l'attrape par le bras et la maintient assez loin pour qu'elle ne puisse pas l'atteindre. On dirait une araignée qui s'est coincé une patte dans une porte. Il la serre si fort que sa peau devient violette. Les larmes lui montent aux yeux et dégoulinent, mais elle continue à se débattre.

— Arrête ! Laisse-la tranquille.

— Si tu le veux vraiment, alors tu dois être ma petite amie, ma jolie. Autrement, elle est cuite.

Camellia rugit, crie et devient folle de rage.

— Laisse-la tranquille !

J'essaie à mon tour de lui donner un coup de poing mais il m'attrape par le poignet, il nous tient toutes les deux. Mes os sont réduits en miettes. Les petits sortent de la cour à toute vitesse, même Stevie, pour venir frapper les jambes de James. Il fait tourner Camellia et se sert d'elle pour faucher Fern et Gabion. Fern saigne du nez, elle hurle en se tenant le visage.

Je capitule :

— D'accord ! D'accord !

Qu'est-ce que je peux faire d'autre ? Je cherche des yeux les adultes mais, comme d'habitude, il n'y en a aucun en vue.

— D'accord, quoi, ma jolie ? demande James.

— D'accord, je serai ta petite amie. Mais compte pas sur moi pour t'embrasser.

Ça semble lui convenir quand même. Il lâche Camellia par terre et lui dit qu'elle ferait mieux de rester là. Il m'entraîne au sommet de la colline et me tire derrière une vieille remise condamnée pour que personne ne puisse y entrer et s'y faire mordre par des serpents. Pour la deuxième fois de la journée, un coup de marteau résonne dans ma poitrine.

Je répète :

— Je t'embrasserai pas.

— Tais-toi.

Derrière la remise, il me pousse par terre et se laisse tomber à côté de moi sans lâcher mon bras. J'ai le souffle court et la gorge nouée. Un goût de bile imprègne ma langue.

Qu'est-ce qu'il compte me faire ? Comme j'ai grandi sur un bateau et que j'ai vu naître quatre enfants après moi, j'en sais un rayon sur ce que les hommes et les femmes fabriquent ensemble. Je ne veux pas que quelqu'un me fasse ça, à moi. Jamais. Je n'aime pas les garçons et je ne les aimerai jamais. L'haleine de James sent la patate pourrie et le seul garçon que j'ai envisagé de laisser m'embrasser, c'était Silas, et ça n'a duré qu'une minute ou deux.

Sa bande se met à chantonner de l'autre côté du bâtiment.

— James a une fi-an-cée ! James a une fi-an-cée ! James et May vont s'em-bra-sser !

Mais James n'essaie pas de m'embrasser. Il reste assis là, et des taches rouges apparaissent sur son cou et ses joues.

— T'es jolie.

Il couine comme un porcelet. C'est drôle, mais je ne ris pas. J'ai trop peur.

— C'est faux.

— Si, très jolie.

Il me lâche le poignet et essaie de me prendre par la main. Je m'esquive et passe mes bras autour de mes genoux, pour me rouler en boule.

— J'aime pas les garçons.

— Je t'épouserai, un jour.

— Je ne veux épouser personne. Je me construirai un bateau et je descendrai le fleuve. Je n'aurai besoin de personne.

— Je pourrai monter sur ton bateau.

— Hors de question.

On reste assis là un petit peu. Les garçons au pied de la colline continuent de chanter : « James a une fiancée ! James a une fiancée ! James et May vont s'embrasser ! »

Il croise les bras sur ses genoux et me regarde.

— C'est de là que tu viens ? Du fleuve ?

— Ouais, c'est ça.

On parle de bateaux. James vient d'une ferme très pauvre du comté de Shelby. Mlle Tann les a ramassés un jour, son frère et lui, sur le bord de la route alors qu'ils allaient à l'école.

Il était en CM1, à l'époque. Il est resté là depuis, sans jamais retourner à l'école une seule fois pendant tout ce temps. Son frère est parti depuis longtemps. Adopté.

James lève le menton.

— Je ne veux pas de nouveaux parents, dit-il. Je sais que je serai bientôt trop grand et je sortirai d'ici. J'aurai besoin d'une femme. On pourrait vivre sur le fleuve, si tu veux.

— Mon papa va venir nous chercher.

Je me sens coupable en disant ça. J'ai pitié de James. Il a l'air de se sentir vraiment seul. Seul et triste. Pourtant, j'ajoute :

— Il va venir bientôt.

James se contente de hausser les épaules.

— Je t'apporterai des biscuits, demain. Tu dois continuer à être ma petite amie.

Je ne réponds pas. Les biscuits me donnent déjà l'eau à la bouche. Je crois que je sais qui allait fouiller dans la cuisine, la nuit.

— Tu ne devrais pas faire ça. Tu risques d'aller au placard.

— J'ai pas peur.

Il pose sa main sur la mienne. Je le laisse faire.

Peut-être que ça ne m'embête pas tant que ça.

Je découvre bientôt qu'être la petite amie de James, c'est pas si mal, finalement. Ce n'est pas dur de parler avec lui et il veut juste me tenir par la main. Personne ne m'embête de la journée. Personne n'est méchant avec Camellia ou Lark ou les petits. James et moi, nous nous promenons dans la cour en nous tenant la main, et il me raconte encore des choses que je dois savoir sur la maison de Mme Murphy. Il me promet encore des biscuits. Il me décrit comment il sortira en douce du dortoir pour aller les chercher cette nuit.

Je lui dis que je n'aime pas les biscuits.

Dans la queue, pour aller au bain, les autres grands ne me regardent pas. Ils savent que cela vaut mieux pour eux.

Mais, le lendemain, James ne vient pas au petit-déjeuner. Mme Pulnik s'est dressée devant la table, tapant une cuiller en bois dans sa grosse main charnue. Elle explique qu'elle a envoyé James dans un endroit où les garçons doivent gagner leur croûte au lieu de la recevoir par la charité de la Société des foyers d'accueil du Tennessee.

— Un garçon assez grand pour courir les filles est assez grand pour trafailler et trop grand pour être désiré par une bonne famille. Mme Murphy refuse ce genre de comportement entre garçons et filles. Chacun de fous connaît les règles.

Elle abat la cuiller de toutes ses forces sur la table et respire si fort que les narines de son large nez aplati se dilatent à chaque expiration. Nous sursautons comme des pantins avec des fils vissés à nos têtes. Elle se penche vers la rangée de garçons attablés. Ils baissent la tête et fixent leurs bols vides.

— Quant à fous, les filles – la cuiller et le bras tressautant se tendent vers nous –, honte à fous pour afoir attiré des ennuis aux garçons. Faites attention, gardez fos jupes baissées et conduisez-fous comme de vraies petites dames.

Elle me regarde durement en ajoutant :

— Sans quoi, je ne feux même pas imaginer ce qui pourrait fous arrifer.

Le sang me monte au cou et au visage. Je me sens coupable parce que James a été renvoyé à cause de moi. Je n'aurais pas dû accepter d'être sa petite amie. Je ne savais pas.

Les dames de service ne font pas descendre Stevie pour le petit-déjeuner. Il n'est pas non plus dans la cour. Les autres enfants m'apprennent qu'il doit rester au lit parce qu'il l'a encore mouillé cette nuit. Un peu plus tard, je le vois à la fenêtre de l'étage, le nez collé à la moustiquaire. Depuis la cour, je lui murmure :

— Sois sage, d'accord ? Sois sage, et tout ira bien.

Plus tard dans l'après-midi, les employées nous alignent tous sur le porche et j'attire mon frère et mes sœurs près de moi parce que j'ai peur. Même les autres enfants n'ont pas l'air de savoir ce qui se passe.

Mme Pulnik et les dames de service nous font défiler devant la citerne d'eau de pluie un par un. Elles essuient les visages, les bras et les genoux crasseux avec des chiffons mouillés avant de nous brosser les cheveux et de nous dire de nous laver les mains. Certains enfants doivent changer de vêtements là, dehors. Quelques-unes reçoivent de nouveaux habits, ou des tabliers à enfiler par-dessus leur tenue de jeu.

Mme Murphy sort de la maison, se campe sur la dernière marche et nous observe. Un battoir à tapis en fil de fer pend à son bras. Je n'ai jamais vu les dames de la cuisine s'en servir pour enlever la terre des tapis, mais je l'ai souvent vu à l'œuvre sur les enfants. Les enfants l'appellent « la sorcière en fil de fer ».

— Aujourd'hui, nous allons faire quelque chose de très spécial, annonce Mme Murphy. Attention, c'est juste pour les petits garçons et les petites filles sages. Quiconque ne se conduit pas parfaitement bien ne sera pas autorisé à y participer. Vous comprenez ?

— Oui, m'dame, dis-je en chœur avec les autres.

— Très bien.

Elle sourit mais son sourire me force à reculer d'un pas.

— Aujourd'hui, reprend-elle, le camion de la bibliothèque va nous rendre visite. Les gentilles dames de la Société de bienfaisance donneront de leur temps pour vous aider à choisir des livres. Il est très important que nous nous montrions sous notre meilleur jour. Chacun d'entre vous pourra avoir un livre, si vous êtes sages.

Elle continue en nous ordonnant d'être polis, de dire « oui, m'dame » et « non, m'dame », de ne pas attraper et tripoter tous les livres et si l'on nous demande si nous sommes heureux ici, nous devons dire que nous sommes reconnaissants envers Mlle Tann car elle nous a trouvés et envers Mme Murphy car elle nous accueille chez elle.

Je n'écoute pas le reste. Je ne pense qu'à une chose, à cette possibilité d'avoir un livre, et je n'aime rien tant que les livres, surtout ceux que je n'ai pas encore lus. Comme nous sommes cinq, nous pouvons avoir cinq livres.

Malheureusement, lorsque les employées ouvrent le portail et que la queue se forme, Mme Murphy nous bloque le passage, à Camellia, moi et les petits.

— Pas vous, dit-elle. Puisque vous n'avez pas encore un coin à vous à l'étage, vous n'avez pas d'endroit pour ranger des livres et nous ne pouvons pas risquer que les biens de la bibliothèque se fassent abîmer.

— Nous en prendrons soin. Je vous le promets.

Normalement, je ne réponds jamais à Mme Murphy, mais, cette fois-ci, je ne peux pas m'en empêcher.

— S'il vous plaît. Est-ce qu'on pourrait au moins avoir un livre ? Je pourrais le lire à mes sœurs et mon frère ? Queenie le faisait...

Je pince les lèvres avant de m'attirer des ennuis. Nous n'avons pas le droit de parler de nos mamans et de nos papas, ici.

Elle soupire et accroche le battoir à tapis à un clou planté dans l'un des piliers du porche.

— Très bien. Mais les petits n'ont pas besoin d'y aller. Vas-y toute seule. Et dépêche-toi.

Je réfléchis un instant à l'idée de laisser les enfants. Camellia les attrape par le bras et les tire vers elle.

— Vas-y, dit-elle en écarquillant les yeux. Trouve-nous quelque chose de bien.

Je leur jette un dernier coup d'œil avant de filer par le portail. Je dois me retenir de traverser la cour à toute vitesse et de débouler entre les magnolias. Une odeur de liberté flotte là-bas. Une bonne odeur. Je dois m'obliger à rester dans la queue et à suivre les autres le long de l'allée, bien sagement.

De l'autre côté de la haie fleurie, il y a un gros camion noir. Deux autres voitures s'arrêtent. Mlle Tann descend de la première et un homme avec un appareil photo de la deuxième. Ils se serrent la main et l'homme tire un calepin et un stylo de sa poche.

Il est écrit *Bibliothèque du comté de Shelby* sur les flancs du gros camion noir et, quand je m'approche, je vois des étagères à l'arrière. Et les étagères sont pleines de livres. Les enfants papillonnent autour d'eux et je dois croiser les mains derrière le dos pour m'empêcher d'y toucher pendant que j'attends mon tour.

— Comme vous pouvez le voir par vous-même, nous fournissons aux enfants de quoi stimuler leur esprit, déclare Mlle Tann, et l'homme le note à toute vitesse dans son calepin, à croire que ces mots risquent de s'envoler s'il ne les attrape pas assez vite. Certains de nos petits protégés n'avaient jamais connu le luxe des livres avant de venir à nous. Nous fournissons de merveilleux livres et jouets dans tous nos foyers.

Je baisse la tête, m'agite sur place et souhaite que la foule se disperse. Si Mlle Tann a d'autres endroits comme celui-ci, je ne sais pas à quoi ils ressemblent, mais il n'y a pas un seul livre chez Mme Murphy et tous les jouets sont cassés. Personne ne se soucie assez de nous pour les réparer. Mlle Tann est venue souvent, pourtant. Elle devrait le savoir.

— Pauvres petits chérubins, lance-t-elle à l'homme. Nous les accueillons lorsqu'ils ne sont pas désirés et quand ils sont mal aimés. Nous leur offrons tout ce que leurs parents ne pouvaient pas ou ne voulaient pas leur fournir.

Je foudroie le sol du regard et serre mes poings dans mon dos. « C'est un mensonge, voilà ce que j'aimerais crier à la face de cet homme. Mon père et ma mère veulent de nous. Ils nous aiment. Comme le père qui est venu voir son petit garçon, Lonnie, et qui a fini effondré sur le perron, pleurant comme un bébé quand on lui a dit que Lonnie avait été adopté. »

— Combien de temps un enfant quelconque reste-t-il dans votre institution ? demande l'homme.

— Oh, nous n'avons pas d'enfants quelconques, glousse Mlle Tann. Ils sont tous exceptionnels. Certains peuvent rester plus longtemps que d'autres, selon l'état dans lequel ils nous arrivent. Certains sont faibles et chétifs, si dénutris qu'ils ne peuvent ni courir ni jouer. Nous les remplumons avec trois repas nourrissants par jour. Les enfants ont besoin de bien manger pour bien grandir. Plein de fruits, de légumes et de viande rouge leur ramènent le rose aux joues.

Pas chez Mme Murphy. Chez Mme Murphy, c'est porridge, un seul petit bol, matin et soir. Nous avons tout le temps faim. La peau de Gabion est blanche comme du lait, et les bras de

Lark et de Fern sont si maigres qu'on peut voir leurs muscles et leurs os.

— Nous contrôlons tous nos foyers pour nous assurer que les enfants sont correctement nourris et traités.

Elle a vraiment l'air de croire à ce qu'elle dit. L'homme hoche la tête et fait : « Mmm Mmm », comme s'il gobait ça tout rond et qu'il trouvait ça délicieux.

« Allez donc voir dans le jardin, à l'arrière, je voudrais lui lancer. Allez voir dans la cuisine. Vous verrez comment c'est vraiment. » J'ai tellement envie de le prévenir ! Mais je sais que, si je le fais, je peux dire adieu à mon livre et bonjour au placard.

— Les enfants se montrent tellement reconnaissants. Nous les tirons du caniveau et...

Quelqu'un me touche le bras, et je sursaute malgré moi. Une dame en robe bleue baisse les yeux vers moi. Son sourire est aussi radieux que le soleil.

— Et toi, qu'est-ce que tu aimes lire ? me demande-t-elle. Quelle sorte de livre ? Tu as attendu si patiemment depuis tout à l'heure...

— Oui, m'dame.

Elle m'entraîne vers les étagères, et j'ai l'impression que mes yeux vont jaillir de ma tête. J'oublie tout sur Mlle Tann, je ne pense plus qu'aux livres. Je suis déjà entrée dans des bibliothèques des villes fluviales mais, à l'époque, on avait aussi nos propres livres sur l'*Arcadie*. Maintenant, on n'a plus rien et, quand on n'a plus le moindre livre, l'idée même d'en toucher un, c'est comme Noël et un anniversaire en même temps. Je balbutie :

— Je... j'aime tous les genres.

Le simple fait de voir ces étagères et toutes ces couleurs et ces mots me fait sourire jusqu'aux oreilles. Je me sens heureuse pour la première fois depuis notre arrivée ici.

— Un gros livre, ce serait peut-être bien, puisqu'on ne peut en prendre qu'un.

— Toi, t'es une futée, répond-elle en me faisant un clin d'œil. Est-ce que tu es une bonne lectrice ?

— Oui, m'dame, très bonne. Quand on vivait...

Je baisse la tête, car j'allais dire : « Quand on vivait sur l'*Arcadie*, Queenie nous faisait toujours la lecture. »

Une employée du foyer se tient à un mètre de moi, et Mlle Tann n'est pas loin non plus. Si elle m'entendait, elle me ferait sortir de là en moins de deux.

— Très bien, reprend la dame. Voyons voir...

— J'aime les aventures. Les histoires avec plein d'aventures.

— Mmm... des aventures de quel genre ?

— Avec des reines et des princesses et des Indiens. Tout un tas de choses.

Mon esprit se remplit aussitôt de contes.

— Un western, peut-être, dans ce cas ?

— Ou le fleuve. Est-ce que vous auriez une histoire qui parle de ça ?

Un livre parlant d'un fleuve, ce serait comme rentrer à la maison. Cela nous ferait tenir le coup, le temps que Briny nous ramène sur l'*Arcadie*.

La dame tape des mains.

— Oh ! Oh, oui, j'ai ça ! s'écrit-elle avant de lever le doigt en l'air. Je sais ce qui sera parfait pour toi.

Après un instant de recherche, elle me tend *Les Aventures d'Huckleberry Finn,* de M. Mark Twain, et je comprends que, celui-là, il était vraiment pour moi. Même si on n'a jamais eu ce livre, Briny nous a raconté des histoires avec Tom Sawyer et Huckleberry Finn et Joe l'Indien. Mark Twain, c'est l'un des écrivains favoris de Briny. Il lisait souvent ses livres quand il était petit. On aurait même pu croire que Tom Sawyer était un ami proche.

La dame dans la robe bleue écrit mon nouveau nom, May Weathers, sur la carte. Puis elle tamponne la date dans le livre et je me rends compte qu'hier, c'était l'anniversaire de Fern. Elle a quatre ans maintenant. Si on était sur l'*Arcadie*, Queenie lui aurait préparé un petit gâteau et on lui aurait tous donné des cadeaux qu'on aurait faits nous-mêmes ou qu'on aurait trouvés sur la rive du fleuve. Ici, chez Mme Murphy, le livre de la bibliothèque fera l'affaire. Quand je retournerai dans la cour, je dirai à Fern que c'est une surprise pour son anniversaire, mais qu'elle ne pourra la garder qu'un petit peu. On fera un gâteau dans la terre, on mettra des fleurs pour le glaçage et des brindilles pour faire les bougies avec des petites feuilles posées en équilibre tout en haut, pour que Fern puisse jouer à les souffler.

La dame de la bibliothèque me serre dans ses bras avant de me congédier, et je me sens si bien que j'ai envie de rester là, contre elle, à respirer l'odeur des livres, mais je ne peux pas.

Je tiens *Huckleberry Finn* très fort contre ma poitrine et je m'élance dans la cour. Maintenant, nous pouvons quitter cet endroit quand nous le voulons. Tout ce que nous avons à faire, c'est aller rejoindre Huckleberry Finn. Il y a de la place sur son radeau pour nous cinq, je parie. On y retrouvera peut-être l'*Arcadie*, quelque part.

Même si je dois retourner dans la maison de Mme Murphy, l'endroit me semble complètement différent.

Maintenant, un fleuve le traverse.

Cette nuit-là, avant de nous coucher, nous ouvrons le livre d'anniversaire de Fern et nous commençons nos aventures avec Huck Finn. Nous avons voyagé au fil du fleuve pendant presque une semaine avec lui quand la voiture noire brillante de Mlle Tann remonte l'allée de la maison, un après-midi. Il fait beau dehors et l'air dans la maison est aussi chaud que de l'huile de friture, si bien que Mme Murphy et elle se retrouvent sur la galerie pour discuter. Je contourne le figuier et vais me glisser sous les azalées pour les écouter.

— Oh, oui, les publicités ont déjà paru dans tous les journaux ! s'exclame Mlle Tann. J'ai eu une idée tellement brillante, il faut bien l'avouer. « Des chérubins blonds comme les blés, pour passer un bel été. Vous n'avez qu'à demander ! » Parfait, non ? Toutes nos petites têtes blondes réunies.

— Comme une réunion de nymphes des bois. Des petits elfes et des petites fées, renchérit Mme Murphy.

— C'est presque aussi irrésistible que le programme « Un bébé pour Noël ». Des clients ont déjà appelé. Une fois qu'ils verront les enfants, ils se les arracheront.

175

— Sans aucun doute.

— Vous préparerez tous les enfants samedi matin, n'est-ce pas ? Je veux les voir bien habillés – jupes bouffantes, rubans et tout le tralala. Des bains pour tout le monde, ils doivent être récurés jusqu'à la moelle. Pas d'ongles noirs ou de crasse derrière les oreilles. Assurez-vous qu'ils savent ce qu'on attend d'eux et ce qui se passera s'ils m'humilient en public. Faites un exemple un peu avant et assurez-vous que tous les autres le voient. Cette fête représente une occasion importante pour asseoir notre réputation de fournisseur des plus beaux spécimens. Avec les nouvelles publicités, nous aurons les meilleures familles du Tennessee et d'une dizaine d'États alentour. Ils viendront voir nos enfants et, dès qu'ils poseront les yeux sur eux, ils ne se contrôleront plus. Il leur faudra l'un d'eux.

— Nous ferons en sorte que les enfants soient préparés comme il se doit. Laissez-moi jeter un dernier coup d'œil à la liste.

Elles arrêtent de parler. Des feuilles de papier crissent. Le vent tourne et agite les branches des azalées et je vois la tête de Mlle Tann. La brise se prend dans ses cheveux courts et gris qui se redressent lorsqu'elle se penche vers Mme Murphy.

Je me colle contre le mur et je ne bouge plus, de crainte qu'elles m'entendent et qu'elles regardent par-dessus la balustrade. Une bourrasque charrie l'odeur d'une chose morte. Je ne vois pas quoi, mais cette bête a sans doute mangé le poison que M. Riggs a disposé par là. Quand la puanteur sera insupportable, il trouvera le cadavre et l'enterrera quelque part.

— May aussi ? s'étonne Mme Murphy, et je dresse l'oreille. On ne peut guère la qualifier de chérubin, à son âge.

Mlle Tann éclate d'un petit rire sec avant de répondre.

— Elle nous aidera avec les plus petits et elle est agréable à regarder, si je me souviens bien.

— Sans doute, répond Mme Murphy d'un ton contrarié. Elle ne fait pas de grabuge, pour sûr.

— J'enverrai des voitures les chercher à une heure ce samedi. Ils ne doivent pas avoir faim, avoir sommeil ou avoir besoin d'aller aux toilettes. Je veux les voir gais, vifs et sûrs de bien se conduire. Voilà ce que j'attends.

— Oui, bien sûr.

— Dieu du ciel, quelle est cette odeur abominable ?

— Des lapins. Ils nous ont empoisonné la vie tout l'été.

Je m'éclipse avant qu'elles se décident à venir inspecter les lieux. M. Riggs n'est nulle part en vue, si bien que je ne mets pas de temps à passer le figuier et à rejoindre la colline. Je ne parle pas de la « fête » à Camellia ni du bain supplémentaire le lendemain. Inutile qu'elle fasse une crise de rage d'avance.

J'ai un mauvais pressentiment : je crois que je n'ai même pas besoin de lui parler du bain supplémentaire, en fait.

Camellia n'est pas blonde.

Il se trouve que j'ai raison. Le samedi, après le petit-déjeuner, je découvre que Camellia n'est pas sur la liste. Où que nous allions, elle ne nous accompagne pas.

— Je m'en fiche bien qu'ils veuillent pas de moi, si ça m'évite un autre bain.

Elle me repousse quand j'essaie de la serrer dans mes bras pour lui dire au revoir.

— Sois sage pendant notre absence, Mellia. N'embête personne, reste à l'écart des grands et ne passe pas devant le figuier, et...

— J'suis pas un bébé.

Camellia relève le menton, mais sa lèvre inférieure tremblote un peu. Elle a peur.

— May ! aboie l'une des employées. En rang, tout de suite !

Elles ont déjà rassemblé tous les enfants de la liste.

Je chuchote à l'oreille de Camellia :

— Nous reviendrons très vite. N'aie pas peur.

— J'ai pas peur.

Elle finit quand même par me serrer dans ses bras.

L'employée me hurle une nouvelle fois dessus et je me dépêche de rejoindre le rang. L'heure et demie qui suit est pleine de savon, de frictions, de brossage de cheveux, de nœuds, de brosse à dents frottée sous les ongles, de rubans et de vêtements neufs couverts de dentelle. On essaie des chaussures tirées d'un placard plein de souliers jusqu'à ce qu'on trouve la bonne pointure.

Lorsque les employées nous emmènent aux voitures qui attendent dans la rue, nous ne sommes plus les mêmes. Nous sommes tous les quatre, avec trois autres filles, un garçon de cinq ans, deux bébés et Stevie, à qui on a dit que s'il mouillait encore son pantalon, il recevrait une correction sur-le-champ.

Nous n'avons pas le droit de parler dans la voiture. Pendant le trajet, c'est l'employée qui parle.

— Les filles, vous vous assiérez gentiment, les jambes serrées comme de jeunes dames. Ne parlez pas sauf si l'on vous pose une question. Vous serez polies avec les invités venus à la fête de Mme Tann. Vous ne direz que du bien de votre séjour dans la maison de Mme Murphy. Il y aura des jouets et des pastels, des gâteaux et des biscuits, aujourd'hui. Vous devrez...

Je perds le fil lorsque la voiture gravit une colline et que le fleuve apparaît. May se volatilise comme un éclat de soleil sur l'eau, et Rill refait surface. Elle s'étire vers la fine ouverture en haut de la vitre, attire l'air à l'intérieur de la voiture et attrape toutes les odeurs familières.

L'espace d'un instant, elle est chez elle.

Lorsque la voiture tourne à un carrefour, le fleuve disparaît. Une chose lourde et triste s'installe en moi. Je pose la tête en arrière sur le siège, et l'employée me dit d'arrêter, parce que j'écrase le nœud dans mes cheveux.

Sur mes genoux, Gabion s'endort. Je le berce tout près de moi, laisse ses cheveux me chatouiller le menton, et je suis quand même de retour chez moi. Ces gens peuvent me contrôler tout entière, sauf là où je vais dans mes pensées.

Ma visite à l'*Arcadie* est de courte durée. Bientôt, nous nous arrêtons devant une grande villa blanche, plus imposante encore que celle de Mme Murphy.

— Tous ceux qui ne seront pas sages le regretteront amèrement, nous met en garde l'employée, le doigt tendu sous nos nez, avant de nous laisser descendre de voiture. Soyez gentils avec les invités. Asseyez-vous sur leurs genoux s'ils vous le demandent. Souriez. Montrez-leur que vous êtes des enfants bien élevés.

Nous entrons, la maison est pleine de gens. D'autres enfants sont là aussi et des bébés. Tout le monde porte de beaux habits et on nous donne des parts de gâteau et des biscuits. Il y a des jouets pour les petits et, en moins de temps qu'il n'en faut pour le dire, Fern, Gabion et même Lark s'éloignent de moi.

Un homme emmène Gabion jouer dehors avec un ballon bleu. Une femme brune s'assoit avec Lark et elles colorient ensemble un livre d'images. Fern rit devant une jolie femme blonde qui se cache derrière ses mains avant de se montrer en disant « Bouh ! ». Cette dame est assise à l'écart dans un fauteuil, elle a l'air triste et fatiguée. Fern la fait rire et, bientôt, la dame porte ma sœur, l'amenant d'un jouet à l'autre, comme si Fern ne savait pas marcher.

Elles finissent par se blottir ensemble dans un fauteuil pour lire un livre et mon cœur se serre. Je pense à Queenie, qui nous lisait souvent des histoires. Je veux que cette femme lâche Fern, qu'elle me la rende.

Un homme entre dans la pièce, chatouille Fern sur le ventre, et la femme sourit avant de dire :

— Oh, Darren, elle est parfaite ! Amelia aurait eu son âge. Assieds-toi et fais-lui la lecture, ajoute-t-elle en tapotant l'accoudoir.

— Continuez, répondit-il en déposant un baiser sur sa joue. Je dois parler à certaines personnes.

Puis il sort de la pièce.

Fern et la dame en sont à leur deuxième livre lorsque l'homme revient. Elles sont si concentrées qu'elles ne remarquent pas qu'il s'assoit à côté de moi sur le canapé.

— Vous êtes sœurs ? m'interroge-t-il.

— Oui, m'sieur.

Je réponds comme on me l'a demandé. « M'dame » et « m'sieur », dès qu'on parle.

Il se penche en arrière et me regarde des pieds à la tête.

— Vous vous ressemblez.

— Oui, m'sieur.

Je baisse les yeux vers mes mains. Mon cœur s'emballe, bondissant dans ma poitrine comme une poule coincée dans la cabine de notre bateau. Qu'est-ce qu'il veut ?

L'homme pose une main sur mon dos. Mes omoplates se referment sur elle. Le duvet sur ma nuque se dresse. Je transpire sous ma robe qui gratte.

— Et quel âge as-tu ? me demande-t-il.

13

Avery

Le cottage est silencieux et baigné par le clair de lune lorsque j'ouvre la porte d'entrée. Je tâtonne pour trouver l'interrupteur, le téléphone coincé entre mon menton et mon épaule en attendant que mon oncle Clifford réponde à la question que je viens de lui poser. Il m'a mis en attente parce qu'il est en train de commander à manger à un drive-in.

Je suis consumée par un souvenir très puissant, le souvenir d'arriver là après la tombée de la nuit pour un court séjour, juste ma grand-mère et moi. Le cottage était exactement comme ça, avec des ombres lunaires sur le sol en forme de frondes de palmier, l'air sentant l'iode, les tapis pleins de sable, l'huile de citron et les meubles qui ont vécu depuis longtemps en bord de mer.

J'agite les doigts. Je sens presque sa main enroulée autour de la mienne. Je devais avoir onze ou douze ans – cet âge ingrat où j'avais arrêté de lui donner la main en public mais là, dans notre endroit magique, ça ne me dérangeait pas.

Debout sur le seuil, je cherche cette impression de confort, sauf que cette visite-ci a un goût étrange, tout en contrastes. Aigre et doux. Familier et inconnu. Les saveurs de la vie.

Oncle Clifford revient en ligne. Après une longue promenade sur la plage et un dîner au Waterfront Restaurant, j'ai décidé que mon oncle était peut-être mon dernier espoir de progresser dans ma quête, pour le moment du moins. Trent Turner m'avait abandonnée en partant en jeep avec l'homme en uniforme. J'avais attendu dans ma voiture mais l'agence immobilière Turner est restée fermée tout l'après-midi.

Jusqu'à maintenant, ce voyage semble être un échec total.

— Qu'est-ce que tu voulais savoir, Avery, à propos de la maison d'Edisto ? s'enquiert oncle Clifford.

— Je me demandais juste si vous y veniez souvent avec mamie Judy, papa et toi. Quand vous étiez petits, je veux dire.

J'essaie de garder un ton décontracté. Je ne veux pas qu'il flaire quelque chose. Oncle Clifford a travaillé pour le FBI dans sa jeunesse.

— Est-ce que mamie Judy avait des amies qu'elle retrouvait ici, ou des gens qu'elle venait voir ?

— Eh bien... laisse-moi réfléchir...

Il rumine un moment avant de finir par lâcher simplement :

— Je crois que nous n'y allions pas si souvent que ça, maintenant que tu en parles. Nous nous y rendions plus souvent quand j'étais enfant. Ensuite, nous préférions aller chez notre grand-mère, sur l'île de Pawleys. La maison était plus grande, il y avait un voilier et il n'était pas rare que des cousins et des cousines viennent jouer avec nous. Le plus souvent, ma mère allait seule à Edisto. Elle aimait écrire là-bas. Tu sais, elle a un peu touché à la poésie et, pendant un moment, elle s'occupait d'une chronique mondaine dans un journal.

Sur le coup, je reste abasourdie.

— Mamie Judy écrivait une chronique mondaine ?

Que l'on peut aussi qualifier de rubrique « Ragots de la semaine ».

— Pas sous son vrai nom, évidemment.

— Sous quel nom alors ?

— Si je te le disais, je serais obligé de te tuer.

— Oncle Clifford !

Alors que mon père est plutôt collet monté, mon oncle a toujours été décontracté et moqueur. Ce n'est pas que quelques cheveux blancs qu'il a donnés à ma tante, Diana, mais toute une chevelure laiteuse qu'elle teint régulièrement comme toute dame du Sud qui se respecte.

— Oh, laisse donc les secrets de ta grand-mère en paix.

Pendant une seconde, je me demande s'il y a un message caché dans sa phrase, puis je devine qu'il ne fait que me taquiner.

— Alors, comme ça, tu es descendue au cottage Myers ?

— Oui. J'ai décidé de m'échapper quelques jours.

— Eh bien, va jeter une ligne dans l'eau pour moi.

— Tu sais que je ne pêche pas. Berk.

Mon pauvre père n'ayant que des filles, il a vainement essayé de faire d'au moins l'une d'entre nous une pêcheuse invétérée.

Même mon oncle sait que c'était une cause perdue.

— Eh bien, tu vois, c'est une chose que tu ne tiens pas de ta grand-mère. Elle adorait pêcher, surtout à Edisto. Quand ton père et moi étions petits, elle nous y emmenait pour retrouver quelqu'un qui avait un petit canot à fond plat. On remontait la rivière et on passait la moitié de la journée à pêcher. Je ne sais plus qui était ce monsieur. Un ami, j'imagine. Il avait un petit garçon blond avec qui j'aimais bien jouer. Son nom commençait par un T... Tommy, Timmie... non... Tr... Trey ou Travis, peut-être.

— Trent ? Trent Turner ?

Le Trent Turner actuel étant le troisième du nom, son père s'appelait Trent aussi, et il doit avoir l'âge de mon oncle.

— C'est possible. Tu me demandes ça pour une raison en particulier ? Il se passe quelque chose ?

Je comprends aussitôt que j'ai posé la question de trop et que j'ai, pas inadvertance, éveillé les soupçons de l'inspecteur qu'il était.

— Non. Pas du tout. Être à Edisto me fait réfléchir à plein de choses. J'aurais aimé venir ici plus souvent avec mamie Judy. J'aurais aimé lui poser des questions pendant qu'elle se rappelait encore le passé, tu vois ?

— Eh bien, c'est un des paradoxes de la vie. On ne peut pas tout avoir. Tu peux prendre un peu de ci et un peu de ça, ou tout ceci et rien de cela. Nous faisons les ajustements qui nous semblent les meilleurs sur le moment. Tu es déjà arrivée loin pour une fille – une femme de trente ans, je veux dire.

Parfois, je me demande si ma famille ne me surestime pas un peu.

— Merci, oncle Clifford.

— De rien. La séance te coûtera cinq dollars.

— Le chèque est déjà parti.

Après avoir raccroché, je repense à notre conversation en vidant le seul sac de courses que j'ai rempli au magasin Bi-Lo, qui, dans mon souvenir, s'appelait Piggly Wiggly.

Y a-t-il le moindre indice dans ce que m'a dit mon oncle ?

Rien ne me saute aux yeux. Rien de concluant. Si le petit garçon dans la barque s'appelait bel et bien Trent, cela me confirme que ma grand-mère avait un lien personnel avec Trent Turner Sr., ce que j'avais déjà deviné. Mais s'ils passaient du temps à pêcher ensemble avec les enfants, cela met à mal ma théorie du chantage. On ne va pas pêcher avec un maître chanteur, et encore moins avec ses enfants en bas âge. On n'emmène pas non plus ses fils si on a une liaison. Surtout pas des enfants assez grands pour se souvenir de la promenade.

Trent Turner Sr. n'était peut-être rien d'autre qu'un ami de longue date. Si ça se trouve, l'enveloppe ne contient que des photos... quelque chose de complètement innocent. Dans ce cas, pourquoi cette promesse entre lui, sur son lit de mort, et son petit-fils, pour s'assurer que ce dernier ne donnerait les paquets à personne d'autre que leurs justes propriétaires ?

J'échafaude des théories tout en emportant mes affaires dans la chambre, où j'ouvre ma valise pour m'installer. Je passe au crible mes théories, comme je le ferais si j'étais de retour dans la salle de réunion, à mon ancien boulot.

Après vérification, plus rien ne tient debout. Et moi non plus, car la journée a été longue. Je suis prête pour une douche et une bonne nuit de sommeil. J'aurais peut-être une idée de génie demain... à moins que je ne retourne voir Trent Turner III et que je lui arrache de force la vérité en lui faisant une prise de catch.

Ces deux possibilités sont aussi vraisemblables l'une que l'autre.

Ce n'est que lorsque je fais couler l'eau de la douche et que je me rends compte qu'il n'y a visiblement pas d'eau chaude dans le cottage que je repense à une chose que m'a dite oncle Clifford. Ma grand-mère venait ici pour écrire.

Est-ce que quelques-uns de ses écrits pourraient être encore là, quelque part ? Est-ce que je pourrais y trouver un indice ?

Je me rhabille en deux secondes. L'idée d'une douche froide n'était pas si tentante que ça de toute façon.

Dehors, les hautes graminées se balancent sur les dunes et la lune se lève au-dessus du bosquet de palmiers. Les vagues martèlent la côte tandis que je fouille les tiroirs, explore les placards, les malles à couvertures et les penderies. J'en suis presque arrivée à la conclusion qu'il n'y a rien à trouver lorsque je me relève après avoir regardé sous le lit de ma grand-mère et que je me rends compte que le petit meuble à côté n'est ni un bureau ni une coiffeuse mais une machine à écrire escamotable. Une vieille machine à écrire noire pend la tête en bas sous le panneau central du meuble. Ayant grandi dans des maisons de famille pleines de meubles anciens, je sais plus au moins comment ce truc fonctionne. Il ne me faut pas très longtemps pour tirer le bon nombre de loquets et faire pivoter le panneau central sur ses gonds. La machine à écrire tourne brusquement et se retrouve à l'endroit.

Je passe le doigt sur les touches. Je vois presque ma grand-mère y pianoter. Je me penche pour étudier le ruban encreur noir. Les touches ont laissé de petites marques à l'arrière. Si c'était un ordinateur, je pourrais peut-être tirer quelque chose du disque dur mais, là, il ne reste rien de lisible. Impossible de dire ce qui a été écrit ni quand.

— Que sais-tu que je ne sais pas ? murmuré-je à la machine tout en farfouillant dans les tiroirs.

Il n'y a rien dans le petit meuble qu'un bête assortiment de stylos et de crayons, de papier machine jauni, une pochette de papier carbone et des rubans correcteurs, blancs crayeux d'un côté et lisses de l'autre. La première bande présente des traces de lettres. En la tenant à la lumière, je déchiffre facilement les mots mal écrits puis corrigés : Palmetto Blvd, Edisto Island...

Ma grand-mère écrivait des lettres, ici, apparemment. Mais, que ce soit intentionnel ou pas, elle a bien effacé ses traces. Il n'y a pas de mots griffonnés, et les feuilles de papier carbone sont intactes, aucun fantôme de mots oublié en chemin. C'est étrange car, à son bureau, dans sa maison d'Aiken, il y avait toujours une pochette remplie de feuilles de papier qui pouvaient être réutilisées pour des petits projets, des pliages ou des dessins d'enfants.

J'appuie sur une touche, je regarde la barre de lettre se lever et frapper le rouleau, n'y laissant qu'une vague esquisse de *K*. L'encre du ruban est sèche.

Le ruban...

Je me retrouve aussitôt penchée sur le corps métallique noir et je m'active pour le soulever afin d'accéder aux bobines. C'est étonnamment simple. Malheureusement, le ruban est presque neuf. Une dizaine de centimètres a été utilisée et pourrait porter l'impression de ce qui a été tapé en dernier, quoi que ce soit. Je le déroule et je le tends à la lumière, les yeux plissés pour mieux voir.

yduJ, séitimA.étiahuossuon-snoissue'ltnemérépseséd issua, tnerT, siamajertê-tuepsnoruaselensuoN.eessenneTud lieucca'dsreyofsedétéicoSaledsevihcraselsnadertua'd revuortestiavuopiuqecednamedemejteeéirartnoc

Au début, c'est du chinois, pour moi, mais j'ai passé suffisamment de temps avec mamie Judy pour savoir comment fonctionne le ruban d'une machine à écrire. Il se déroule à mesure que les touches sont frappées. Les lettres sont forcément dans un ordre logique.

Les premières lettres de la ligne prennent soudain tout leur sens. « Judy. » Le prénom de ma grand-mère écrit à l'envers, de droite à gauche car les premières lettres qui apparaissent sur le ruban sont les dernières frappées. Un autre mot jaillit de la mélasse, « Tennessee », juste après, ou avant, le point.

Trois autres mots commençant par une majuscule : « Société foyers accueil ».

J'attrape un crayon et un bout de papier pour décoder le reste.

... contrariée et je me demande ce qui pouvait se trouver d'autre dans les archives de la Société des foyers d'accueil du Tennessee. Nous ne le saurons peut-être jamais, Trent, aussi désespérément l'eussions-nous souhaité.

Amitiés,
Judy

J'essaie d'assembler les derniers morceaux de l'histoire en fixant ma propre écriture. Les foyers sont pour les orphelins et les enfants abandonnés attendant d'être adoptés. La jeune femme sur la photo de May Crandall était enceinte. Était-ce une parente de ma grand-mère... qui s'était retrouvée en mauvaise posture ?

Des possibilités prennent vie dans ma tête – une jeune fille aux yeux étincelants venant d'une bonne famille, un homme de réputation douteuse, un mariage clandestin scandaleux – ou pire, pas de mariage du tout. Une grossesse embarrassante. Son fiancé l'avait peut-être abandonnée... et si elle avait été contrainte de retourner dans sa famille ?

À cette époque, les filles étaient envoyées à la campagne pour accoucher de bébés qu'elles abandonnaient pour qu'ils soient adoptés par d'autres. Même maintenant, parmi les connaissances de ma mère, des femmes échangent parfois des murmures à propos d'une telle « partie chez sa tante pour quelque temps ». C'est peut-être ce que Trent Turner essaie de garder secret.

Une chose est sûre – la dernière lettre écrite sur cette machine était adressée à un Trent Turner et, même si je ne peux pas savoir si c'est récent, il ne fait plus aucun doute que le contenu de l'enveloppe mystérieuse répondra à de nombreuses questions.

À moins qu'il n'en soulève d'autres.

Sans réfléchir, je traverse la maison à toutes jambes, j'attrape mon téléphone et je compose le numéro de Trent Turner, que j'ai mémorisé.

La sonnerie retentit deux fois avant que je jette un coup d'œil à la pendule et que je me rende compte qu'il est presque minuit. Vraiment pas une heure acceptable quand on appelle un quasi-étranger. Ma mère serait horrifiée.

Si tu veux que cet homme coopère, ce n'est pas la bonne solution, Avery, me dis-je lorsqu'une voix pâteuse, ensommeillée, répond : « 'soir, Nrent Nurner à l'appareil », et me confirme que je l'ai, en effet, tiré du lit. C'est sans doute pour ça qu'il a répondu sans vérifier qui appelait.

— La Société des foyers d'accueil du Tennessee, lancé-je aussitôt parce que j'ai calculé que je n'aurai que deux secondes et demie avant que ses idées s'éclaircissent et qu'il raccroche.

— Quoi ?

— La Société des foyers d'accueil du Tennessee. Quel est le rapport avec votre grand-père et ma grand-mère ?

— Mademoiselle Stafford ?

Malgré l'adresse très formelle, son ton rauque, à peine réveillé, donne une touche intime à sa phrase, presque comme une conversation sur l'oreiller. S'ensuit un profond soupir, et j'entends des ressorts de matelas grincer.

— Avery. Appelez-moi Avery, s'il vous plaît. Je vous en supplie, vous devez me le dire. J'ai trouvé quelque chose. Je dois savoir ce que ça signifie.

Encore un long soupir. Il se racle la gorge mais sa voix reste éraillée et somnolente.

— Vous avez une idée de l'heure qu'il est ?

Je jette un coup d'œil penaud vers la pendule, comme si ça pouvait excuser mon impolitesse.

— Toutes mes excuses. Je n'avais pas fait attention avant de composer le numéro.

— Vous auriez pu raccrocher.

— J'avais peur que, si je le faisais, vous ne décrocheriez plus jamais.

Un petit ricanement guttural me dit que j'ai raison.

— C'est pas faux.

— S'il vous plaît, écoutez-moi. Je vous en prie. J'ai fouillé le cottage de ma grand-mère toute la soirée et j'ai trouvé quelque chose, et vous êtes le seul à pouvoir me dire ce que ça signifie. C'est juste que... je dois savoir ce qui se passe et comment je dois y faire face. S'il y a eu un scandale quelque part dans le passé de notre famille, il est bien possible que ce ne soit plus important maintenant, sauf peut-être pour quelques membres bien conservées de l'arrière-garde des commères de service, mais je ne peux pas en être sûre avant de savoir de quoi il retourne.

— Je ne peux vraiment rien vous dire.

— Je comprends que vous ayez fait une promesse à votre grand-père, mais...

— Non.

Il semble bien réveillé, tout à coup – et maître de lui.

— Enfin, je ne peux pas vous le dire. Je n'ai jamais ouvert une seule de ces enveloppes. J'ai aidé mon grand-père à les transmettre aux personnes à qui elles étaient adressées. C'est tout.

Est-ce qu'il dit la vérité ? J'ai dû mal à l'imaginer. Je suis du genre à décoller précautionneusement le scotch de l'emballage pour jeter un coup d'œil aux cadeaux de Noël à la seconde où ils apparaissent sous le sapin. Je n'aime pas les surprises.

— Quel est le lien, dans tout ça ? Le rapport avec la Société des foyers d'accueil du Tennessee ? Les foyers de l'enfance, ce sont pour les orphelins. Est-ce que ma grand-mère cherchait quelqu'un qui avait été adopté ?

Dès que j'émets cette hypothèse, j'ai peur d'en avoir trop dit. Je me hâte d'ajouter :

189

— C'est juste une théorie. Je n'ai aucune raison de penser que c'est vrai.

Je ferais mieux d'éviter d'ouvrir la boîte de Pandore en public. Je ne sais pas si je peux faire confiance à Trent Turner, même s'il faut être sacrément intègre pour vivre pendant des mois avec des enveloppes scellées. M. Turner l'Ancien devait savoir que son petit-fils avait une volonté de fer.

Le silence s'éternise tant que je me demande si Trent n'a pas raccroché. J'ai peur de parler, peur que, quoi que je dise, cela fasse pencher la balance d'un côté ou de l'autre.

Je ne suis vraiment, vraiment pas du genre à implorer, et pourtant je finis par murmurer :

— Je vous en supplie. Je suis désolée qu'on ait pris un mauvais départ, cet après-midi, mais je ne sais vraiment pas quoi faire d'autre.

Il inspire bruyamment. Je vois presque son torse se gonfler.

— Venez.

— Quoi ?

— Venez chez moi avant que je change d'avis.

Je suis tellement stupéfaite que j'en reste coite. Je ne sais pas trop si je suis impatiente ou morte de trouille... ou complètement folle pour ne serait-ce qu'envisager d'aller chez un inconnu au beau milieu de la nuit.

D'un autre côté, il est connu pour être un homme d'affaires respectable, dans l'île.

Un homme d'affaires qui sait que j'ai déterré au moins une partie d'un secret.

Le secret dont son grand-père lui a confié la garde sur son lit de mort.

Et s'il y avait de mauvaises intentions, derrière cette invitation de minuit ? Personne ne saura où je suis. À qui puis-je le dire ?

Je ne vois personne à qui je pourrais me confier sur cette affaire, là, tout de suite.

Je vais laisser un message... ici, dans le cottage...

Non... attends. Je vais m'envoyer un e-mail. Si je suis portée disparue, c'est la première chose qui sera inspectée.

Cette idée me semble un peu idiote et mélodramatique, et puis, plus tant que ça...

— Le temps de retrouver mes clefs de voiture...

— Pas besoin. Je vis à quatre maisons de vous.

— Vous êtes dans le quartier ? m'étonné-je en tirant les rideaux de la cuisine pour essayer de voir quelque chose à travers l'écran de houx et de chênes.

Depuis tout ce temps, il était presque mon voisin ?

— Ça va plus vite par la plage. Je vais allumer l'éclairage extérieur.

— J'arrive tout de suite.

Je fouille dans la maison pour trouver une lampe de poche et des piles. Heureusement, quel que soit le membre de ma famille venu là en dernier, il m'a laissé les fournitures de base. Mon téléphone sonne alors que je tape l'e-mail que je compte m'envoyer, décrivant où je vais et l'heure de mon départ. Je sursaute au moins d'un mètre avant d'être prise de sueurs froides. Trent a déjà changé d'avis...

Mais le numéro affiché est celui d'Elliot. Je suis trop tendue pour calculer l'heure qu'il est à Milan en ce moment, mais il doit travailler, sans aucun doute.

— J'étais occupé quand tu as appelé hier, désolé.

— C'est ce que j'ai pensé. La journée a été chargée ?

— Plutôt, répond-il comme toujours – dans sa famille, les femmes ne s'intéressent pas au monde du travail. Comment ça se passe, à Edisto ?

Franchement, chez nous, les nouvelles vont plus vite que sur CNN.

— Comment sais-tu que je suis ici ?

— Ma mère me l'a dit, soupire-t-il. Comme ta sœur, Courtney et les garçons séjournent en ce moment chez tes parents, elle est passée à Drayden Hill pour sa dose de pouponnage. Elle refait une fixation sur ses futurs petits-enfants.

Il a l'air excédé, ce que je peux comprendre.

— Elle m'a rappelé que j'ai déjà trente et un ans et elle cinquante-sept, et qu'elle ne veut pas être une vieille grand-mère.

— Oh, oh.

Parfois, je me demande ce que ça me fera d'avoir Bitsy en belle-mère. Je l'adore, et elle n'a que de bonnes intentions mais, à côté d'elle, Pomme d'amour est un monument de subtilité.

— Est-ce qu'on peut envoyer ta sœur et les triplés chez elle pour quelques jours ? demande-t-il, désabusé. Ça lui fera peut-être passer l'envie d'être grand-mère.

Même si je comprends la blague, elle touche une corde sensible. J'adore mes neveux, même si ce sont de petits Cro-Magnon.

— Tu peux toujours demander.

Elliot et moi n'avons parlé bébé que comme une possibilité dans notre avenir, pourtant, il craint déjà que les naissances multiples soient héréditaires, dans ma famille. Il ne se croit pas capable de s'occuper de plus d'un enfant à la fois. De temps en temps, j'ai peur que, pour Elliot, avoir des enfants un jour, ce ne soit plutôt jamais. Mais je sais qu'on réglera ça quand le moment sera venu. Comme tous les couples, non ?

— Alors, combien de temps penses-tu rester à la mer ? demande-t-il pour changer de sujet.

— Deux ou trois jours. Si je reste plus, Leslie enverra quelqu'un à ma recherche.

— Tu sais, elle ne pense qu'à ton bien. Tu dois être vue. C'est pour ça que tu es rentrée chez toi.

Je voudrais lui rétorquer : « Je suis surtout rentrée pour m'occuper de mon père. » Avec Elliot, rien n'est gratuit. Je ne connais personne qui soit aussi fixé sur des objectifs que lui.

— Je sais. Mais j'apprécie de pouvoir faire une pause. Tu as l'air d'en avoir besoin toi aussi. Repose-toi pendant que tu es là-bas, d'accord ? Et ne t'inquiète pas pour ta mère et son obsession des petits-enfants. Demain, elle aura une nouvelle lubie.

Nous nous disons au revoir puis je finis mon e-mail de pré-caution adressé à moi-même. Si on n'entend plus parler de moi, quelqu'un finira par vérifier ma boîte mail.

Minuit, mardi soir. Je vais quatre maisons plus bas en par-tant du cottage d'Edisto parler à Trent Turner d'une affaire qui concerne mamie Judy. Je devrais être de retour dans une heure. Je laisse ce message juste au cas où.

Même si ça semble crétin, je l'envoie quand même avant de m'éclipser.

Dehors, la nuit est profonde et tranquille tandis que je suis le sentier à travers les dunes, la lampe de poche braquée devant moi pour guetter d'éventuels serpents. Le long de la côte, les lumières sont éteintes dans la plupart des cottages ; on ne voit que l'éclat de la pleine lune et une grappe de lumières qui semblent flotter à l'horizon sur la mer. Des feuilles et des hautes herbes murmurent autour de moi et, sur la plage, des crabes pâles détalent de travers dans le sable. Je fais glisser le faisceau lumineux sur eux, prenant bien soin de ne pas gâcher leur festin en marchand sur l'un d'eux.

La brise se glisse sur ma nuque et dans mes cheveux, et j'ai envie de marcher, de me détendre, de profiter du chant apaisant de la mer. J'ai des disques de musique de méditation qui ressemblent à ça, mais je prends rarement le temps de les écouter pour de vrai. Là, je me dis que c'est une honte. J'avais oublié à quel point cet endroit est paradisiaque, une rencontre parfaite entre la terre et la mer, épargnée par les gratte-ciel, les feux de camp et les véhicules tout-terrain.

J'arrive au cottage de Trent Turner plus tôt que je ne l'aurais voulu. Mon pouls s'accélère lorsque j'emprunte un petit che-min bien délimité dans les broussailles, puis une longueur de caillebotis qui mène à un portail. Ce cottage doit être de la même époque que celui de ma grand-mère. Il se dresse sur de courts pilotis, au milieu d'un grand terrain qui accueille aussi un cabanon, sur le côté. Une allée de pierre mène aux marches de la galerie. Des papillons de nuit tourbillonnent autour de l'ampoule qui pendouille au-dessus du perron.

Trent ouvre la porte sans me laisser le temps de frapper. Il porte un T-shirt délavé déchiré à l'encolure et un bas de jogging qui lui descend sur les hanches. Ses pieds bronzés sont nus et il arbore une coiffure saut du lit du plus bel effet.

Les bras croisés, il s'adosse au chambranle de la porte pour m'étudier.

Je me sens empotée, comme une adolescente le soir de son premier rendez-vous pour aller au bal du collège. Je ne sais plus où me mettre.

— Je commençais à me demander, dit-il.

— Si j'allais venir ?

— Si votre appel n'était pas juste un cauchemar.

Malgré ses mots, ses lèvres esquissent un sourire et j'en déduis qu'il plaisante.

Et pourtant, je rougis un peu. C'est tellement impoli de ma part.

— Je suis vraiment désolée. C'est juste que... je dois savoir. Quel était le rapport entre votre grand-père et ma grand-mère ?

— Le plus vraisemblable, c'est qu'il travaillait pour elle.

— Pour faire quoi ?

Son regard se déporte au-dessus de mon épaule, vers le petit cabanon sur le côté du jardin. Je sens qu'il débat avec lui-même. Doit-il ou non briser la promesse faite sur le lit de mort de son grand-père ?

— On engageait mon grand-père pour retrouver...

— Retrouver quoi ?

— Des gens.

14

Rill

Le soir tombe lorsque la fête se termine et que les employées commencent à rassembler les enfants pour les remettre dans les voitures et les ramener au foyer. À ce moment-là, je ne veux presque pas partir. Tout l'après-midi, on a eu des biscuits, de la crème glacée, des rouleaux de réglisse, du gâteau, du lait, des sandwichs, des livres de coloriage, de nouvelles boîtes de pastels, des poupées pour les filles et des voitures en fer-blanc pour les garçons.

J'ai tellement mangé que je peux à peine bouger. Après trois semaines de privations, cet endroit a des allures de paradis.

Je regrette que Camellia rate tout ça mais, d'un autre côté, je ne sais pas si elle aurait pu le supporter. Elle n'aime pas qu'on la câline... ou qu'on la touche. Je vole un biscuit pour elle et le glisse dans la poche avant de ma robe chasuble en espérant que personne ne nous fouille avant de partir.

Les gens nous appellent tous « ma chérie », « ma puce » et « Oh, mon trésor ! » Tout comme Mlle Tann, le temps qu'on reste là-bas. Comme le jour de la visite du camion de la bibliothèque, elle raconte des salades. Ses yeux scintillent et elle sourit, comme si ça l'amusait de jouer la comédie.

Une fois encore, je me tais pour ne pas rétablir la vérité.

— Ils sont parfaits, à tous points de vue, répète-t-elle en boucle aux invités. Des spécimens au physique merveilleux et aussi à l'esprit avancé pour leur âge. Nombre d'entre eux viennent de parents doués pour la musique et les arts plastiques. Ce sont des ardoises vierges qui attendent juste qu'on les remplisse. Ils pourront devenir tout ce que vous voulez.

Elle s'adresse soudain au couple qui n'a pas lâché Gabion de tout l'après-midi :

— C'est un adorable petit bonhomme, n'est-ce pas ?

Ils ont joué à la balle, aux voitures et l'homme a lancé Gabby en l'air, ce qui le faisait rire aux éclats.

Maintenant qu'il est l'heure de partir, la femme ne semble pas vouloir lâcher Gabby. Elle s'avance jusqu'à la porte d'entrée, et mon petit frère s'accroche à son cou de la même façon que Fern s'accroche au mien.

— A veux rester, gémit Gabby.

— Nous devons partir.

Je fais passer Fern sur ma hanche pendant que Mme Pulnik essaie de nous pousser vers la sortie. Je n'en veux pas à Gabby de faire un caprice. Moi aussi, l'idée de retourner chez Mme Murphy me fait horreur. Je préférerais continuer à regarder Fern lire d'autres livres avec la gentille dame mais celle-ci est partie un peu plus tôt avec son mari. Avant de me la redonner, elle a embrassé Fern sur le front en disant :

— On se reverra bientôt, ma chérie.

— Gab... dis-je avant de me reprendre pour ne pas prononcer le nom qui me vaudra une calotte sur la tête chez Mme Murphy si Mme Pulnik m'entend. Robby, tu ne peux pas rester ici. Viens, allez. Nous devons découvrir ce qui est arrivé à Huckleberry Finn et à Jim une fois qu'ils sont partis sur le fleuve vers l'Arkansas, tu te souviens ?

Je tends un bras vers lui sans lâcher Fern de l'autre. Gabby refuse de venir et la femme refuse de le lâcher.

— Nous lirons le livre dès que nous serons de retour chez Mme Murphy. Dis au revoir à la gentille dame.

— Silence ! s'écrie Mlle Tann en me foudroyant du regard.

Je me recule et laisse retomber mon bras si vite qu'il me claque la cuisse.

Mlle Tann sourit à la femme, puis entortille un doigt dans les cheveux de Gabby. Elle redevient gentille aussi vite qu'elle était devenue méchante.

— Notre petit Robby n'est-il pas à croquer ? Tellement charmant ! On dirait que vous vous entendez à merveille avec lui.

— Oui, en effet.

Le mari de la dame s'approche. Il redresse le col de sa veste d'un coup sec.

— Nous devrions peut-être discuter un instant, dit-il. Il est très certainement possible de trouver un arrangement pour que...

— Tout à fait, le coupe-t-elle. Mais je dois vous prévenir, ce petit amour est vraiment très populaire. J'ai déjà eu plusieurs demandes le concernant. Ces yeux bleus adorables bordés de cils sombres et ses boucles blondes ! Quelle rareté ! Comme un petit angelot. Il ferait chavirer le cœur de la plupart des mères.

Ils regardent tous mon frère. L'homme tend la main et pince doucement la joue de Gabby, qui pousse un rire de bébé très mignon. Il n'a pas gloussé comme ça depuis que la police nous a arrachés de l'*Arcadie*. Je suis contente qu'il soit heureux, ne serait-ce qu'une journée.

— Faites sortir les autres enfants, ordonne Mlle Tann d'une voix grave et sèche avant de murmurer à l'oreille de Mme Pulnik : Mettez-les dans la voiture. Attendez cinq minutes avant de laisser le conducteur démarrer.

Elle ajoute d'un ton encore plus bas :

— À dire vrai, je ne pense pas que nous aurons besoin de vous.

Mme Pulnik se racle la gorge et lance d'une voix amicale et joyeuse que nous n'entendons jamais chez Mme Murphy :

— Allez, tout le monde aux foitures ! Fenez, les enfants !

Lark, Stevie et les autres se précipitent dehors. Fern donne des coups de pied dans ma jambe et gigote contre ma hanche comme si elle essayait de faire sortir de l'écurie un poney têtu.

— Mais Ga... Robby...

197

Des racines ont poussé sous mes pieds et, au début, je ne comprends même pas pourquoi. Ces gens veulent juste tenir Gabby encore un peu et lui faire quelques bisous de plus. Ils aiment jouer avec les petits garçons. J'ai gardé Gabby, Lark et Fern à l'œil toute la journée, dès que je pouvais échapper aux quelques hommes qui voulaient savoir qui j'étais et pourquoi j'étais là, puisque j'étais plus âgée que tous les autres. J'ai filé de pièce en pièce, de fenêtre en fenêtre, pour m'assurer que je savais où étaient les petits et que personne n'était méchant avec eux.

Mais, dans un coin de ma tête, je pensais à la sœur de Stevie, qui est partie de la maison de Mme Murphy sans jamais revenir. Je sais ce qui arrive aux orphelins, ce que sont Sherry et Stevie, mais pas nous. Nous, on a un papa et une maman qui vont venir nous chercher.

Est-ce que la femme qui jouait avec Gabion le sait ? Est-ce que quelqu'un lui a dit ? Elle ne le prend pas pour un orphelin, n'est-ce pas ?

Je fais un pas de plus vers mon frère.

— Donnez-le-moi. Je peux le porter.

La femme me tourne le dos en disant :

— Il est bien, là.

— Dehors ! me crache Mme Pulnik.

Des doigts s'enfoncent douloureusement dans mon bras et je sais ce qui va se passer si je n'obéis pas.

Je touche le petit genou de Gabby en murmurant :

— Tout va bien. La dame veut juste te dire au revoir.

Il lève sa petite main dodue et l'agite vers moi.

— Au 'voir.

Son sourire me montre toutes ses dents. Je me souviens du jour où chacune d'elles est sortie.

— Aux foitures.

Les ongles pointus de Mme Pulnik s'enfoncent dans ma peau. Elle me tire si fort par le bras que je trébuche sur le seuil en sortant et manque faire tomber Fern.

— Oh, bonté divine, est-ce que c'est sa sœur ? s'inquiète la dame qui porte Gabion.

— Certainement pas ! ment de nouveau Mlle Tann. Les plus petits s'attachent aux plus grands, au foyer. C'est tout. On ne peut rien y faire. Ils oublient tout aussi vite, bien évidemment. La seule parente de ce chérubin était une petite sœur. Tout juste née. Adoptée par une famille très influente, pas moins. Vous voyez donc que ce n'est pas un petit garçon ordinaire. Vous avez choisi le plus raffiné. La mère était diplômée de l'université, une femme extrêmement intelligente. Décédée durant l'accouchement, malheureusement, et les enfants ont été abandonnés par leur père. Mais cela vaut mieux pour eux. Et ce petit bonhomme-là ne serait-il par adorable, à gambader sur vos plages de Californie ? Bien sûr, une adoption hors État requiert des frais particuliers...

Ce sont les derniers mots que j'entends avant que Mme Pulnik me traîne sur les marches du perron en sifflant dans sa barbe ce que Mme Murphy me fera si je ne suis pas le mouvement. Sa poigne me tord tellement le bras que je suis certaine qu'elle va me le casser.

Je m'en fiche bien. Je ne sens plus rien – ni l'herbe séchée par le soleil d'été qui crisse sous mes pieds, ni les chaussures rigides que les employées m'ont données ce matin. Ni la brise chaude et moite de ce début de soirée ni la robe trop serrée qui me tire la peau lorsque Fern donne des coups de pied, se tortille et tend les bras par-dessus mon épaule en gémissant :

— Gabby... Gabby...

Ma peau est glacée, comme si j'étais tombée dans le fleuve en plein hiver et que tout mon sang s'était réfugié au plus profond de moi pour m'empêcher de geler à mort. Mes bras et mes jambes m'ont l'air d'appartenir à quelqu'un d'autre. Ils bougent, mais juste parce qu'ils savent ce qu'ils sont censés faire, pas parce que je le leur ordonne.

Mme Pulnik nous jette, Fern et moi, dans la voiture avec les autres enfants et grimpe à côté de moi. Je reste assise, raide, les yeux braqués sur la grande maison, et j'attends que la porte s'ouvre et que quelqu'un fasse traverser le jardin à Gabby. Je le souhaite tellement que ça me fait mal au cœur.

— Où est Gabby ? gémit Fern dans mon oreille, et Lark m'observe avec ses grands yeux tristes et muets.

Elle n'a pas dit grand-chose depuis qu'on est arrivés chez Mme Murphy et elle ne dit rien non plus à cet instant, mais je l'entends quand même. « Tu dois récupérer Gabion », me dit-elle.

Je l'imagine en train de traverser la cour.

J'espère.

J'observe.

J'essaie de réfléchir.

Qu'est-ce que je devrais faire ?

La montre de Mme Pulnik s'impatiente. Tic, tic, tic, tic.

Les paroles de Mlle Tann fusent dans ma tête à toute vitesse, comme des araignées d'eau quand on jette une pierre dans le fleuve. Elles partent dans toutes les directions à la fois.

« Décédée durant l'accouchement... »

Ma mère est morte ?

« ... les enfants ont été abandonnés... »

Briny ne va pas venir nous chercher ?

« La seule parente de ce chérubin était une petite sœur. Tout juste née. »

L'un des jumeaux n'est pas mort à l'hôpital ? J'ai une nouvelle petite sœur ? Mlle Tann l'a donnée à quelqu'un ? Est-ce que c'est un mensonge ? Est-ce que tout ça n'est qu'un gros mensonge ? Mlle Tann peut mentir si facilement qu'on dirait qu'elle-même croit ce qu'elle dit. La maman de Gabby n'est pas allée à l'université. Queenie est intelligente, mais elle n'a été à l'école que jusqu'au collège, avant de rencontrer Briny et de partir vivre sur le fleuve avec lui.

Ce sont des mensonges, me dis-je. Tout ce qu'elle raconte, un gros mensonge. Forcément.

Elle essaie de rendre ce couple heureux, mais ils devront nous rendre Gabion, parce que Mlle Tann sait que notre père va venir nous chercher dès qu'il le pourra. Briny ne nous abandonnerait jamais. Il ne laisserait pas une femme comme Mlle Tann prendre ma nouvelle petite sœur, si j'en ai vraiment une. Jamais de la vie. Il préférerait encore mourir.

Est-ce que Briny est mort ? Est-ce que c'est pour ça qu'il ne vient pas nous chercher ?

La voiture démarre et je m'élance vers la vitre, poussant Fern de mes genoux. Elle glisse sur la banquette pendant que j'attrape la poignée de la portière. Je vais courir jusqu'à la maison et je dirai la vérité à ces gens. Je leur dirai que Mlle Tann est une menteuse. Je m'en fiche de ce qu'on me fera, après.

Mais, avant que je puisse tenter quoi que ce soit, Mme Pulnik m'attrape par le gros nœud chic que l'une des employées m'a attaché dans les cheveux pour me faire belle ce matin. Fern gigote pour ne plus se trouver entre nous et atterrit par terre avec Stevie et Lark.

— Tu fas rester sage ! me crache-t-elle dans l'oreille de son souffle chaud et puant – l'odeur du whisky de Mme Murphy. Sinon, Mme Murphy te mettra au placard ! Et pas seulement toi. On fous y accrochera tous les cinq, comme des chaussures pendant par leurs lacets. Il fait froid dans le placard. Et tout noir. Tu crois que les petits seront contents, dans l'obscurité ?

Mon cœur bat follement quand elle me tire la tête en arrière. Ma nuque craque. Mes cheveux sont arrachés. Un éclair blanc de douleur m'aveugle un instant.

— C'est compris ?

Je fais de mon mieux pour acquiescer.

Elle me pousse contre la portière et ma tête rebondit sur la vitre.

— Je n'imaginais pas que toi, tu me causerais du souci.

Un torrent de larmes me monte aux yeux, je cille de toutes mes forces pour les retenir. Je ne pleurerai pas. Hors de question.

La banquette s'incline, je suis comme aspirée vers le corps trapu de Mme Pulnik. Elle pousse un soupir ronronnant, comme un chat sur une chaise au soleil.

— Chauffeur, ramenez-nous à la maison. C'est l'heure.

201

Je m'écarte d'elle et regarde par la vitre aussi longtemps que je le peux jusqu'à ce que la maison blanche avec ses grandes colonnes disparaisse.

Dans la voiture, personne ne parle. Fern me regrimpe sur les genoux et nous restons assises, aussi immobiles que des statues.

Sur le trajet du retour, je guette le fleuve. Un rêve fugitif se glisse dans mon esprit pendant que Fern se pend à mon cou, que Lark se colle contre mon genou, que Stevie se blottit entre mes pieds, ses doigts crispés sur les boucles de mes chaussures. J'imagine que, lorsque nous passerons devant le fleuve, l'*Arcadie* y sera, et Briny verra la voiture.

Dans ma rêverie, il remonte la berge en courant, force le chauffeur à s'arrêter. Il ouvre la portière, nous sort tous de là, même Stevie. Lorsque Mme Pulnik essaie de s'interposer, il lui donne un coup de poing dans le nez, comme il le ferait si quelqu'un essayait de l'arnaquer dans une salle de billard. Briny nous kidnappe, à la manière du père de Huck Finn, dans l'histoire, mais le père de Huck était méchant, alors que Briny est gentil.

Ensuite, il retourne à la grande maison blanche, reprend Gabion à Mlle Tann et nous emmène tous très loin.

Mais mon rêve ne se réalise pas. Le fleuve apparaît et disparaît. L'*Arcadie* n'est nulle part en vue et, bientôt, l'ombre du foyer de Mme Murphy engloutit la voiture. Sous ma peau, je suis vide et froide, comme les cavernes d'Indiens où Briny nous a emmenés camper, un jour, quand on avait grimpé en haut des falaises. Il y avait des os dans les cavernes. Des os morts de gens disparus. Il y a des os morts en moi.

Rill Foss ne peut pas respirer ici. Elle ne vit pas ici. Juste May Weathers. Rill Foss vit sur le fleuve. C'est la princesse du royaume d'Arcadie.

Ce n'est que lorsque nous marchons sur le trottoir vers la maison de Mme Murphy que je pense à Camellia. Je me sens coupable d'avoir imaginé que Briny nous secourait dans la voiture, qu'il nous emmenait loin, sans elle.

J'ai peur de ce qu'elle dira quand je lui raconterai que Gabion n'est pas avec nous – que j'espère qu'il reviendra plus tard. Camellia répondra que j'aurais dû me battre plus fort, que j'aurais dû mordre et griffer et hurler comme elle l'aurait fait. Et elle aurait peut-être raison. Je mérite peut-être qu'elle me le dise. Je suis peut-être trop trouillarde, j'ai vraiment pas envie de finir dans le placard. Je veux pas qu'il y mettent mes petites sœurs non plus.

Quand nous entrons dans la maison, une peur panique m'envahit. Le genre de terreur qui nous prend sur un fleuve en crue au moment du dégel, quand on voit un bloc de glace foncer droit vers le bateau. Parfois, il est si gros qu'on sait qu'on n'a aucune chance de le repousser avec une gaffe. Il va nous percuter, et violemment, et si son bord entaille notre coque, on coule.

Je suis à deux doigts de lâcher les petits, de faire demi-tour et de m'enfuir du foyer avant que la porte se referme sur nous. La maison pue l'humidité, les toilettes sales, le parfum et l'odeur de whisky de Mme Murphy. La puanteur me saisit à la gorge et je ne peux plus respirer, si bien que je suis contente qu'on nous dise d'aller jouer dehors parce que les autres ne sont pas encore rentrés pour le dîner.

— Et fous ne defez pas salir les fêtements ! beugle Mme Pulnik.

Je cherche Camellia dans les coins où je lui ai dit de rester, des endroits sûrs. Je ne la trouve nulle part. Les grands ne répondent pas quand je leur demande où elle est. Ils haussent juste les épaules et continuent à jouer avec des marrons ramassés sous les arbres près de la clôture du jardin.

Camellia ne joue ni au sable, ni sur les balançoires, ni à la dînette à l'ombre des arbres. Tous les autres enfants sont là, sauf Camellia.

Pour la deuxième fois de la journée, j'ai l'impression que mon cœur va être arraché de ma poitrine. Et s'ils l'avaient emmenée je ne sais où ? Et si elle avait piqué une crise après notre départ, et qu'elle s'était attiré des ennuis ?

Je hurle :

— Camellia !

Je tends l'oreille, mais je n'entends que les voix des autres enfants. Ma sœur ne répond pas.

— Camellia !

Je me dirige vers le côté de la maison, dans la direction des azalées, lorsque je la vois enfin. Elle est assise par terre, dans le coin de la galerie, les jambes ramassées contre sa poitrine, le visage enfoui dans ses genoux. Ses cheveux noirs et sa peau sont recouverts d'une couche de terre grise. On dirait qu'elle s'est battue avec quelqu'un pendant mon absence. Il y a des égratignures sur son bras, et elle s'est écorché un genou.

C'est peut-être pour ça que les grands ont refusé de me dire où elle était. C'est sans doute avec eux qu'elle a eu des problèmes.

Je laisse les petits à côté des plaqueminiers et je leur dis de rester là et de ne pas s'éloigner, puis je grimpe les marches menant à la galerie et remonte la longue allée jusqu'à Camellia. Mes chaussures rigides claquent contre le bois, clac, clac, clac, mais ma sœur ne fait pas un geste.

— Camellia ?

Je salirais ma robe si je m'asseyais, du coup, je m'accroupis à côté d'elle. Elle dort peut-être.

— Camellia ? Je t'ai apporté quelque chose. C'est dans ma poche. Allons sur la colline où personne ne nous verra, et je te le donnerai.

Elle ne répond pas. Je touche ses cheveux, ce qui la fait sursauter. Un petit nuage gris s'élève quand ma main glisse vers son épaule. Ça sent la cendre, mais pas vraiment la cendre de cheminée. Je connais cette odeur, sauf que je n'arrive pas à la replacer.

— Dans quoi tu t'es fourrée, pendant qu'on était partis ?

Quand je la touche de nouveau, elle baisse l'épaule et lève la tête. Sa lèvre est enflée et il y a quatre bleus ronds sur son menton. Ses yeux sont rouges et gonflés, comme si elle avait pleuré, mais c'est surtout ce que j'y vois qui m'inquiète le plus.

C'est comme si je regardais par la fenêtre dans une pièce vide. Il n'y a rien à l'intérieur que de l'obscurité.

Une bouffée de la même odeur monte de nouveau d'elle et, tout à coup, je sais. De la cendre de charbon. À chaque fois qu'on amarrait l'*Arcadie* près d'un chemin de fer, on allait ramasser du charbon tombé des trains. « Pour se chauffer et cuisiner. En toute gratuité », disait toujours Briny.

Est-ce que Briny est là ?

Dès que cette idée m'effleure, je comprends à quel point je me trompe. À quel point c'est horrible. Une chose épouvantable est arrivée pendant mon absence.

— Qu'est-ce qu'il y a ? je demande à ma sœur en tombant à genoux, trop effrayée pour me soucier de ma robe, même si des petites échardes se plantent dans mes jambes. Camellia, qu'est-ce qu'il s'est passé ?

Sa bouche bée mais aucun bruit n'en sort. Une larme s'échappe de son œil et trace une rivière rose à travers la poussière de charbon.

— Dis-moi.

Quand je me penche pour la voir mieux, elle tourne la tête et regarde de l'autre côté. Sa main, serrée en poing, nous sépare. Je la prends dans la mienne, je force ses doigts à s'ouvrir pour voir ce qu'elle tient et, aussitôt, je sens remonter dans ma gorge tous les biscuits et la crème glacée avalés pendant la fête. Des bonbons à la menthe, ronds et sales, sont collés si fort à la paume de ma sœur qu'ils ont fondu dans sa peau.

Je ferme les yeux, je secoue la tête, je ne veux pas savoir mais je sais quand même. J'ai beau me débattre, mon esprit me traîne jusqu'au sous-sol de Mme Murphy, dans le coin sombre derrière l'escalier où de la cendre recouvre le bac à charbon et la chaudière. Je vois des bras maigres, forts, se débattre, des jambes qui remuent dans tous les sens. Je vois une grosse main qui se referme sur une bouche hurlante, les doigts sales et graisseux serrant si fort qu'ils impriment quatre bleus ronds.

Je veux courir dans la maison, crier, hurler. Je veux frapper Camellia pour s'être entêtée à aller près des azalées alors que je lui avais dit de s'en tenir éloignée, je veux l'attraper et la serrer tout contre moi et tout arranger. Je ne sais pas exactement ce que Riggs lui a fait, mais je sais que c'est grave. Je sais aussi que, si nous le disons, il fera tomber ma sœur d'un arbre pour qu'elle se brise le crâne. Peut-être qu'il me fera la même chose. Dans ce cas, qui s'occupera des petits ? Qui attendra le retour de Gabion ?

J'attrape ma sœur par la main, d'une tape, je fais tomber les bonbons, qui rebondissent sur les lattes de la galerie et tombent dans les parterres de fleurs, où ils disparaissent sous une tige de jasmin.

Elle ne résiste pas quand je la fais lever.

— Viens. Si elles te voient dans cet état quand la cloche du dîner sonnera, elles penseront que tu t'es battue et t'enfermeront dans le placard.

Je la fais descendre de la galerie comme un sac de blé et je la traîne jusqu'à la citerne d'eau de pluie et, peu à peu, j'en verse sur sa peau pour la rincer du mieux que je peux.

— Tu dois leur dire que tu es tombée de la balançoire.

Même si je tiens son visage entre mes mains, elle refuse de me regarder.

— Tu m'entends ? Si quelqu'un t'interroge sur tes écorchures, tu dis que t'es tombée de la balançoire, et c'est tout.

Là-bas, sur les marches, Fern, Lark et Stevie nous attendent, aussi muets que des souris.

— Restez là… et laissez Camellia tranquille, leur dis-je. Elle se sent pas bien.

— Elle a bobo au ventre ? demande Fern en se glissant près de nous, et Lark l'imite, mais Camellia les repousse de toutes ses forces.

Lark me dévisage, déroutée. D'habitude, elle est la seule que Camellia apprécie.

— Laissez-la tranquille, je vous dis.

— On voit sa culotte ! On voit sa culotte ! s'époumone l'un des grands au milieu de la cour.

Ils commencent toujours à se rapprocher à cette heure, pour être les premiers servis au dîner. Je ne sais pas pourquoi. On reçoit tous la même ration, à chaque repas.

Je rabaisse la robe de Camellia sur ses genoux en crachant vers lui :

— Tais-toi, Danny Boy !

Danny Boy, c'est une chanson irlandaise, du coup, les employées l'appellent comme ça parce qu'il est irlandais. Et roux, avec un millier de taches de rousseur, comme James. C'est lui qui commande leur meute, depuis que James est parti. Mais Danny Boy est mauvais jusqu'au trognon.

Il s'approche tout près, les pouces passés dans la corde qui retient son pantalon trop grand.

— Ça alors, on t'a fait toute belle et proprette ? J'parie que même ces jolis vêtements ont pas suffi à te trouver de nouveaux parents.

— Nous n'avons pas besoin de nouveaux parents. On en a déjà.

— Qui voudrait de toi, de toute façon ? lance-t-il avant d'apercevoir le bras et la jambe égratignés de Camellia et de se rapprocher. Qu'est-ce qu'elle a ? On dirait qu'elle s'est battue.

Je me dresse devant lui. Si je dois aller au placard pour protéger ma sœur, tant pis.

— Elle est tombée et elle s'est fait un peu mal. C'est tout. Ça te défrise ?

La cloche sonne pour annoncer le dîner, et nous nous mettons en rang avant que ça puisse dégénérer.

En fait, ce soir, ce n'est pas le placard, qui m'inquiète, c'est Camellia. Elle ne dit rien de tout le repas et elle ne touche pas à son assiette mais, quand c'est l'heure d'aller au bain, elle reprend vie et fait une scène épouvantable. Elle hurle comme une bête, griffe, donne des coups de pied et laisse de longues zébrures rouges sur le bras de Mme Pulnik.

Les employées doivent se mettre à trois pour l'immobiliser et la traîner jusqu'à la salle de bains. Entre-temps, Mme Pulnik m'a attrapée par les cheveux.

— Pas un mot, ou tu en subiras les conséquences.

Fern, Lark et Stevie se serrent les uns contre les autres, adossés au mur.

Dans la salle de bains, Camellia rugit et pousse des cris aigus. Des éclaboussures fusent. Une bouteille se brise. Des brosses de bain tombent sur le sol. La porte vibre sur ses gonds.

— Riggs ! hurle Mme Pulnik dans l'escalier. Apportez-moi ma corde. Ma corde pour le placard !

Et, juste comme ça, Camellia disparaît. La dernière fois que je la vois, une employée la traîne dans le couloir, enveloppée dans un drap comme une chenille pour qu'elle ne puisse plus donner de coups de pied ou de poing.

Cette nuit-là, nous ne sommes plus que trois. Je ne sors pas notre livre pour lire, et mes petites sœurs ne me supplient pas pour entendre la suite de l'histoire. Lark et Fern et moi, nous nous blottissons dans un lit de camp et je fredonne l'une des vieilles chansons de Queenie jusqu'à ce que mes sœurs s'endorment. Je finis par m'assoupir aussi.

Un peu avant l'aube, Fern mouille le lit pour la première fois depuis ses deux ans et demi. Je ne la gronde même pas. Je me contente de nettoyer de mon mieux et j'entrouvre autant que possible le soupirail du sous-sol. J'enroule la couverture et les sous-vêtements de Fern mouillés et je les glisse sous les buissons où, je l'espère, personne ne les trouvera. Je me faufilerai plus tard dans les azalées pour les étendre afin que tout soit sec avant la nuit.

C'est un peu plus tard, quand je m'escrime à disposer la couverture sur les branches, que le vent fait frémir les feuilles et qu'elles s'écartent suffisamment longtemps pour que je voie quelque chose. Sous le lampadaire à gaz de la rue, il y a des gens qui regardent la maison. Dans le clair-obscur de l'aube, je ne vois ni les visages ni les vêtements, juste la silhouette voûtée d'un vieil homme et celle d'un jeune garçon maigre.

Ils ressemblent à Zede et Silas.

Les feuilles retombent et ils disparaissent aussi vite qu'ils étaient apparus.

15

Avery

L'enveloppe est étonnamment ordinaire. Le genre en papier
kraft qu'on utilise au bureau. Elle n'a pas l'air de contenir
grand-chose – quelques feuilles de papier, pliées en trois. Elle
est cachetée, et le nom de ma grand-mère est inscrit au dos
d'une écriture tremblante qui dépasse dans la marge et dégouline du bord.

— La maladie de Parkinson de mon grand-père lui donnait
vraiment du souci, vers la fin, m'explique Trent.

Il se frotte le front, fronce les sourcils devant l'enveloppe,
comme s'il se demandait encore s'il avait vraiment eu raison
de briser sa promesse en me la remettant.

Je sais qu'il serait plus sage que je l'ouvre avant qu'il change
d'avis, mais la culpabilité me retient. Trent a l'air d'un homme
qui a failli à sa mission. Et c'est à cause de moi.

Je comprends trop bien la loyauté qu'on peut éprouver pour
sa famille. C'est justement cela qui m'a conduite ici, au beau
milieu de la nuit.

— Merci, dis-je, comme si ça pouvait l'aider.

Il se masse un sourcil du bout du doigt avant de hocher la
tête, comme à contrecœur.

— Je préfère vous prévenir, ça peut empirer les choses, au
lieu de les arranger. Si mon grand-père a passé tant de temps
à aider des gens à en retrouver d'autres, c'est qu'il y avait une
raison. Quand ma grand-mère et lui se sont mariés et ont repris
les affaires familiales à Charleston, il est allé à la fac de droit

pour pouvoir s'occuper lui-même de ses contrats immobiliers...
mais il avait aussi une autre motivation. À dix-huit ans, il avait
découvert qu'il avait été adopté. Personne ne le lui avait jamais
dit. Son père adoptif était sergent dans la police de Memphis
et, même s'ils n'avaient jamais été très proches, lorsque mon
grand-père a appris qu'on lui avait menti toute sa vie, ça a été
la goutte qui a fait déborder le vase. Il s'est enrôlé dans l'armée
le lendemain et n'a plus jamais reparlé à son père adoptif. Il a
recherché sa famille biologique pendant des années sans jamais
la trouver. Ma grand-mère a toujours pensé qu'il aurait mieux
valu qu'il ne tombe jamais sur son dossier d'adoption. À dire
vrai, elle regrettait que les parents adoptifs de mon grand-père
ne l'aient pas détruit.

— Les secrets ont leur façon à eux de refaire surface.

C'est un brin de sagesse que mon père m'a répété bien des
fois. « Les secrets nous rendent aussi vulnérables, face à nos
ennemis, qu'ils soient politiques ou autres ».

Quoi qu'il puisse y avoir dans cette enveloppe, je m'en porterai mieux en le sachant.

Pourtant, mes doigts tremblent quand je les glisse sous le
rabat.

— Je comprends pourquoi votre grand-père se dévouait
pour aider les autres à trouver des informations et des parents
perdus de vue.

Mais quel est le rapport avec ma grand-mère ?

Le rabat se décolle peu à peu, à mesure que je tire. Je m'y
attelle lentement, comme ma mère ouvre un cadeau d'anniversaire, en prenant soin de ne pas déchirer le papier.

— Bon, quand faut y aller, faut y aller.

J'en sors avec précaution une enveloppe plus petite qui a été
ouverte par le passé. Les papiers qu'elle contient ont été pliés
ensemble, comme une brochure ou une facture, mais je vois
bien qu'il s'agit de documents administratifs officiels.

Assis en face de moi, Trent baisse les yeux vers ses mains
lorsque je déplie le contenu sur la table.

— Je voudrais vraiment...

Inutile que je le remercie de nouveau. Cela ne l'empêchera pas de se débattre avec sa conscience.

— Je veux que vous sachiez que vous pouvez compter sur moi pour que j'utilise au mieux ces informations. Je ne les laisserai pas provoquer un scandale familial. Je respecte l'inquiétude de votre grand-père, étant donné le genre de recherches qu'il faisait pour les autres.

— Il était bien placé pour en connaître les conséquences.

Un bruit dans la maison nous fait tourner la tête alors que j'aplatis les documents sur la table. Je reconnais le claquement nocturne de petits petons sur le sol couvert de sable. Je m'attends presque à voir l'un de mes neveux, debout dans le couloir mais, à la place, je découvre un petit blondinet de trois ou quatre ans, aux yeux bleus bouffis de sommeil, avec la fossette la plus mignonne du monde au milieu du menton. Je sais de qui il la tient.

Trent Turner a un fils. Est-ce qu'il y a une Mme Turner qui dort là, quelque part ? Cette question s'accompagne d'une pointe de déception saugrenue. Je me surprends à chercher une alliance au doigt de Trent avant de retourner mon attention vers le petit garçon et de penser : Arrête ça. Avery Stafford, qu'est-ce qui cloche chez toi ?

C'est dans des moments pareils que je me demande vraiment ce qui ne va pas. Pourquoi est-ce que je ne me sens pas comme une femme qui a fusionné avec son âme sœur, pour toujours et à tout jamais, fin de l'histoire ? Mes deux sœurs sont tombées folles amoureuses de leurs maris et n'ont jamais eu l'air de remettre leurs sentiments en question. Tout comme ma mère. Et ma grand-mère.

Le petit garçon me scrute tandis qu'il contourne la table en bâillant et en se grattant le front du dos de la main. Son geste semble exagéré. On dirait une actrice de film muet qui s'entraîne à tomber en pâmoison.

— Tu n'es pas censé être au lit, Jonah ? demande son père.

— Si, si...

— Et tu t'es levé parce que... ?

Trent a beau essayer de paraître bourru, son visage attendri ne berne personne. Jonah prend appui sur ses genoux avec ses deux mains, lève une jambe et commence à l'escalader comme une cage à écureuil.

Trent le hisse sur ses genoux et Jonah tend le cou pour murmurer :

— Y a pedrodatile dans mon placard.

— Un ptérodactyle ?

— Oui.

— Jonah, il n'y a rien du tout dans ton placard. C'est juste le film que les grands enfants t'ont laissé regarder chez tata Lou, tu te souviens ? Tu as déjà fait un cauchemar, à cause de ça. Un dinosaure n'aurait même pas la place d'entrer dans ton placard, de toute façon. Il n'y a pas de dinosaure là-dedans.

— Si, y en a, renifle l'enfant.

Accroché au T-shirt de son père, il se tortille pour m'observer dans un bâillement sonore.

Je ne devrais pas m'en mêler. Je risque d'aggraver les choses. Cela dit, j'ai déjà connu ce problème de dinosaures à Drayden Hill ou en vacances, avec les enfants de mes sœurs.

— Mes nièces et mes neveux ont eu le même souci que toi. Eux aussi, ils avaient peur des dinosaures, mais tu sais ce qu'on a fait ?

Jonah secoue la tête, et Trent m'adresse un regard perplexe, sous ses sourcils blonds froncés. Il a un front vraiment très souple.

Deux paires d'yeux bleus identiques m'invitent à exposer ma solution au problème des visites nocturnes de sauriens.

Heureusement, j'en ai une.

— Le lendemain, on a été au magasin pour acheter des lampes de poche – des lampes de poche trop classe. Avec une lampe de poche trop classe près du lit, quand tu te réveilles la nuit, que tu crois voir quelque chose, tu peux allumer la lampe et la pointer ici ou là pour vérifier. Et tu sais ce qui se passe à chaque fois, quand tu te sers de ta lampe de poche ?

Jonah attend, tout ouïe, sa petite bouche charnue entrouverte, mais son père connaît visiblement la réponse. Il a l'air de vouloir se frapper le front, l'air de dire : « Pourquoi n'y ai-je pas pensé avant ? »

— À tous les coups, quand on braque la lumière, il n'y a rien.

— À tous yé coups ? répète Jonah, sceptique.

— Oui. Promis.

Jonah se tourne vers son père pour avoir confirmation et ils échangent un doux regard empreint de confiance. C'est un père impliqué, à l'évidence. Le soir, il pourfend quelques monstres avant de border son fils.

— On ira chercher une lampe de poche demain au magasin. Ça te dit ?

Je remarque qu'il ne dit pas : « Maman ira t'acheter une lampe demain. » Je remarque aussi qu'il n'ordonne pas à son fils d'être un grand garçon, qu'il n'insiste pas pour aller recoucher de force le pauvre gamin. Il se contente de faire pivoter Jonah contre une épaule et pose la main sur la table, les doigts tendus vers les documents pressés sous ma propre main.

Jonah glisse un pouce dans sa bouche et se blottit contre le torse de son père.

Je baisse les yeux vers les papiers, surprise qu'ils aient temporairement quitté mes pensées. Jonah est irrésistiblement mignon.

La page du dessus est une photocopie granuleuse d'un formulaire quelconque. Feuille d'historique, peut-on lire en en-tête, écrit en lettres noires imposantes. Au-dessous, le sujet a reçu un numéro de dossier : « 7501 ». « ÂGE : nouveau-né. SEXE : M. » Le nom du bébé est indiqué comme étant « Shad Arthur Foss, église fréquentée inconnue ». Dans un coin de la feuille, un tampon indique « octobre 1939 », et le document vient visiblement d'un hôpital de Memphis, dans le Tennessee. « NOM DE LA MÈRE : Mary Anne Anthony. NOM DU PÈRE : B. A. Foss. » Pour les deux parents, pour toute adresse, il y a écrit : « Indigents, campement au bord du fleuve. Ils avaient tous les deux la fin de la vingtaine à la naissance du bébé. »

L'employée responsable du document, Mlle Eugenia Carter, résume la situation du nouveau-né en quelques mots, au-dessous d'un titre de rubrique plein de termes sans doute médicaux. « CAUSE POUR REMISE À LA SFA du TENNESSEE : né hors mariage – parents inaptes. CIRCONSTANCE DE LA REMISE : papiers signés par la mère et le père à la naissance. »

— Ces noms ne me disent rien, marmonné-je en décollant la feuille des autres avant de la poser sans bruit sur la table.

D'accord, la famille est grande, mais je n'ai jamais vu de Foss ou d'Anthony sur un faire-part de mariage, et je n'en ai jamais rencontré non plus à un enterrement.

— Je ne comprends vraiment pas comment tout ça peut avoir un rapport avec ma grand-mère. À part que cela coïncide à peu près avec son année de sa naissance.

L'âge de mamie Judy change à chaque fois qu'on le lui demande. Elle n'admet rien et trouve bien grossier quiconque l'interroge sur le sujet.

— Ce Shad Arthur Foss est peut-être quelqu'un qu'elle a connu plus tard, à l'école ? Qu'elle aurait pu vouloir aider à retrouver des informations sur sa naissance ?

La page suivante est une copie d'une fiche de renseignements sur le nouveau-né Foss.

DATE DE NAISSANCE : 1er septembre 1939
POIDS À LA NAISSANCE : prématuré, 1,8 kg
POIDS ACTUEL : 3,1 kg
ENFANT : Le bébé est né prématurément et ne pesait qu'un kilo et huit cents grammes. Il s'est développé normalement à tout point de vue. Tests de Kahn et Wasserman négatifs, frottis de la mère négatif. Aucune maladie infantile ni vaccin.
Mère : 28 ans, Américaine d'origine polonaise-hollandaise. Certificat d'études, yeux bleus, cheveux blonds, environ 1,70 m et 52 kg. Religion catholique. Considérée comme très séduisante et intelligente.
Père : 29 ans, Américain d'origine écossaise-irlandaise et cajun-française. Certificat d'études, yeux marron, cheveux noirs, environ 1,85 m et 80 kg. Pas de religion connue.

Pas de maladies héréditaires dans les deux familles et, malgré les erreurs extra-maritales de ces deux jeunes individus, les familles de la mère et du père sont travailleuses et respectées dans leurs communautés. Aucun membre de ces familles n'est intéressé par la garde des enfants.

Je fais glisser sur la table le deuxième document vers Trent, qui inspecte le premier. Sur la troisième page, on peut lire :

ACTE DE REMISE D'ENFANT SIGNÉ
PAR LES PARENTS OU LES TUTEURS

AU PROFIT DE LA SOCIÉTÉ
DES FOYERS D'ACCUEIL DU TENNESSEE

AIDER UN ENFANT À TROUVER UN FOYER,
TEL EST NOTRE CREDO

La triste histoire du petit Shad est racontée de nouveau en lettres d'imprimerie inégales sur des lignes pointillées à côté de questions telles que « Bonne santé ? Robuste ? Difforme ? Handicapé ? Malade ? Est-ce que l'enfant a eu l'appendicite ? Est-ce qu'il est faible d'esprit ? Est-ce qu'il est adoptable ? »

Le formulaire confiant le petit Shad à l'adoption est signé, scellé devant témoins. L'enfant est transféré au foyer d'accueil de Memphis, pour observation, en vue d'un placement.

— Je ne comprends vraiment pas ce que tout cela veut dire.

Mais une chose est sûre, ma grand-mère ne serait jamais venue si souvent à Edisto pour rencontrer Trent Turner Sr. si ce n'était pas important. J'ai aussi du mal à croire qu'elle se serait donné tant de mal juste pour aider un ami. C'était une affaire personnelle.

— Est-ce qu'il reste d'autres dossiers comme celui-là ? Est-ce que votre grand-père a laissé d'autres choses ?

Trent détourne le regard comme pour décider de ce qu'il peut me dire, luttant de nouveau avec sa conscience. Il finit par lâcher :

— Juste quelques enveloppes scellées comme celle-ci, avec un nom dessus. Mon grand-père a pu transmettre la plupart des documents à qui de droit avant de décéder. Les paquets restants doivent concerner des gens qui avaient dû mourir sans qu'il le sache.

Trent s'interrompt pour changer Jonah de position – il s'est endormi sur son épaule.

— Il a suivi certaines affaires pendant cinquante ou soixante ans, depuis le début de ses recherches, en fait. Pourquoi il décidait de s'occuper de tel ou tel cas, je ne sais pas. Je ne lui ai jamais demandé. Je me souviens vaguement que des clients venaient le voir avec des photos et s'asseyaient à la table, dans le petit cabanon dehors, où ils pleuraient et parlaient, mais cela n'était pas si fréquent. Il menait le plus gros de ses affaires à Charleston. Si j'ai pu avoir une vague idée de son activité, c'est parce que je venais ici, à Edisto, avec lui, dès que j'en avais l'occasion. De temps en temps, il recevait des gens ici – pour plus de discrétion, j'imagine. J'ai l'impression qu'il avait parfois à faire à des personnes très influentes.

Il m'adresse un regard entendu et je sais qu'il me met dans le même sac. Je frémis.

— Je ne vois toujours pas ce que tout cela a à voir avec ma grand-mère. Est-ce qu'il y a quelque chose dans les papiers de votre grand-père qui serait lié à une certaine « May Crandall » ? Ou peut-être à quelqu'un appelé Fern... ou Queenie ? Il pourrait s'agir d'amis de ma grand-mère.

Il pose le menton sur les cheveux tout doux de Jonah.

— Ces noms ne me disent rien mais, comme je vous l'ai expliqué tout à l'heure, je n'ai pas vu ses documents depuis sa mort. J'ai fermé son bureau et je n'y ai pas remis les pieds.

D'un mouvement de l'épaule, il m'indique le petit cabanon comme endormi sous le halo d'une lampe de jardin.

— Je me suis juste chargé des enveloppes, comme il me l'avait demandé. Quoi qu'il reste dans son bureau, je me suis dit qu'il pensait que ce n'est plus important. Il était très respectueux de la vie privée des gens, vu ce qu'il avait traversé en découvrant la vérité sur sa naissance. Il n'avait jamais voulu prendre la responsabilité d'altérer l'histoire familiale de quelqu'un d'autre de la même façon. Sauf si on lui demandait précisément ce genre d'informations.

— Cela veut donc dire que ma grand-mère est bel et bien venue le voir ?

— Étant donné ce que je sais des méthodes de travail de mon grand-père, oui.

Il se mordille la lèvre, pensif. Je me surprends à le fixer, en perdant presque le fil de la conversation.

— Si quelqu'un d'autre avait cherché à retrouver votre grand-mère – un parent perdu de vue, disons –, mon grand-père aurait donné les papiers à cette personne dès qu'il aurait trouvé votre grand-mère, puis il aurait fermé le dossier. Il laissait toujours ses clients décider de prendre contact ou non. Le fait qu'il n'ait pas fermé le dossier et qu'il ait écrit Judy Stafford dessus signifie que votre grand-mère cherchait quelqu'un... une personne qu'il n'a jamais réussi à trouver.

Mon esprit tourne à toute vitesse, malgré l'heure tardive.

— Est-ce qu'il serait possible que je voie le reste ?

Je sais que ma demande est déplacée, mais j'ai peur que Trent change d'avis s'il a le temps de réfléchir à tout ça. Une leçon de tribunal. Si vous avez besoin que votre témoin change de direction, demandez une pause. Sinon, continuez à le presser dans la direction que vous suivez.

— Croyez-moi, il vaut mieux éviter d'entrer là-dedans la nuit. C'est un vieux cabanon d'esclaves qui a été placé sur la propriété, il ferme donc très mal. On ne sait pas ce qui peut vivre dedans à l'heure actuelle.

— J'ai grandi dans des écuries. Je n'ai pas peur de grand-chose.

Il a un sourire en coin, ce qui fait apparaître une fossette.

— Pourquoi est-ce que cela ne me surprend pas ? demande-t-il avant de remonter Jonah sur son épaule. Laissez-moi juste le temps de le recoucher.

Nos regards se croisent et, l'espace d'un instant, nous… nous perdons dans les yeux l'un de l'autre. C'est peut-être la lumière tamisée des lampes anciennes ou le côté intime du cottage, mais j'éprouve quelque chose que je ne veux pas du tout ressentir. Une émotion qui se glisse en moi, languide et tiède, comme un bassin d'eau de mer laissé par la marée un soir d'été quand l'atmosphère s'est rafraîchie.

Je plonge un orteil dans l'eau, je ris doucement, je me sens rougir, je baisse les yeux avant de jeter un autre coup d'œil à la dérobée vers Trent. Son sourire s'épanouit et une étrange sensation se propage en moi jusqu'à mes doigts de pied. Comme un éclair crépitant au loin sur l'eau – quelque chose d'imprévisible et de dangereux.

J'en reste ébahie un instant, j'oublie où je suis et pourquoi je me trouve là.

La tête de Jonah roule sur l'épaule de son père et le charme est rompu. Je m'éveille comme un patient le lendemain d'une anesthésie. Mon esprit est embrumé. Mes idées mettent un moment à s'éclaircir et me forcent enfin à détourner les yeux. Quelque part dans le processus, je jette un coup d'œil vers mon annulaire où, à cet instant, il n'y a plus de bague de fiançailles parce que, avant que ma soirée ne prenne un tournant aussi fou, je l'avais enlevée pour éviter de la badigeonner de crème après ma douche.

Mais qu'est-ce qui se passe ? Je n'ai jamais rien connu de pareil. Jamais. Je ne suis pas du genre à avoir des absences. Je ne me laisse pas subjuguer par des gens. Je ne me conduis pas de manière inconvenante avec des inconnus. L'importance capitale de ne pas faire ce genre de chose a été gravée en moi depuis ma naissance, ce que la fac de droit a bien renforcé.

— Je ferais mieux d'y aller.

Comme fait exprès, mon téléphone vibre dans ma poche – intrusion du monde réel. Ma chaise grince quand je la recule. Le bruit semble prendre Trent de court. Est-ce qu'il avait vraiment l'intention de me laisser entrer dans le bureau de son grand-père cette nuit ? Ou envisageait-il quelque chose de plus... intime ?

J'ignore le téléphone et je remercie Trent de m'avoir donné l'enveloppe avant d'ajouter :

— On pourrait peut-être se voir demain ?

Au grand jour, tout sera plus clair. J'ajoute :

— Pour regarder ce qu'il reste d'autre ?

Je prends un risque, dans tous les cas. D'ici demain, Trent aura eu le temps de repenser à tout cela. Mais, là, cette nuit, les risques sont d'une autre nature.

— Je vous ai dérangé bien trop longtemps. C'était vraiment impoli de ma part d'appeler à cette heure-ci. Je suis désolée... J'étais si... désespérée de savoir.

Il réprime un bâillement, ferme les yeux puis force ses paupières à se rouvrir.

— Aucun problème. Je suis un oiseau de nuit.

— Ça se voit.

Ma plaisanterie lui arrache un éclat de rire.

— Demain, dit-il, comme une promesse. Après le travail, par contre. J'ai une journée bien remplie. Je vais demander à ma tante si elle peut garder Jonah quelques heures de plus.

Cet engagement me soulage. J'espère juste qu'il le respectera toujours après une bonne nuit de sommeil.

— On se voit demain soir, dans ce cas. Appelez-moi pour me dire vers quelle heure. Oh, et ne laissez pas Jonah chez sa tante à cause de moi. J'ai trois neveux, des triplés de deux ans. J'adore les petits garçons.

Après avoir récupéré les papiers de mamie Judy et ma lampe de poche, je fais un pas vers la porte avant de m'arrêter, cherchant du regard un crayon et un bout de papier.

— Je devrais vous donner mon numéro.

— Je l'ai déjà, répond-il avec une grimace. Sur mon portable, au moins... deux cents fois.

Sa réponse devrait m'embarrasser mais nous rions tous les deux. Il se tourne vers le couloir.

— Laissez-moi recoucher Jonah, je vais vous raccompagner jusqu'à la plage et vérifier que vous rentrez bien chez vous.

Ma tête dit aussitôt « Non », mais je dois tout de même me forcer à articuler quand je lui réponds :

— Pas la peine. Je connais le chemin.

Par la fenêtre, je vois le paysage illuminé par le clair de lune, l'eau qui scintille à travers les palmiers qui bordent le jardin du cottage. Les hibiscus et le jasmin frémissent dans la brise marine. C'est un mariage parfait. Du genre que seule cette région de Caroline du Sud peut créer.

Trent me jette un coup d'œil.

— On est au beau milieu de la nuit. Laissez-moi au moins me conduire en gentleman.

J'attends pendant qu'il va recoucher Jonah. Puis nous traversons la galerie à l'arrière pour descendre les marches. Le vent venu de la mer soulève mes cheveux et les fait tourbillonner, effleure au passage ma peau et se glisse dans mon T-shirt. Au pied des marches, je regarde vite fait le petit cabanon d'esclaves, j'étudie les vieilles fenêtres aux croisillons de bois, six en tout, qui courent sur toute la façade. Est-ce que des réponses sont cachées derrière le verre voilé par le sel ?

— Il date des années 1850, déclare Trent, comme pour chercher un sujet de discussion.

Nous ressentons peut-être tous les deux la pression étrange qu'exerce cet endroit, exigeant de nous bien plus qu'une conversation polie.

— Mon grand-père l'a déplacé lui-même jusqu'ici lorsqu'il a acheté ce terrain. Il s'en servait au début comme bureau professionnel. Ce lopin a été sa première transaction immobilière. Il a acquis le terrain adjacent à la propriété Myers et l'a divisé pour y faire construire cette maison-ci et les deux qui se dressent entre elles.

Encore un lien entre Trent Turner Sr. et ma grand-mère. À l'évidence, ils se connaissaient depuis longtemps. Est-ce qu'elle l'avait engagé pour l'aider à trouver quelqu'un car elle savait qu'il s'occupait de ce genre de chose ? Ou bien est-ce cette activité qui l'a conduit à ma grand-mère ? Est-ce elle qui lui a suggéré d'acheter la propriété à côté de son cottage ? Est-ce que le Trent Turner actuel est aussi perdu que moi au milieu de ces histoires de famille ? Est-ce qu'une génération a vécu des vies entremêlées qui, pour une raison obscure, ont été dissimulées à la génération suivante ?

Ces questions me nouent le cerveau lorsque nous nous arrêtons au sentier de la plage, où les hautes herbes luisent tels des brins de verre filé au clair de lune.

— C'est une belle nuit, dit-il.

— Oui, c'est vrai.

— Méfiez-vous. La marée monte. Vous allez vous mouiller les pieds.

Du menton, il me désigne l'océan et je ne peux pas m'empêcher de suivre son regard. Une procession de vagues semble dessiner un chemin jusqu'à la lune tandis que, dans le ciel, le manteau étoilé brille d'un impossible éclat. Depuis combien de temps ne me suis-je pas assise dans le noir pour profiter d'une nuit pareille ? Tout à coup, j'éprouve une envie irrépressible. D'eau, de ciel et de journées qui ne sont pas divisées en carrés minuscules dans un agenda.

Est-ce que ma grand-mère ressentait la même chose ? Était-ce pour cette raison qu'elle venait ici si souvent ?

— Je vous remercie encore... de m'avoir laissée interrompre votre soirée.

Je fais un pas en arrière, du sable à l'herbe. Quelque chose se glisse devant mon pied, et je pousse un petit cri.

— Vous feriez mieux d'allumer la lampe.

La dernière chose que je voie avant de m'entourer d'une sphère de lumière artificielle, c'est Trent qui m'adresse un grand sourire.

Je tourne les talons et je m'éloigne, en sachant qu'il m'observe.

Mon téléphone vibre de nouveau et, quand je le sors de ma poche, c'est comme un portail vers un autre monde. Je ne mets pas de temps à le franchir. J'ai besoin de quelque chose de familier, de sûr, sur lequel me concentrer, après cet étrange moment sur la plage avec Trent.

Mais pourquoi Abby m'appelle-t-elle ? Du bureau, à Baltimore ? Pourquoi essayer de me joindre à cette heure indue ?

Quand je réponds, elle est hors d'haleine.

— Avery, te voilà ! Tout va bien ? J'ai reçu un e-mail tordu de ta part, tout à l'heure.

Je m'esclaffe :

— Oh, Abby, je suis désolée. Je voulais me l'envoyer à moi-même.

— Tu dois te rappeler où tu vas, maintenant ? Voilà où t'a mené ta vie dans la haute société de la Caroline du Nord ?

Abby est une habitante typique de Washington, une battante qui a grimpé tous les échelons depuis le logement social de ses parents jusqu'à la fac de droit. C'est aussi une avocate fédérale incroyable. Nos déjeuners et nos cogitations sur les affaires en cours me manquent beaucoup.

Si je devais me confier à quelqu'un à propos des informations autour de mamie Judy, ce serait elle, mais il est plus sûr de l'interroger sur ce qui se passe au bureau.

— Longue histoire. Dis-moi, pourquoi es-tu encore levée à cette heure ?

— Je bosse. Demain, le juge a ordonné la production de plusieurs pièces. Pour blanchiment d'argent, faux et usage de faux. Une grosse affaire. Ils ont engagé Bracken et Thompson.

— Waouh... les grands pontes.

Parler boutique me ramène direct chez moi, à Baltimore. Quelles que soient les idioties qui me sont passées par la tête chez Trent, elles disparaissent aussitôt, ce qui m'arrange bien.

— Dis-moi où vous en êtes.

Mes sens se mettent en alerte d'une façon qui n'a rien à voir avec la nuit ou le coup d'œil par-dessus mon épaule qui m'apprend que Trent m'observe toujours.

Abby se lance dans les détails de l'enquête et mon esprit se concentre sur l'affaire. Une vérité indéniable me frappe soudain.

Mon ancienne vie me manque.

16

Rill

— On se lève, c'est le matin ! On dirait que le soleil a enfin décidé de se montrer aujourd'hui ! déclare Mlle Dodd en déverrouillant la porte du sous-sol.

Mlle Dodd est nouvelle, elle est là depuis deux jours. Elle est plus jeune que les autres et plus gentille aussi. Si j'arrive à lui parler seule à seule, je lui demanderai des nouvelles de Camellia. Personne ne veut me dire où est ma sœur. Mme Pulnik m'ordonne de la fermer et d'arrêter d'embêter les employées avec ça.

Danny Boy prétend que Camellia est morte. Il m'assure qu'il s'est réveillé un soir et a entendu Mme Murphy dire à Riggs que Camellia était morte après avoir été mise dans le placard et ce qu'il devait faire d'elle. Danny Boy raconte que Riggs a porté son corps jusqu'au camion pour aller le jeter dans les marais. Il l'a vu de ses yeux. Il dit que ma sœur est partie pour toujours et que c'est bon débarras.

Je ne crois pas un mot de ce que dit Danny Boy. Il est mauvais jusqu'au trognon.

Mlle Dodd me dira la vérité.

Pour l'instant, elle est surtout embêtée par la puanteur qui flotte dans la chambre. Il y fait humide lorsqu'il pleut, et, par-dessus le marché, Fern mouille le lit toutes les nuits depuis qu'ils ont pris Camellia et Gabion. Je supplie Fern de se retenir, mais ça ne change rien.

— Par tous les cieux, quelle pestilence ! s'écrie-t-elle en nous toisant d'un air inquiet. Ce n'est pas un endroit pour des enfants.

Je me place entre elle et le lit de camp mouillé. J'y ai empilé les couvertures parce que c'est tout ce que j'ai trouvé pour cacher la vérité.

— J'ai... j'ai renversé le pot de chambre.

Elle regarde dans le coin de la pièce. Le ciment est sec sous le pot.

— Est-ce que quelqu'un a eu un petit accident au lit ?

Les larmes me montent aux yeux et Lark recule vers le mur en entraînant Fern avec elle. J'attrape le tablier de Mlle Dodd tout en tournant la tête parce que je m'attends à recevoir une gifle. Malgré tout, je dois l'empêcher de monter prévenir Mme Pulnik.

— Ne le dites pas.

Les cils châtains de Mlle Dodd papillonnent au-dessus de ses yeux gris vert doux.

— Au nom de saint François, et pourquoi pas ? Nous allons nettoyer la tache et tout ira bien.

— Fern va avoir des ennuis.

J'imagine que Mlle Dodd ne sait pas encore ce qui arrive aux enfants qui mouillent leurs lits, ici.

— Oh, doux Jésus, bien sûr que non.

— S'il vous plaît...

Je sens la panique monter en moi comme un raz-de-marée.

— S'il vous plaît, ne le dites pas.

Je ne peux pas perdre Fern et Lark. Je ne sais pas vraiment ce qui est arrivé à Camellia et, après quatre jours, je me doute que ces gens ne vont pas non plus nous rendre Gabby. J'ai perdu mon frère. Camellia a disparu. Lark et Fern sont tout ce qu'il me reste.

Mlle Dodd prend mon visage entre ses deux mains et me tient la tête tout doucement.

— Chhhh. Calme-toi, maintenant. Je vais m'assurer que ce sera nettoyé. Ne t'inquiète pas, ma puce. Nous garderons ça pour nous.

Mes larmes coulent de plus belle. Personne ne m'a tenue de cette façon depuis Queenie.

— Calme-toi, répète-t-elle avant de jeter un coup d'œil nerveux en arrière. On ferait mieux de monter avant qu'ils viennent nous chercher.

Je hoche la tête en lâchant un « Oui, m'dame » étranglé. Le pire, ce serait que j'attire des ennuis à Mlle Dodd. Je l'ai entendue dire à une des cuisinières que son père était mort l'année dernière et que sa mère était malade de l'hydropisie, et elle a quatre petits frères et sœurs qui vivent dans une ferme au nord, dans le comté de Shelby. Mlle Dodd a marché et a fait de l'auto-stop jusqu'à Memphis pour trouver du travail afin de leur envoyer de l'argent.

Mlle Dodd a besoin de ce travail.

Moi, j'ai besoin de Mlle Dodd.

Je rassemble Fern et Lark et nous franchissons la porte avant Mlle Dodd. Riggs traîne près de la chaudière, curieux comme un chien de cuisine. Comme toujours, je baisse la tête et l'observe du coin de l'œil.

— Monsieur Riggs, lance Mlle Dodd juste avant que nous atteignions les marches. Je me demandais si vous pouviez m'accorder une faveur ? Pas besoin d'en parler à qui que ce soit.

— Pour sûr, m'dame.

Avant que j'aie le temps de l'interrompre, elle demande :

— Est-ce que vous pourriez mélanger un peu de Javel et d'eau pour frotter le lit de camp près de la porte ? Laissez-moi le seau quand vous aurez fini. Je laverai le reste plus tard.

— Oui, m'dame. Je-je le fe-ferai pour vous, bafouille-t-il, et ses dents tordues dépassent de son sourire, longues et jaunes comme celles d'un castor. J'imagine que celles-là vo-vont bientôt mon-monter à l'étage.

Il agite le manche de la pelle vers nous.

— Le plus tôt ce sera, le mieux cela vaudra.

Mlle Dodd ne sait pas à quel point elle se trompe. Une fois à l'étage, il n'y aura plus de porte verrouillée entre nous et Riggs.

— Une chambre au sous-sol ne convient pas à de jeunes enfants, ajoute-t-elle.

— Non, m'dame.

— Et s'il y avait le feu à la maison, elles pourraient se trouver prises au piège.

— En cas de f-feu, je dé-dé-défoncerais la porte, ça oui.

— Vous avez bon cœur, monsieur Riggs.

Mlle Dodd ne sait pas la vérité, sur Riggs. C'est sûr.

— M-merci, m'dame.

— Et pas besoin de parler du nettoyage à qui que ce soit, lui rappelle-t-elle. Ce sera notre petit secret.

Riggs se contente de sourire et nous observe, ses yeux blancs sur les bords, fous comme ceux d'un ours en hiver. Quand on voit un ours en hiver, il faut être très prudent. Il a faim, il veut trouver de la nourriture pour ne plus avoir faim. Il se fiche de savoir ce que c'est.

Le regard de Riggs ne me quitte pas pendant le petit-déjeuner et même plus tard dans la journée quand le jardin est assez sec pour qu'on nous laisse sortir. En traversant la galerie, je jette un coup d'œil dans le coin et je pense à Camellia en me demandant : Est-ce que Danny Boy disait vrai ? Est-ce que ma sœur est morte ?

Ce serait ma faute. Je suis la plus âgée. J'étais censée protéger tout le monde. C'est la dernière chose que Briny m'ait dite avant de partir en vitesse pour traverser le fleuve. « Surveille les petits, Rill. Prends soin de tout le monde, jusqu'à ce qu'on revienne. »

Même les noms résonnent étrangement dans mon esprit, maintenant. Les gens m'appellent toujours May. Peut-être que Rill est encore sur le fleuve, quelque part avec Camellia et Lark, Fern et Gabion. Ils se laissent peut-être porter par le courant paresseux de l'été, regardant les bateaux et les barges passer, et les éperviers tournoyer au-dessus de l'eau, guettant un poisson à pêcher.

Rill n'est peut-être qu'une histoire que j'ai lue, comme Huck Finn et Jim. Peut-être que je ne suis pas, que je n'ai jamais été, Rill.

Je me tourne, dévale les marches et traverse le jardin à toute vitesse, ma robe claquant sur mes jambes. J'écarte les bras, la tête en arrière, je vole au vent et, l'espace d'un instant, je retrouve Rill. Je suis elle. Je suis sur l'*Arcadie*, notre petit bout de paradis.

Je ne m'arrête pas de courir quand j'arrive au portail où les grands ont leur tunnel. Ils sont occupés à embêter deux nouveaux enfants arrivés pendant la pluie de la veille. Des frères, je crois. Je m'en fiche, de toute façon. Si Danny Boy essaye de m'arrêter, je serre mon poing et je l'assomme, comme Camellia le ferait. Je le ferai rouler dans la poussière contre le grillage et je lui grimperai sur le ventre pour passer par-dessus la clôture et être libre.

Je ne m'arrêterai pas de courir avant d'être arrivée à la berge du fleuve.

Je contourne le vieil appentis en cavalant toujours aussi vite que possible et je saute contre les barreaux de fer, j'essaie d'arriver suffisamment haut pour me hisser par-dessus, mais je n'y parviens pas. Bien avant le sommet, je glisse et tombe lourdement. J'agrippe les barreaux, je les secoue, je crie, je hurle comme une bête sauvage se débattant dans une cage.

Je continue jusqu'à ce que les barreaux soient tout glissants de sueur et de larmes, et tachés par mon sang. Les barreaux ne cèdent pas. Ils ne s'ébranlent pas d'un pouce. Ils tiennent bon alors que je m'effondre au sol en m'abandonnant aux larmes.

Quelque part, derrière le bruit de mes sanglots, j'entends Danny Boy dire :

— La jolie fille a perdu la boule, pour sûr.

J'entends Fern et Stevie qui pleurent, Fern qui m'appelle et les grands qui les malmènent, qui les font tomber chaque fois qu'ils essaient de passer le portail. Je dois y aller. Je dois les aider mais, plus que tout, j'ai juste envie de disparaître. Je veux me retrouver seule dans un endroit où personne ne pourra me trouver. Où personne ne pourra me voler ceux que j'aime.

Danny Boy tord le bras de Stevie derrière son dos et le force à dire « Je me rends », avant de continuer quand même jusqu'à ce que le cri de Stevie me poignarde le ventre. Il crève l'endroit

227

que je voudrais aussi dur que la pierre. Comme Excalibur, le cri de Stevie me transperce.

Sans réfléchir, je retraverse la cour et j'attrape Danny Boy par les cheveux, si fort que sa tête bascule en arrière.

— Lâche-le ! Laisse-le partir et ne lui fais plus jamais mal. Sinon je te briserai la nuque comme celle d'un poulet. Je le jure.

Sans Camellia pour se bagarrer à notre place, tout à coup, je suis elle.

— Je te briserai la nuque, et c'est toi que je balancerai dans les marais.

Un autre garçon lâche Fern et recule. Il me fixe, les yeux écarquillés. Quand je vois mon ombre, je comprends pourquoi. Mes cheveux volent dans tous les sens. Je ressemble à Méduse, des mythes grecs.

— Bagarre ! Bagarre ! hurle un enfant avant de venir profiter du spectacle.

Danny Boy relâche Stevie. Il ne veut pas se prendre une raclée devant tout le monde. Stevie tombe tête la première et se relève la bouche pleine de terre. Il crache et pleure, je pousse Danny Boy au loin pour prendre les mains de Stevie et de Fern. Nous sommes de l'autre côté de la colline quand je me rends compte qu'il manque quelqu'un. Mon cœur se serre.

— Où est Lark ?

Fern s'enfonce un poing dans la bouche comme si elle craint de se faire gronder. Elle a peut-être peur de moi, après ce qu'elle vient de voir.

— Où est Lark ?

— 'adame, bredouille Stevie, le premier mot que je l'entends prononcer depuis qu'on est arrivés ici. 'adame.

Je m'agenouille dans l'herbe humide et je les regarde bien en face, tous les deux.

— Quelle madame ? Quelle madame, Fern ?

— La madame l'a sortie sur la galerie, murmure Fern à travers ses doigts, les larmes aux yeux. Comme ça.

Elle attrape Stevie par le bras et le soulève avant de le traîner au sol sur quelques pas. Stevie hoche la tête pour me dire que c'est ce qu'il a vu, lui aussi.

— Une madame ? Pas Riggs ? Ce n'est pas Riggs qui l'a attrapée ?

Ils font non de la tête, tous les deux.

— 'adame, répète Stevie.

J'ai l'esprit toujours embrumé par des larmes séchées et un reste de haine. Est-ce que Lark s'est attiré des ennuis ? Est-ce qu'elle était malade ? Impossible. Au petit-déjeuner, elle était comme d'habitude. Ils n'emmènent pas les enfants à l'infirmerie sauf s'ils sont brûlants de fièvre ou qu'ils vomissent.

Je pointe le terrain de jeux du doigt en leur ordonnant :

— Allez là-bas, tous les deux. Asseyez-vous sur la bascule et n'en descendez pas, quoi qu'il arrive, sauf si je viens vous chercher ou si vous entendez la cloche. Compris ?

Ils ont l'air de mourir de peur, tous les deux, mais ils hochent la tête et se prennent la main. Je les regarde marcher jusqu'à la bascule, puis je me dirige vers la maison. Quand je passe devant le portillon, je fais savoir à Danny Boy que, s'il les embête, il aura affaire à moi.

Mon courage me quitte aussi vite qu'il était venu quand je traverse le jardin. Je fixe la maison en espérant voir Mlle Dodd. Un marteau me cogne dans les tympans quand je grimpe sur la pointe des pieds les marches de la galerie et que j'entre dans la buanderie. Selon qui me verrait là, je pourrais avoir de gros ennuis si on croit que j'essaie de voler de la nourriture.

Les femmes de couleur sont occupées à la lessiveuse et à l'essoreuse quand je passe devant la porte. Est-ce qu'elles savent ce qui est arrivé à Lark ? Est-ce qu'elles me le diraient si elles le savaient ? D'habitude, nous nous passons devant sans rien dire, comme s'il valait mieux pour tout le monde que nous nous ignorions.

Elles ne lèvent pas les yeux et je ne demande rien. Il n'y a personne dans la cuisine, et je me dépêche de sortir de la pièce pour ne pas m'y faire surprendre.

Les portes battantes grincent quand je passe la tête dans le hall d'entrée de la maison de Mme Murphy. Il est presque trop tard quand je l'entends parler et que je vois la porte de son bureau ouverte. Mlle Tann y est aussi. Je reconnais sa voix et, à son ton mielleux, je comprends qu'elle parle à quelqu'un d'autre que Mme Murphy.

— Je pense que vous la trouverez charmante. Parfaite à tout point de vue. La mère avait commencé l'université avant la crise. Une jeune femme très intelligente et considérée comme très jolie. C'est héréditaire, assurément. Cette petite est une vraie Shirley Temple et n'aura même pas besoin d'une indéfrisable. Elle parle peu mais elle a de très bonnes manières. Elle ne vous mettra jamais dans l'embarras en public, ce qui, je le sais, est important dans votre profession. J'aurais préféré que vous nous permettiez de vous l'amener chez vous. Ce n'est pas notre procédure normale de laisser les nouveaux parents venir dans nos foyers.

— J'apprécie que vous ayez fait preuve de souplesse, répond un homme à la voix grave, comme un commandant d'armée. Il est difficile pour nous de nous rendre où que ce soit sans être reconnus.

— Nous comprenons parfaitement, susurre Mme Murphy – je ne l'ai jamais entendue parler de façon si aimable. Votre visite est un véritable honneur. Dire que vous êtes là, chez moi !

— Vous avez choisi l'une de nos meilleures pupilles, déclare Mlle Tann en se rapprochant de la porte. Et tu te conduiras comme la meilleure, n'est-ce pas, Bonnie ? Tu feras tout ce que ta nouvelle maman et ton nouveau papa te demanderont. Tu es une petite fille très chanceuse. Et tu nous en es très reconnaissante, n'est-ce pas ?

Bonnie, c'est le nouveau nom de Lark.

Je tends l'oreille pour savoir si elle répond, mais je n'entends rien.

— Bien, je suppose que nous devons te laisser partir, même si tu vas beaucoup nous manquer, dit Mlle Tann.

Un homme et une femme sortent dans le hall, avec Lark. L'homme est très beau, comme un prince dans un livre de contes de fées. La femme est magnifique, avec une coiffure sophistiquée et du joli rouge à lèvres. Lark porte une robe blanche à frous-frous. On dirait une ballerine miniature.

Ma gorge se noue. J'ouvre la porte de la cuisine en grand. Tu dois les arrêter, me dis-je. Tu dois leur montrer que Lark est ta sœur et qu'ils ne peuvent pas la prendre.

Une main m'attrape par le bras et me tire en arrière, et la porte se referme en claquant. Je trébuche, je chancelle tandis que quelqu'un me traîne à travers la cuisine, la buanderie, jusqu'à la galerie à l'arrière. Je ne sais même pas qui me tient jusqu'à ce que Mlle Dodd me fasse pivoter et me redresse en me tenant par les épaules.

— Tu n'as pas le droit d'aller là-bas, May ! s'écrie-t-elle, les yeux exorbités, la peau blême – elle semble presque aussi apeurée que moi. Tu connais les règles ! Si tu embêtes Mme Murphy et Mlle Tann, tu le paieras cher.

La boule qui me noue la gorge se brise comme un œuf frais pondu. Qui s'écoule, poisseux, chaud, épais.

— M-ma sœur...

— Je sais, ma chérie, répond-elle en me prenant le visage entre les mains. Mais tu dois penser à son bien. Elle a une maman et un papa qui sont des stars de cinéma.

Elle inspire comme si elle venait de gagner le gros lot à la tombola de la foire.

— Je sais que tu seras triste un moment, pourtant, c'est ce que l'on pouvait espérer de mieux. Des parents tout neufs et une maison toute neuve. Une toute nouvelle vie.

— On a déjà des parents !

— Chut ! Calme-toi.

Mlle Dodd m'entraîne dans le jardin, loin de la porte. Quand j'essaie de me libérer, elle me cramponne.

— Tais-toi. Tu ne peux pas faire une scène. Je sais que tu voudrais que tes parents reviennent vous chercher, mais ils ne peuvent pas. Ils ont signé un acte de remise à la Société des foyers d'accueil du Tennessee. Vous êtes tous orphelins, maintenant.

— C'est faux !

Je hurle. Je ne peux pas m'en empêcher. Je lui sors toute la vérité – tout sur l'*Arcadie*, et Queenie, et Briny et mon frère et mes sœurs. Je lui parle de Camellia et du placard, et les employées qui racontent des versions différentes de ce qui lui est arrivé, et Danny Boy qui m'a dit qu'on l'avait jetée dans les marais.

Mlle Dodd reste plantée là, bouche bée. Elle me tient si fort par les épaules que ma peau s'étire et me brûle.

— Tu me jures devant Dieu que c'est la vérité ? demande-t-elle quand je me retrouve à court de mots.

Je ferme les yeux très fort, hoche la tête et ravale mes larmes et ma morve.

— Chhh, souffle-t-elle en me serrant contre elle. Ne dis rien de plus. À personne. Reste là, va jouer avec les autres enfants. Sois sage et ne dis rien. Je vais voir ce que je peux apprendre sur cette histoire.

Quand elle me relâche, je lui attrape la main.

— Ne le dites pas à Mme Murphy. Elle m'enlèvera Fern. Fern, c'est tout ce qu'il me reste.

— Je ne dirai rien. Je ne te laisserai pas non plus. Je vais découvrir ce qui est arrivé à ta sœur. Dieu m'en soit témoin, nous allons arranger ça, mais tu vas devoir être très forte.

Elle me fixe droit dans les yeux et je vois du feu en elle. Même si ce feu est réconfortant, je sais ce que je viens de lui demander. Si Mme Murphy peut faire disparaître Camellia, elle pourra faire pareil avec Mlle Dodd.

— N-ne les laissez pas vous faire du mal, mademoiselle Dodd.

— Je suis plus futée qu'il n'y paraît.

Elle me chasse vers le jardin et, en un rien de temps, nous avons une amie, ici. Quelqu'un écoute enfin notre histoire.

Cette nuit-là, Fern pleure et fait une crise interminable en réclamant Lark. Même quand j'essaie de lui lire quelques pages du livre, elle ne veut pas se calmer et je finis par ne plus la supporter. Je l'attrape, je lui serre les bras, je la soulève et plante mes yeux dans les siens.

— Arrête ! je hurle, et ma voix résonne dans la petite pièce. Arrête, espèce d'idiote ! Elle est partie ! Ce n'est pas ma faute ! Arrête, ou tu vas avoir une fessée !

Je lève la main, et ce n'est que lorsque ma sœur cligne, cligne, cligne des yeux que je vois ce que je suis en train de faire.

Je la lâche sur le lit, me détourne, m'attrape les cheveux et tire jusqu'à ce que ça me fasse mal. Je veux me les arracher tous. Jusqu'au dernier. Je veux connaître une douleur que je comprends au lieu d'une agonie que je ne comprends pas. Je veux une douleur qui ait un début et une fin, pas une qui dure encore et encore et qui tranche jusqu'à l'os.

La douleur me change en quelqu'un que je ne connais même pas.

Elle me transforme en l'une d'elles. Je le vois sur le visage de ma sœur. Ça me blesse plus que tout le reste encore.

Je tombe sur le lit de camp que Mlle Dodd a fait nettoyer pour nous. Il sent la Javel, maintenant. Lorsque trois bonbons à la menthe roulent de sous l'oreille sale, je les jette vers le pot de chambre.

Fern vient s'asseoir près de moi et me tapote le dos comme le faisait maman pour calmer un bébé. Ce jour, cet endroit, et tout ce qui s'est passé ici me traverse l'esprit. Je le vois comme un film du cinématographe, comme ceux qu'on peut regarder pour cinq cents lorsque la foire traverse les villes fluviales et braque ses projecteurs brillants sur le flanc d'un bâtiment ou d'une grange. Mais les images qui bougent dans ma tête ondulent, floues, trop rapides.

Je finis par sombrer plus loin encore, et tout devient noir et silencieux.

Au milieu de la nuit, je me réveille, et Fern est blottie contre moi. Une couverture nous recouvre toutes les deux. Elle est de travers et un peu bouchonnée, du coup, je comprends que c'est Fern qui a dû la mettre là.

Je la serre en rêvant de l'*Arcadie*, et c'est un joli rêve. Nous sommes tous réunis, de nouveau, et le jour est si doux, c'est comme des gouttes de nectar tombées d'un chèvrefeuille. Je tends la langue et savoure, savoure.

Je me perds dans l'odeur du feu de bois et du brouillard matinal si épais qu'il dissimule la rive opposée et transforme le fleuve en océan. Je cours sur les bancs de sable avec mes sœurs, je me cache dans les hautes herbes et j'attends qu'elles me trouvent. Leurs filets de voix se prennent dans la brume, si bien que je ne sais pas si elles sont près ou loin.

Sur l'*Arcadie*, Queenie fredonne une chanson. Je m'assieds dans l'herbe, immobile comme une statue, pour écouter la voix de ma maman.

> *Quand le merle au printemps*
> *Sur le saule pleureur,*
> *Perché et bercé, je l'entends chanter,*
> *Il chante Aura Lee,*
> *Aura Lee, Aura Lee,*
> *Jeune fille aux cheveux d'or,*
> *Le soleil se lève avec toi...*

Je suis tellement absorbée par la chanson que je n'entends même pas la porte du sous-sol se déverrouiller avant que le bouton de porte tourne. Je m'assieds d'un coup, je vois qu'il fait déjà jour. De fins rayons de soleil se glissent à travers les azalées et tombent en diagonale dans la chambre.

Dans le coin, Fern se lève du pot et remonte ses sous-vêtements. Après la nuit passée, elle a peut-être trop peur pour remouiller les draps.

— C'est bien, Fern, je lui murmure avant de refaire le lit.

— Pas besoin de ça. Toi, tu n'iras nulle part aujourd'hui.

La voix sur le seuil n'est pas celle de Mlle Dodd. C'est celle de Mme Murphy. Elle me cingle comme un fouet et m'ébranle tout entière. Elle n'était jamais descendue jusqu'ici.

— Comment oses-tu ? crache-t-elle en pinçant les lèvres si fort que ses pommettes ressortent.

L'air siffle à travers ses dents tordues. Après trois pas rapides, elle m'attrape par les cheveux.

— Comment oses-tu profiter de mon hospitalité, de ma gentillesse, pour me calomnier ? Tu croyais vraiment que cette petite péquenaude, cette petite vaurienne t'aiderait vraiment ? Oh, bien sûr, elle a été assez stupide pour croire tes mensonges. Mais tout ce que tu as gagné, c'est de lui faire perdre son travail, et Mlle Tann ira chercher les petits frères et les petites sœurs Dodd avant peu. On les a signalés à l'assistance sociale du comté de Shelby, et les papiers sont en cours de préparation. C'est ça que tu voulais ? Ça que tu avais en tête quand tu lui as déversé dans les oreilles ces horribles histoires concernant M. Riggs ? Mon propre cousin, non moins ! Mon cousin, qui nettoie le bazar que vous autres sangsues mettez dans le jardin, qui répare vos jouets et entretient la chaudière pour que ces petits chéris n'attrapent pas un rhume pendant les nuits froides !

Elle adresse un rictus haineux à Fern, qui a reculé aussi loin que possible dans le coin.

— Je... je... je n'ai pas...

Qu'est-ce que je peux faire ? Où est-ce que je peux aller ? Je pourrais essayer de m'enfuir par la porte, mais elle a piégé Fern.

— Ne perds pas ton temps à le nier. Honte. Honte à toi. Honte à toi pour tes mensonges. Je t'ai donné bien plus que les poux du fleuve que tu mérites. Eh bien, voyons comment tu te sentiras après avoir passé un peu de temps toute seule pour réfléchir à tes erreurs.

Elle me pousse fort et je tombe en arrière sur le lit. Elle attrape Fern avant que je puisse me relever.

Ma sœur hurle et tend la main vers moi.

— Arrêtez ! crié-je en me levant d'un bond. Vous lui faites mal !

— Estime-toi heureuse que je ne fasse pas pire. On devrait peut-être la faire payer pour tes crimes ? crache-t-elle en me poussant hors de son chemin. Donne-moi encore du souci, et je te jure que je le ferai.

Je veux me battre, mais je me retiens. Je sais que, sinon, ça retombera sur Fern.

— Sois sage, dis-je à ma petite sœur. Sois une bonne fille.

La dernière chose que je vois d'elle, ce sont ses pieds glissant dans la cendre de charbon lorsque Mme Murphy la traîne hors de la chambre. Le loquet tourne et j'écoute les cris de Fern qui s'éloignent de plus en plus. À la fin, ils disparaissent pour de bon.

Je me laisse tomber sur le lit de camp, j'attrape la couverture qui est encore chaude là où elle nous couvrait, Fern et moi, je pleure jusqu'à ce qu'il ne me reste plus de larmes, et je suis incapable de faire autre chose que de regarder le plafond.

J'attends toute la journée, mais personne ne vient me chercher. J'entrouvre le soupirail du sous-sol et j'entends les enfants jouer dehors. Le soleil monte dans le ciel, puis progresse vers l'ouest. Pour finir, la cloche du dîner retentit.

Peu après, les poutres du plafond vibrent sous les pas des enfants qui montent se coucher.

J'ai faim et j'ai soif mais, ce qui me manque le plus, c'est Fern. Ils ne vont pas la faire dormir ailleurs, pas vrai ? Juste à cause de ce que j'ai dit ?

Et pourtant, si, ils le font.

Quand le silence est revenu dans la maison, je me recouche. Mon estomac gargouille et me fait mal comme si un rat me le rongeait de l'intérieur. Dans ma gorge, j'ai l'impression que quelqu'un m'a griffée jusqu'à ce que la chair soit à vif.

Je dors, me réveille, dors, me réveille.

Le matin, Mme Pulnik vient m'apporter un seau d'eau et une louche.

— Ne bois que des petites gorgées. Tu ne ferras personne pendant quelque temps. Et tu es prifée de nourriture.

Elle ne m'apporte à manger que trois jours plus tard. J'ai tellement faim que je me suis mise à dévorer les bonbons à la menthe que Riggs glisse sous la porte, même si je me déteste de le faire.

Les jours se suivent et se ressemblent. Je lis jusqu'à la fin *Huckleberry Finn*, quand Huck décide qu'il préfère encore s'enfuir en territoire indien plutôt que de se faire adopter.

Je ferme les yeux et je m'imagine que je m'enfuis moi aussi en territoire Indien. J'ai un beau, un grand cheval bai, avec des balzanes et une liste blanche, comme Tony le Super Cheval, dans les films de Tom Mix. Ma monture est plus rapide que tout, et on galope, on galope, on galope.

Je recommence le livre depuis le début et me retrouve dans le Missouri, sur les bords du grand fleuve. Je voyage sur le radeau d'Huckleberry Finn pour passer le temps.

La nuit, lorsque le vent écarte les branches, je regarde par le soupirail, guettant Zede ou Silas ou Briny sous le lampadaire. Un soir qu'il y a du vent, je les vois. Une femme est avec eux. Elle est trop trapue pour être Queenie. Je crois que c'est Mlle Dodd.

Ils disparaissent aussi vite qu'ils étaient apparus. Je me demande si je ne suis pas en train de perdre la tête.

Un jour, Mme Pulnik vient me prendre mon livre en m'accusant d'avoir attiré des ennuis à Mme Murphy auprès des dames de la Société de bienfaisance. Elle me traite de voleuse et me frappe fort au visage parce que je ne lui ai pas rappelé que j'avais encore un ouvrage de la bibliothèque.

Je ne sais pas comment je vais tenir sans *Huckleberry Finn*. Je perds le compte des jours, mais il se passe longtemps avant que Mme Pulnik me fasse enfin sortir de la chambre et m'emmène au bureau de Mme Murphy. Je pue presque autant que le pot de chambre et mes cheveux sont emmêlés en grosses touffes crasseuses. La lumière est si vive là-haut que je trébuche, que je me cogne dans les meubles, au point que j'avance à tâtons.

Mme Murphy n'est qu'une ombre floue derrière son bureau. Je plisse les yeux pour la voir mieux, avant de me rendre compte que ce n'est pas Mme Murphy. C'est Mlle Tann. Mme Murphy se tient derrière elle, près de la fenêtre.

Mme Pulnik me pousse en avant. Mes jambes se dérobent sous moi et je tombe brusquement à genoux. Mme Pulnik m'attrape la robe et les cheveux et me maintient à terre.

Mlle Tann se lève et se penche par-dessus le bureau.

— Je crois que c'est exactement là qu'est ta place. Par terre, à genoux, pour implorer le pardon de tout le mal que tu as causé. Pour tous les mensonges que tu as racontés sur cette pauvre Mme Murphy. Tu n'es qu'une sale petite ingrate, n'est-ce pas ?

— O-oui, m'dame, dis-je dans un murmure.

Je dirais n'importe quoi pour sortir de cette pièce au plus vite.

Mme Murphy plante ses poings sur ses hanches.

— Tous ces mensonges, sur mon cousin ! Ces mensonges horribles, épouvantables...

— Tsss ! la coupe Mlle Tann, la main levée, et Mme Murphy ferme sa bouche. Oh, je crois que May sait bien ce qu'elle a fait. Je crois qu'elle cherchait juste à attirer l'attention sur elle. Est-ce donc cela, ton problème, May ? Tu aimes faire l'intéressante ?

Je ne sais pas quoi répondre, alors je reste là, à genoux, le cœur au bord des lèvres, le menton tremblant. Mme Pulnik me presse encore plus fort contre le sol. La douleur me descend de la racine des cheveux et remonte depuis mes genoux. Un torrent de larmes monte en moi, mais je ne peux pas le leur montrer.

— Réponds-moi !

La voix de Mlle Tann emplit la pièce comme un coup de tonnerre. Elle contourne le bureau de sa démarche claudiquante et se dresse devant moi en agitant le doigt. Ses yeux sont du gris froid des orages d'hiver.

— O-oui, m'dame... n-n-non, m'dame.

— Alors, oui ou non ?

J'ouvre la bouche, rien ne sort.

Ses doigts se referment sur mon menton. Elle me fait lever la tête et se penche vers moi. Elle sent le talc et a mauvaise haleine.

— On n'a plus la langue si bien pendue, maintenant, n'est-ce pas ? Tu as peut-être compris le mal que tu as fait ?

Je parviens à hocher un peu la tête.

Un sourire pince ses lèvres et ses yeux prennent un éclat glouton, comme si elle sentait ma peur et qu'elle aimait ça.

— Tu aurais peut-être dû y penser avant cette histoire ridicule à propos de ta sœur imaginaire et de ce pauvre M. Riggs.

Le sang me cogne dans la tête. J'essaie de comprendre ce qu'elle vient de dire, sans succès.

— Il n'y a jamais eu de... Camellia. Nous le savons très bien, toi et moi, n'est-ce pas, May ? Vous étiez quatre quand vous êtes arrivés ici. Deux petites sœurs et un petit frère. Juste quatre. Et nous avons merveilleusement bien travaillé en trouvant des foyers pour eux, jusqu'à présent. De bons foyers. Et, pour cela, tu nous es infiniment reconnaissante, n'est-ce pas ?

Elle fait un geste vers Mme Pulnik. Son poids disparaît de mes épaules. Mlle Tann me relève par le menton jusqu'à ce que je me tienne debout devant elle.

— Je ne veux plus entendre ce genre de sornettes de ta part. C'est compris ?

J'acquiesce en me détestant de le faire. C'est injuste. Tout ce que j'ai dit à Mlle Dodd était vrai. Mais je ne peux pas retourner au sous-sol. Je dois retrouver Fern et m'assurer qu'ils ne lui ont pas fait de mal. Fern, c'est tout ce qu'il me reste.

— Bien.

Mlle Tann me lâche, place une main sur l'autre devant elle et se balance sur ses talons tandis que sa robe virevolte autour de ses genoux.

Mme Murphy rit dans sa barbe.

— Eh bien, ces petits mioches des rues ont tout de même un peu de cervelle dans leurs têtes vides.

Les lèvres de Mlle Tann s'étirent en un rictus qui fait froid dans le dos.

— Même les plus récalcitrants peuvent être matés. Tout dépend des moyens employés pour leur inculquer la leçon.

Elle me lorgne des pieds à la tête en louchant, puis la pendule sonne sur le manteau de la cheminée.

— Je dois vraiment poursuivre mes affaires, dit-elle avant de me passer devant et de sortir en laissant un nuage poudreux parfumé dans la pièce.

J'essaie de ne pas l'inspirer mais il s'immisce dans mes narines.

Mme Murphy s'assied à son bureau et prend quelques papiers comme si elle avait oublié que j'étais là.

— Dorénavant, tu me seras reconnaissante pour mon hospitalité.

— O-oui, m'dame. E-est-ce que je peux voir Fern, maintenant ? m-madame Murphy ?

J'avais presque trop peur pour demander, pourtant, je me suis forcée, il le fallait.

Elle ne lève pas les yeux lorsqu'elle me répond :

— Ta sœur est partie. Elle a été adoptée. Tu ne la reverras plus jamais. Tu peux aller jouer dehors avec les autres enfants, maintenant.

Elle feuillette les papiers et prend un stylo.

— Madame Pulnik, assurez-vous que May prenne un bain avant que vous la montiez à l'étage jusqu'à son nouveau lit, ce soir. Je ne supporte pas son odeur.

— J'y feillerai.

Mme Pulnik referme sa main sur mon bras, je le sens à peine. Lorsqu'elle me laisse dehors, je reste assise longtemps sur les marches de la galerie. Les autres enfants me passent devant et me regardent comme une bête curieuse.

Je ne leur prête aucune attention.

Stevie s'approche et essaie de grimper sur mes genoux, mais je ne supporte pas qu'il soit près de moi. Cela me rappelle trop Fern.

— Va jouer avec les camions, lui dis-je, avant de m'éloigner dans le jardin, jusqu'à la clôture derrière la salle paroissiale, où je me glisse sous un nid de vignes sauvages pour me cacher.

À travers les feuilles, je regarde les fenêtres du dortoir des filles, à l'étage, et je me demande : Si je saute de là, cette nuit, est-ce que je mourrai ?

Je ne peux pas vivre sans Fern. Depuis sa naissance, c'est comme si nos cœurs étaient cousus.

Maintenant, mon cœur a disparu.

Je pose la tête sur le sol, je sens quelques rayons de soleil sur ma nuque et je laisse le sommeil m'envahir en espérant que je ne me réveillerai pas.

Quand je m'éveille enfin, quelqu'un me touche le bras. Je m'écarte en sursaut et me ramasse sur moi-même, pensant que c'est Riggs. Sauf que le visage qui m'observe me fait penser que je suis encore en train de rêver.

Forcément.

— Silas ?

Il pose un doigt sur ses lèvres.

— Chut ! murmure-t-il.

Je tends la main entre les barreaux, tremblante. Je dois m'assurer qu'il est réel.

Ses doigts se referment sur les miens. Il me serre fort.

— On vous a enfin trouvés, dit-il. Une dame à l'hôpital a forcé tes parents à signer des papiers juste après la naissance des bébés. On a dit à ton père que, s'il signait, la facture du docteur pour Queenie serait payée pour lui et que les bébés seraient enterrés comme il fallait. Mais les papiers n'étaient pas pour ça. Ça leur donnait le droit d'aller vous chercher sur l'*Arcadie*. Quand Briny et Zede ont été voir la police, on leur a dit que Briny vous avait confiés à la Société des foyers d'accueil du Tennessee – et qu'il n'y avait rien à y faire, que c'était comme ça. On vous cherche depuis des semaines. Cette femme, Mlle Dodd, elle a fini par nous trouver et nous dire où vous étiez tous. Je venais là dès que je pouvais, pour surveiller cet endroit, en espérant que t'y étais encore.

— Elles m'avaient enfermée... J'ai eu des problèmes.

Je n'arrive pas à croire à ce qui se passe. Ça doit être mon imagination.

— Où sont Queenie et Briny ?

— Ils préparent l'*Arcadie*. Pour qu'il soit prêt à reprendre le fleuve. Il est resté amarré longtemps.

Je m'assieds contre les barreaux. Ma peau est chaude et rouge. La sueur dégouline sous la chemise de nuit en haillons que je porte depuis des semaines, maintenant. Que pensera Briny quand il saura la vérité ?

— Ils ont pris tout le monde. Tout le monde sauf moi. Je n'ai pas réussi à faire ce que Briny voulait. Je n'ai pas réussi à faire en sorte qu'on reste ensemble.

— Ça va aller, murmure Silas, qui me caresse les cheveux pendant que je pleure, ses doigts coincés dans mes mèches emmêlées. Je vais te faire sortir de là. Je vais venir ce soir et couper un des barreaux... là-bas, sous le houx, où les feuilles sont bien épaisses. Tu peux venir là, cette nuit ? Tu peux sortir en douce ?

J'étrangle un hoquet, je renifle et je hoche la tête. Si James arrivait à descendre aux cuisines pour voler de la nourriture, alors je peux le faire aussi. Et si j'arrive aux cuisines, je peux sortir dans la cour.

Silas étudie la clôture.

— Donne-moi un peu de temps. Deux heures après la nuit noire, pour que je découpe ce barreau sans me faire voir. Ensuite, tu viens. Le moins de temps ils auront pour voir que t'es plus là, le mieux ce sera.

On prépare le plan, puis il me dit qu'il ferait mieux d'y aller avant qu'on le repère. J'ai toutes les peines du monde à lui lâcher la main, à ressortir des vignes et à m'éloigner de lui.

Ce n'est que pour quelques heures de plus, me dis-je. Juste la fin de la journée, puis le dîner, un dernier bain et je serai chez moi. Chez moi, sur l'*Arcadie*.

Mais quand je retraverse le jardin, je vois Stevie, qui me cherche partout, et je me dis : Et lui, alors ?

Danny Boy sort des buissons pour harceler Stevie au portillon.

— Tu le laisses tranquille.

Je vais me planter juste devant lui et je le regarde de haut. Je crois que j'ai grandi pendant que j'étais enfermée au sous-sol. Et j'ai maigri aussi, ça, c'est sûr. Le poing que j'agite sous le nez de Danny Boy semble si osseux qu'on le jurerait brandi hors d'une tombe.

— J'vais pas me battre contre toi. Tu pues de trop.

Danny Boy a du mal à avaler sa salive. Il se dit peut-être que, si j'ai survécu des semaines au sous-sol, je suis trop coriace pour lui. Il craint peut-être qu'on lui inflige la même chose s'il est surpris en pleine bagarre.

Il ne nous embête pas, ni Stevie ni moi, tout le reste de la journée.

Quand nous nous mettons dans la queue le soir, je garde la première place du rang, pour Stevie et moi. Ça ne plaît pas à Danny Boy, mais il n'a pas le courage de m'arrêter. Il se contente de se moquer de mes cheveux et de mon odeur.

— Il paraît que ta petite sœur stupide revient demain, crache-t-il dans mon dos quand on entre dans la maison. Il paraît que ces gens n'en voulaient pas, en fin de compte, parce qu'elle est trop débile pour pas pisser dans son lit.

C'est sans doute encore des mensonges, pourtant, une petite lueur d'espoir s'allume tout de même en moi. Je ne l'écrase pas du talon. Au contraire, je l'alimente et souffle dessus tout doucement. Après dîner, je prends mon courage à deux mains et je demande à une employée si c'est vrai que ma sœur Fern revient. Elle me le confirme. Depuis tout le temps qu'elle est partie, Fern n'a pas cessé de faire des crises, de me réclamer et se faire dessus.

— À croire que tout le monde est têtu comme un âne, chez vous, dit l'employée. Quelle honte. Elle risque de ne plus retrouver de famille, maintenant.

J'essaie de ne pas avoir l'air ravie, pourtant je le suis. Une fois que Fern sera revenue, nous pourrons nous enfuir toutes les deux, par contre, je vais devoir faire attendre Silas une autre nuit. Ce soir, je sortirai en douce pour l'avertir.

Je dois juste trouver le moyen de m'éclipser sans me faire attraper par les surveillantes. Elles risquent de m'avoir à l'œil puisque ce sera ma première nuit à l'étage. Mais ce ne sont pas les surveillantes qui m'inquiètent le plus ; c'est Riggs. Lui aussi, il doit savoir où je vais dormir ce soir.

Et il sait qu'il n'y a pas de verrou sur la porte.

17

Avery

Si vous avez du temps à tuer, l'île d'Edisto n'est pas un mauvais choix.

Le vent venu de la mer s'infiltre dans les moustiquaires et taquine l'ourlet de la robe portefeuille toute simple que j'ai enfilée en fin de journée. J'ai oublié de prendre le chargeur de mon portable avant de partir de chez moi. Maintenant, la batterie est à moitié vide, et il n'y a aucun chargeur compatible sur l'île. Plutôt que de répondre à des e-mails ou de farfouiller sur internet à la recherche d'éléments en rapport avec les révélations de cette nuit, j'ai été obligée de me distraire à l'ancienne.

Faire du kayak dans l'estuaire valait bien une deuxième douche à peine tiède, même si cela m'a aussi valu une tache indélébile sur mon short, due au résidu noirâtre sur le siège du kayak de location, mélange de moisissure et de vase. J'ai l'impression d'avoir redécouvert le moi de mon enfance.

Mon excursion à la rame a ravivé des souvenirs enfouis depuis longtemps d'une virée à Edisto avec mon père quand j'étais en sixième. Je travaillais sur un projet sur les écosystèmes des eaux noires du littoral. En bonne petite perfectionniste, j'avais voulu collecter mes propres échantillons et prendre des photos plutôt que de me contenter de celles publiées dans des livres. Mon père avait cédé. Nos deux jours passés ici nous ont fourni quelques-uns de nos rares moments père-fille qui n'étaient pas liés à un concours hippique ou à une opération de communication. Je chéris encore ce souvenir, même toutes ces années plus tard.

Je me souviens aussi que c'est Elliot qui m'avait aidée à fabriquer le décor pour ma présentation. On avait récupéré des éléments dans un placard rempli de vieux matériel de campagne, repeint les pancartes et discuté sans fin sur la meilleure façon de faire tenir toutes seules ces pancartes. Nous étions aussi peu doués l'un que l'autre pour le bricolage.

« Je ne sais pas pourquoi tu n'as pas acheté un truc tout fait », s'était-il plaint après notre deuxième échec cuisant. À ce moment-là, il était déjà tard et on se trouvait encore dans l'écurie de mon père, avec de la peinture jusqu'aux coudes, entourés de bouts de bois mal cloués.

— Parce que je veux indiquer sur mon devoir que la présentation a été faite à partir de matériaux recyclés. Je veux pouvoir dire que je l'ai fait moi-même.

— Je ne vois pas la différence…

Le reste de la dispute s'est perdu, et bien heureusement, dans les méandres du temps. Je me souviens en revanche qu'on était si bruyants que le palefrenier de mon père avait fini par venir nous voir avec des supports en bois utilisés pour les obstacles hippiques. Il y avait ajouté des colliers de serrage et du ruban adhésif résistant. Ensuite, Elliot et moi avions fait le reste.

Le souvenir de ce projet scientifique me fait rire. Je jette un coup d'œil à ma montre en pensant contacter Elliot pour le lui raconter, mais je ne veux pas être coincée au téléphone quand l'appel de Trent Turner arrivera. Je commence à m'inquiéter en voyant l'heure. Il est cinq heures passées, et je n'ai pas eu de nouvelles. Il finit plus tard, ce soir ?

Il a peut-être changé d'avis et ne veut plus me laisser voir le reste des dossiers de son grand-père.

Une autre heure passe tout doucement. Je suis aussi anxieuse qu'un hamster dans une cage trop petite. Je m'assieds. Me relève. Je me déplace dans le cottage en vérifiant que mon portable capte correctement.

N'y tenant plus, je me faufile jusqu'à la plage et je guette discrètement le moindre signe de vie autour du cottage de Trent. Quand mon téléphone sonne, j'ai fini par arriver à mi-chemin, jetant des coups d'œil derrière les dunes et à travers les hautes herbes.

Je suis tellement surprise par la sonnerie que je sursaute, trébuche dans le sable et manque de faire tomber mon portable.

— J'ai cru que je n'arriverais pas à vous joindre, déclare Trent lorsque je finis par décrocher. J'ai frappé trois fois et personne n'a répondu. Je me suis dit que vous aviez peut-être changé d'avis.

J'essaie de dissimuler mon excitation, en vain.

— Pas du tout ! Je suis là. Dans le jardin.

Il a dit qu'il avait frappé ? Il est à ma porte ?

— Je vais faire le tour.

Je me tourne vers le cottage Myers et je me rends compte à quel point je suis loin. Il va se douter de ce que je trafiquais.

— Attention, je crois que des orties poussent sur le portillon.

— Non, ça n'en a pas l'air.

Je fonce droit vers mon jardin, mais je cours dans le sable et ma longue robe s'enroule autour de mes jambes, mes tongs claquent à chaque pas. J'aperçois une chemise bleue près de la haie de palmiers de ma grand-mère juste à temps pour ralentir et avancer d'un pas nonchalant sur le caillebotis.

Malgré tout, Trent me décoche un regard perplexe.

— Vous m'avez l'air un peu trop chic… pour aller farfouiller dans le bureau de mon grand-père. Je vous ai dit que c'était le bazar, là-dedans, non ? Et qu'il y fait très chaud.

— Oh… vous parlez de ça ? dis-je en baissant les yeux vers ma robe. C'est tout ce qui restait dans ma valise. J'ai fait du kayak ce matin et j'ai bousillé mes autres vêtements. Je suis une vraie loque.

— Je vous assure que non.

J'essaie de savoir s'il se montre juste gentil ou si c'est un compliment, mais je n'arrive pas à trancher. Je comprends pourquoi il a du succès dans l'immobilier. Il suinte le charme par tous les pores.

— Vous êtes prête ?

— Oui, c'est parti.

Je referme le portillon à l'arrière du jardin et nous descendons ensemble vers la plage. Il s'excuse d'être rentré si tard.

— Il y a eu un peu d'agitation chez tata Lou, aujourd'hui. D'une façon ou d'une autre – aucun des cousins ne tient vraiment à confesser les détails –, Jonah s'est enfoncé un Choco Pop dans le nez. J'ai dû jouer au chirurgien pour lui enlever ça.

— Vous l'avez eu ? Il va bien ?

— Vive le poivre ! me lance-t-il dans un grand sourire. L'obstruction a été levée par injection d'air comprimé dans les voies nasales. Autrement dit, il a éternué. Quant à savoir si tata Lou réussira à confesser l'un des cousins pour savoir qui est le responsable, c'est pas gagné. Ils sont sept. Que des garçons, et Jonah est le plus petit, de trois ans – du coup, il apprend la vie à la dure.

— Le pauvre lapin. Je compatis. Je sais qu'être le plus jeune, ce n'est pas toujours facile. Il n'y a que des filles, dans notre famille, et c'était assez dur comme ça. Si vous devez aller le chercher...

— Vous rigolez ? J'aurais affaire à une vraie mutinerie si je faisais ça. Il adore être chez sa tante. Deux sœurs de ma mère et une cousine à elles habitent dans la même rue, et mes parents y sont aussi une partie de l'année, si bien qu'il y a toujours de l'animation et de bonnes choses à manger, sans parler des copains de jeu. C'est la raison principale qui m'a convaincu d'emménager ici et de racheter l'agence immobilière après la mort de la mère de Jonah. Je devais réduire mes heures de travail au plus raisonnable, mais je souhaitais aussi que Jonah soit entouré par sa famille. Je ne voulais pas qu'il grandisse dans un appartement, seul avec moi.

Mille questions se forment dans ma tête. La plupart me semblent beaucoup trop personnelles.

— Où habitiez-vous, avant ?

Je connais déjà la réponse. J'avais fait des recherches sur lui quand je craignais encore une affaire de chantage.

— New York.

Vu son pantalon en toile, son polo, ses mocassins décontractés et son léger accent texan, c'est dur de l'imaginer tiré à quatre épingles dans le costume noir habituel des businessmen new-yorkais.

— Je bossais dans l'immobilier pour les entreprises.

J'ai la drôle d'impression que, lui et moi, nous sommes un peu pareils. Nous nous ajustons tous les deux à un nouvel environnement, une nouvelle vie. J'envie la sienne.

— Un gros changement, j'imagine ? Vous vous plaisez, ici ?

— C'est un rythme beaucoup plus lent... répond-il avec une pointe de quelque chose, du regret, peut-être. Mais oui, c'est chouette, ici.

— Je suis désolée, pour votre femme.

Même si je m'interroge sur les détails, je ne demanderai rien. Son petit côté séducteur n'est peut-être que le résultat d'une solitude bien naturelle quelques mois à peine après une perte si terrible. Je ne veux surtout pas lui donner de faux espoirs. Je porte ma bague de fiançailles mais, comme c'est une émeraude de taille princesse, les gens ne comprennent pas toujours sa signification.

— Nous n'étions pas mariés.

Je rougis aussitôt, je m'en veux d'avoir tiré des conclusions. Ces temps-ci, on ne sait jamais quoi penser.

— Oh... désolée. Je veux dire...

— Ce n'est rien, me rassure-t-il dans un sourire. C'est compliqué, voilà tout. Nous étions collègues... et amis. Après son divorce, on a franchi quelques lignes, qu'on n'aurait jamais dû dépasser. Je me doutais que Jonah était de moi, pourtant Laura m'assurait que non. Puis elle a déménagé dans le nord de l'État pour redonner une chance à son mariage. J'ai laissé tomber. Je n'ai su la vérité pour Jonah qu'après l'accident de voiture qui l'a tuée. Jonah souffrait de blessures internes et il avait besoin d'un donneur pour une transplantation de rein.

La sœur de Laura a pris contact avec moi parce qu'ils espéraient que je serais compatible. C'était le cas, et voilà comment tout est devenu clair.

— Oh.

Je n'ai rien trouvé de mieux à dire.

Il surprend mon regard. Nous nous arrêtons de parler au moment de prendre le sentier qui tourne vers sa maison, et je sens que le reste de l'histoire va arriver.

— Jonah a deux demi-frères dont il ne se souvient déjà presque plus. Je crois qu'il n'aura pas la chance de les connaître, sauf s'ils décident de se mettre en relation une fois adultes. Après le jugement me confiant la garde de Jonah, leur père a décrété qu'ils ne devaient rien avoir à faire avec moi ou Jonah. Ce n'est pas ce que j'aurais souhaité, mais c'est comme ça. Du coup, je comprends les gens que mon grand-père aidait mieux que vous ne pourriez le croire.

— Je vois pourquoi.

Je suis surprise par sa totale franchise. La profondeur de son chagrin et de sa déception est évidente. Il n'essaie même pas de masquer le fait qu'il est en conflit avec certaines de ses décisions ou qu'une erreur de jugement passée a provoqué une situation remplie de choix difficiles. Ces réalités affecteront Jonah jusqu'à la fin de sa vie.

Je viens d'un monde où l'on n'admettrait jamais si ouvertement de telles choses, et encore moins à un quasi-inconnu. Dans le monde que je connais, une apparence flatteuse et une réputation intacte comptent plus que tout. Trent me pousse à me demander si je ne me suis pas trop habituée aux contraintes qui vont avec l'obligation de préserver une bonne image publique.

Que ferais-je si je me retrouvais sans une situation pareille ?

— Jonah m'a tout l'air d'un chouette petit garçon, dis-je.

— Il l'est vraiment. Je ne peux pas m'imaginer vivre autrement, maintenant. Tous les parents ressentent ça, sans doute.

— J'en suis certaine.

Il attend que je m'engage sur le sentier puis me suit. Je me prends une toile d'araignée dans la figure en entrant dans le jardin, puis une deuxième. Je me souviens aussitôt pourquoi mes cousines et moi, on se battait toujours pour savoir qui devait passer en premier sur les sentiers quand on faisait des promenades à cheval dans les bois de Hitchcock. Je décolle les fils soyeux de ma peau, puis j'attrape une fronde de palmier séchée pour l'agiter devant moi.

— Vous n'êtes pas aussi snob que je le pensais, glousse Trent.

— Je vous ai dit que j'avais grandi dans des écuries.

— Je ne vous croyais pas vraiment. Je pensais que le bureau de mon grand-père risquait de vous effrayer quand vous le verriez.

— Aucun risque, dis-je avant de voir par-dessus mon épaule qu'il sourit. Vous l'espériez ?

Le sentier débouche sur le jardin et son sourire disparaît dès que nous nous approchons du petit cabanon bas de plafond et que nous grimpons les marches du perron.

— Je ne sais pas trop. J'aurais préféré que mon grand-père soit encore là pour prendre lui-même ces décisions.

L'inquiétude creuse des lignes profondes sur son front bronzé tandis qu'il tire les clefs de sa poche et qu'il baisse les yeux vers elles.

— Je comprends. Vraiment. Je me suis demandé plus d'une fois si je devais vraiment farfouiller dans le passé de ma grand-mère, mais je ne peux pas m'en empêcher. Pour moi, la vérité est plus importante que tout.

Il glisse la clef dans la serrure et déverrouille la porte.

— Vous parlez comme une journaliste plutôt que comme une femme politique. Vous feriez mieux de vous méfier, Avery Stafford. Ce genre d'idéalisme se retournera contre vous dans la sphère politique.

Sa remarque me hérisse le poil.

— Et vous, vous parlez comme quelqu'un qui a fréquenté le mauvais genre d'hommes politiques.

Il ne dit rien d'autre que ce que Leslie m'a répété cent fois. Elle a peur que je sois trop intello et pas assez réaliste pour comprendre l'implication d'une candidature aux élections sénatoriales. Elle oublie que, ma vie durant, j'ai dû écouter des inconnus m'offrir leurs avis sur tout, depuis nos vêtements jusqu'aux coûts de nos études dans les écoles privées où nous allions. En fait, pas seulement des inconnus, mais aussi des amis.

— Dans ma famille, le service public est toujours du service public.

Son visage est impassible, si bien que je ne peux pas deviner s'il est d'accord avec moi ou non.

— Dans ce cas, vous n'allez pas aimer ce que vous allez découvrir en rapport avec la Société des foyers d'accueil du Tennessee. Ce n'est pas une histoire très jolie, quel que soit l'angle d'approche.

— Pourquoi ?

— C'était une institution extrêmement respectée, et la femme qui la dirigeait, Georgia Tann, opérait dans des cercles d'influence, tant sociale que politique. Elle était très estimée du grand public. Les gens admiraient son œuvre. Elle a changé la façon dont on percevait les orphelins, souvent considérés comme des cas irrécupérables. En réalité, à Memphis, cette Société des foyers d'accueil était pourrie jusqu'à la moelle. Pas étonnant que mon grand-père n'ait jamais voulu parler de ce qu'il faisait dans cette petite cabane. Les histoires sont tristes, voire horribles, et il y en a littéralement des milliers. Ces gamins étaient vus comme de la marchandise. Georgia Tann a fait fortune en faisant payer des sommes colossales pour l'adoption, le transport et la remise de ces enfants hors de l'État. Elle arrachait des gamins à des familles pauvres et les vendait à des célébrités ou à des hommes politiques. Elle avait les forces de l'ordre et les juges pour enfants dans sa poche. Elle dupait de jeunes mères à la maternité en leur faisant signer des papiers officiels alors qu'elles étaient encore sous sédatifs. Elle leur racontait que leurs bébés étaient morts alors que c'était faux.

Il tire une feuille de papier pliée de sa poche arrière et me la tend.

— Et ce n'est pas tout. J'ai imprimé ça, au bureau, entre deux rendez-vous.

C'est un scan d'un vieil article de journal. Le titre n'y va pas par quatre chemins : « La baronne de l'adoption : une tueuse en série parmi les plus prolifiques ? »

Trent s'immobilise, la main sur la poignée. Il attend que j'aie parcouru l'article.

— Personne n'entrait là sauf mon grand-père et, de temps en temps, des clients – pas même ma grand-mère. Il faut dire qu'elle ne s'intéressait pas au sujet. Je vous ai déjà dit que, pour elle, il ne servait à rien de remuer le passé. Elle avait peut-être raison. Sur la fin, mon grand-père a dû arriver lui aussi à cette conclusion. Il m'a dit de vider l'endroit et de détruire tout ce qui s'y trouvait encore. Je préfère vous prévenir. Je n'ai aucune idée de ce qui nous attend de l'autre côté de cette porte.

— Je comprends. Mais je suis... j'étais avocate dans le Maryland. Il en faut beaucoup pour me choquer.

Pourtant, le titre lui-même de l'article est choquant. Je sens que Trent ne me laissera pas entrer tant que je n'aurai pas lu toute l'histoire – tant que je n'aurai pas été prévenue. Il veut que je comprenne que ce que nous allons découvrir n'aura rien à voir avec de belles histoires mièvres de pauvres orphelins trouvant enfin des familles aimantes.

Je retourne à l'article et commence à parcourir le texte :

Jadis considérée comme la « mère de l'adoption moderne » et consultée par non moins qu'Eleanor Roosevelt pour réformer les politiques d'adoption aux États-Unis, Georgia Tann a en effet facilité l'adoption de milliers d'enfants des années 1920 jusqu'aux années 1950. Elle a aussi dirigé un réseau qui, sous sa surveillance, a laissé mourir ou provoqué la mort d'au moins cinq mille enfants et nourrissons.

« Bon nombre de ces enfants n'étaient pas orphelins, explique Mary Sykes qui, avec sa sœur encore bébé, a été volée sur le seuil de la maison de leur mère célibataire, à seulement quatre ans, pour être confiée à la Société des foyers d'accueil du Tennessee. La plupart d'entre eux avaient des parents aimants qui souhaitaient les élever. Bien souvent, les enfants étaient littéralement enlevés en plein jour et, malgré tous les efforts de leurs parents biologiques pour les récupérer légalement, on ne leur permettait jamais de gagner leurs procès. » Mme Sykes a vécu trois ans dans une grande maison blanche gérée par Georgia Tann et son réseau d'employées.

La jeune sœur de Mary, qui n'avait que six mois lorsqu'une dame qui se réclamait des services sociaux les a arrachées à la maison familiale, n'a survécu que deux mois dans ce foyer.

« On ne donnait pas de nourriture ni de soins corrects aux nourrissons, se rappelle Mme Sykes. Je me souviens de m'être assise par terre dans une salle pleine de berceaux, la main passée à travers les barreaux, pour tapoter le bras de ma sœur. Elle était trop faible, trop déshydratée ne serait-ce que pour pleurer. Personne ne voulait l'aider. Une fois qu'il est devenu clair que son état était irréversible, une employée l'a mise dans un carton et l'a emportée. Je ne l'ai jamais revue. J'ai entendu dire plus tard que, si les bébés tombaient trop malades ou s'ils pleuraient trop, on les abandonnait dans une poussette au soleil. J'ai moi-même des enfants, et même des petits-enfants, et des arrière-petits-enfants, maintenant. Je ne peux pas m'imaginer qu'on puisse faire de telles choses, et pourtant, c'est arrivé. Nous étions attachés aux lits et aux chaises ; nous étions battus, on nous maintenait la tête sous l'eau à l'heure du bain ; nous étions agressés sexuellement. C'était la maison des horreurs. »

En l'espace de trente ans, des enfants sous la protection de la SFAT ont massivement été déclarés disparus, leurs papiers se volatilisaient avec eux, ne laissant aucune trace de leurs vies. Si des membres de leurs familles biologiques venaient chercher des informations ou saisir les tribunaux, on leur disait simplement que les enfants avaient été adoptés et que les archives étaient scellées.

Opérant sous la protection de Boss Crump, l'homme politique le plus influent de Memphis à l'époque, le réseau de Georgia Tann était visiblement intouchable. »

Le reste de l'article décrit en détail la vente d'enfants à des parents fortunés et des stars de Hollywood, le chagrin des familles biologiques, les descriptions de maltraitance et d'agressions sexuelles. Les dernières lignes sont une citation d'un homme qui gère un site internet appelé Les Agneaux perdus.

« La branche de Memphis de la SFAT avait des informateurs partout – dans les bureaux des services sociaux, les cliniques rurales, dans les quartiers pauvres et les bidonvilles. Les bébés étaient souvent donnés à des travailleurs sociaux et des officiels qui auraient pu se mettre en travers de la route de Tann. Des parents adoptifs recevaient parfois des lettres de chantage, ils étaient menacés de se voir retirer la garde de leurs enfants adoptés. Georgia Tann cultivait la protection de Boss Crump et des juges aux affaires familiales. Au final, elle a pu altérer bien des vies selon son bon plaisir. Elle s'est prise pour Dieu, sans jamais éprouver le moindre regret. Elle a fini par mourir d'un cancer avant qu'on puisse la forcer à répondre de ses actes. Des gens puissants voulaient que l'affaire soit classée sans suite, ce fut donc le cas. »

— C'est...

Les mots me manquent. Je m'apprête à dire « incroyable », mais ce n'est pas le bon terme.

— ... épouvantable. C'est dur d'imaginer qu'une telle chose ait pu se produire, à si grande échelle... pendant des années.

— La SFAT n'a été forcée de fermer qu'en 1950.

Trent partage visiblement mon mélange d'effroi, d'étonnement et de rage. L'histoire de Mary Sykes touchant sa sœur mourante me rappelle mes nièces et mes neveux, et le lien qui les unit les uns aux autres. Courtney avait l'habitude de grimper dans le berceau des triplés et de s'endormir avec eux si elle les entendait pleurer la nuit.

— Je n'arrive pas... à m'imaginer.

J'ai déjà travaillé sur des affaires d'abus sexuels sur enfants et de corruption – ici, c'est l'échelle qui me sidère. Des dizaines et des dizaines de personnes devaient être au courant.

— Comment est-ce que tant de personnes ont pu fermer les yeux ?

Je comprends soudain. J'ai de la famille dans le Tennessee. Des membres influents de la vie politique. Ils détenaient des positions clefs aux niveaux national, judiciaire et fédéral. Est-ce qu'ils étaient au courant ? Est-ce qu'ils ont fermé les yeux ? Est-ce la raison pour laquelle mamie Judy était en contact avec Trent Turner Sr. ? Est-ce qu'elle essayait de redresser les torts familiaux ?

Elle ne voulait peut-être pas que le grand public découvre que sa famille avait été mêlée à ces actes monstrueux, voire qu'elle les avait encouragés...

Je me sens pâlir et je tends le bras pour prendre appui contre le mur. J'ai froid malgré la chaleur estivale.

Alors qu'il s'apprête à ouvrir la porte, Trent me lance d'un air inquiet :

— Vous êtes sûre ?

Il n'a pas l'air tellement plus rassuré que moi. On dirait deux gamins se défiant d'entrer en territoire interdit. Est-ce qu'il espère que je vais changer d'avis et nous éviter à tous deux les détails qui nous attendent, quels qu'ils soient ?

— La vérité remonte toujours à la surface, tôt ou tard. Je suis du genre à croire qu'on s'en tire mieux si on est prévenu assez tôt.

Malgré mes belles paroles, je m'interroge. Toute ma vie, j'ai été certaine que nous étions au-dessus de tout soupçon. Que notre famille était un livre ouvert. C'était peut-être naïf de ma part. Et si, pendant toutes ces années, j'avais eu tort ?

Trent regarde ses chaussures, dégage du pied un coquillage du seuil. Il rebondit contre un tracteur rouge en plastique qui semble particulièrement poignant à cet instant.

— J'ai peur de découvrir que l'adoption de mon grand-père était comme celles décrites par l'article, quand des enfants étaient donnés à des officiels pour les faire taire. Le père adoptif de mon grand-père était sergent dans la police de Memphis. Ils n'étaient pas de ceux qui pouvaient dépenser une fortune en frais d'adoption...

Il laisse sa phrase en suspens comme s'il ne voulait pas ajouter plus de mots à cette histoire, mais ses yeux reflètent ma propre peur. Portons-nous la culpabilité des péchés des générations passées ? Et, si c'est le cas, pouvons-nous supporter ce fardeau ?

Trent ouvre la porte et, peut-être, dévoile le mystère.

À l'intérieur, le cabanon est bas de plafond et rempli d'ombres. La peinture blanche s'écaille sur les murs en bardeaux et les fenêtres se sont tordues dans leurs châssis. L'air sent la poussière et la moisissure, et quelque chose d'autre qu'il me faut un instant pour identifier. Du tabac à pipe. Ce parfum me rappelle aussi mon grand-père Stafford. Son bureau dans la maison de Lagniappe Street a toujours eu cette odeur, même aujourd'hui.

Trent allume la lumière et l'ampoule clignote obstinément dans un abat-jour Ikea qui jure avec le reste de la décoration.

Nous entrons dans la pièce unique. Elle contient un grand bureau semblant venir d'une vieille bibliothèque, deux grands casiers, une petite table en bois et deux chaises dépareillées. Un vieux téléphone à cadran est toujours posé sur le bureau. À côté, une boîte de thé pleine de crayons à papier, une agrafeuse, une perforatrice trois trous, un cendrier qui n'a pas été vidé, une lampe de bureau col de cygne et une machine à écrire électrique d'un vert olive délavé. Les étagères qui longent le mur du fond ploient sous le poids des dossiers, des classeurs vieillissants, des feuilles volantes, des magazines et des livres.

Trent soupire, se passe la main dans les cheveux. Il semble trop grand pour cet espace réduit. Sa tête n'est qu'à vingt centimètres des poutres qui, je le vois maintenant, ont été taillées à la main et crantées – sans doute récupérées sur des épaves. Je lui lance :

— Ça va ?

Il hoche la tête puis hausse les épaules en me montrant un chapeau, un vieux parapluie au pommeau sculpté en forme de dragon et une paire de mocassins bleus. Les trois attendent près du portemanteau, dans l'espoir, dirait-on, que leur propriétaire revienne.

— On a l'impression qu'il est ici, non ? La plupart du temps, son odeur, c'était celle de cet endroit.

Trent ouvre les persiennes et la lumière du soleil illumine les affiches qui couvrent les murs.

— Regardez, murmuré-je, la gorge asséchée par la poussière.

Il y a littéralement des dizaines de photos, certaines arborant les couleurs vives de la modernité, d'autres dans des teintes passées de vieux Polaroid, d'autres en nuances de noirs et de gris, bordées de blanc, portant des dates telles que : juillet 1941, décembre 1936, avril 1952...

Trent et moi, nous nous tenons côte à côte, fixant le mur, chacun perdu dans ses pensées, impressionnés et horrifiés tout à la fois. J'observe ces images – des visages d'enfants juxtaposés à des visages d'adultes. Les ressemblances sont évidentes. Ce sont des mères, des pères, des enfants, sans doute des parents biologiques séparés les uns des autres. Les portraits des enfants sont accrochés près de photos plus récentes des adultes qu'ils sont devenus.

Je plonge les yeux dans le regard d'une belle jeune femme au sourire radieux, qui tient un bébé sur sa hanche. Une robe trop grande et un tablier pendouillent sur sa silhouette, lui donnant l'air d'une fillette déguisée. Elle ne peut pas avoir plus de quinze ou seize ans.

Que pourrais-tu me dire ? Que t'est-il arrivé ?

Près de moi, Trent observe quelques photos. Il y en a encore plus sous celles affichées au mur, des couches et des couches d'images. Trent Sr. était un homme consciencieux.

— Il n'y a rien d'écrit au dos, déclare-t-il. J'imagine que cela explique pourquoi il n'a pas pris la peine de me dire de m'en occuper. Impossible de savoir qui sont ces gens sans les connaître.

Mes pensées prennent une triste tournure, se teintent d'une émotion diffuse. Mon attention est attirée par une photo de quatre femmes, posant bras dessus bras dessous sur une plage. Même si la photo est en noir et blanc, j'imagine les couleurs vives de ces robes bain de soleil des années soixante et de leurs chapeaux à large bord. Je perçois même les reflets dorés du soleil sur leurs longues boucles blondes.

L'une de ces femmes est ma grand-mère. Elle tient son chapeau en place. Le bracelet libellule pend à son poignet.

Les trois autres femmes lui ressemblent. Les mêmes boucles blondes, les mêmes yeux clairs, bleus, sans doute. On pourrait facilement les croire de la même famille, alors que je n'en reconnais aucune.

Chacune d'elles porte un bracelet libellule semblable à celui de ma grand-mère.

Dans le fond, un peu flous, des petits garçons sont accroupis près de la trace laissée par la marée haute, les genoux pointés vers le haut tandis qu'ils s'occupent avec des seaux et construisent des châteaux de sable.

Est-ce que l'un d'eux est mon père ?

Je tends la main vers la photo et Trent s'étire pour me l'attraper. Lorsqu'il ôte la punaise, un petit cliché clair tombe, voletant comme un cerf-volant perdu dans le vent. L'image m'est familière avant même que je me baisse pour la ramasser.

Un agrandissement de cette scène se trouve dans un cadre nacré, sur la table de nuit de May Crandall, à la maison de retraite.

Une voix résonne dans l'air, mais je suis si concentrée que je ne me rends presque pas compte que c'est la mienne :

— J'ai déjà vu cette photo.

18

Rill

Dans la maison, il fait un noir d'encre. Pas de lampe allumée et les rideaux empêchent les rayons de la lune d'entrer dans le dortoir. Autour de moi, des enfants gigotent dans leurs lits, gémissent et grincent des dents dans leur sommeil. Après avoir été enfermée si longtemps toute seule dans le sous-sol, être avec les autres est rassurant mais, en vérité, l'endroit est loin d'être sûr. Ces filles racontent de sacrées histoires. Elles disent que Riggs vient parfois la nuit et prend celle qu'il veut – la plupart du temps, des petites qu'il peut porter facilement.

Je suis trop grande pour qu'on me porte. Je l'espère. Mais je n'ai aucune envie de le découvrir.

Silencieuse comme une ombre, je me glisse de sous ma couverture et je traverse le parquet sur la pointe des pieds. J'y ai déjà marché très prudemment ce soir pour me coucher dans mon nouveau lit. Je sais quelles lattes grincent. Combien de pas me séparent de la porte, puis de l'escalier, quel est le chemin le plus sûr pour passer devant le petit salon à côté de la cuisine où les employées sommeilleront dans leurs fauteuils. James m'a raconté comment il descendait à la cuisine la nuit pour voler les biscuits de Mme Murphy. Je sais comment il s'y est pris pour ne jamais se faire attraper.

Pourtant, tout ce qu'il avait découvert ne l'a pas sauvé, au bout du compte, du coup, je dois être prudente si je veux sortir en douce pour prévenir Silas que j'attends ici le retour de Fern. Dès qu'elle sera arrivée, je la prendrai dans mes bras et nous nous faufilerons dans la nuit, et Silas nous ramènera chez nous, sur le fleuve, et tous ces moments terribles seront enfin finis.

Et si Briny et Queenie ne voulaient plus de moi, après ce que j'ai fait ? Ils me haïront peut-être autant que je me hais. Peut-être qu'en regardant la fille maigre et triste que je suis devenue ils verront juste quelqu'un dont personne ne veut.

Je fais taire mon esprit, parce qu'un esprit, ça peut nous rendre fous si on le laisse faire. Je dois rester concentrée, faire bien tout ce qu'il faut pour ne pas être surprise.

Ce n'est pas aussi dur que je le craignais. J'arrive au pied de l'escalier en un rien de temps. Un petit cercle lumineux vient du salon près de la cuisine. Quelqu'un ronfle à l'intérieur. Près de la porte, une paire de pieds chaussés de gros souliers blancs est ouverte en éventail comme des ailes de mouche. Je ne regarde même pas à qui ils appartiennent. Je me contente de longer le mur près du poêle, en restant dans l'ombre comme James me l'avait dit. Mes orteils testent chaque nouvelle latte, très prudemment. L'ourlet effiloché de ma chemise de nuit se prend dans la façade rugueuse du poêle. J'imagine que cela fait du bruit, mais en fait, non.

La porte moustiquaire dans la buanderie grince un peu quand je tire dessus pour l'ouvrir. Je m'arrête, le souffle coupé, je tends l'oreille en guettant des bruits dans la maison.

Il n'y a rien.

Aussi silencieuse qu'un courant d'air, je sors. Dehors, les planches de la galerie sont humides de rosée, comme le pont de l'*Arcadie*. Au-dessus de moi, les sauterelles et les criquets stridulent si fort qu'on croirait entendre le pouls de la nuit, et un million d'étoiles brillent tels des feux de camp lointains. La demi-lune pend lourdement dans le ciel, comme si elle se balançait sur le dos. Sa jumelle chevauche la surface ridée de la citerne d'eau de pluie.

Tout à coup, je me retrouve chez moi. Enveloppée dans une couverture de nuit et d'étoiles. Cette couverture fait partie de moi, et je fais partie d'elle. Personne ne peut me toucher. Personne ne peut nous différencier l'une de l'autre.

Des crapauds-buffles croassent et des oiseaux noirs piaillent tandis que je traverse le jardin en courant, la fine robe blanche effleurant mes jambes, aussi légère que des soies d'asclépiade. Près de la clôture du fond, je m'approche des buissons de houx et je pousse le cri d'un engoulevent.

Un écho me répond. Je souris, j'inspire le parfum lourd et sucré du jasmin et je me précipite vers ce bruit en me frayant un chemin dans le tunnel des grands jusqu'à la clôture. Silas est de l'autre côté. Dans l'ombre, je ne vois pas son visage, juste le contour de son chapeau de paille et de ses jambes noueuses pliées comme celles d'une grenouille. Il tend la main vers moi à travers les barreaux.

— Allons-y, murmure-t-il avant de refermer ses doigts autour d'un barreau comme s'il comptait l'arracher à mains nues. J'ai découpé celui-là presque jusqu'au bout. Ça devrait...

Je lui attrape la main pour l'arrêter. S'il détache le barreau, les grands verront le trou au matin en venant à leur cachette.

— Je ne peux pas.

Pourtant, tout mon corps me hurle : « Vas-y ! Cours ! »

— Je ne peux pas partir tout de suite. Fern revient demain. Les gens qui l'avaient prise ne veulent plus d'elle. Je dois attendre demain soir, pour pouvoir l'emmener.

— Tu dois t'enfuir maintenant. Je reviendrai chercher Fern plus tard.

Des doutes fusent dans ma tête, de-ci de-là.

— Non. Une fois qu'ils sauront que je suis partie, qu'ils auront vu le trou dans la clôture, nous n'arriverons jamais à la faire sortir d'ici. Je pourrai encore m'éclipser demain soir. Et il y a aussi un petit garçon, Stevie. Il vient du fleuve, lui aussi. Je ne peux pas le laisser là.

Comment ferai-je pour le récupérer ? Je sais où il dort, mais de là à le prendre dans la chambre des petits, de récupérer Fern et de sortir sans que personne nous voie...

Cela semble impossible.

Et pourtant, la simple présence de Silas renforce ma détermination. Et me donne du courage. J'ai l'impression de pouvoir tout faire. Je trouverai un moyen. Je ne peux pas laisser Fern ou Stevie ici. Leur place est sur le fleuve. Leur place est avec nous. Mme Murphy et Mlle Tann m'ont déjà volé suffisamment de choses. Je veux tout récupérer. Je veux redevenir Rill Foss.

Avant que ce soit fini, je retrouverai toutes mes sœurs et mon petit frère et je les ramènerai à la maison, sur l'*Arcadie*. Voilà ce que je ferai.

Silas tend la main et son long bras maigre s'enroule autour de moi. Je me penche vers lui, son chapeau tombe. Son front se pose contre ma joue, ses cheveux noirs comme l'aile d'un corbeau me chatouillent le visage.

— Je ne veux pas que tu retournes là-bas.

Il glisse sa main sur mes cheveux, doucement, tendrement. Mon pouls s'accélère.

Je dois me retenir de ne pas défoncer la clôture, là, tout de suite.

— Ce n'est que pour un jour de plus.

— Je serai là demain soir, promet-il.

Il m'embrasse sur la joue. Une nouvelle émotion me traverse dans un frémissement et je dois fermer les yeux pour lutter contre elle.

Le laisser là est la chose la plus difficile que j'aie jamais faite de toute ma vie. Pendant que je m'éloigne à quatre pattes, il applique de la boue sur les barreaux pour que personne ne voie les coupures fraîches dans le métal. Si l'un des grands s'adosse à la clôture pendant qu'ils sont dans leur tunnel, j'espère que le barreau ne cédera pas.

Je suis de retour dans la maison, en haut de l'escalier – sans même respirer, j'ai l'impression. À l'étage, je jette un coup d'œil dans le couloir, je guette le moindre bruit avant de contourner la rambarde contre laquelle nous faisons la queue pour le bain. Il n'y a rien que les ombres projetées par le clair de lune qui s'invite par la fenêtre de l'escalier et des ronflements. L'un des petits parle dans son sommeil. Je me fige, mais il se tait aussitôt.

Plus que quinze pas et je serai de retour dans ma chambre. J'ai réussi. Personne ne saura où j'ai été. Demain, ce sera encore plus facile maintenant que je l'ai déjà fait une fois. James avait raison. Ce n'est pas difficile de s'en tirer, ici, quand on est futé.

Je peux tous les berner. Cette idée enfle en moi. Elle me donne l'impression que je leur ai pris quelque chose, quelque chose qu'ils m'avaient volé. Une impression de pouvoir. Voilà ce que je ressens, maintenant. Quand nous serons tous sains et saufs sur l'*Arcadie,* que le fleuve nous emportera loin d'ici, j'oublierai cet endroit. Je ne dirai à personne ce qui s'est passé. Ce sera comme si ce n'était jamais arrivé.

Un affreux cauchemar peuplé d'affreuses personnes.

Je suis si absorbée dans mes pensées que je marche où il ne faut pas. Une latte grince sous mon pied. Je retiens un hoquet, baisse les yeux et décide que la meilleure chose à faire, c'est de me dépêcher au cas où l'une des employées arriverait. Si je suis au lit, elles ne pourront pas savoir qui c'était...

Je ne vois pas M. Riggs avant de lui rentrer presque dedans. Il sort de la chambre des petits. Il recule d'un pas, et moi aussi. Son épaule se cogne dans le mur et il souffle :

— Ouille.

Je me tourne pour m'enfuir mais il m'attrape par la chemise de nuit et les cheveux. Sa grosse main se referme sur mon nez et ma bouche. Je sens une odeur de sueur, de whisky, de tabac et de cendre de charbon. Il me tire la tête en arrière si loin que je me dis : Il va me briser la nuque, tout de suite. Il va me briser la nuque et me pousser dans l'escalier et dire que je suis tombée. Ça finira comme ça...

Du coin de l'œil, j'essaie de l'observer. Il regarde partout, comme pour décider où il peut m'emmener. Je ne peux pas le laisser me descendre au sous-sol. Sinon, je suis morte. Je le sais. Fern va revenir demain, et je ne serai plus là.

Il jette un coup d'œil dans l'escalier et chancelle. Sa botte m'écrase l'orteil, et des étoiles explosent devant mes yeux pendant que je gémis. Il plaque sa main plus fort encore, au point que je ne peux plus respirer. J'entends ma colonne vertébrale craquer. Je me tortille, je pousse, je me débats pour me libérer, mais il m'écrase un peu plus contre lui avant de me soulever pour m'emmener au fond du couloir vers les ombres près de la porte de la salle de bains. Ses doigts cherchent la poignée à tâtons pour l'ouvrir. Je gémis, je me débats, j'essaie de me libérer jusqu'à ce qu'il pousse un grognement guttural sourd et me coince contre le mur pour pouvoir accéder à la porte. Son ventre m'écrase la poitrine, des points noirs tourbillonnent devant mes yeux et mes poumons brûlent par manque d'air.

Son visage s'approche de mon oreille.

— T-toi et moi, on p-p-peut être amis. Je p-p-peux te donner des b-b-bonbons et des b-b-biscuits. Tout ce que t-tu veux. On peut être les m-m-meilleurs amis du m-monde.

Il frotte sa joue contre mon menton et mon épaule, et ses moustaches m'irritent quand il me renifle les cheveux avant de fourrer sa tête dans l'encolure de ma chemise de nuit.

— T-tu sens comme d-dehors. T-t'as retrouvé un des g-grands en b-bas ? T-t'as un n-nouveau petit c-copain ?

Sa voix résonne comme si elle venait de très loin, comme les cornes de brume sur le fleuve par les matins froids. Mes genoux se dérobent sous moi. J'ai des fourmis dans les pieds, je ne les sens plus. Je ne sens plus le mur non plus, ni lui. Mes côtes tressautent comme les branchies d'un poisson pendu sur un enfiloir.

Je vois des fées, des étincelles. Elles dansent follement dans les ténèbres.

Non ! me dis-je. *Non !* Mais je n'ai plus d'arme pour me défendre. Mon corps n'est plus. Je vais peut-être étouffer et mourir. Je l'espère.

Tout à coup, il me relâche – un courant d'air frais m'effleure là où était son corps et une goulée d'oxygène me remplit le ventre. Je glisse le long du mur et m'effondre, étourdie, avant de cligner des yeux en essayant de me redresser.

La voix sèche d'une employée résonne dans l'escalier.

— Monsieur Riggs ? Que faites-vous ici à cette heure de la nuit ?

Ma vue s'éclaircit et je le vois dressé devant moi, pour qu'elle ne puisse pas m'apercevoir. Je recule dans l'ombre, blottie en boule contre le mur. Si on me surprend ici, c'est moi qui aurai des problèmes, pas lui. Ils vont encore m'enfermer... voire pire.

— J-j'ai entendu le tonnerre, y a pas longtemps. F-faut f-fermer les fenêtres.

L'employée arrive sur le palier. Le clair de lune l'illumine et je vois qu'il s'agit de la nouvelle qui est arrivée depuis le départ de Mlle Dodd. Je ne sais pas grand-chose sur elle, ni si elle est gentille ou méchante. Elle a une voix méchante. Elle n'aime pas que Riggs traîne là-haut, c'est clair et net. Si elle lui cherche des ennuis, elle ne restera pas longtemps chez Mme Murphy.

— Je n'ai rien entendu, répond-elle en se tournant d'un côté puis de l'autre, vers les portes des chambres.

— J'étais d-dehors q-quand j'ai entendu. Y avait des ch-chats errants qui m-miaulaient. J'ai s-sorti mon f-fusil pour les t-tuer.

— Dieu du ciel ! Vous auriez réveillé toute la maisonnée. Ces chats ne font de mal à personne, tout de même.

— C-cousine Ida, elle aime p-pas qu-qu'y ait des trucs qui rôdent.

Cousine Ida, c'est Mme Murphy. Il le précise pour remettre l'employée à sa place.

— Je vais m'occuper moi-même des fenêtres.

Elle ne va pas redescendre, et je ne sais pas si je suis rassurée ou pas. Si elle s'approche encore, elle me verra. Si elle part, Riggs me traînera jusqu'à la salle de bains.

— Inutile de déranger votre sommeil, monsieur Riggs, alors que je suis payée pour surveiller les enfants la nuit.

Il s'écarte de moi et se rapproche d'elle d'une démarche chaloupée. Il lui bloque le passage en haut de l'escalier. Les deux ombres ne font plus qu'une. Il murmure quelque chose.

— Monsieur Riggs ! s'écrie-t-elle tandis qu'une main sort de l'ombre avant d'y replonger – un claquement de peau contre peau s'ensuit. Avez-vous bu ?

— J'ai v-v-vu comment v-vous me regardiez.

— Je n'ai rien fait de tel !

— S-soyez g-gentille, ou je d-dirai à c-cousine Ida. Elle aime p-pas qu'on m-m-m'embête.

Elle se glisse contre le mur et le dépasse, il la laisse faire.

— Vous... vous avez intérêt à ne pas m'approcher ou... ou c'est moi qui irai tout dire. Je dirai que vous vous êtes enivré et que vous êtes comporté comme un malotru avec moi.

De son pas lourd, il s'approche des marches.

— V-vous feriez mieux d-d'aller voir les p'tits g-garçons d'abord. Qu-quelqu'un s'est levé d-de son lit, là-d-dedans.

Il descend bruyamment l'escalier. Les planches grincent et chantent.

Les bras croisés sur sa poitrine, l'employée le regarde partir avant de gagner la chambre des petits. Je me lève sur des jambes tremblantes et me précipite jusqu'à mon lit, où je tire les couvertures jusqu'à mon cou et m'enroule dedans. Et j'ai bien fait de me dépêcher, car l'employée visite notre chambre ensuite, peut-être parce qu'elle a vu que Riggs était tout près de la porte.

Elle avance dans le dortoir en soulevant des couvertures et nous inspecte les unes après les autres comme pour vérifier quelque chose. Quand elle arrive à mon lit, je me force à respirer lentement et profondément, et je me retiens de toutes mes forces de trembler lorsqu'elle soulève la couverture pour mettre sa main sur ma peau. Elle se demande peut-être pourquoi j'étais enroulée dedans alors qu'il fait une chaleur moite. Elle sent peut-être l'odeur de la nuit sur moi, comme Riggs.

Elle reste devant mon lit un moment.

Elle finit par partir et je reste allongée, les yeux ouverts dans l'obscurité. Encore un jour, me dis-je. Tu dois tenir encore un jour.

Je me le répète, encore et encore, comme une promesse. Il le faut. Autrement, je trouverai un moyen d'arracher la moustiquaire de la fenêtre et je sauterai en espérant que c'est assez haut pour que j'en meure.

Je ne peux pas vivre comme ça.

Je m'endors en sachant que c'est la vérité.

Au matin, je me réveille dans un état de nerfs épouvantable. Je me rendors, me réveille, me rendors, attendant que les voix des employées nous disent de nous lever et de nous habiller.

Je sais que je ne dois pas bouger avant. Mme Pulnik m'a bien fait comprendre les règles de l'étage avant de me montrer mon nouveau lit et la petite caisse en dessous où ranger mes affaires.

Mais je n'aurai pas besoin de cette caisse très longtemps. Je nous ferai sortir d'ici ce soir, tous les trois – Fern, Stevie et moi – par tous les moyens. Si je dois attraper un couteau de cuisine et poignarder quelqu'un pour passer, je le ferai, me dis-je. Je ne laisserai personne m'arrêter.

Ce n'est qu'en descendant pour le petit-déjeuner que je comprends que, ces promesses, je vais avoir du mal à les tenir. Dès qu'elle s'est levée, ce matin, Mme Pulnik a repéré des empreintes sableuses dans la cuisine. Elles sont sèches, du coup, elle devine qu'elles datent de cette nuit. Elles s'effacent avant d'arriver à l'escalier, si bien qu'elle ne sait pas où la piste menait, mais les traces sont suffisamment grandes pour qu'elle soit certaine qu'il s'agit de l'un des grands. Elle les a tous alignés et leur fait poser le pied l'un après l'autre sur l'empreinte pour découvrir le coupable.

Elle n'a pas encore remarqué que j'avais de grands pieds. Debout près de ma place à table avec les autres filles, je resserre les orteils en espérant qu'elle ne regardera pas vers moi.

Peut-être qu'un garçon aura la même pointure que moi, me dis-je, et je sais que c'est mal parce que j'attirerais des ennuis à un innocent. De gros ennuis. Mme Murphy, qui est aussi dans le réfectoire, semble plus échauffée qu'une marmite sur un poêle. Elle tient un parapluie dont on a arraché toute la toile. Elle a l'intention de fouetter quelqu'un avec. Ensuite, ce sera sans doute le placard.

Je ne dois pas finir dans le placard.

Mais est-ce que je peux laisser quelqu'un se faire punir à ma place sans rien faire alors que c'est ma faute ? Ce serait comme si je donnais moi-même ces coups de parapluie.

Du coin de l'œil, j'aperçois Riggs au fond de la buanderie, près de la porte de derrière. Il profite du spectacle. Il hoche la tête et me sourit, et mon sang se fige.

Debout, dans un coin, la nouvelle employée surveille la scène, et ses yeux sombres papillonnent dans toutes les directions. Elle n'a jamais rien vu de tel.

— C'est... c'est peut-être moi, balbutie-t-elle. M. Riggs m'a prévenue qu'il y avait des chats errants, dehors, et je suis sortie pour les chasser.

Mme Murphy l'entend à peine.

— Ne vous mêlez pas de ça ! hurle-t-elle. Et vos pieds sont trop petits. Qui essayez-vous donc de couvrir ? Qui ?

— Personne.

Ses yeux se braquent un instant vers moi.

Mme Murphy et Mme Pulnik essayent de suivre son regard. Le temps ralentit.

Ne bouge pas. Ne bouge pas, me dis-je. *Pas un geste.* Je reste figée.

— C-c'est p't'être m-moi, hier s-soir. Y-y a de la b-boue autour de la c-citerne d'eau de p-pluie, lance Riggs maintenant que tout le monde regarde de mon côté de la table.

Au début, je crois qu'il veut m'aider, puis je comprends qu'il veut juste éviter que je sois enfermée ce soir, là où il ne pourra pas me trouver.

Mme Murphy agite la main vers lui.

— Tais-toi donc. Franchement, tu es bien trop gentil avec ces petits ingrats. On leur donne un doigt et ils nous prennent le bras, soupire-t-elle avant de faire claquer le parapluie sur sa main en étudiant les filles de mon côté de la table. Bien... Si ce n'est pas un des garçons... qui cela peut-il être ?

La fille qui était dans le lit en face du mien la nuit dernière, Dora, penche la tête en arrière, s'affaisse sur elle-même et s'évanouit.

Personne ne bouge.

— Pas elle, j'imagine, déclare Mme Murphy. Dans ce cas, qui ?

Le parapluie tourbillonne en l'air comme une baguette magique.

— Écartez-vous de la table, les filles, ordonne-t-elle, l'œil brillant. Voyons qui peut bien être notre petite Cendrillon.

Le téléphone sonne, et tout le monde sursaute. Puis nous restons immobiles comme des statues, même les employées, pendant que Mme Murphy décide ou non de décrocher. Lorsqu'elle s'y résout, elle manque arracher le téléphone du mur, mais sa voix se fait toute mielleuse dès qu'elle reconnaît son interlocutrice.

— Oh, bonjour, Georgia. Quel bonheur d'avoir de vos nouvelles de si bon matin.

Elle marque une pause et reprend :

— Oui, bien sûr. Certainement. Je suis levée depuis des heures. Laissez-moi regagner mon bureau pour reprendre votre appel en privé.

Les mots qui résonnent dans le téléphone sont débités aussi vite que le *pan-pan-pan* des mitrailleuses Gatling des cow-boys dans les westerns.

— Oh, je vois. Bien sûr.

Mme Murphy pose son parapluie et place la main sur son front, ses lèvres étirées montrant ses dents d'une façon qui me rappelle Queenie la dernière nuit où je l'ai vue.

— Eh bien, nous pourrons y parvenir pour dix heures, mais je ne pense pas que ce soit souhaitable. Voyez-vous...

Une réponse fuse dans le combiné, rapide et sonore.

— Oui, je comprends. Nous ne serons pas en retard, siffle-t-elle à travers ses dents et, lorsqu'elle raccroche brutalement le combiné, elle me montre du doigt, les yeux plissés et la bouche en cul-de-poule.

— Emmenez-la, nettoyez-la et passez-lui une robe du dimanche. Quelque chose de bleu pour rappeler ses yeux... et avec un tablier. Mlle Tann la veut en ville, à l'hôtel, pour dix heures.

L'expression de Mme Pulnik reflète celle de Mme Murphy. La dernière chose dont elles aient envie, là, tout de suite, c'est de me donner un bain, de me coiffer et de m'enfiler une robe.

— Mais... elle...

— Ne me défiez pas ! hurle Mme Murphy avant de flanquer une torgnole à Danny Boy, parce qu'il est le plus près d'elle.

Tout le monde se crispe lorsqu'elle agite son doigt dans la pièce.

— Qu'est-ce que vous regardez, vous tous ?

Les enfants ne savent pas s'ils doivent s'asseoir ou rester où ils sont. Ils attendent jusqu'à ce que Mme Murphy ouvrent les portes battantes à la volée. Puis ils se glissent sur leurs chaises tandis que les gonds continuent de grincer.

— Je fais m'occuper de toi moi-même, déclare Mme Pulnik en m'attrapant par le bras et en me serrant fort.

Je sais qu'elle va se venger sur moi, d'une façon ou d'une autre.

Mais je sais aussi que, quoi que Mlle Tann ait prévu, ce sera peut-être pire. Il y a des histoires qui circulent sur ce qui arrive aux enfants lorsque les employées les emmènent à l'hôtel.

— Et ne lui faites pas de bleus ! ordonne Mme Murphy depuis le hall d'entrée.

Juste comme ça, je suis sauvée et, en même temps, pas du tout. Mme Pulnik me tire les cheveux et me tord de partout. Elle met tout en œuvre pour que l'heure suivante soit la plus douloureuse possible, et elle y parvient. Le temps qu'on me fasse enfin sortir pour rejoindre Mme Murphy dans la voiture, ma tête m'élance et mes yeux sont rouges de toutes les larmes que l'on m'a interdit de verser.

Dans la voiture, Mme Murphy ne dit pas un mot, ce qui m'arrange. Je me blottis contre la portière et je regarde par la vitre, effrayée et meurtrie. Je ne sais pas ce qu'il va m'arriver, mais je sais que ce ne sera rien de bon. Ici, rien de bon ne peut arriver.

Sur la route du centre-ville, nous passons devant le fleuve. Je vois des remorqueurs, des barges et un grand bateau-théâtre. La musique de son orgue à vapeur s'invite dans la voiture, et je me souviens comme Gabion aimait danser sur le pont de l'*Arcadie* quand les bateaux-théâtres passaient devant nous. Il nous faisait tous rire, encore et encore. Mon cœur s'étire vers l'eau, espérant voir l'*Arcadie*, ou le bateau du vieux Zede, ou n'importe quel bateau-maison, mais il n'y a rien. Sur la berge, un campement a été déserté. Il n'y a plus que quelques restes de feu de camp, des zones d'herbe piétinée et une pile de bois flotté que quelqu'un a ramassé et jamais brûlé. Les bateaux-logements sont tous partis.

Une idée me frappe soudain : on doit être presque en octobre. Bientôt, les érables et les copalmes vont changer de couleur, avec des touches de rouge et de jaune bordant leurs feuilles. Les vagabonds du fleuve ont déjà commencé le long et lent voyage vers le sud, là où les hivers sont doux et où l'eau regorge de gros poissons-chats.

Briny est toujours là, me dis-je mais, tout à coup, j'ai l'impression que je ne le reverrai plus jamais, ni Fern, ni aucun de ceux que j'aime. Ce sentiment m'engloutit tout entière, et ma seule défense est de laisser mon esprit quitter mon corps. Je n'y suis plus lorsque le chauffeur gare la voiture devant un haut bâtiment. J'entends à peine Mme Murphy me décrire les horreurs qu'il m'arrivera si je ne me conduis pas comme il faut. J'ai à peine mal lorsqu'elle me pince à travers ma robe et tourne la peau sur mes côtes en me disant que j'ai intérêt à faire tout ce qu'on me demande là-dedans, et que je n'ai pas le droit de dire non à qui que ce soit, ni de pleurer, ni de faire une scène.

— Tu seras bien gentille comme un petit chaton, m'ordonne-t-elle en me pinçant plus fort, son visage collé au mien. Ou tu le regretteras... et ton petit protégé aussi, Stevie. Tu ne voudrais pas qu'il lui arrive quoi que ce soit, n'est-ce pas ?

Elle me fait sortir sur le trottoir et m'entraîne à sa suite. Autour de nous, des hommes en costume avancent d'un pas pressé. Des femmes se promènent en tenant des paquets de couleurs vives. Une maman en manteau rouge sort de l'hôtel en poussant un landau et nous jette un coup d'œil en passant. Elle a un visage doux, je veux courir vers elle. Je veux m'accrocher à son manteau et tout lui raconter.

« Aidez-moi ! » lui dirai-je.

Mais je ne peux pas. Je sais qu'ils se vengeront sur Stevie si je fais ça. Et sans doute sur Fern aussi, une fois qu'ils l'auront ramenée chez Mme Murphy. Quoi qu'il arrive, je dois être sage aujourd'hui. Je dois faire tout ce qu'on me dit, afin qu'on ne m'enferme pas quand on rentrera ce soir.

Je me redresse et je me dis que c'est la dernière fois. C'est la dernière fois qu'ils me forceront à faire quoi que ce soit.

Quoi qu'on me veuille, je jouerai le jeu.

Mais mon cœur tressaute et mon ventre se noue comme un poing. Un homme en uniforme nous tient la porte. On dirait un soldat ou un prince. Je veux qu'il me sauve comme le font les princes dans les contes de fées.

— Bonjour, dit Mme Murphy, souriante, avant de lever le menton et d'entrer.

À l'intérieur de l'hôtel, les gens rient, discutent et déjeunent au restaurant. C'est un bel endroit, comme un château, mais j'ai du mal à voir sa beauté, à cet instant. Il ressemble trop à un piège.

Le liftier reste immobile comme une statue près des boutons. Il n'a même pas l'air de respirer lorsque la petite cabine nous emmène là-haut, tout là-haut. Quand nous sortons, l'homme me jette un regard triste. Est-ce qu'il sait où on m'emmène... et ce qu'il va se passer ?

Mme Murphy m'entraîne dans un couloir, puis toque à une porte.

— Entrez, lance une femme et, quand nous obéissons, nous voyons Mlle Tann vautrée sur un divan comme un chat paressant au soleil.

Derrière elle, les rideaux sont ouverts et une grande baie vitrée nous montre toute la ville de Memphis. Nous sommes au-dessus des toits. Je n'ai jamais été si haut de toute ma vie.

Je serre les poings et les cache dans mon tablier froissé en essayant de ne pas bouger.

Mlle Tann tient un verre à moitié plein. Elle semble patienter là depuis longtemps. Peut-être vit-elle à l'hôtel ?

Elle fait tournoyer le liquide marron, le soulève vers une porte en face du divan.

— Mettez-la dans la chambre, et ce sera tout, madame Murphy. Fermez la porte quand vous partirez... et ordonnez-lui bien de

273

rester assise sagement. Je parlerai avec lui ici, d'abord, pour m'assurer que tout est en règle selon notre... arrangement.

— Rester ne m'embête pas, Georgia.

— Comme vous voulez, répond-elle en me suivant des yeux lorsque Mme Murphy m'entraîne vers la porte en me soutenant par le bras, ce qui m'oblige à marcher de travers.

— Franchement, il y avait de meilleurs choix, mais je peux comprendre pourquoi il la veut.

— Moi, je ne comprends pas comment quiconque pourrait vouloir d'elle.

Dans la chambre, Mme Murphy me fait asseoir sur le lit, fait bouffer la robe à volants autour de moi, si bien que je ressemble à une poupée qu'on pose sur les oreillers. Elle tire mes cheveux par-dessus mon épaule et les laisse retomber en longues boucles, puis elle m'ordonne de ne pas bouger d'un pouce.

— Pas un, répète-t-elle en se dirigeant vers la porte, qu'elle referme derrière elle.

Je les entends parler dans la pièce d'à côté, Mlle Tann et elle. Elles discutent de la vue en buvant un verre. Puis il n'y a plus que les bruits lointains de la ville. Des coups de klaxon. Un tramway fait sonner sa cloche. Un vendeur de journaux alpague les passants.

Je ne sais pas combien de temps se passe avant que quelqu'un frappe à la porte de la suite. Mlle Tann va ouvrir en parlant de son ton mielleux, et j'entends la voix d'un homme, mais je ne comprends pas ce qu'ils se disent avant qu'ils s'approchent de ma porte.

— Bien sûr, elle est tout à vous... si vous êtes certain de toujours vouloir d'elle, évidemment, susurre Mlle Tann.

— Oui, et j'apprécie que vous ayez modifié nos arrangements en si peu de temps. Ma femme est accablée depuis des années, parfois au point de rester des semaines d'affilée au lit, où elle s'enferme loin de moi. Que puis-je faire d'autre ?

— En effet. Et je comprends que la fille puisse convenir à vos besoins, mais j'ai d'autres enfants qui sont plus...

accommodantes, suggère Mlle Tann. Nous avons beaucoup de filles plus âgées. À votre disposition.

Pitié, pensé-je. Choisissez quelqu'un d'autre. Et je comprends une nouvelle fois que j'ai de mauvaises pensées. Je ne devrais pas souhaiter qu'il arrive de mauvaises choses à d'autres enfants.

— Non, je la veux elle, spécifiquement.

Je serre les couvertures. De la sueur poisse la paume de mes mains et imprègne le tissu. J'y enfonce mes ongles.

Sois sage. Quoi qu'il se passe, sois sage.

Silas revient ce soir...

— Que puis-je faire d'autre ? répète l'homme. Ma femme est si fragile. L'enfant n'arrête pas de faire des crises. Je ne peux pas me permettre tout ce raffut en permanence dans la maison. Je suis compositeur, vous savez, et cela me gêne dans mon travail. Je dois rendre des partitions pour plusieurs films avant fin novembre, et le temps commence à manquer.

— Oh, monsieur, je peux vous garantir que vous aurez davantage de soucis avec cette fille, et non moins, intervint Mme Murphy. Je pensais... je croyais que vous la vouliez seulement pour... J'étais loin de me douter que vous comptiez l'emmener pour de bon, sinon je serais intervenue plus tôt.

— Peu importe, madame Murphy, rétorque Mlle Tann. La fille est suffisamment âgée pour se plier à tout ce que M. Sevier peut attendre d'elle.

— Oui... oui, bien sûr, Georgia. Pardonnez mon interruption.

— La fille est parfaite, à tout point de vue, je peux vous l'assurer, monsieur. Immaculée.

L'homme dit quelque chose que je ne comprends pas, puis Mlle Tann lui répond :

— Très bien, dans ce cas. J'ai ses papiers pour vous et, bien sûr, comme avec l'autre adoption, il faudra compter un an pour que la procédure soit finalisée, mais je doute que cela soit problématique, surtout pour un client de votre... stature.

La conversation s'interrompt. Des feuilles de papier crissent.

— Je veux juste que Victoria soit de nouveau heureuse, soupire l'homme. J'aime ma femme profondément, et ces dernières années ont été épouvantables. Les docteurs disent que le seul espoir qu'elle surmonte sa mélancolie, c'est qu'elle trouve une raison irrésistible de regarder vers l'avenir plutôt que vers le passé.

— De telles situations sont, évidemment, la raison même de notre existence, monsieur Sevier.

La voix de Mlle Tann tremblote, comme si elle se retenait de pleurer.

— Ces pauvres enfants perdus et les familles qui ont besoin d'eux me donnent l'élan nécessaire et la motivation pour le travail éprouvant que je fais. Jour et nuit, je supporte mon labeur et les débuts tristes de ces petits êtres pour pouvoir les sauver, leur accorder une existence, et ajouter de la vie à d'innombrables foyers vides. Bien sûr, venant moi-même d'une bonne famille, j'aurais pu choisir un chemin plus aisé, mais quelqu'un doit se sacrifier pour protéger ceux qui ne peuvent se protéger eux-mêmes. C'est une vocation. C'est ma vocation, et je l'accomplis sans attendre d'accolades ou de gains personnels en retour.

L'homme soupire, comme impatient.

— Je vous en suis très reconnaissant, bien sûr. Est-ce qu'il faut autre chose pour conclure notre affaire ?

— Rien du tout.

Des pas résonnent dans la pièce, ils s'éloignent de la porte au lieu de s'en rapprocher.

— Tous les papiers sont en ordre. Vous vous êtes déjà acquitté du paiement des frais. Elle est à vous, monsieur Sevier. Elle attend, là, dans la chambre, et nous vous laissons seuls pour que vous puissiez faire connaissance... de la façon qu'il vous conviendra.

— Je vous encourage à vous montrer ferme avec elle. Elle...

— Venez, madame Murphy.

Elles partent, et je reste assise sans bouger sur le lit, guettant l'arrivée de l'homme. Il s'approche de la porte et s'arrête de l'autre côté. Je l'entends inspirer, puis expirer bruyamment.

Je serre fort la robe au-dessus de mes genoux, tremblante comme une feuille.

La porte s'ouvre et il se dresse là, à quelques pas.

Je connais son visage. Il s'était assis à côté de moi sur le canapé le jour de la fête et m'avait demandé quel âge j'avais.

C'était sa femme qui avait fait la lecture à Fern.

19

Avery

Le conducteur devant moi ralentit, mais je suis tellement occupée à regarder deux adolescentes faire trotter leurs chevaux au bord de la route que je freine *in extremis*. La voiture tourne sur la route qui mène au centre équestre. Je me demande si c'est là que vont les ados avec leurs chevaux. C'est la saison des derbys. Plus jeune, je serais allée participer à la course ou au moins la regarder mais, dernièrement, j'ai à peine le temps de me plaindre que la vie d'adulte ne laisse aucune place aux activités qui me passionnaient avant, comme l'équitation.

À cet instant, mon esprit est déjà à plusieurs kilomètres de là, dans la chambre de May Crandall à la maison de retraite. J'ai demandé à Ian, le stagiaire sympa, de passer quelques coups de fil discrets pour déterminer où elle se trouvait et quel était son état de santé. Elle est de retour dans sa chambre et elle se sent suffisamment bien pour redonner du fil à retordre au personnel.

Derrière moi, Trent klaxonne et lève la main, comme pour me dire : « Fais un peu attention », mais il sourit derrière ses lunettes de soleil.

Si nous n'étions pas dans des voitures séparées, je lui rétorquerais : « C'est toi qui as insisté pour venir. Je t'ai prévenu que les choses seraient imprévisibles. »

Il se contenterait sans doute de rire et de me dire qu'il ne raterait ça pour rien au monde.

Nous sommes comme deux collégiens qui sèchent les cours pour la première fois. Ni lui ni moi ne sommes là où nous devrions être ce matin, mais, après la découverte de la photo dans le bureau de son grand-père hier soir, nous ne pouvions renoncer à ce voyage. Même un appel matinal raté de Leslie et une demi-douzaine de demandes de clients à l'agence de Trent n'ont pu changer le plan que nous avons échafaudé spontanément la nuit dernière. D'une façon ou d'une autre, nous allons découvrir ce que nos grands-parents cachaient et comment mon histoire et la sienne sont liées... et ce que May Crandall vient faire là-dedans.

J'ai intentionnellement évité de répondre aux appels de Leslie, et Trent a collé un mot sur la porte de son agence – depuis, nous sommes en cavale, après un départ à l'aube.

Un peu plus de deux heures plus tard, nous voilà à Aiken. Nous comptons passer voir May Crandall après son petit-déjeuner. Selon ce que nous découvrirons, nous irons peut-être dans la maison de ma grand-mère, sur Lagniappe Street.

J'essaie de me concentrer sur la conduite tandis que nous louvoyons dans des rues tranquilles bordées d'arbres, les magnolias endormis et les hauts pins projetant leurs ombres sur ma voiture comme pour dire : « Pourquoi se presser ? Ralentis. Profite de ta journée. »

Pendant une fraction de seconde, je me détends en me disant que ce n'est qu'une matinée de fin d'été comme les autres. Mais, dès que la maison de retraite apparaît au coin de la rue, l'illusion s'évanouit. Comme pour enfoncer le clou, mon téléphone sonne de nouveau et le nom de Leslie apparaît sur l'écran pour la quatrième fois. Ce n'est pas le bon moment, mais ça me rappelle que, dès que notre visite à May Crandall sera terminée – et quoi qu'elle nous apporte –, je devrai me manifester. Les problèmes du présent se rappellent à moi. Littéralement.

Je me rassure en me disant que, si ces appels concernaient la santé de mon père, ce serait l'une de mes sœurs, et non Leslie, qui m'aurait appelée. C'est donc sûrement lié au boulot. Quelque chose a dû sortir depuis que j'ai parlé à Ian hier soir, ou alors il m'aurait avertie. Leslie a sans doute organisé une opération de com' immanquable, et elle veut que je rentre plus tôt de mes mini-vacances à Edisto. Elle ne se doute pas que je suis déjà là.

L'idée de replonger dans l'arène politique me serre un peu le ventre. Je ne veux vraiment pas y penser. Je mets mon téléphone sur vibreur et je le fourre dans mon sac sans jeter un œil à la ribambelle de textos. J'ai sans doute des e-mails en souffrance, aussi. Leslie n'apprécie pas du tout qu'on l'ignore.

Dès que je me gare sur le parking, je ne pense plus du tout à elle. J'attrape la pochette qui abrite les photos anciennes du panneau d'affichage et les papiers trouvés dans l'enveloppe de mamie Judy, et je descends de voiture.

Trent me rejoint sur le trottoir en lançant :

— Si jamais un jour on doit prendre des routes de campagne ensemble, c'est moi qui conduirai.

— Pourquoi, tu ne me fais pas confiance ?

Un étrange petit frisson me glisse le long du dos mais, aussi sec, je le chasse d'un haussement d'épaules. Être de retour à Aiken me rappelle brutalement que, même si je trouve Trent charmant, il n'y aura jamais rien d'autre qu'une amitié entre nous.

Je me suis assurée de mentionner mon fiancé dans la conversation avant qu'on parte d'Edisto, juste pour que les choses soient claires.

— J'ai confiance en toi, oui. En ta conduite... ça reste à voir.

— Je n'ai même pas failli lui rentrer dedans.

On s'envoie des piques tout en avançant vers le bâtiment et je ris sans savoir pourquoi quand nous arrivons à la porte. L'odeur de désodorisant et le silence oppressant me dégrisent aussitôt.

L'expression de Trent se transforme, elle aussi,. Son sourire disparaît.

— Ça me rappelle des souvenirs.

— Tu es déjà venu ici ?

— Non, mais ça ressemble beaucoup à l'endroit où nous avons placé ma grand-mère après son attaque. Même si nous n'avions pas le choix, c'était dur pour mon grand-père.

Pendant soixante ans, ils n'avaient jamais été séparés plus d'une nuit ou deux.

— C'est tellement difficile, quand on en arrive au point où il n'y a plus de bonne solution.

Il connaît la situation de mamie Judy. C'est venu dans la conversation hier soir, pendant qu'on discutait sur le seuil du petit cabanon à propos des photos et de leur signification possible.

Une aide-soignante en blouse colorée passe devant nous. Elle nous salue et semble se demander si elle me reconnaît. Puis elle s'éloigne. Tant mieux. La dernière chose dont j'ai besoin, c'est que quelqu'un m'identifie ici. Si cela remonte jusqu'à Leslie et mon père, je subirai un interrogatoire et je n'ai aucune idée de ce que je pourrai dire.

Devant la porte de May Crandall, je me rends compte que je ne sais pas trop quoi lui dire, à elle aussi. Est-ce que je dois débouler dans sa chambre avec mes photos et lui demander : « Quel est le lien entre vous et ma grand-mère ? Qu'est-ce que Trent Turner Sr. a à voir avec vous ? »

Est-ce que je devrais plutôt la jouer subtile ? Je ne la connais pas assez pour savoir comment elle va réagir à notre venue. J'espère que la présence de Trent pourra apporter une touche de magie. Après tout, May connaissait sans doute son grand-père.

Et si c'était trop pour elle, notre venue à tous les deux ? Elle sort tout de même d'une hospitalisation. Je ne veux pas lui causer d'autres problèmes. En fait, revenir ici me fait comprendre que j'aurais dû faire quelque chose pour l'aider. Je pourrais peut-être parler à Andrew Moore, de l'Association de défense des droits des seniors. Il pourrait peut-être me suggérer quelques organisations qui s'occupent des personnes âgées comme May, dont les familles sont éloignées.

Trent s'arrête sur le seuil et me montre l'étiquette sur la porte.

— On dirait bien que c'est là.

— Je suis nerveuse, admets-je. Je sais qu'elle a été malade. Je ne sais pas si elle est suffisamment remise pour...

— Qui traîne devant ma porte ? lance soudain May, ce qui fait taire mes inquiétudes aussitôt. Allez-vous-en ! Je n'ai besoin de rien. Je refuse que vous échangiez des messes basses à mon sujet !

Un chausson fuse dans l'entrebâillement de la porte, puis une brosse à cheveux le suit et s'écrase bruyamment dans le couloir.

Trent ramasse les projectiles.

— Elle vise bien.

— Laissez-moi tranquille ! insiste May.

Trent et moi échangeons un coup d'œil incertain. Je me penche vers la porte, évitant d'être dans la ligne de mire, au cas où elle aurait d'autres munitions à portée de main.

— May ? Écoutez-moi une seconde, s'il vous plaît. C'est Avery Stafford. Vous vous souvenez ? Nous nous sommes rencontrées il y a quelques semaines ? Vous aimiez bien mon bracelet libellule. Ça vous dit quelque chose ?

Silence.

— Vous disiez que ma grand-mère était une de vos amies. Judy. Judy Myers Stafford ? Nous avions discuté toutes les deux de la photo sur votre chevet.

J'ai l'impression que tout mon monde a été chamboulé depuis ce jour-là.

— Alors ? crache May au bout d'un moment. Vous entrez ou quoi ?

De l'autre côté de la porte, j'entends des draps frotter et des couvertures se soulever. Je ne sais pas si elle se prépare à nous recevoir ou à nous bombarder de plus belle.

— Vous avez fini de balancer des trucs ?

— J'imagine que vous ne partiriez pas, même si je continuais.

Malgré sa réponse acerbe, je perçois une note d'intérêt dans son ton. Elle m'invite à entrer, alors je m'exécute, laissant Trent en sécurité dans le couloir.

Elle est assise dans son lit, vêtue d'une robe de chambre bleue assortie à ses yeux. Même calée par des coussins, il y a un quelque chose de régalien dans la façon dont elle m'observe, comme si elle était habituée, même longtemps avant ses années d'hospice, à être servie au lit.

— J'espérais que vous vous sentiriez suffisamment bien pour discuter avec moi, aujourd'hui. J'ai parlé de vous à ma grand-mère. Elle a mentionné une Queen... ou Queenie, mais c'est tout ce dont elle se souvenait.

— Elle en est à ce point ? s'écrie May, choquée.

— J'en ai bien peur, dis-je, désolée de lui annoncer une telle nouvelle. Mamie Judy n'est pas malheureuse. C'est juste qu'elle a oublié beaucoup de choses. C'est dur pour elle.

— Et pour vous aussi, j'imagine ?

La déduction soudaine de May m'ébranle.

— Oui, en effet. Ma grand-mère et moi, nous avons toujours été proches.

— Pourtant, elle ne vous a jamais parlé des personnes sur cette photo ?

Cette question cache une insinuation : que cette femme et ma grand-mère étaient intimes. Je ne suis pas certaine de pouvoir me résigner à ne jamais connaître la vérité si May refuse de me la dire.

— J'ai le sentiment qu'elle le ferait, maintenant, si elle le pouvait. Mais j'espère que, puisqu'elle ne peut pas, vous me parlerez.

— Cela n'a rien à voir avec vous.

May se détourne un peu de moi, comme si elle craignait que je la regarde droit dans les yeux.

— J'ai l'impression que si. Et peut-être que...

Son attention se porte vers le couloir.

— Qui c'est, devant ma porte ? Qui d'autre nous écoute ?

— Je suis venue avec quelqu'un. Il m'a aidée à essayer de comprendre ce que ma grand-mère n'a pas pu me dire. C'est juste un ami.

Trent entre et traverse la pièce, la main tendue, affichant le genre de sourire qui pourrait vendre des cornets de glace à des Esquimaux.

— Trent, dit-il en se présentant. Enchanté de faire votre connaissance, madame Crandall.

Elle accepte ses salutations et serre sa main entre les deux siennes, le maintenant un peu penché au-dessus de son lit pendant qu'elle se tourne vers moi.

— Juste un ami, vous disiez ? J'en doute.

J'ai un petit mouvement de recul.

— Trent et moi avons fait connaissance il y a quelques jours à peine, quand je suis descendue à Edisto.

— Un endroit charmant, Edisto.

Elle se concentre sur Trent, les yeux plissés.

— Oui, en effet, dis-je en me demandant pourquoi elle le scrute comme ça. Ma grand-mère y a passé pas mal de temps, au fil des ans. Mon oncle Clifford m'a appris qu'elle aimait s'y retirer pour écrire. Il semblerait que le grand-père de Trent et elle aient eu des affaires en commun, là-bas.

Comme si j'interrogeais un témoin à la barre, je guette les moindres changements dans son attitude. Elle essaie de les dissimuler, mais ils sont bien là et ils sont évidents – un peu plus à chaque phrase.

Elle se demande ce que je sais, précisément.

— Je ne crois pas avoir entendu votre nom de famille, lance-t-elle à Trent.

La pression semble monter dans la pièce tandis qu'elle attend sa réponse et, lorsqu'il se présente plus formellement, elle hoche la tête en souriant.

— Mmm... Oui, vous avez ses yeux.

Je ressens le petit frisson qui me prend lorsque je sais qu'un témoin s'apprête à craquer. Souvent, il ne faut qu'une toute petite chose – l'apparition surprise d'un visage familier, un lien vers un fait du passé dissimulé, les bribes d'un secret gardé trop longtemps.

Les doigts de May relâchent la main de Trent en tremblant. Elle effleure sa mâchoire. Des larmes perlent sur ses cils.

— Vous lui ressemblez. Lui aussi, c'était un bel homme.

Son sourire pincé laisse deviner qu'elle devait faire tourner les têtes, à son époque – une femme qui n'avait aucun mal à évoluer dans un monde masculin.

Trent rougit même un peu. C'est mignon. J'apprécie cet échange malgré moi.

May agite un doigt vers moi.

— Celui-là, il faut le garder. Croyez-en ma vieille expérience.

C'est à mon tour de rougir.

— Malheureusement, je suis déjà fiancée.

— Mais je ne vois pas encore d'alliance, rétorque May avant de me prendre la main pour examiner de près ma bague de fiançailles. Et je sais reconnaître l'étincelle, entre deux personnes. Rien d'étonnant. J'ai enterré trois maris, jusqu'ici.

Trent laisse échapper un léger éclat de rire, puis il baisse la tête et sa frange blonde comme le sable glisse sur son front.

— Et je n'ai rien à voir avec leurs morts, au cas où vous vous poseriez la question, nous informe May. J'ai aimé profondément chacun d'eux. L'un était professeur, le deuxième, pasteur, et le dernier était un artiste qui avait trouvé sa vocation sur le tard. Le premier m'a appris à réfléchir, le deuxième à savoir et le troisième à ouvrir les yeux. Tous les trois m'ont guidée. J'étais musicienne, voyez-vous. Je travaillais à Hollywood et j'ai aussi voyagé avec de grands orchestres. C'était à la belle époque, bien avant cette idiotie digitale.

Mon téléphone vibre dans mon sac, ce qui arrache un froncement de sourcils à May.

— Ces maudits bidules ! Le monde irait mieux si ces choses n'avaient jamais été inventées.

Je fais taire le téléphone pour de bon. Si May est enfin prête à me raconter l'histoire de la photo sur son chevet, je ne tolérerai pas la moindre distraction. D'ailleurs, c'est le moment idéal pour remettre le témoin sur les rails.

J'ouvre l'enveloppe et en tire les photos trouvées dans le cabanon chez Trent.

— En fait, nous nous posions des questions sur ces clichés. Et aussi sur la Société des foyers d'accueil du Tennessee.

Son visage se durcit aussitôt. Elle me décoche un regard embrasé.

— J'aurais préféré ne jamais réentendre ces mots.

Trent referme ses mains sur celle de May et baisse les yeux vers leurs doigts entrelacés.

— Je m'excuse, madame Crandall... si nous remuons des souvenirs douloureux. Mon grand-père ne m'avait jamais rien dit. Enfin, je savais qu'il avait été adopté très jeune et qu'il avait coupé les ponts avec ses parents adoptifs en l'apprenant. Mais je ne savais pas grand-chose de la Société des foyers d'accueil du Tennessee – jusqu'à récemment. Peut-être que, de temps en temps, j'avais entendu des gens mentionner ce nom à mon grand-père, lorsque des visiteurs passaient chez nous. J'avais conscience qu'il aidait ces gens d'une façon ou d'une autre, et qu'il se sentait obligé de les recevoir en privé – dans son bureau ou sur son bateau. Ma grand-mère n'avait jamais aimé entendre parler boulot dans la maison, que ce soit de l'immobilier ou autre chose. Je ne savais rien du passe-temps de mon grand-père, ou plutôt de sa deuxième profession, enfin, bref, jusqu'à ce que je l'aide à s'occuper des derniers dossiers, avant sa mort. Il m'a demandé de ne pas lire les documents, et je lui ai obéi. Jusqu'à ce qu'Avery arrive à Edisto, il y a quelques jours.

May en reste bouche bée, les larmes aux yeux.

— Il est parti, c'est cela ? Je savais qu'il était très malade.

Trent confirme qu'il a perdu son grand-père quelques mois plus tôt et May l'attire pour déposer un baiser sur sa joue.

— C'était un homme bien et un très bon ami.

— Avait-il été adopté par le truchement de la Société des foyers d'accueil du Tennessee ? demande-t-il. Est-ce que c'est pour ça qu'il s'y intéressait ?

Un hochement de tête résigné lui répond.

— Oui, effectivement. Et moi aussi. C'est là que nous nous sommes rencontrés. Bien sûr, il n'avait que trois ans, à l'époque. Il était si mignon, si charmant... Il ne s'appelait pas comme ça. Il n'a repris son nom que bien plus tard, lorsqu'il a découvert qui il était vraiment. Il avait une sœur dont il a été séparé au cours de notre passage au foyer. Elle avait deux ou trois ans de plus, et je crois qu'il a espéré toute sa vie que, en reprenant son nom de naissance, cela l'aiderait à la retrouver. C'est le plus ironique, dans cette histoire. L'homme qui a permis à tant d'entre nous de reprendre contact n'a jamais réussi à localiser sa propre sœur. Elle fait peut-être partie de ceux qui n'ont pas survécu. Ils ont été si nombreux...

Elle laisse sa phrase en suspens, la voix brisée. Elle se redresse dans le lit et s'éclaircit la gorge.

— Je suis née sur le Mississippi, dans un bateau construit par mon père. Queenie, c'était ma mère, Briny, mon père. J'avais trois petites sœurs, Camellia, Lark et Fern, et un frère, Gabion. C'était le plus jeune...

Elle ferme les yeux et je les vois bouger sous ses fines paupières veinées de bleu lorsqu'elle poursuit son histoire. À croire qu'elle rêve, qu'elle regarde les images défiler. Elle nous raconte le jour où ils ont été arrachés à leur bateau, par la police, pour finir dans un orphelinat. Elle décrit des semaines de peur et d'incertitude, des employées cruelles, la séparation d'avec ses sœurs et son frère, les mêmes horreurs que celles que nous avons lues, Trent et moi.

Son histoire nous brise le cœur et nous fascine tout à la fois. Nous nous tenons de chaque côté du lit et nous écoutons en osant à peine respirer.

— Au foyer, j'ai perdu la trace de mon frère et de deux de mes sœurs, conclut-elle. Mais Fern et moi avons eu de la chance. On nous a gardées ensemble. Adoptées ensemble.

Elle regarde par la fenêtre et, l'espace d'un instant, je me demande si elle nous a dit tout ce qu'elle comptait nous dire. Elle finit par retourner son attention vers Trent.

— La dernière fois que j'ai vu votre grand-père enfant, j'avais peur qu'il soit l'un de ceux qui ne survivraient pas à son séjour là-bas. Il était tellement timide... Il s'attirait toujours les foudres des employées, sans le faire exprès. Je le considérais presque comme mon petit frère, quand je suis partie. Jamais je n'aurais pensé le revoir un jour. Lorsqu'un certain Trent Turner m'a contactée des années plus tard, je l'ai pris pour un imposteur. Je n'ai pas reconnu son nom, évidemment. Georgia Tann rebaptisait les enfants – pour empêcher leurs familles biologiques de les retrouver, sans doute. Je peux vous dire que je me souviens d'elle comme d'une femme horrible et cruelle – croyez-moi, l'étendue de ses crimes ne sera peut-être jamais révélée. Peu de ses victimes ont pu accomplir ce que votre grand-père a fait – réclamer un nom de naissance et une filiation. Il a même retrouvé sa mère biologique avant qu'elle meure et s'est remis en contact avec d'autres parents. Il est redevenu Trent mais, lorsqu'il était petit, je le connaissais sous le nom de Stevie.

Son attention se perd de nouveau, semblant emporter son esprit avec elle. Je bouge un tout petit peu la photo des quatre femmes, je lance quelques suppositions. Au tribunal, on m'accuserait d'influencer le témoin mais, ici, c'est juste pour aider l'histoire à se révéler.

— Est-ce que ce sont vos sœurs, sur la photo, avec vous et ma grand-mère ?

Je sais que les trois femmes à gauche sont sœurs ou cousines. C'est évident, même si leurs chapeaux ombrent leurs visages. Je suis toujours troublée par leur ressemblance avec ma grand-mère. La couleur des cheveux. Les yeux clairs qui ont l'air de voir au-delà de la photo. En revanche, les traits du visage, du moins autant que je puisse le voir, sont différents. Ceux des trois sœurs sont affirmés, comme taillés à la serpe. Leur menton est large et carré, leur nez droit et leurs yeux en amande remontent un peu sur les côtés. Elles sont belles. Ma grand-mère est jolie, aussi, mais ses traits sont plus discrets, plus aquilins, et ses grands yeux bleus lui mangent presque le visage. Ils sont lumineux, même en noir et blanc.

May prend la photo et la tient entre ses mains tremblantes. Sa contemplation paraît durer une éternité. Je dois me retenir de l'interroger. Que se passe-t-il dans sa tête ? À quoi pense-t-elle ? Que se rappelle-t-elle ?

— Oui. Nous trois – Lark, Fern et moi. De vraies naïades.

Elle émet un petit rire malicieux et tapote la main de Trent.

— Je crois que votre grand-mère s'inquiétait un peu lorsque nous venions dans le coin. Elle s'en faisait pour rien. Trent l'aimait tendrement. Nous lui étions si reconnaissantes de nous avoir aidées à nous retrouver... Edisto, c'était un endroit spécial, pour nous. C'est là-bas que nous avons été réunies pour la première fois.

— Et que vous avez rencontré ma grand-mère ?

J'attends désespérément une réponse simple à tout cela. Une qui ne pèsera pas sur ma conscience. Je ne veux pas découvrir que ma grand-mère tentait par je ne sais quel moyen de faire pénitence pour l'implication de notre famille dans les affaires de la Société des foyers d'accueil, que mes grands-pères faisaient partie des nombreux hommes politiques qui avaient protégé Georgia Tann et son réseau, qui fermaient les yeux devant ses atrocités parce que des familles influentes ne voulaient pas que les crimes de cette femme soient révélés ni que leurs propres adoptions soient annulées.

— C'est là que vous êtes devenues amies, toutes les deux ?

Son doigt suit la bordure blanche de la photo. Elle regarde ma grand-mère. Si seulement je pouvais me faufiler dans sa tête ou, mieux encore, dans la photo elle-même.

— Oui, c'est ça. Nous nous étions croisées à plusieurs reprises lors de réceptions ou autres avant de faire vraiment connaissance mais, je dois l'avouer, je m'étais fait une idée totalement fausse d'elle. Au fil du temps, elle est devenue une amie très proche. Et elle s'est montrée très généreuse en nous prêtant à moi et mes sœurs son cottage d'Edisto de temps en temps, pour que nous puissions nous retrouver au calme. Cette photo a été prise au cours de l'une de nos visites. Votre grand-mère nous avait rejointes. C'était une journée magnifique sur la plage, à la fin de l'été.

L'explication m'apaise et j'aimerais m'en contenter mais elle ne me dit pas pourquoi les mots « Société des foyers d'accueil du Tennessee » se trouvaient sur le ruban de la machine à écrire de ma grand-mère... ni pourquoi elle était en relation avec Trent Turner Sr.

— Le grand-père de Trent a laissé une enveloppe pour mamie Judy, dis-je. À en croire son carnet de rendez-vous, je crois que, avant qu'elle tombe malade, elle avait prévu de venir la récupérer. Dans l'enveloppe, j'ai trouvé des documents de la Société des foyers d'accueil du Tennessee. Des rapports médicaux et un acte de remise au foyer pour un nourrisson appelé Shad Arthur Foss. Pour quelle raison aurait-elle pu demander ces papiers ?

Ma question la prend au dépourvu. Il y a bien autre chose dans cette histoire, mais elle refuse de lâcher le morceau.

Ses paupières papillonnent, puis se ferment.

— Je suis vraiment... vraiment... fatiguée tout à coup. Toute cette... cette conversation... C'est plus que je n'en fais... pendant... une semaine.

— Est-ce que ma grand-mère avait un lien avec la Société des foyers d'accueil du Tennessee ? Est-ce que ma famille était mêlée à tout ça ?

Si je ne le découvre pas aujourd'hui, j'ai comme l'impression que je ne le saurai jamais.

— Il faudra le lui demander directement.

May s'enfonce dans ses coussins et pousse un soupir exagéré.

— C'est impossible. Je vous l'ai déjà dit. Elle ne se rappelle plus grand-chose. S'il vous plaît, dites-moi juste la vérité. Arcadie. Est-ce que ce nom a un rapport avec tout ça ?

Je serre un peu plus fort la barre du lit.

Trent pose sa main sur la mienne.

— Il vaut peut-être mieux qu'on en reste là aujourd'hui, souffle-t-il.

Je vois que May se referme sur elle-même, que l'histoire s'efface comme un dessin à la craie sur un trottoir par un jour de pluie.

Je m'accroche aux couleurs dégoulinantes.

— Je veux juste savoir si ma famille était... responsable d'une façon ou d'une autre. Pourquoi ma grand-mère s'intéressait-elle tant à tout ça ?

May tâtonne sur la barre du lit jusqu'à trouver mes doigts. Elle me les serre, comme pour me réconforter.

— Non, bien sûr que non, mon petit. Ne vous inquiétez pas. À une époque, Judy m'aidait à écrire mon histoire. C'est tout. Puis j'ai changé d'avis. J'ai découvert que, dans la vie, les événements du passé sont un peu comme les endives. C'est souvent amer. Il vaut mieux ne pas mâcher trop longtemps. Votre grand-mère écrivait très bien, mais c'était difficile pour elle d'entendre le récit de notre vie au foyer. Son talent la destinait à des récits plus joyeux, je pense.

— Elle vous aidait à écrire votre histoire ? C'est tout ?

Était-ce possible ? Pas de gros secret de famille, juste mamie Judy qui mettait ses compétences au service d'une amie, pour faire la lumière sur une vieille injustice dont les effets se faisaient encore ressentir ? Mon soulagement est tel que je sens tout mon corps se relâcher.

Tout concorde, à présent.

— Il n'y a rien de plus, soupire May. J'aimerais pouvoir vous en dire davantage.

Sa dernière phrase m'alerte comme un filet de fumée solitaire venu d'un feu qu'on avait soi-disant éteint. Les témoins qui ne disent pas la vérité ont du mal à s'arrêter à un oui ou non absolu.

Qu'est-ce qu'elle aimerait me dire d'autre ? Est-ce qu'il y a vraiment autre chose ?

May cherche la main de Trent, la serre, puis la relâche.

— Je suis désolée pour votre grand-père. Pour nombre d'entre nous, il a été un ange gardien. Avant l'ouverture des archives des services d'adoption de l'État en 1996, nous avions peu de moyens de savoir où se trouvaient nos parents – et qui nous étions vraiment. Mais votre grand-père savait s'y prendre. Sans lui, Fern et moi n'aurions jamais retrouvé notre sœur. Elles sont parties toutes les deux, maintenant – Lark et Fern. J'apprécierais beaucoup que vous évitiez de déranger leurs familles, même maintenant... et la mienne aussi. La première fois que nous avons été réunies, nous étions déjà des jeunes femmes, avec nos vies, nos maris, nos enfants. Nous avons choisi de ne pas faire intrusion dans nos existences respectives. Savoir que les autres se portaient bien, ça nous suffisait. Votre grand-père le comprenait. J'espère que vous respecterez nos volontés.

Elle ouvre les yeux et se tourne vers moi pour ajouter :

— Tous les deux.

Soudain, tous les signes de fatigue ont disparu. Le regard qu'elle me lance est profond, exigeant.

— Bien sûr, répond Trent.

Mais je devine que ce n'est pas l'accord de Trent qu'elle attend.

— Je n'avais pas l'intention de déranger qui que ce soit.

À présent, c'est moi qui tourne autour du pot... car je ne peux pas faire de promesses intenables.

— Je voulais juste savoir comment ma grand-mère s'était retrouvée mêlée à tout ça.

— Et maintenant, vous le savez, alors tout va bien.

Elle souligne son affirmation par un hochement de tête résolu. Je ne sais pas qui elle essaie de convaincre – moi ou elle-même.

— J'ai fait la paix avec mon passé. C'est une histoire que j'espère ne jamais devoir raconter de nouveau. Comme je l'ai dit plus tôt, j'ai même fini par renoncer à la partager avec votre grand-mère. Pourquoi libérer tant de laideur dans le présent ? Nous traversons tous des épreuves. Les miennes sont peut-être différentes de beaucoup, mais j'en suis venue à bout, comme Lark et Fern et, je l'imagine, même si nous n'avons jamais réussi à le trouver, mon frère aussi. Je préfère l'espérer. C'est lui, la raison principale qui me poussait à vouloir écrire notre histoire il y a des années, quand j'ai amadoué votre grand-mère pour qu'elle m'assiste dans ce projet. J'imaginais sans doute qu'un livre ou un article de journal l'atteindrait peut-être s'il était encore en vie et, dans le cas contraire, s'il faisait partie des trop nombreux enfants qui avaient simplement disparu sous l'autorité de la Société des foyers d'accueil du Tennessee, cela lui fournirait une sorte de mémorial. Et pour mes parents biologiques aussi. Il n'y a pas de pierre tombale qu'on puisse aller fleurir pour eux. Du moins, pas à ma connaissance.

— Je suis vraiment... désolée pour tout ce que vous avez dû traverser.

Elle acquiesce, ferme les yeux, me tient à distance.

— Je ferais bien de me reposer. Bientôt, ils vont venir me tâter, m'examiner ou me traîner jusqu'à cette maudite salle de kinésithérapie. J'ai presque quatre-vingt-dix ans. Pourquoi aurais-je besoin de tonus musculaire ?

— Je croirais entendre mon grand-père, ricane Trent. Si on l'avait écouté, on l'aurait placé dans une barque et laissé dériver sur le fleuve Edisto.

— Une idée fort charmante. Vous voulez bien me trouver un bateau ? Ensuite, je me débrouillerai pour rentrer chez moi à Augusta, puis je me laisserai flotter le long du fleuve Savannah.

Les yeux toujours clos, elle esquisse un sourire. Peu après, sa respiration s'approfondit, ses paupières tressautent dans leurs cadres plissés. Le sourire demeure. Je me demande si elle est redevenue cette petite fille qui parcourait les eaux boueuses du Mississippi à bord du bateau de fortune construit par son père.

J'essaie de m'imaginer à sa place, après avoir vécu deux vies, après avoir été, littéralement, deux personnes différentes. Je n'y arrive pas. Je n'ai jamais rien connu d'autre qu'une vie passée à l'abri, derrière la muraille protectrice de mon nom de famille, soutenue, nourrie, aimée par mes proches. À quoi ressemblait la vie de May avec ses parents adoptifs ? Je n'y pense qu'à cet instant, mais elle n'a pas vraiment raconté cette partie de son histoire. Elle a juste dit que, après un passage éprouvant au foyer, sa sœur et elle avaient été confiées à une famille.

Pourquoi s'est-elle arrêtée là ? Le reste était-il trop intime ?

Même si elle a répondu à la question que j'étais venue lui poser, et bien qu'elle m'ait demandé de ne pas creuser davantage, je ne peux pas m'empêcher de vouloir en savoir plus.

Trent semble penser comme moi. Ce qui ne m'étonne pas. L'histoire de sa famille est liée à celle de May.

Nous nous attardons quelques minutes, lui d'un côté du lit, moi de l'autre, et nous l'observons, perdus dans nos propres pensées. Nous finissons par reprendre les photos et sortons de la chambre à contrecœur. Nous ne disons pas un mot avant d'être à l'abri d'éventuelles oreilles indiscrètes.

— J'ignorais tout de cette partie de l'histoire de mon grand-père.

— Ce doit être difficile, de le découvrir maintenant.

Trent fronce les sourcils.

— C'est bizarre de penser à ce qu'il a vécu enfant. Je ne l'en admire que plus – pour ce qu'il a fait de sa vie, pour la personne qu'il était. Mais ça me rend dingue aussi. Je me demande à quoi aurait ressemblé sa vie s'il ne s'était pas trouvé au mauvais endroit au mauvais moment, si ses parents n'avaient pas été pauvres, si quelqu'un avait mis fin aux activités de la Société des foyers d'accueil du Tennessee avant qu'elle s'empare de lui. S'il avait grandi avec sa famille biologique, aurait-il été le même ? Est-ce qu'il aimait la rivière parce qu'il venait d'un fleuve, ou parce que l'homme qui l'a élevé allait pêcher le week-end ? May a dit qu'il avait rencontré d'autres membres de sa famille biologique. Qu'est-ce qu'il a ressenti ? Pourquoi est-ce qu'il ne nous en a jamais présenté un seul ? Il y a tant de questions que j'aimerais pouvoir lui poser...

Nous nous arrêtons juste devant la porte d'entrée, aussi peu pressés l'un que l'autre de nous séparer, de retourner à nos voitures respectives. La raison de notre rencontre a été balayée par l'histoire de May. L'heure des adieux devrait sonner, mais j'ai l'impression que des liens nous unissent et qu'ils ne doivent pas être tranchés.

— Tu penses que tu vas essayer d'en retrouver... des membres de la famille de ton grand-père ?

Il glisse les mains dans les poches de son jean, puis hausse les épaules, les yeux baissés vers le trottoir.

— C'est si loin, je n'en vois pas l'intérêt. Ce ne serait que de lointains parents, maintenant. Ce qui explique peut-être que mon grand-père n'ait pas pris la peine de nous les présenter. Malgré tout, je vais peut-être faire quelques recherches. J'aimerais connaître certains détails... au moins pour Jonah, mes nièces et mes neveux. Ils se poseront peut-être des questions un jour. Je ne veux plus de secrets.

La conversation s'étiole. Trent s'humecte les lèvres, comme s'il voulait dire quelque chose, mais qu'il n'était pas certain d'avoir le droit de le faire.

Lorsque nous reprenons la parole, nous parlons en même temps.

— Merci...

— Avery, je sais que nous...

Bizarrement, ça nous amuse tous les deux. Nos rires relâchent un peu la tension.

— Les dames d'abord.

Il indique mon visage de la main, comme pour inviter les mots à sortir de ma bouche. Je ne sais pas quoi dire. Après tout ce qu'on a traversé ces deux derniers jours, je n'arrive pas à croire que ça va se finir comme ça. Nous sommes liés ou, du moins, c'est l'impression que j'ai.

Je suis peut-être juste idiote.

— J'allais te remercier pour tout ce que tu as fait. Pour ne pas m'avoir laissée rentrer bredouille. Je sais que briser la promesse faite à ton grand-père a été difficile. Je ne...

Nos regards se croisent. Le reste de la phrase se volatilise. J'ai les joues en feu. Je ressens de nouveau une espèce d'alchimie entre nous. Je pensais que c'était l'attrait du mystère mais, maintenant que l'énigme est résolue, la pointe de fascination est toujours là.

Une idée soudaine me traverse, complètement imprévue et déplacée : Et si je commettais une erreur avec Elliot. Et je comprends à cet instant que cette idée ne jaillit pas de nulle part. J'avais juste évité la question, jusque-là. Est-ce que nous nous aimons vraiment, Elliot et moi ? Ou est-ce que nous sommes juste des trentenaires décidés à se caser ? Sommes-nous unis par une longue et profonde amitié ou par la passion ? Même si nous nous sommes répété que nous ne laisserions pas nos familles nous forcer la main, est-ce que nous les avons tout de même laissées faire ? Une bribe de coaching politique de Leslie me revient soudain en tête. Et tout m'apparaît comme évident.

« Si nous avions vraiment besoin de renforcer notre image, Avery, il n'y aurait rien de tel que l'annonce providentielle d'un mariage imminent. Cela mis à part, il n'est pas avantageux pour une jolie jeune femme d'être célibataire à Washington, même si elle pense maîtriser à la perfection son apparence en société. Les loups doivent savoir qu'il n'y a rien à attendre de ce côté-là. »

J'essaie de chasser cette idée, mais c'est comme une brindille coincée dans le toupet d'un cheval. Des mèches s'enroulent tout autour. Je ne m'imagine plus faisant machine arrière, maintenant. Tout le monde, tout le monde attend qu'on annonce bientôt une date officielle. L'inverse serait... impensable. Pomme d'amour et Bitsy auraient le cœur brisé. Socialement et politiquement, j'aurais l'air d'une cruche, de quelqu'un incapable de se décider, qui ne connaît même pas ses propres sentiments.

Et si c'était mon cas ?

— Avery ? me lance Trent, les yeux plissés, la tête penchée.

Il se demande à quoi je pense. Et je ne peux vraiment pas lui répondre.

— À ton tour.

Je ne me fais pas confiance pour en dire davantage, vu que mon esprit a décidé de faire du hors-piste dans des contrées folles.

— Ce n'est plus important, maintenant.

J'insiste :

— C'est pas juste. Qu'est-ce que tu voulais dire ?

Il se rend sans se défendre davantage.

— Je suis désolé qu'on soit partis d'un mauvais pied, le jour de ton arrivée. En temps normal, je ne parle pas de cette façon aux clients.

— Eh bien, je n'étais pas vraiment une cliente, alors tu es tout excusé.

En fait, il s'est plutôt bien comporté, vu mon insistance. Je suis bien une Stafford, finalement. J'ai tendance à croire que j'obtiendrai toujours ce que je veux.

Ce qui, je le comprends en frémissant, me rapproche des parents adoptifs qui ont par inadvertance financé le business de Georgia Tann. Je ne doute pas qu'il y ait eu parmi eux des gens bien intentionnés, et que certains enfants aient vraiment eu besoin d'un nouveau foyer, mais d'autres, surtout ceux qui savaient que des sommes exorbitantes étaient lâchées en échange de fils et de filles sur demande, devaient avoir une idée de ce qui se passait. Ils partaient simplement du principe que l'argent, le pouvoir et leur statut social leur en donnaient le droit.

À cette idée, je me sens soudain coupable. Je repense à tous les privilèges que l'on m'a accordés, y compris un fauteuil au Sénat pratiquement servi sur un plateau.

Ai-je vraiment le droit à tout ça, juste parce que je suis née dans la bonne famille ?

Mal à l'aise, Trent replonge les mains dans ses poches. Il jette un coup d'œil vers sa voiture, puis se retourne vers moi.

— Donne-moi des nouvelles de temps en temps. Passe-moi un coup de fil la prochaine fois que tu viens à Edisto.

Cette idée m'enchante.

— J'aimerais vraiment savoir si tu découvres autre chose sur la famille de ton grand-père... si tu découvres quoi que ce soit, je veux dire. Enfin, je ne veux pas te mettre la pression. Je ne voudrais pas paraître indiscrète.

— Pourquoi t'arrêter en si bon chemin ?

Je toussote en faisant mine d'être vexée mais nous savons tous les deux que c'est la vérité.

— C'est l'avocate en moi qui parle, désolée.

— Tu dois être une bonne avocate.

— J'essaie.

Je me sens pousser des ailes, portée par cette fierté qui nous gagne lorsque quelqu'un d'autre salue notre travail. C'est un accomplissement que je ne dois qu'à moi-même.

— J'aime redresser des torts.

— Ça se voit.

Une voiture se gare sur une place voisine. Cette intrusion nous rappelle que nous ne pouvons pas rester là éternellement. Trent regarde longuement la maison de retraite.

— On dirait qu'elle a eu une sacrée vie.

— C'est vrai.

L'idée que May, l'amie de ma grand-mère, croupisse dans cet endroit jour après jour me fend le cœur. Pas de visiteurs. Personne à qui parler. Des petits-enfants éloignés, pris dans une situation familiale compliquée. Ce n'est la faute de personne. Juste la réalité. Je vais vraiment contacter Andrew Moore pour voir s'il peut me suggérer des associations qui pourraient l'aider.

Un klaxon retentit dans la rue et, tout près, une portière claque. La vie suit son cours, et Trent et moi devrions l'imiter.

Son torse se gonfle avant de se relâcher. Son souffle m'effleure l'oreille lorsqu'il se penche pour déposer une bise sur ma joue.

— Merci, Avery. Je suis content de connaître la vérité.

Son visage s'attarde près du mien. Je sens un mélange de parfum, iode, shampooing pour bébé et une touche d'odeur de vase. Ou alors c'est mon imagination.

— Moi aussi.

— Donne-moi des nouvelles, répète-t-il.

— Promis.

Du coin de l'œil, j'aperçois une femme qui s'approche de nous. Chemisier blanc, escarpins, jupe noire. Ses pas ultra-rapides semblent déplacés, ils n'ont rien à faire là, dans cette journée. Le feu me monte aussitôt aux joues et je m'écarte si vite de Trent qu'il me jette un coup d'œil dérouté.

Leslie m'a retrouvée. J'aurais dû y penser, avant de demander à Ian de vérifier l'état de santé de May. Le menton de Leslie disparaît dans les plis de son cou lorsqu'elle nous observe, Trent et moi. J'imagine trop bien ce qu'elle pense. En fait, je n'ai même pas besoin de l'imaginer. Je le vois. L'échange dont elle a été témoin prête à confusion.

— Merci encore, Trent, dis-je pour dissiper l'impression qu'elle doit avoir. Sois prudent sur la route.

Je recule d'un pas, les mains jointes devant moi.

Son regard fouille le mien.

— De rien, répond-il, tête penchée, yeux plissés.

Il ne se doute pas que quelqu'un se tient derrière lui, ni que le monde réel est revenu jusqu'à nous avec la force d'une tornade.

— On t'a cherchée partout, déclare Leslie pour signaler sa présence sans perdre de temps en présentations. Ton portable ne marche pas ce matin, ou alors tu te cachais ?

Trent s'écarte et son regard passe de l'attachée de presse de mon père à moi.

— J'étais en vacances, dis-je. Tout le monde savait où j'étais.

— À Edisto ? rétorque-t-elle avec une pointe de sarcasme.

Clairement, je ne suis plus à Edisto, à cet instant. Elle braque un autre regard soupçonneux vers Trent. Je balbutie :

— Oui... eh bien... je...

Mon esprit pédale dans la semoule. Des perles de sueur coulent sous la robe à motif floral que j'ai achetée le matin même pour avoir quelque chose de propre à porter aujourd'hui. Je finis par lâcher :

— C'est une longue histoire.

— J'ai bien peur qu'on n'ait pas de temps pour ça aujourd'hui. On a besoin de toi, à la maison.

Elle veut faire comprendre à Trent que nous avons des choses à faire et qu'il n'est plus le bienvenu ici. Ça marche. Il me lance un dernier coup d'œil perplexe, puis prend congé en expliquant qu'il doit aller voir quelqu'un pendant qu'il est à Aiken.

— Prends soin de toi, Avery, dit-il en partant vers sa voiture.

— Trent... merci encore !

Il lève la main d'une façon qui me fait comprendre que, quoi qu'il se passe ici, il ne veut pas y être mêlé.

J'aimerais lui courir après et au moins m'excuser pour les manières brusques de Leslie, mais je ne peux pas. Cela ne soulèverait que de nouvelles questions.

— Je crois que mon téléphone était éteint, dis-je pour désamorcer l'interrogatoire de Leslie. Désolée. Qu'est-ce qui se passe ?

Elle bat doucement des cils, le menton relevé.

— Nous en parlerons dans un instant. Je voudrais d'abord qu'on discute de ce que je viens de voir, rétorque-t-elle en agitant la main vers Trent qui, je l'espère, est assez loin pour ne pas l'entendre. Parce que, ça, c'était perturbant !

— Leslie, c'est un ami. Il m'a aidée à retracer une partie de notre histoire de famille. C'est tout.

— Une histoire de famille ? Vraiment ? Ici ? Et quel genre d'histoire ? renifle-t-elle, frustrée.

— Je préfère ne pas en parler.

Les yeux de Leslie lancent des éclairs. Ses lèvres se pincent en une ligne fine. Elle inspire, bat de nouveau des cils et lève un regard échauffé vers moi.

— Eh bien, laisse-moi te dire une chose. Ce que je viens de voir, quoi que ce soit, c'est exactement le genre de truc que tu ne peux pas te permettre. Tu ne dois rien faire qui puisse être mal interprété, utilisé ou retourné contre nous, Avery. Rien. Tu dois être aussi innocente que l'agneau qui vient de naître, et ce que j'ai vu n'avait pas du tout l'air innocent. Tu imagines ce que ça aurait donné sur une photo ? Nous tous, toute l'équipe, on mise tout sur toi. Au cas où on aurait besoin de toi.

— Je sais. Je comprends.

— La dernière chose dont cette famille ait besoin, c'est d'une nouvelle controverse.

— Compris.

J'enrobe mes paroles dans un vernis de confiance en moi mais, en mon for intérieur, je suis perdue. Gênée. Contrariée de devoir discuter avec Leslie à cet instant. J'hésite entre l'apaiser et courir après Trent. J'ai peur ne serait-ce que de lever les yeux pour voir s'il est arrivé à son véhicule.

Un moteur rugit tout à coup, ce qui répond à ma question. J'entends la voiture de Trent reculer, puis s'éloigner. C'est sans doute mieux comme ça, me dis-je. Non, c'est mieux comme ça. J'avais planifié toute ma vie, avant d'aller à Edisto. Pourquoi tout remettre en question à cause... d'une vieille histoire de famille, des choses qui n'ont plus d'importance, un homme avec qui je n'ai aucun lien à part une histoire que même ceux qui l'ont vécue veulent oublier ?

— La situation a évolué, déclare Leslie.

Il me faut un instant pour intégrer ses paroles, alors même que je la regarde.

— *The Sentinel* vient de publier un gros dossier sur les maisons de retraite détenues par des grands groupes et leurs responsabilités esquivées. Ce n'est qu'une question de jours avant que les médias nationaux ne reprennent l'info. L'article a souligné des exemples de Caroline du Sud. Il compare les prix de Magnolia Manor et des établissements visés par certains procès pour maltraitance. Il y a des images des victimes et de leurs familles. Le dossier s'appelle « La vieillesse à deux vitesses », et il est illustré par une photo prise de loin de ton père et de ta grand-mère se promenant dans les jardins de Magnolia Manor.

Je la fixe, bouche bée, alors que la colère bouillonne en moi.

— Comment osent-ils ! Pour qui se prennent-ils ?! Ils n'ont pas le droit de harceler ma grand-mère.

— C'est la politique, Avery. La politique et le sensationnalisme. Ils ne reculeront devant rien.

20

Rill

L'homme s'appelle Darren, et la femme Victoria, mais ils nous ont dit que nous devons les appeler « père » et « mère », pas Darren et Victoria, ni M. et Mme Sevier. Ça ne m'embête pas trop. J'ai jamais appelé quiconque « père » ou « mère », si bien que ces mots ne sont pas réservés à quelqu'un, pour moi. Ce sont juste des mots. Un point, c'est tout.

Nos parents, ce sont Queenie et Briny, et nous irons les rejoindre coûte que coûte, dès que j'aurai trouvé un moyen. Ce ne sera pas aussi difficile que je le pensais. La maison des Sevier est grande et pleine de pièces que personne n'utilise et, dehors, il y a une longue galerie qui fait le tour de la maison et domine de grandes prairies et des bois, et tout ça descend, descend jusqu'à la meilleure chose du monde – l'eau. Ce n'est pas une rivière ; c'est un lac, long et étroit, qui débouche sur une zone de marais qui s'appelle Dedmen's Slough... et ce marais descend jusqu'au Mississippi. Je le sais parce que j'ai demandé à Zuma, qui fait le ménage ici et la cuisine, et qui habite au-dessus du vieux hangar à charrettes, où M. Sevier gare ses voitures. Il en a trois. Je n'avais jamais rencontré quelqu'un qui avait trois voitures.

Le mari de Zuma, Hoy, et leur fille, Hootsie, vivent là-bas avec elle. Hoy s'occupe du jardin, d'un poulailler, des chiens de chasse de M. Sevier qui aboient et hurlent toute la nuit, et d'un poney que, comme nous le répète Mme Sevier depuis deux semaines maintenant, nous pouvons monter si nous le voulons.

J'ai répondu qu'on n'aimait pas les poneys, même si c'est faux. J'ai fait comprendre à Fern qu'elle n'avait pas intérêt à me contredire.

Le mari de Zuma est effrayant – grand et noir comme un diable – et, après avoir vécu chez Mme Murphy, je ne veux pas qu'un jardinier nous entraîne dans un coin, moi ou Fern, où que ce soit. Je ne veux pas non plus qu'on se retrouve seule avec M. Sevier. Lui aussi, il a essayé de nous emmener voir le poney, mais seulement parce que Mme Sevier l'a forcé. Il ferait n'importe quoi pour empêcher sa femme d'aller errer sur le sentier qui descend jusqu'au jardin où deux bébés mort-nés et trois qui n'ont jamais pu naître ont tous des tombes surmontées de petits agneaux de pierre. Lorsque Mme Sevier s'y rend, elle s'allonge sur le sol et pleure. Puis elle rentre à la maison, se met au lit et n'en bouge plus. Il y a de vieilles cicatrices sur ses poignets. Je sais pourquoi elles y sont, mais je ne le dis pas à Fern, bien sûr.

— Va juste t'asseoir sur ses genoux et laisse-la te coiffer et jouer à la poupée avec toi. Assure-toi qu'elle est heureuse, dis-je à Fern. Pas de pleurs et pas de pipi au lit. Tu m'entends ?

C'est la seule raison pour laquelle les Sevier m'ont fait venir ici – parce que Fern n'arrêtait pas de pleurer, de mouiller son lit et de faire des scènes.

Dans l'ensemble, Fern se conduit bien, maintenant. Malgré tout, certains jours, rien ne peut aider Mme Sevier. Certains jours, elle ne veut pas le moindre contact avec les vivants. Elle ne veut que les morts.

Lorsqu'elle garde le lit à l'étage et pleure ses bébés perdus, M. Sevier va se cacher dans sa salle de musique, et nous sommes coincées avec Zuma, qui pense que notre arrivée lui donne trop de travail. Mme Sevier avait l'habitude d'acheter de petites choses pour la fille de Zuma, Hootsie, qui a dix ans, deux ans de moins que moi. Maintenant, c'est nous que Mme Sevier gâte. Ça, ça ne plaît pas non plus à Zuma. Elle a réussi à extorquer suffisamment d'informations à Fern pour savoir d'où nous venons et elle ne comprend pas pourquoi des gens aussi raffinés que M. et Mme Sevier voudraient de deux

« chie dans l'eau » comme nous. Elle ne se prive pas de nous le dire, mais jamais quand Mme Sevier pourrait l'entendre, bien sûr.

Zuma n'ose pas nous frapper, même si elle aimerait bien. Quand Hootsie fait du cinéma, Zuma lui donne une sacrée fessée déculottée. Des fois, Zuma agite sa grande cuiller en bois vers nous quand personne regarde et dit :

— Vous autres, vous devriez être sacrément reconnaissantes. Vous devriez lui embrasser les pieds, à Mme Sevier, parce qu'elle vous a laissées entrer dans cette jolie maison. Je sais ce que vous êtes, et vous z'avez pas intérêt à l'oublier non plus. Vous z'êtes là juste le temps que la dame, elle ait son propre bébé. Le monsieur, il pense que si elle arrête de s'inquiéter toujours pour ça, ça arrivera. Et là, vous déguerpirez comme des rats que vous êtes. Dehors avec les poubelles. Vous z'êtes là que pour le moment. Vous croyez pas chez vous. J'ai déjà vu ça, je vous préviens. Vous resterez pas longtemps.

Elle a raison, inutile que je la contredise. Au moins, on nous donne à manger, ici, et vraiment beaucoup. Il y a des robes à frous-frous, même si elles grattent et qu'elles sont trop raides à force d'être amidonnées, des rubans pour les cheveux, et des pastels, des livres et des chaussures à brides toutes neuves. Il y a un petit service à thé en porcelaine et des biscuits pour le goûter. On n'a jamais eu de service à thé, alors Mme Sevier doit nous montrer comment faire.

Il n'y a pas de queue à l'heure du bain. Nous ne sommes pas obligées de nous déshabiller pendant que d'autres nous regardent. Personne ne nous frappe à la tête. Personne ne menace de nous attacher et de nous suspendre dans le placard. Personne ne se fait enfermer au sous-sol. Du moins, jusqu'à maintenant et, comme le dit Zuma, nous ne resterons pas suffisamment longtemps pour savoir si cela pourrait arriver.

Une chose dont je suis sûre, par contre, c'est que, lorsque les Sevier en auront assez de nous, nous ne retournerons pas chez Mme Murphy. La nuit, quand je suis en sécurité dans la chambre près de Fern, je regarde en bas, au-delà des pâturages, et je vois l'eau à travers les arbres. Je guette les lanternes glissant sur le lac, et j'en aperçois quelques-unes. Parfois, je vois des lumières, même au loin sur l'eau, flottant comme des étoiles tombées du ciel. Tout ce que j'ai à faire, c'est trouver un moyen d'embarquer sur un bateau avec Fern, et nous pourrons traverser les marais de Dedmen's Slough jusqu'au fleuve. Ensuite, le voyage sera facile jusqu'à l'endroit où la Wolf rejoint le Mississippi à Mud Island, et c'est là que Queenie et Briny nous attendront.

Je dois juste trouver un bateau et j'y arriverai. Après notre départ, les Sevier n'auront aucune idée de ce qui nous est arrivé. Mlle Tann ne leur a pas révélé que nous venions du fleuve, et je parie que Zuma ne dira rien non plus. Nos nouveaux parents pensent que notre vraie maman a été à l'université et que notre papa était professeur. Ils pensent qu'elle est morte après avoir attrapé une pneumonie et que lui a perdu son travail et ne pouvait plus nous garder. Ils pensent aussi que Fern n'a que trois ans, alors qu'elle en a quatre.

Je ne détrompe pas les Sevier. J'essaie surtout d'être bien sage pour que rien ne se produise avant que Fern et moi puissions nous enfuir.

— Vous voilà, dit Mme Sevier lorsqu'elle nous trouve en bas, à table dans la salle à manger, en train d'attendre le petit-déjeuner.

Elle fronce les sourcils en voyant que nous avons déjà enfilé les vêtements sortis pour nous la veille au soir. Fern porte des culottes bleues à carreaux avec un petit chemisier qui se boutonne dans le dos. Il a des manches ballon et laisse voir son ventre sous la dentelle en bas du chemisier. Moi, j'ai une robe violette à jabot légère, un peu serrée au niveau du buste. J'ai dû rentrer mon ventre pour la boutonner, ce qui est étonnant, mais je grandis, j'imagine. Queenie dit que, chez les Foss, les enfants ont toujours des poussées de croissance.

Soit je suis en pleine poussée, soit c'est parce que nous mangeons beaucoup plus qu'un peu de bouillie, ici. Tous les matins, nous nous asseyons autour d'un repas copieux et, au déjeuner,

Zuma nous apporte des sandwichs sur un plateau. Le soir, nous prenons encore un grand repas, sauf si M. Sevier est occupé dans sa salle de musique. Dans ce cas, on nous sert de nouveau des sandwichs sur un plateau et Mme Sevier joue à des jeux de société avec nous, ce que Fern adore.

— May, je t'ai déjà dit que vous n'êtes pas obligées de vous lever si tôt et que tu n'as pas besoin d'habiller la petite Beth.

Elle croise les bras sur sa robe de chambre soyeuse si chic qu'elle a l'air d'appartenir à la reine Cléopâtre. Fern et moi avons des robes de chambre assorties. Mère a demandé à Zuma de les coudre juste pour nous, en cadeau. Nous ne les avons jamais enfilées. Je me dis qu'il vaut mieux qu'on ne s'habitue pas aux choses luxueuses, puisqu'on ne va pas rester longtemps.

En plus, il y a deux petites bosses qui pointent sur mon buste, et la robe de chambre, trop fine, trop brillante, les fait ressortir, alors que je ne veux pas qu'on les voie.

— Nous avons attendu... un petit peu.

Je baisse les yeux. Elle ne comprend pas que, toute notre vie, nous nous sommes levées à l'aube. On ne peut pas faire autrement, sur un bateau. Quand le fleuve se réveille, on se réveille avec lui. Les oiseaux parlent, et les bateaux sifflent et les vagues s'écrasent sur la coque les unes après les autres si on est amarrés près d'une voie de navigation large. Il faut surveiller les lignes, remonter les poissons, alimenter la chaudière. Il y a plein de choses à faire.

— Il est temps que tu apprennes à dormir jusqu'à une heure correcte.

Mme Sevier me regarde en secouant la tête, et je ne sais pas si elle fait semblant ou si elle ne m'aime pas beaucoup.

— Tu n'es plus à l'orphelinat, May. Tu es ici chez toi.

— Oui, m'dame.

— Oui, mère.

Elle pose une main sur ma tête et se penche pour embrasser Fern sur la joue avant de faire mine de lui grignoter l'oreille. Fern glousse et pousse des petits cris ravis.

— Oui, mère.

Ça ne vient pas naturellement, mais je m'améliore. La prochaine fois, je m'en souviendrai.

Elle s'assied au bout de la table et fixe le grand couloir, le menton posé sur la main, les sourcils froncés.

— J'imagine que vous n'avez pas vu père ce matin ?

— Non... mère.

Fern se ratatine sur sa chaise et jette un coup d'œil inquiet vers Mme Sevier. Nous savons tous où il est. Nous entendons une mélodie résonner dans le couloir. Il n'est pas censé entrer dans sa salle de musique avant le petit-déjeuner. Nous les avons déjà entendus se disputer à ce sujet.

— Dar-ren ! hurle-t-elle, ses ongles pianotant sur la table.

Fern se bouche les oreilles et Zuma arrive précipitamment en tenant un bol de porcelaine dont le couvercle cliquette et manque de tomber avant qu'elle le rattrape. Elle écarquille tellement les yeux que le blanc se voit tout autour de ses iris, puis elle se rend compte que Mme Sevier n'est pas fâchée contre elle.

— J'vais le chercher, m'dame, déclare-t-elle en posant le bol sur la table avant de beugler en direction de la cuisine : Hootsie, apporte les plateaux avant qu'y sont tout froids !

Elle repart à toute vitesse, raide comme un piquet, et me jette un regard furieux quand mère tourne la tête. Avant notre arrivée, Zuma n'avait pas besoin de salir toute cette vaisselle pour le petit-déjeuner. Elle n'avait qu'un plateau à préparer, qu'elle montait à la chambre de Mme Sevier. C'est Hootsie qui me l'a dit. Avant notre arrivée, Hootsie restait parfois à l'étage toute la matinée avec la dame, et regardait des numéros de *Life* et des livres d'images avec elle en essayant de la distraire pour que son mari puisse travailler.

Maintenant, Hootsie doit aider à la cuisine, et c'est notre faute.

Elle glisse un pied sous la table et m'écrase les orteils lorsqu'elle apporte les œufs.

Aussitôt, Zuma revient dans le couloir avec M. Sevier. C'est la seule à pouvoir le faire sortir de sa salle de musique lorsque la porte est fermée. Elle l'a élevé depuis qu'il était tout petit et elle s'occupe encore de lui comme s'il était toujours un enfant. Il l'écoute, elle, plus que sa femme.

— Y faut que vous mangiez ! dit-elle en le suivant dans le couloir, ses mains entrant et sortant des ombres matinales. Moi qu'ai fait toute cette cuisine, et v'là que c'est déjà à moitié froid.

— Je me suis réveillé tôt avec une mélodie en tête. Il fallait que je la transcrive avant qu'elle s'enfuie.

Il s'arrête au bout du couloir, une main sur le ventre, une autre en l'air. Il improvise une petite gigue comme un comédien sur scène. Puis il s'incline devant nous.

— Bonjour, mesdames.

Après avoir froncé les sourcils, Mme Sevier les haussent et son front se plisse.

— Tu sais que nous nous étions mis d'accord, Darren. Pas avant le petit-déjeuner, et tous les repas doivent être pris à table, ensemble. Comment les filles pourraient-elles apprendre à vivre en famille si tu vas t'enfermer tout seul à toute heure ?

Au lieu de s'arrêter à sa chaise, il contourne la table et l'embrasse en plein sur les lèvres.

— Comment va ma muse, ce matin ?

— Oh, arrête ! se plaint-elle. Tu essaies juste de m'amadouer !

— Est-ce que j'y arrive ?

Il nous fait un clin d'œil, à Fern et moi. Fern glousse, moi, je fais comme si je n'avais rien vu.

Soudain, j'ai comme un poids sur ma poitrine, je baisse les yeux vers mon assiette et je revois Briny embrassant Queenie de la même façon quand il traversait la cabine pour aller sur le pont arrière.

Le repas ne sent plus bon du tout, tout à coup, même si mon estomac grogne. Je ne veux pas manger la nourriture de ces gens, ni rire de leurs blagues ni les appeler mère et père. J'ai une maman et un papa, et je veux rentrer à la maison pour les retrouver.

Fern ne devrait pas rire et s'amuser avec eux. Ce n'est pas juste.

Je passe la main sous la table pour lui pincer la jambe, et elle pousse un petit cri.

Nos parents adoptifs se penchent vers nous pour essayer de comprendre ce qui s'est passé. Fern ne dit rien.

Zuma et Hootsie apportent les autres plats et nous déjeunons pendant que M. Sevier nous explique sa nouvelle musique et la façon dont la mélodie parfaite lui est arrivée au beau milieu de la nuit. Il parle de partitions, de pauses et de notes et de plein d'autres choses. Mme Sevier soupire et regarde par la fenêtre, mais je ne peux pas m'empêcher de l'écouter. Je n'ai jamais entendu quelqu'un me raconter comment les musiciens écrivent leurs compositions sur le papier. Tous les airs que je connais, je les ai entendus quand Briny jouait de la guitare ou de l'harmonica, ou même du piano dans les salles de billard. La musique se glisse très profondément en moi et me fait éprouver des tas de choses.

Maintenant, je me demande si Briny savait que des gens écrivent des airs sur du papier, comme une histoire, et que ces airs se retrouvent dans des films, comme le raconte M. Sevier. Justement, sa nouvelle musique est pour un film. Au bout de la table, il agite les mains en l'air et parle fort, tout excité, en décrivant une scène où les pillards du hors-la-loi Quantrill traversent le Kansas et brûlent une ville entière.

Il fredonne l'air en tambourinant sur la table, les couverts vibrent et je sens les chevaux qui galopent et les coups de feu qui pétaradent.

— Qu'en penses-tu, chérie ? demande-t-il à Mme Sevier une fois qu'il s'arrête.

Elle joint les deux mains et Fern l'imite.

— Un chef-d'œuvre, répond-elle. Bien sûr que c'est un chef-d'œuvre. Tu n'es pas d'accord, Bethie ?

Je n'arrive pas à m'habituer à ce qu'ils appellent Fern Beth – ils pensent que c'est son vrai prénom, évidemment.

— Chéd'œufs !

Fern essaie de répéter le mot « chef-d'œuvre », la bouche pleine de miettes.

Ils rient tous les trois, pendant que je fixe mon assiette.

— C'est tellement bon de la voir heureuse, soupire mère en se penchant pour écarter une mèche du visage de Fern afin d'éviter que des miettes s'y collent.

— Oui, en effet, répond M. Sevier.

Il regarde sa femme mais elle ne le sait pas. Elle est trop occupée à chouchouter Fern.

Mme Sevier enroule les cheveux de Fern autour de son doigt pour transformer les petites bouclettes en grosses anglaises comme celles de Shirley Temple. Mme Sevier la préfère comme ça. La plupart du temps, je me fais une tresse, qui me tombe dans le dos, pour qu'elle n'ait pas l'idée de faire la même chose avec moi.

— Je craignais que nous n'atteignions jamais cette étape, dit-elle à son mari.

— Ce genre de chose prend du temps.

— J'avais tellement peur de ne jamais être mère.

Les yeux de M. Sevier s'illuminent, comme s'il était heureux. Il regarde de l'autre côté de la table.

— Elle est à nous, maintenant.

« Non, c'est faux ! voudrais-je hurler. Tu n'es pas sa mère. Tu n'es pas notre mère. Ces bébés morts au fond du jardin, ceux-là sont à toi. » Je hais Mme Sevier, parce qu'elle veut Fern. Je hais ces bébés parce qu'ils sont morts. Je hais M. Sevier parce qu'il nous a amenées ici. S'il nous avait laissées tranquilles, nous serions déjà de retour sur l'*Arcadie,* Fern et moi. Personne n'entortillerait les cheveux de ma sœur pour faire des boucles à la Shirley Temple et personne ne l'appellerait Beth.

Je serre les dents si fort que la douleur me remonte jusqu'en haut du crâne. Je suis contente. Ce n'est qu'une petite douleur et je sais d'où elle vient. Je peux y mettre fin quand je veux. Celle dans mon cœur est bien plus grande. Et je ne peux pas la soulager, malgré tous mes efforts. Ça me fait tellement peur que je ne peux plus respirer.

Et si Fern décide qu'elle aime plus ces gens que moi ? Et si elle oubliait Briny et Queenie et l'*Arcadie* ? Nous n'avions pas de robes coquettes, pas de trottinettes sur le pont, pas d'ours en peluche, pas de pastels, pas de petite dînette en porcelaine, là-bas. Tout ce que nous avions, c'était le fleuve, mais le fleuve nous nourrissait, nous emportait, nous libérait.

Je dois m'assurer que Fern n'oublie pas. Elle ne peut pas devenir Beth.

— May ?

Alors que Mme Sevier me parlait, je n'ai rien écouté. J'affiche un sourire de façade et lève les yeux vers elle.

— Oui... mère ?

— J'ai dit que j'allais emmener Beth à Memphis pour lui faire essayer des chaussures spéciales, aujourd'hui. Il est important que nous corrigions sa jambe qui tourne en dedans avant qu'elle ne grandisse. Une fois que la croissance est trop avancée, c'est trop tard, m'a-t-on dit. Ce serait bien dommage, alors que cela peut être guéri.

Elle penche un peu la tête. On dirait un aigle guettant un poisson. Joli à voir, mais le poisson ferait mieux de se méfier. Je suis contente que mes pieds soient sous la table, comme ça, elle ne voit pas ma jambe droite. Nous avons tous le pied droit tourné un peu en dedans. Ça nous vient de Queenie. Briny dit que c'est notre marque de fabrique, en tant que membres de la lignée royale du royaume d'Arcadie.

Je redresse malgré moi ma jambe, au cas où elle aurait l'idée de vérifier.

— Elle devra porter une attelle la nuit, m'annonce Mme Sevier.

Près d'elle, M. Sevier ouvre le journal et le scrute tout en mangeant son bacon.

— Oh... je marmonne.

J'enlèverai l'attelle de la jambe de Fern, pendant la nuit. Voilà ce que je ferai.

— Je pensais l'y emmener seule.

Les paroles de Mme Sevier semblent très prudentes, ses yeux bleus se rivent à moi sous ses boucles blondes qui me rappellent

311

Queenie même si je ne le veux pas. Queenie est beaucoup plus jolie. C'est vrai.

— Beth doit s'habituer à passer du temps avec sa nouvelle mère, à ce que nous soyons juste toutes les deux… sans faire de scène.

Elle sourit à ma sœur qui, armée d'une petite fourchette pour bébé en argent, est occupée à pourchasser dans son assiette une des fraises en conserve de Zuma. Les Sevier n'aiment pas qu'on mange avec les doigts.

Mme Sevier frappe dans ses mains pour attirer l'attention de son mari, qui baisse un peu son journal et pointe son nez par-dessus.

— Darren, Darren, regarde-la. Comme elle est mignonne !

— Ne la lâche pas, soldat ! dit-il. Quand tu auras capturé celle-là, tu pourras en avoir une autre.

Fern pique la fraise, la met tout entière dans sa bouche et sourit pendant que du jus lui dégouline par les commissures.

Nos nouveaux parents rigolent. Mme Sevier tapote les joues de Fern avec une serviette de table, pour qu'elle ne salisse pas sa blouse.

J'hésite à la supplier de me laisser les accompagner chez le docteur qui s'occupe des pieds. J'ai peur de la laisser éloigner Fern de moi. Elle lui achètera des tas de trucs, et Fern l'aimera bien. Mais je ne veux pas aller à Memphis. La dernière chose dont je me souvienne de cet endroit, c'est de m'y être fait emmener par Mme Murphy et donner à mon nouveau père dans une chambre d'hôtel.

Si je reste à la maison pendant que Mme Sevier est absente, je pourrais sans doute sortir et explorer les alentours. La plupart du temps, elle n'aime pas qu'on traîne dehors. Elle a peur qu'on touche des orties ou qu'on se fasse mordre par un serpent. Elle ne peut pas savoir que nous, les enfants du fleuve, connaissons déjà toutes ces choses à l'âge où l'on apprend à marcher.

— Tu commenceras bientôt l'école, m'annonce ma mère, contrariée que je n'aie pas répondu tout de suite, pour le docteur. Beth est encore trop jeune, bien sûr. Elle a encore deux ans à passer à la maison avant d'entrer à l'école... si nous l'y inscrivons. Je la garderai peut-être avec moi un an de plus. Cela dépendra...

Une main aux doigts fins se pose sur son ventre et s'y déploie doucement. Elle ne le dit pas mais elle espère qu'il y a un bébé.

J'essaie de ne pas y penser. Et de ne pas penser à l'école non plus. Une fois qu'ils m'y enverront, Mme Sevier passera toute la journée avec Fern. Fern l'aimera plus que moi, c'est sûr. Je dois nous faire partir d'ici avant que ça arrive.

Mme Sevier s'éclaircit la gorge et son mari rebaisse son journal.

— Qu'y a-t-il à ton programme aujourd'hui, chéri ? demande-t-elle.

— De la musique, quelle question ! Je veux finir la nouvelle partition pendant que l'air est encore frais dans ma tête. Puis j'appellerai Stanley et je lui jouerai un morceau au téléphone... pour qu'il me dise si cela convient bien au film.

Elle soupire, et des rides se pressent au coin de ses yeux.

— Je pensais que tu pourrais demander à Hoy de sortir la carriole et d'atteler le poney, pour que vous puissiez faire un tour, tous les deux.

Son regard glisse de son mari à moi.

— Ça te plairait, May ? Si tu es avec père, tu n'auras pas peur du poney. Il est très doux. J'en avais un comme lui quand j'étais petite, à Augusta. Je l'aimais plus que tout au monde.

Mes muscles se crispent et je me sens pâlir. Je n'ai pas peur du poney. Mais de M. Sevier. Même s'il ne m'a rien fait, après avoir vécu chez Mme Murphy, je sais ce qui peut arriver.

— Je ne veux pas vous embêter.

J'ai les mains moites, je les essuie sur ma robe.

— Mmm... fait M. Sevier, les sourcils froncés, comme si cette idée ne lui plaisait pas plus qu'à moi, ce qui m'arrange. Nous verrons comment se passe la journée, chérie. La production du film a pris déjà tellement de retard, mon délai est plus court que d'habitude, et avec le chaos qui a régné dans la maison ces dernières semaines à cause de...

Sa femme relève le menton et secoue imperceptiblement la tête.

— Eh bien, nous verrons comment évolue la journée.

Je regarde par terre et plus personne ne parle de la carriole. Nous terminons le petit-déjeuner, puis M. Sevier disparaît dans sa salle de musique aussi vite qu'il le peut. Bientôt, Fern et Mme Sevier s'en vont aussi. Je prends mes pastels et un livre, puis je vais m'asseoir à l'arrière de la maison, là où une grande terrasse domine les bois, puis le lac. Des notes de piano s'échappent du studio de M. Sevier. Elles se mêlent au chant des oiseaux et, les yeux fermés pour les écouter, j'attends que Zuma et Hootsie regagnent le hangar pour pouvoir me glisser dans la maison et l'explorer un peu...

Je m'assoupis et je rêve que Fern et moi sommes sur la jetée où M. Sevier va s'asseoir pour pêcher. Nous sommes assises sur l'une de ces grosses valises qu'ils entreposent dans le placard, près des balais et des serpillières de Zuma, et que nous avons remplie de jouets à partager avec Camellia, Lark et Gabion. Nous attendons que Briny et Queenie viennent nous chercher.

L'*Arcadie* arrive en vue au bout du lac. Il avance tout doucement à contre-courant. Puis, tout à coup, le vent se lève et l'emporte au loin. Je regarde par-dessus mon épaule et je vois une grosse voiture noire traverser le champ derrière nous en rebondissant sur les bosses. Le visage de Mlle Tann est plaqué contre la vitre. Ses yeux brûlent de colère. J'attrape Fern et m'élance vers l'eau pour que nous puissions nous échapper à la nage.

Nous commençons à courir, mais plus nous fonçons, plus la jetée s'allonge.

La voiture arrive à monter sur la jetée et s'arrête juste derrière nous. Une main m'attrape par la robe et les cheveux.

— Tu n'es qu'une petite souillon ingrate, n'est-ce pas ? dit Mlle Tann.

Je me réveille en sursaut. Hootsie se tient devant moi, avec un verre de thé et un plateau contenant mon déjeuner. Elle les pose brutalement sur la table en osier. La boisson déborde, éclabousse le plateau et l'assiette.

— Ça sera comme de la nourriture du fleuve, maintenant, pas vrai ? Bien ramolli.

Elle me jette un sourire moqueur.

Je prends le sandwich trempé et le mords à belles dents en lui rendant son sourire. Hootsie ne s'imagine pas ce qu'on a vécu avant de venir ici. Je suis capable de manger du porridge avec des charançons dedans sans sourciller. Un peu de thé renversé sur un sandwich ne va pas me décourager. Ni Hootsie, malgré tous ses efforts. Elle n'est pas très coriace. Et des enfants coriaces, j'en ai connu.

Elle soupire en relevant le nez puis s'en va. Après mon repas, je pose la serviette sur l'assiette pour ne pas attirer les mouches. Puis je longe la galerie qui fait le tour de la maison vers la salle de musique. Même si le silence est revenu, je reste prudente lorsque j'arrive au bout de la maison et que je tourne à l'angle. Aucun signe de M. Sevier. Je m'en assure avant de m'approcher davantage.

Quand je me glisse par la porte moustiquaire, il fait sombre dans la salle de musique car les rideaux ont été tirés à fond. Dans un coin, un projecteur dessine un carré de lumière blanche sur le mur. Ça me rappelle le cinématographe itinérant qui s'arrêtait parfois dans les villes fluviales. Je m'approche et vois mon ombre, longue et fine, avec des petits bouts de lumière bouclée qui brillent entre mes cheveux. Je repense à Briny, qui faisait des marionnettes avec ses mains derrière les fenêtres éclairées de l'*Arcadie*, de temps en temps. J'en essaie une, mais je ne me souviens plus comment faire.

À côté du projecteur, une aiguille sautille sur un disque tournoyant posé sur un phonographe. Un petit bruit de grattement sort par le côté de la malle qui le contient. J'avance vers lui, regarde dans la boîte et observe le disque noir tourner. Nous en avions eu un, brièvement, sur le pont arrière de notre bateau, sauf qu'il marchait avec une manivelle. Briny l'avait trouvé dans une vieille maison près du fleuve où plus personne n'habitait.

Il l'a échangé contre du bois de chauffage, un peu plus tard.

Je me dis que je ne devrais pas toucher celui-là, mais je ne peux pas m'en empêcher. C'est le plus bel objet que j'aie jamais vu. Il doit être tout neuf.

Je soulève la boule d'argent qui tient l'aiguille et la décale d'un cheveu pour entendre juste les dernières notes de musique. Puis je remonte un peu plus loin, et encore un peu plus loin. Le volume est très bas, j'espère que personne d'autre n'entend.

Au bout d'une minute, je m'approche du piano et je repense à Briny, quand lui et moi, on s'asseyait côte à côte au piano dans les salles de billard ou sur les bateaux-théâtres quand ils étaient déserts. Il m'apprenait à jouer des morceaux. Parmi tous les enfants Foss, j'étais la meilleure pour les mémoriser ; c'est ce que Briny disait.

Les dernières notes s'échappent du phonographe et l'aiguille dérape.

Je rejoue la mélodie au piano, tout doucement. J'appuie à peine sur les touches. Ce n'est pas trop compliqué de retrouver l'air. Il me plaît, alors je recule encore l'aiguille pour en apprendre un peu plus. Cette partie est plus difficile, elle me demande davantage de travail mais je finis par la retrouver.

— Eh bien, bravo !

Je me lève d'un bond et vois M. Sevier debout, une main sur la porte moustiquaire. Il la lâche et applaudit. Je m'éloigne à toute vitesse du piano en cherchant une issue par où m'enfuir.

— Je suis désolée. J'aurais pas dû…

Les larmes me nouent la gorge. Et s'il était furieux et qu'il le disait à Mme Sevier et qu'ils se débarrassaient de moi avant que Fern et moi ayons le temps de partir sur le fleuve pour rentrer chez nous ?

Il entre et laisse la moustiquaire se refermer.

— Ne t'inquiète pas. Tu ne risques pas d'abîmer le piano. En revanche, Victoria tenait vraiment à ce que nous sortions en carriole pendant son absence. J'ai demandé à Hoy d'atteler le poney. J'ai fait venir des ouvriers pour construire un petit cottage au bord du lac – un endroit tranquille où travailler

quand la maison est trop bruyante. Nous descendrons en carriole pour jeter un œil au chantier, puis nous ferons le tour de
la propriété. À notre retour, je te montrerai comment...

Il fait quelques pas supplémentaires dans la pièce.

— Tu sais quoi ? À bien y réfléchir, le poney ne se fâchera
pas si on le fait attendre un peu. Il est du genre patient.
Recommence, dit-il en faisant tournoyer sa main vers le piano.

Les larmes s'échappent dans ma gorge. Je ravale ce qu'il en
reste tandis qu'il s'approche du phonographe.

— Voilà. Je vais repositionner l'aiguille. Qu'as-tu retrouvé
pour l'instant ?

— Je ne sais pas, réponds-je dans un haussement d'épaules.
Pas grand-chose. Je dois écouter vraiment longtemps d'abord.

Il remonte plus loin que moi mais je réfléchis très vite et je
retrouve le passage presque sans fautes.

— Tu as déjà joué, avant ? me demande-t-il.

— Non, m'sieur.

Il recule un peu plus l'aiguille et je recommence tout. Je me
trompe juste une fois, sur la nouvelle partie.

— Impressionnant.

Ce n'est pas vrai, mais ça fait plaisir à entendre. En même
temps, je m'interroge : Que veut-il ? Il n'a pas besoin de moi
pour jouer du piano. Il est lui-même très doué. Encore meilleur
que le disque sur le phonographe.

— Encore, dit-il en faisant de nouveau tournoyer sa main.
Juste de mémoire.

Je m'exécute, mais il y a quelque chose qui cloche.

— Oups, fait-il. Tu entends ça ?

— Oui, m'sieur.

— C'est un dièse, voilà le problème, m'explique-t-il en me
montrant le clavier. Je peux te montrer si tu veux.

Je hoche la tête et me retourne vers le piano pour placer
mes doigts sur les touches.

— Non, comme ça.

Il se penche derrière moi et me montre comment étirer ma
main.

— Le pouce, sur le do du milieu. Tu as des doigts fins et souples. De vraies mains de pianiste.

Ce sont les mains de Briny, mais M. Sevier ne le sait pas.

Il appuie sur mes doigts, un par un. Les touches jouent la mélodie. Il me montre comment faire le dièse où je me trompais.

— Voilà, comme ça, dit-il. Tu entends la différence ?

Je hoche la tête.

— Oui ! Je l'entends !

— Tu sais quelle note vient ensuite ? Dans la mélodie, je veux dire.

— Oui, m'sieur.

— Parfait.

Avant que j'aie le temps de réfléchir, il s'assied à côté de moi.

— Tu joues la mélodie, je m'occupe des accords. Tu verras comment les deux vont s'assembler. C'est comme ça qu'on crée un morceau, comme celui que tu as entendu sur le disque.

J'obéis tandis qu'il joue les notes les plus basses de son côté, et notre musique est comme celle du disque ! Je la sens monter du piano et se glisser dans mon corps. Maintenant, je sais ce que ressentent les oiseaux quand ils chantent.

À la fin, je lui demande :

— Est-ce qu'on peut recommencer ? Même une autre partie ?

J'en veux encore, encore, encore.

Il relance le disque, m'aide à trouver les bonnes touches et, ensuite, nous jouons ensemble. Il rit lorsque nous avons fini, et moi aussi.

— Il faudra envisager de te faire prendre des cours, dit-il. Tu as du talent.

Je le scrute pour voir s'il se moque de moi. Du talent ? Moi ?

Je cache mon sourire derrière ma main, puis je me retourne vers le clavier et mes joues prennent feu. Est-ce qu'il le pense vraiment ?

— Je ne le dirais pas si ce n'était pas vrai, May. Je ne sais peut-être pas grand-chose sur l'éducation des petites filles, mais, en musique, je m'y connais.

Il se penche pour essayer de voir mon visage.

— Je comprends que ce soit difficile pour toi, de venir ici, dans une nouvelle maison, à ton âge... mais je crois que, toi et moi, on peut être amis.

Aussitôt, je me retrouve dans le couloir, chez Mme Murphy, dans le noir, et Riggs m'a coincée entre le mur et son ventre, et il m'écrase, m'étouffe, et mon corps ne sent plus rien. L'odeur du whisky, de la cendre de charbon remonte dans mon nez et il murmure : « T-toi et moi, on p-p-peut être amis. Je p-p-peux te donner des b-b-bonbons et des b-b-biscuits. Tout ce que t-tu veux. On peut être les m-m-meilleurs amis du m-monde. »

D'un bond, je me lève du tabouret en écrasant les touches si fort qu'elles jouent toutes en même temps. Le bruit se mêle au claquement de mes semelles sur le sol.

Je ne m'arrête pas de courir avant d'être à l'étage, roulée en boule en bas de mon armoire, mes pieds arc-boutés contre la porte pour que personne ne puisse entrer.

21

Avery

Les Stafford ne sont jamais aussi redoutables que lorsqu'ils sont assiégés. Depuis trois semaines maintenant, nous nous protégeons à l'abri des barricades, repoussant la presse, dont l'objectif principal est de nous dépeindre comme une famille criminellement élitiste parce que nous avons choisi un établissement haut de gamme pour ma grand-mère, qui a les moyens de payer les frais, par ailleurs. Ce n'est pas comme si nous demandions aux contribuables de financer les coûts... Et c'est précisément ce que j'aimerais dire à chaque journaliste qui nous accoste avec un micro pendant nos déplacements entre les réunions publiques, les rassemblements, les événements mondains... et même à l'église.

Alors que je reviens à Drayden Hill après avoir accompagné mes parents à l'église, puis à un brunch, j'aperçois mes sœurs dans l'enclos d'une des juments qui a pouliné, avec les triplés d'Allison. Dans la carrière, Courtney a sorti un vieux hongre gris de bon caractère pour un petit galop. Elle le montre à cru et, alors que je me gare, j'imagine le rythme des foulées de Doughboy, ses muscles qui se tendent et se relâchent, les ondulations de son large dos.

— Hé, tata Avy ! Tu viens faire une promenade avec moi ? me lance Courtney, pleine d'espoir, lorsque je m'approche de la clôture. Tu pourras me ramener à la maison plus tard.

Je m'apprête à lui répondre : « Laisse-moi juste le temps d'enfiler un jean », mais la mère de Courtney me prend de court.

— Court', tu dois préparer tes affaires pour la colonie !

— Rhooo, pff, rumine ma nièce avant de repartir pour un nouveau tour de piste.

Je me glisse dans l'enclos et traverse tant bien que mal le paddock avec mes talons hauts. Près de la clôture du fond, les garçons s'amusent à glisser des fleurs et des brins d'herbe entre les barres de bois pour donner à manger aux poulains de l'année. Allison et Missy prennent des rafales de photos avec leurs iPhones. Les petits shorts en crépon de coton et les nœuds papillon des garçons n'ont plus l'air aussi immaculés qu'à l'église.

Missy s'accroupit et serre l'un de nos neveux dans ses bras tout en l'aidant à tenir une fleur sauvage.

— Ah, là, là... cette époque me manque, dit-elle, nostalgique.

Ses propres enfants, de grands ados, sont partis en tant que moniteurs de colonie à Asheville, là où nous avions passé une partie de nos vacances d'enfance. Court' doit les rejoindre demain pour un séjour plus court.

— Ces trois hooligans sont à louer quand tu veux, répond Allison, une lueur d'espoir dans les yeux, avant de glisser une mèche de son épaisse chevelure auburn derrière son oreille. Et quand je dis, quand tu veux, c'est sincère ! Tu n'es même pas obligée de prendre les trois, juste un ou deux.

Nous rions ensemble. C'est un joli moment, la tension se relâche. Ces dernières semaines ont mis tout le monde sur les nerfs.

— Comment était papa, pendant le brunch ?

Comme toujours, Missy revient à des questions pratiques.

— Pas trop mal, j'imagine. Ils sont restés après, pour discuter avec des amis. Avec un peu de chance, maman le persuadera de se reposer une fois qu'ils rentreront à la maison. Nous avons un dîner ce soir.

Mon père est déterminé à suivre le rythme, même si la controverse autour de mamie Judy l'épuise. Il a du mal à supporter que sa mère soit devenue une cible au cours de la dernière bataille politique en date. Le sénateur Stafford peut encaisser les attaques directes mais, lorsque sa famille se retrouve au milieu des tirs croisés, sa pression artérielle monte en flèche.

Les jours où il doit porter la pompe à chimio attachée à sa jambe, on a l'impression qu'il est prêt à s'effondrer sous le poids supplémentaire.

— Nous partirons avant qu'ils reviennent, dans ce cas, déclare Allison en jetant un coup d'œil vers l'allée. Je voulais juste prendre quelques images des poulains et des garçons dans leurs habits du dimanche. Leslie pensait que quelques photos sur le thème « bébés animaux + bébés Stafford » serait un bon moyen de faire diversion sur les réseaux sociaux. Quelque chose d'inoffensif et de mignon.

— En tout cas, ça marcherait sur moi, dis-je en embrassant un de mes neveux sur la tête.

En échange, il lève les bras vers moi et me tapote le visage avec ses mains pleines de terre.

— Hé, tata Avy, regarde ça ! lance Courtney en s'apprêtant à sauter un petit obstacle avec Doughboy.

— Courtney ! hurle sa mère. Pas sans selle et sans ta bombe ! Je m'esclaffe :

— Voilà une fille selon mon cœur.

— Elle te ressemble beaucoup trop, glousse Missy en me donnant un coup d'épaule.

— Je ne vois pas du tout de quoi tu veux parler.

Le nez droit d'Allison se fronce quand elle répond :

— Ben, voyons !

— Sois sympa, Al. Laisse-la rester, dis-je, prenant malgré moi le parti de Courtney. D'ailleurs, j'ai un peu de temps libre et une promenade à cheval me tente bien. Je la ramène chez vous dans une heure... ou deux. Elle pourra faire sa valise ensuite.

Ma nièce franchit un nouvel obstacle avec Doughboy.

— Courtney Lynne ! la gronde Allison.

Je m'apprête à protester que ce ne sont que de petits sauts et que, par ailleurs, Courtney monte comme une cavalière éméraite, mais je suis distraite par l'arrivée d'une voiture qui avance jusqu'au paddock. Je reconnais aussitôt la BMW argentée décapotable. Et j'ai l'impression de recevoir un haltère de cinq kilos dans le ventre.

— Bitsy est là ? demande Missy.

— On dirait bien, malheureusement.

Je ne devrais pas dire ça, surtout de ma future belle-mère, mais la dernière chose dont j'ai besoin aujourd'hui, c'est d'être harcelée une nouvelle fois par Bitsy et ses idées pour notre mariage. Elle veut bien faire, sauf qu'elle me tombe dessus à la moindre occasion.

Le poids se soulève lorsque je vois quelqu'un d'autre descendre de voiture – un homme grand, brun et irrésistiblement beau.

— Tiens, tiens, regarde qui est venu voir sa dulcinée. Je ne savais pas que ton mec était dans le coin, minaude Missy avant d'agiter les bras. Salut, Elliot !

J'en reste bouche bée.

— Il ne devait... Il ne m'avait pas dit qu'il venait à Aiken. Quand nous avons parlé hier, il était à Washington pour une réunion, et il avait prévu de prendre l'avion aujourd'hui pour la Californie.

— On dirait qu'il a changé d'avis. C'est romantique, non ? susurre Allison en me poussant vers le portail de l'enclos. Tu ferais bien d'aller lui faire un câlin.

— Et un bisou, renchérit Missy. Et tout ce qui te passera par la tête !

— C'est fini, oui, toutes les deux ?

C'est peut-être à cause de toutes ces années d'enfance où mes sœurs nous ont taquinés, Elliot et moi, parce qu'elles pensaient que nous sortions ensemble alors que c'était faux, mais j'ai soudain le cou et les joues en feu lorsque Elliot agite la main et se dirige vers le portail du paddock. Il est à tomber dans son costume gris ajusté. Oui, il est habillé pour le travail. Que fait-il ici ?

Tout à coup, je ne peux plus attendre, il faut que je sache. J'enlève mes chaussures et je cours dans l'herbe pour aller me jeter dans ses bras. Il me soulève un instant, me repose et m'embrasse. Tout est merveilleux. C'est doux, familier et

323

rassurant, et je me rends compte que c'est exactement ce dont j'ai besoin en ce moment.

— Qu'est-ce que tu viens faire à Aiken ?

Je suis encore sous le choc de son arrivée imprévue – ravie, mais étonnée.

Ses yeux brun profond scintillent. Il est content de m'avoir fait une telle surprise.

— J'ai changé de vol pour pouvoir passer quelques heures ici avant de partir pour Los Angeles.

— Tu pars à L.A. aujourd'hui ?

Je m'en veux de paraître déçue, mais j'avais déjà commencé à prévoir des choses.

— Ce soir. Désolé de ne pas avoir pu prévoir une visite plus longue. Enfin, c'est mieux que rien, non ?

J'entends soudain une voiture dans l'allée. J'entraîne Elliot vers les écuries. C'est sans doute mes parents qui reviennent du brunch. S'ils nous voient, nous n'aurons pas une seconde à nous.

— Allons marcher un peu. Je te veux rien qu'à moi.

Avec un peu de chance, mes parents ne remarqueront pas la voiture garée près du monospace d'Allison.

Elliot baisse les yeux vers mes pieds nus.

— Tu n'as pas besoin de chaussures ?

— Je piquerai des bottes d'équitation dans la sellerie. Si je retourne à la maison, tout le monde saura que tu es là, et ma mère voudra papoter avec toi.

Une idée en amenant une autre, je l'interroge :

— Ta mère sait que tu es en ville ?

Bitsy nous tuera tous les deux si Elliot repart sans être passé chez elle.

— T'inquiète pas. J'ai déjà été la voir. On a pris un petit-déjeuner tardif.

Ce qui explique pourquoi Bitsy n'était pas au brunch, tout à l'heure.

— Ta mère savait que tu venais, et tu ne me l'as pas dit ?

Je m'en veux d'être jalouse, mais je n'y peux rien. Elliot débarque en ville et la première personne qu'il va voir, c'est Bitsy ?

Il m'attire contre lui et m'embrasse d'une façon qui me laisse comprendre qui il aime le plus.

— Je voulais te faire une surprise, dit-il tandis que nous longeons les écuries. Et la voir en premier pour en être débarrassé. Tu sais comment elle est.

— Je comprends.

Comme toujours, il a géré la situation avec Bitsy de la meilleure façon possible. Il nous a épargné une visite ensemble, qui aurait tourné en discussion intense à propos de couleur de tulle et je ne sais quoi.

— Est-ce qu'elle t'a barbé avec le mariage ?

— Un peu, admit-il. Je lui ai répondu que toi et moi allions en parler.

Je me retiens de lui dire que, dans le langage de Bitsy : « Nous allons en parler » signifie « Oui, nous ferons comme tu voudras ». En fait, sa mère est bien la dernière personne dont nous voulons nous préoccuper.

Il ouvre la sellerie et me tient la porte avant d'entrer pour accrocher sa veste à une patère.

— Comment va ton père, en ce moment ?

Je lui donne les dernières nouvelles tout en cherchant une paire de bottes à ma taille. Je les enfile et glisse mon pantalon de tailleur à l'intérieur.

— Magnifique, me taquine-t-il en étudiant ma tenue.

Elliot n'est pas du genre « pantalon rentré dans des bottes ».

— Si tu veux, je peux aller chercher quelque chose de mieux à la maison pendant que Pomme d'amour te parle de l'avantage des mariages printaniers...

Il glousse avant de se frotter les yeux, et je vois qu'il est fatigué. Cela me touche d'autant plus qu'il a fait une escale ici.

— C'est tentant mais... non. Allons marcher un peu, ensuite on pourra peut-être s'échapper pour faire un tour en voiture.

— Chouette. J'envoie un texto à Allison et Missy pour leur demander de ne pas dire à nos parents que tu es là.

Je me dépêche de taper le SMS pendant que nous nous dirigeons vers les sentiers. Comme toujours, la conversation se fait naturellement entre Elliot et moi. Sa main se glisse dans la mienne et nous parlons de ses affaires, des problèmes de famille, de son voyage à Milan, de politique. Nous nous racontons tout ce que nous n'avions pas eu le temps de nous dire au téléphone. Ça fait du bien, comme rentrer chez soi après un long voyage.

Les rythmes de la conversation, de notre promenade, sont ceux que nous avons appris avec le temps. Nous savons tous les deux où nous allons : jusqu'à un petit lac approvisionné par une source, où nous nous assiérons sous un kiosque entouré de pins qui, aussi loin que je me rappelle, a toujours été là. Nous y sommes presque lorsque je me retrouve à lui raconter l'histoire de May Crandall, de la Société des foyers d'accueil du Tennessee, et l'étrange mise en garde de mamie Judy contre la mystérieuse « Arcadie ».

Elliot s'arrête au pied du kiosque. Il s'appuie contre une colonne, les bras croisés sur la poitrine, et me fixe comme s'il venait de me pousser des cornes.

— Avery, d'où ça sort, tout ça ?

— Tout... quoi ?

— Toute cette histoire... je ne sais pas... ces fouilles presque archéologiques dans le passé ? Ces choses qui n'ont rien à voir avec nous ? Tu n'es pas assez occupée avec ton père, le tapage autour des plaintes contre les maisons de retraite et Leslie qui essaie sans cesse de te mener à la cravache ?

Je ne sais pas si je dois me vexer ou prendre la réaction d'Elliot comme la voix de la raison.

— Justement. Et si cette histoire avait bel et bien quelque chose à voir avec nous ? Et si mamie Judy s'intéressait tant à la Société des foyers d'accueil du Tennessee parce que notre famille y était liée d'une façon ou d'une autre ? Et si mes ancêtres avaient soutenu la législation qui avait légalisé toutes ces adoptions et scellé les archives ?

— Si c'était le cas, pourquoi voudrais-tu en savoir plus ? Qu'est-ce que ça peut faire, des décennies après les faits ?

Il plisse le front, et ses sourcils semblent se rejoindre en un nœud noir.

— Parce que... eh bien... parce que c'était important pour ma grand-mère, pour commencer.

— C'est exactement pour ça que tu dois te méfier de cette histoire.

J'en reste ébahie pendant une seconde. Je commence à m'échauffer sous le chemisier en soie sans manches que je portais à l'église. Tout à coup, mon fiancé parle beaucoup trop comme sa mère. Même son intonation me rappelle Bitsy. Au fil du temps, ma grand-mère et elle s'étaient retrouvées plus d'une fois sur des fronts opposés concernant plusieurs affaires de la ville, souvent avec Pomme d'amour coincée au milieu.

— Qu'est-ce que tu veux dire, exactement ?

C'est peut-être la fatigue, ou alors Bitsy l'a mis en rogne au petit-déjeuner, mais je suis choquée lorsqu'il agite la main en l'air et la laisse retomber contre sa jambe dans un claquement.

— Avery, tu sais bien que Judy Stafford a toujours été trop franche. Ce n'est un secret pour personne. Ne fais pas comme si je suis le premier à le dire, ajoute-t-il en me fixant d'un air calme exaspérant. Elle a plus d'une fois failli ruiner la carrière de ton grand-père... sans parler de celle de ton père.

Outrée, je lui rétorque :

— Elle pensait qu'il fallait dire tout haut ce qui n'allait pas.

— Elle adorait surtout la controverse.

— C'est faux.

Je suis tellement énervée que mon sang palpite dans mon cou mais, surtout, j'éprouve comme un déchirement. Je me sens trahie de ne découvrir que maintenant ce qu'il pense de ma famille mais je me dis surtout : Elliot est enfin là, et nous nous disputons ?

Il tend la main, me frotte doucement le bras avant de me serrer les doigts.

— Hé... Avy, murmure-t-il d'un ton apaisant. Je ne veux pas qu'on se fâche. Je te donne juste mon avis, en toute franchise. Parce que je t'aime et que je veux ce qu'il y a de mieux pour toi.

Nos regards se croisent et c'est comme si je voyais à travers lui jusqu'à son cœur. Il est complètement sincère. Il m'aime vraiment. Et il a le droit de penser ce qu'il veut. Ce qui me gêne, c'est que son avis soit si différent du mien.

— Moi non plus, je ne veux pas qu'on se fâche.

Notre désaccord se termine comme tous les autres – sur l'autel du compromis.

Il porte ma main à ses lèvres et l'embrasse.

— Je t'aime.

Dans ses yeux, je vois toutes ces années, tous ces voyages, toutes ces expériences partagées. Je vois le garçon qui était mon ami et l'homme qu'il est devenu.

— Je sais. Je t'aime aussi.

— J'imagine qu'on devrait parler mariage, soupire-t-il dans une grimace qui me laisse deviner que l'interrogatoire subi au petit-déjeuner n'a pas dû être de la tarte. J'ai promis à ma mère qu'on le ferait.

Il sort son téléphone pour vérifier l'heure, puis nous nous dirigeons vers notre endroit habituel sous le kiosque. Nous nous y asseyons, mais il fait trop chaud pour que nous nous y attardions, et encore moins pour décider quoi que ce soit. Pour finir, nous récupérons discrètement sa voiture pour aller dîner en ville dans notre petit restaurant préféré où nous faisons ce que nous avons toujours fait durant notre enfance, notre adolescence, nos années d'université : discuter longuement de ce que nous voulons et essayer de le séparer de ce que tous les autres attendent de nous.

Même si nous n'avons pas vraiment trouvé de conclusion lorsque Elliot doit filer à l'aéroport, nous avons eu le temps de tout nous raconter, et nous sommes sur la même longueur d'onde, ce qui est le plus important.

Pomme d'amour m'accueille à la porte quand je rentre à la maison. Elle scrute l'allée. D'une façon ou d'une autre, elle a découvert la visite d'Elliot et elle est déçue qu'il ne m'accompagne pas.

— Il est occupé, maman, dis-je pour l'excuser. Il a un avion à prendre.

— J'aurais pu lui faire préparer l'une des chambres d'amis. Il est toujours le bienvenu.

— Il le sait, maman.

Elle marque une pause, un doigt pianotant sur la porte, en fixant l'allée d'un air désespéré. Elle a sans doute rafraîchi tout l'État avec l'air conditionné de la maison lorsqu'elle referme enfin la porte, résignée au fait qu'Elliot ne viendra pas.

— Bitsy a appelé. Elle m'a dit qu'elle avait évoqué l'organisation de votre mariage – ou plutôt votre manque d'organisation – avec Elliot ce matin et qu'il a promis que vous en discuteriez tous les deux. Je me disais juste que, une fois que vous auriez profité d'un dîner en tête à tête, vous viendriez tous les deux à la maison.

— On a discuté de certaines possibilités. Mais nous n'avons encore rien décidé.

Elle se mordille la lèvre, soucieuse.

— Je ne veux pas que tout ce qui se passe en ce moment soit... une distraction pour vos projets. Je ne veux pas que vous vous sentiez obligés de repousser votre avenir.

— Maman, ce n'est pas le cas du tout.

— Vraiment ?

Elle a l'air si déçue et désespérée que j'en ai mal pour elle. Un mariage prochain serait une bonne nouvelle, un événement qui redonnerait foi en l'avenir. Ce serait aussi le genre d'annonce publique qui indiquerait subtilement que le clan Stafford est assez confiant pour continuer à vivre normalement.

Elliot et moi, nous sommes peut-être égoïstes de tenir tout le monde en haleine, comme ça. Est-ce que ça nous tuerait vraiment de fixer une date et un lieu – et peut-être même un jardin plein d'azalées au printemps ? Toute la famille en serait incroyablement heureuse. Et si on est sûr de se marier avec la bonne personne, qu'est-ce que ça peut faire, où et quand cela arrive ?

— Nous nous déciderons bientôt, promis.

Malgré ma réponse rassurante, dans le recoin le plus sombre de mon esprit, j'entends encore ces mots : « Avery, tu sais bien que Judy Stafford a toujours été trop franche. Ce n'est un secret pour personne. » Ce que Elliot ne comprend pas – ou ce qu'il ne veut pas voir, peut-être –, c'est que ma grand-mère et moi, nous nous ressemblons beaucoup.

— Tant mieux, se réjouit Pomme d'amour, et ses rides soucieuses s'apaisent au coin de ses yeux. Mais je ne veux pas te presser.

— Je sais.

Elle pose ses mains fraîches de part et d'autre de mon visage et me fixe d'un air d'adoration.

— Je t'aime, ma Belette.

Ce surnom d'enfant me fait rougir.

— Je t'aime aussi, maman.

— Elliot est un homme chanceux. Je suis certaine qu'il s'en rend compte chaque fois que vous êtes ensemble.

Elle verse une larme, ce qui me fait pleurer un peu aussi. Ça fait du bien de la voir si... heureuse.

— Bon. Tu ferais mieux d'aller te changer ou nous serons en retard pour la récolte de fonds de la chorale de ce soir. Le concert commencera à sept heures avec un chœur d'enfants venus d'Afrique. Il paraît qu'ils sont fabuleux.

— Compris, maman.

Je me promets de reparler du mariage à Elliot dès qu'il reviendra de L.A. Le fait que, demain, j'aie prévu d'aller voir mamie Judy à Magnolia Manor renforce un peu plus ma détermination. Je veux que ma grand-mère soit là pour profiter de la cérémonie. Depuis mon enfance, j'ai imaginé ce jour avec elle près de moi. Et nous ne savons pas combien de temps il nous reste.

Je rumine quelques idées pendant la soirée. J'essaie de former une image mentale d'un mariage dans un jardin. Elliot et moi, des centaines d'amis et de connaissances, une parfaite journée de printemps. Ça pourrait être vraiment charmant, une version moderne d'une vieille tradition. Mamie Judy et mon grand-père se sont mariés dans les jardins de Drayden Hill.

Elliot serait d'accord, peu importe qu'il résiste d'instinct à l'idée que sa mère ou la mienne régisse nos vies. Si j'ai vraiment envie de me marier dans un jardin, il le voudra aussi.

Le lendemain matin, je file jusqu'à Magnolia Manor avec un nouveau programme en tête. Je vais demander à mamie Judy des détails de son propre mariage. Elle se souvient peut-être de quelques moments favoris que nous pourrions recréer.

Comme si elle sentait que, cette fois-ci, je suis venue pour une raison importante, elle m'accueille avec un sourire radieux et un regard qui semble indiquer qu'elle me reconnaît.

— Oh, te voilà ! Assieds-toi là, près de moi. J'ai quelque chose à te dire.

Elle essaie de tirer l'autre fauteuil à oreilles près d'elle, sans succès. Je l'avance un peu, puis je m'assieds au bord pour que nos genoux se touchent.

Elle m'agrippe la main et me fixe si intensément que je suis clouée sur place.

— Je veux que tu détruises tout ce qu'il y a dans le placard de mon bureau. Celui de la maison de Lagniappe Street.

Son regard se rive au mien lorsqu'elle ajoute :

— J'imagine que je ne sortirai jamais d'ici pour m'en charger moi-même. Et je ne voudrais pas qu'on lise mes carnets quand je ne serai plus là.

Je me prépare pour supporter l'inévitable montée de chagrin.

— Ne dis pas ça, mamie. Je t'ai vue en salle de kinésithérapie, l'autre jour. L'instructeur a dit que tu t'en sortais très bien.

Je fais comme si je n'avais rien entendu sur ses carnets. Je ne supporte pas cette idée. Ce serait comme dire adieu à la guerrière hyperactive qu'elle était.

— Il y a des noms et des numéros de téléphone, là-dedans. Je ne peux pas les laisser tomber dans de mauvaises mains. Allume un feu dans le jardin et jette-les dedans.

Là, je me demande si son esprit n'a pas pris la clef des champs. Pourtant, elle semble lucide. Allumer un feu dans le jardin... au milieu de la ville, dans une rue cossue bordée de maisons anciennes soigneusement préservées ? Les voisins appelleraient la police illico.

J'imagine déjà les gros titres dans les journaux.

— Ils penseront que tu fais brûler des feuilles, ajoute-t-elle en me glissant un clin d'œil de conspiratrice. Ne t'en fais pas, Beth.

Là, je me rends vraiment compte que nous ne sommes pas dans la même réalité. J'ignore qui est Beth. Je suis presque soulagée que ma grand-mère ne sache pas à qui elle parle. Voilà une excuse parfaite pour ne pas obéir à son désir de nettoyage de placard.

— Je vais voir ce que je peux faire, mamie, dis-je.

— Merveilleux. Tu as toujours été bonne avec moi.

— C'est parce que je t'aime.

— Je sais. N'ouvre pas les boîtes. Contente-toi de les brûler.

— Les boîtes ?

— Celles qui contiennent mes vieux articles sur les potins mondains. Ce ne serait pas très convenable qu'on se souvienne de moi en tant que Miss Térieuse, tu sais.

Elle a beau se couvrir la bouche, feindre d'être embarrassée par son passé de chroniqueuse mondaine, je sais qu'il n'en est rien. À voir son expression, c'est évident. J'agite le doigt devant elle en protestant :

— Tu ne m'avais jamais dit que tu écrivais de genre de chroniques.

— Vraiment ? lance-t-elle en feignant l'innocence. C'était il y a si longtemps...

— Tu ne racontais rien qui ne soit pas vrai, dans tes articles, j'espère ? dis-je pour la taquiner.

— Bien sûr que non. Mais les gens n'apprécient pas toujours qu'on dise la vérité, n'est-ce pas ?

Miss Térieuse disparaît de la conversation aussi vite qu'elle y était apparue. Ma grand-mère me parle de gens morts depuis des années alors que, dans son esprit, elle a déjeuné avec eux hier.

Je l'interroge sur son mariage. En réponse, elle m'offre un méli-mélo de souvenirs issus de ses propres noces et de celles auxquelles elle a assisté au fil du temps, y compris celles de mes sœurs. Mamie Judy adore les mariages.

Elle ne se souviendra même pas du mien.

Après cette conversation, je me sens triste et vidée. Il y a toujours ici et là des étincelles de lucidité pour me redonner espoir, mais les vagues de la démence les emportent rapidement au large.

Et nous sommes vraiment loin de la côte lorsque je l'embrasse pour lui dire au revoir, en la prévenant que mon père passera la voir dans la journée, avec un peu de chance.

— Oh, et qui est donc ton père ? demande-t-elle.

— Wells, ton fils.

— Je crois que tu dois faire erreur. Je n'ai pas de fils.

Alors que je sors du bâtiment, je sens que j'ai désespérément besoin de parler à quelqu'un pour me décharger de tout ça. Je prends mon téléphone, consulte ma liste de contacts préférés et arrête mon doigt sur le numéro d'Elliot. Après la façon dont il a critiqué ma grand-mère hier, j'ai l'impression que ce serait presque déloyal de lui dire à quel point elle perd la tête.

Ce n'est que lorsque mon téléphone sonne et qu'un nom s'affiche sur l'écran que je comprends qu'il y a bien quelqu'un à qui je pourrais en parler. Je repense à son expression, lorsqu'il évoquait les promesses faites à son grand-père sur son lit de mort, les promesses qui ont protégé les secrets de May Crandall et de ma grand-mère et, d'instinct, je sais qu'il me comprendra.

Une part de moi-même se retrouve aussitôt à Edisto, même si nous ne nous sommes pas reparlé depuis notre au revoir à la maison de retraite quelques semaines plus tôt. Je m'étais dit que je ne reprendrais pas contact avec lui, qu'il valait mieux tourner la page.

Dès que je réponds, j'ai l'impression, au ton de sa voix, qu'il ne sait pas trop pourquoi il a appelé. Je me demande s'il s'est dit la même chose que moi : qu'il n'y a pas de place pour une amitié entre nous. L'arrivée de Leslie sur le parking l'avait démontré.

— Je me disais juste... finit-il par balbutier. En fait, j'ai vu quelques articles dans la presse sur l'affaire de la maison de retraite. Je pensais à toi.

Une douce sensation m'envahit. Et me prend complètement au dépourvu. Je ne dois pas le laisser paraître dans ma voix.

— Oooh, ne m'en parle pas. Si ça continue, je vais me défouler sur quelqu'un, façon Tortues Ninjas.

— J'ai du mal à te croire.

— T'as raison, j'imagine. Pourtant, j'aimerais bien. C'est tellement... exaspérant. Je sais que mon père est un personnage public important, mais nous sommes encore des êtres humains, tu vois ce que je veux dire ? Je pensais que certains sujets resteraient hors champ... comme le cancer, par exemple. Ou la démence d'une grand-mère qui lutte pour se rappeler qui elle est. J'ai l'impression que, ces derniers temps, les gens sont prêts à appuyer là où ça fait le plus mal. Ce n'était pas comme ça, quand j'étais petite. Même en politique, les gens avaient...

Je cherche mes mots et, le mieux que je trouve, c'est :

— ... un peu de décence.

— Nous vivons dans une société du spectacle, répond Trent d'un ton sobre. Tout est permis.

Je m'apprête à râler de plus belle sur les attaques visant ma famille avant de me raviser.

— Désolée, dis-je. Je n'avais pas l'intention de te barber avec ça. J'ai peut-être besoin d'un autre séjour à la mer.

Je comprends un peu tard à quel point mes paroles peuvent paraître aguicheuses.

— Que dirais-tu d'un déjeuner, à la place ?

— Pardon ?

— Comme je suis à Aiken, je me demandais si tu étais libre à midi. J'ai fait quelques recherches dans les papiers de mon grand-père et j'ai discuté avec des gens qui l'aidaient. L'un d'eux travaillait au tribunal du comté de Shelby, dans le Tennessee, lorsque les registres d'adoption étaient encore scellés. De ce que j'ai pu voir, il a fourni plein d'informations à mon grand-père.

Je me retrouve aussitôt dans le petit cabanon d'Edisto. Je sens l'odeur du tabac, je revois les vieilles coupures de journaux, les panneaux d'affichage en liège tout secs, la peinture qui s'écaille, les photos passées.

— Des informations pour que ton grand-père puisse aider des adoptés à retrouver des membres de leur famille ? Alors... tu reprends le flambeau ?

— Pas vraiment. J'ai juste un peu farfouillé ici et là, pour May Crandall. En me disant que je découvrirais peut-être quelque chose sur le petit frère qu'elle n'a jamais retrouvé, Gabion.

J'en reste un instant sans voix. Ce type est profondément intègre. Il est aussi plus altruiste que moi. J'ai été tellement accaparée par mes problèmes familiaux que j'ai toujours repoussé mon coup de fil au service juridique de l'Association de défense des droits des seniors pour améliorer la situation de May. Je comprends maintenant que c'était délibéré. J'ai eu peur de m'impliquer à cause de la controverse autour de l'article : « La vieillesse à deux vitesses ». Si l'on apprend que je l'ai aidée, nos adversaires politiques pourraient m'accuser de l'instrumentaliser pour redorer notre image abîmée.

Je ne peux pas non plus risquer qu'on me voie déjeuner avec Trent. Pourtant, je n'arrive pas à me résoudre à le lui dire, si bien que je continue à tourner autour du pot.

— C'est vraiment gentil de ta part. Qu'est-ce que tu as trouvé ?

— Rien de significatif, jusqu'à maintenant. Il y a une adresse en Californie sur les papiers du tribunal. Je leur ai écrit pour savoir s'ils avaient des informations concernant un garçon de deux ans adopté par l'intermédiaire de la Société des foyers d'accueil du Tennessee en 1939... ou au moins pour savoir qui vivait à cette adresse à la fin des années trente. Mais j'ai peu d'espoir.

— Et tu es venu jusqu'ici pour l'annoncer à May ?

— Non... je ne voudrais pas lui faire une fausse joie, j'attendrai de voir si ça donne quelque chose. En fait, je suis venu chercher de la confiture. Quand on s'est vus la dernière fois, je suis passé voir ma tante, à la sortie d'Aiken. Elle préparait de la gelée de mûres. Les pots sont prêts, maintenant.

— Deux heures et demie de route pour ça, ça fait beaucoup, ris-je.

— Toi, tu n'as jamais goûté la confiture de ma tante. En plus, Jonah adore aller là-bas. Mon oncle Bobby a toujours un âne.

— Jonah est avec toi ?

Ce déjeuner me semble soudain envisageable si nous sommes tous les trois. Même si quelqu'un nous surprenait, personne ne penserait à mal si Jonah est là. Je passe en revue la ribambelle de choses prévues pour l'après-midi en essayant de calculer si je peux décaler quelques trucs pour pouvoir m'échapper suffisamment longtemps.

— Tu sais quoi ? J'adorerais déjeuner avec vous deux.

— Je pense que j'arriverai à arracher Jonah à oncle Bobby et sa mule. Dis-moi quand et où. Tu as des préférences ? Nous sommes assez flexibles... sauf à l'heure de la sieste. Ça pourrait être sanglant.

Sa remarque me fait glousser de nouveau.

— Il dort à quelle heure ?

— Vers deux heures.

— Très bien. Et si on se retrouvait de bonne heure ? Onze heures, peut-être ? Ou c'est trop tôt ?

Je ne sais pas du tout si la maison de sa tante est très loin de la ville mais, s'il y a une mule, c'est forcément loin de là où je me trouve. Il n'y a plus de fermes autour de Magnolia Manor depuis des années. Dans le quartier, ce sont plutôt des jardins impeccables.

— Tu choisis le restaurant et je vous y rejoindrai. Rien de trop chic, d'accord ? Et quelque chose d'un peu excentré, ce serait parfait.

Mes critères font rire Trent.

— On ne fait pas dans le chic. Plutôt dans le genre fast-food avec aire de jeux. Tu n'en connaîtrais pas un, par hasard ?

Mon esprit fait un bond dans le temps, vers un souvenir cher à mon cœur.

— En fait, si. Il y en a un avec un terrain de jeux pas loin de la maison de ma grand-mère. Elle nous y emmenait quand on était gosses.

Je lui indique le chemin et tout est réglé. L'avantage, c'est que, si on se retrouve à onze heures, personne ne remarquera mon absence à la maison.

Je suis une femme adulte, me dis-je en faisant demi-tour pour me diriger vers le quartier de ma grand-mère. Je ne devrais pas me sentir comme une adolescente filant en douce, tout ça parce que je prévois d'aller déjeuner avec un... un ami.

J'ai quand même le droit d'avoir une vie privée, non ?

Je me perds dans mon débat mental pendant un moment, mes pensées changeant de direction comme ma propre voiture. J'ai peut-être été trop gâtée, dans le Maryland, à vivre dans mon petit monde anonyme, à un poste qui était à moi et rien qu'à moi, sans dépendre d'employés, de bureaux à Washington liés à un État particulier, d'électeurs, de donateurs et d'un réseau politique tout entier.

Je n'avais peut-être jamais réalisé à quel point être une Stafford est épuisant, surtout ici, dans notre berceau électoral. L'identité collective est si envahissante qu'elle ne laisse pas de place pour une identité individuelle.

Jadis, j'aimais ça... pas vrai ? J'appréciais les petits avantages qui en découlaient. Chaque voie que j'empruntais était aussitôt défrichée pour moi.

Mais, maintenant, j'ai goûté au plaisir d'escalader mes propres sommets, à ma façon.

Est-ce que cette vie ne me convient plus ?

Cette idée me tranche en deux, laissant une moitié de mon identité de chaque côté. Suis-je la fille de mon père ou juste moi ? Dois-je sacrifier l'une pour être l'autre ?

Ce n'est sans doute qu'une... une réaction aux derniers jours hyperstressants.

Je m'arrête à un stop et je regarde la rue de mamie Judy, par-delà le creux dans la route où, enfants, nous sautions dans les flaques lorsqu'il pleuvait, par-delà la haie bien taillée et la boîte aux lettres surmontée d'une tête de cheval.

Il y a un taxi stationné dans l'allée de ma grand-mère. Dans une ville de la taille d'Aiken, un taxi dans une allée privée, ce n'est pas commun.

J'hésite à l'intersection et je fixe le taxi un moment. Il ne bouge pas. Le chauffeur ne sait peut-être pas que la maison est inoccupée, maintenant ? Il a dû s'arrêter à la mauvaise adresse.

Je m'engage dans l'allée à mon tour en m'attendant à ce qu'il s'en aille mais il ne bouge pas. En fait, on dirait qu'il... sommeille sur le siège conducteur ? Il ne remue pas quand je le dépasse et me gare devant lui.

Même s'il est assez âgé pour avoir une licence de chauffeur de taxi, il semble jeune, presque adolescent. Il n'y a pas de passager à l'arrière et personne autour de la maison, pour ce que j'en vois. J'en viens presque à croire que c'est lié à l'horrible article, un journaliste venu prendre des photos en douce pour montrer comment vivent les riches... Mais pourquoi se déplacerait-il en taxi ?

Le chauffeur fait un bond lorsque je tapote sur la vitre à moitié ouverte. Bouche bée, il cligne des yeux pour s'éclaircir la vision.

— Hum... je crois que je me suis endormi, admet-il. Désolé, m'dame.

— Je pense que vous vous trompez d'endroit.

Il regarde autour de lui en réprimant un bâillement tandis que ses cils sombres papillonnent dans le soleil de cette fin de matinée.

— Non, m'dame. La réservation est pour dix heures trente.

Je vérifie l'heure à ma montre.

— Vous attendez là depuis presque une demi-heure... dans l'allée ?

Qui aurait pu envoyer un taxi attendre dans l'allée de ma grand-mère ?

— On a dû vous donner la mauvaise adresse.

J'imagine un pauvre client faisant les cent pas devant chez lui.

Le chauffeur ne semble pas du tout inquiet. Il se redresse dans son fauteuil et jette un coup d'œil vers l'ordinateur de bord.

— Non, m'dame. C'est un abonnement. Tous les mardis à dix heures trente. Prépayé, du coup, mon père... enfin, je veux dire mon patron me dit de venir attendre ici, puisque c'est déjà payé.

— Tous les mardis ?

Je feuillette mentalement l'emploi du temps de ma grand-mère lorsqu'elle vivait encore ici avec une aide à plein-temps. Le jour où on l'a retrouvée perdue et désorientée dans un centre commercial, elle était dans un taxi.

— Depuis combien de temps ça dure – ces réservations du mardi ?

— Euh... je devrais peut-être... appeler le bureau, vous pourriez parler à...

— Non, c'est bon.

J'ai peur que le patron ne réponde pas à mes questions. Le gamin derrière le volant, lui, n'a pas l'air très méfiant.

— Quand vous veniez chercher ma grand-mère le mardi, vous l'emmeniez où ?

— Jusqu'à Augusta, devant une propriété au bord de l'eau. Je l'y ai conduite quelques fois, mais mon père et mon grand-père l'ont fait pendant... des années. Nous sommes une entreprise familiale. Depuis quatre générations.

Sa dernière phrase m'émeut presque, on dirait qu'il l'a lue directement sur leur plaquette commerciale.

— Des années ?

Je suis tellement déroutée que ce mot n'est même plus approprié pour décrire mon état. Rien dans les carnets de ma grand-mère n'indique un abonnement hebdomadaire pour un taxi le mardi. Elle n'avait pas de rendez-vous hebdomadaires, à part ses réunions du club de bridge et ses visites chez le coiffeur. À Augusta, en plus ? C'est à trente minutes de route. Qui pouvait-elle bien aller voir si régulièrement à Augusta ? Et en taxi ? Pendant des années ?

— Et elle allait tout le temps au même endroit ?

— Oui, m'dame. Autant que je le sache.

Il a l'air très mal à l'aise, maintenant. D'un côté, il se rend compte que je lui fais subir un interrogatoire. De l'autre, il ne veut pas perdre ce qui est manifestement une manne financière. Je n'imagine même pas le prix du trajet jusqu'à Augusta.

Ma main se pose sur le bord de la vitre. C'est peut-être idiot, mais je veux m'assurer qu'il ne quitte pas les lieux du crime pendant que je trie toutes ces informations. « Une propriété au bord de l'eau... »

Tout à coup, une idée surgit dans mon esprit.

— Au bord de l'eau... vous voulez dire au bord du fleuve ?

Le fleuve Savannah traverse Augusta. Quand Trent et moi avions discuté avec May, elle avait évoqué cette ville. Elle nous disait vouloir rentrer chez elle et dériver sur le Savannah.

— Euh, c'est possible que ça donne sur le fleuve. Le portail est tout... envahi par la végétation, vous voyez ? Je la dépose devant et j'attends. Je ne sais pas ce qui se passe une fois qu'elle y entre.

— Elle reste combien de temps ?

— Quelques heures. Mon vieux avait l'habitude de descendre jusqu'au pont pour pêcher pendant qu'il l'attendait. Ça ne la dérangeait pas. Quand elle était prête à repartir, elle le prévenait en appuyant sur le klaxon du taxi.

Je le fixe, abasourdie. Je n'arrive même pas à associer tout ça avec la grand-mère que je connaissais. La grand-mère que je pensais connaître.

Est-ce qu'elle allait là-bas pour écrire l'histoire de May Crandall, finalement ? Ou bien y a-t-il autre chose ?

Je lance soudain :

— Vous pourriez m'y emmener ?

Le chauffeur hausse les épaules. Il descend de voiture pour m'ouvrir la portière à l'arrière.

— Bien sûr. La course est payée.

Mon cœur s'emballe. J'ai la chair de poule. Si je monte dans cette voiture, où vais-je atterrir ?

Mon téléphone vibre, ce qui me rappelle que j'allais quelque part avant ce détour. C'est un texto de Trent m'annonçant que Jonah et lui nous gardent une table. Le fast-food est déjà plein, ce matin.

Au lieu de lui répondre par messagerie, je m'éloigne du taxi pour l'appeler. Je m'excuse de ne pas être au rendez-vous et je lui demande :

— Est-ce que tu peux... est-ce que tu veux bien m'accompagner quelque part ?

Dite à haute voix, l'explication de la situation semble encore plus bizarre.

Heureusement, Trent n'en conclut pas que j'ai perdu la tête. En fait, il est intrigué. Nous décidons que le taxi fera un détour par le restaurant pour que Trent et Jonah puissent le suivre dans leur propre voiture.

— En attendant, je te prends un burger, suggère Trent. Ils ont des milk-shakes réputés dans le monde entier, ici. Jonah a déjà confirmé. Tu en veux un ?

— Merci, c'est tentant.

Mais je ne suis pas certaine que je pourrai manger quoi que ce soit.

Durant le court trajet jusqu'au fast-food, j'arrive à peine à me concentrer, je suis sur les nerfs. Trent attend sur le parking avec Jonah déjà ceinturé à l'arrière. Il me tend un sac et un milk-shake, puis me dit qu'il sera juste derrière moi.

— Tout va bien ? s'inquiète-t-il.

Nos regards se croisent un instant et je me perds dans le bleu profond de ses yeux. Je me sens m'y détendre, je me dis : Trent est là. Tout ira bien.

Cette idée m'ôte presque le poids de la terreur que je sens monter en moi. Presque.

Et je comprends suffisamment cette sensation pour savoir que je ne devrais pas l'ignorer. C'est le sixième sens qui se réveille chaque fois que j'apprends quelque chose de pratiquement impensable à propos de gens impliqués dans une affaire en cours – le voisin de confiance était responsable de la disparition de l'enfant ; cette élève de 4ᵉ à l'air si innocente stockait des bombes artisanales ; le père de quatre enfants propre sur lui dont l'ordinateur était rempli de photos dégoûtantes. Cet instinct me prépare pour quelque chose ; mais je ne sais pas quoi.

— Ça va, dis-je. J'ai juste peur de voir où ce taxi va nous emmener... et ce que nous allons y découvrir.

Trent pose une main sur mon bras, et ma peau s'embrase sous ses doigts.

— Tu veux monter avec nous ? On peut suivre le taxi tous les trois.

Il jette un coup d'œil vers sa voiture, où Jonah me fait de grands signes depuis son siège auto pour attirer mon attention. Il voudrait partager ses frites avec moi.

— Non. Merci. Je voudrais encore parler au chauffeur pendant le trajet.

En vérité, je pense qu'il m'a dit tout ce qu'il savait mais je veux l'occuper pour éviter qu'il contacte la compagnie. Son père pourrait voir d'un autre œil le fait que j'utilise l'abonnement de ma grand-mère pour me faire déposer à une destination mystérieuse. Il pourrait être assez futé pour y voir une atteinte à la vie privée.

— Et je ne veux pas risquer qu'il nous sème.

Les doigts de Trent s'attardent un instant sur mon bras quand il me relâche... ou alors c'est juste mon imagination.

— On sera juste derrière toi, d'accord ?

J'acquiesce et je fais coucou à Jonah, qui m'offre un sourire plein de frites, puis nous partons. Il n'y a pas beaucoup de monde sur la route, si bien que le chauffeur peut discuter avec moi au cours des trente-cinq minutes de trajet. Il me dit qu'il s'appelle Oz et que, lorsqu'il emmenait ma grand-mère, elle lui donnait toujours des biscuits, des chocolats ou des bonbons récupérés à la fin de soirées. Pour cette raison, il se souvient très bien d'elle. Il est désolé d'apprendre qu'elle est en maison de retraite. Il n'est visiblement pas au courant de la campagne médiatique. Il est trop occupé à travailler, car il assure la plupart des courses de son père, qui a des problèmes de santé.

— Je m'inquiétais pour elle, la dernière fois que je l'ai amenée ici, admet-il lorsque nous quittons l'autoroute pour emprunter les chemins sinueux ruraux, signe que nous nous rapprochons sans doute de notre destination.

Des murailles de buissons, de lierre et de grands pins se resserrent autour de nous à mesure que nous louvoyons sur le chemin.

— Elle se déplaçait sans mal mais elle avait l'air un peu perdue, poursuit-il. Quand je lui ai demandé si je pouvais l'accompagner jusqu'au portail, elle a refusé. Elle m'a dit qu'il y avait une voiturette de golf qui l'attendait de l'autre côté, comme toujours, et que je ne devais pas m'inquiéter. Alors je l'ai laissée faire. C'était la dernière fois que je l'ai conduite ici.

Je reste silencieuse, à l'arrière de la voiture, en essayant de visualiser ce qu'Oz me raconte. J'ai beau essayer, c'est hors de ma portée.

— La semaine suivante, mon père s'est fait opérer du cœur. On a pris un chauffeur intérimaire pendant plus d'un mois. Le premier mardi après ma reprise, quand je suis venu la prendre, il n'y avait personne. C'est comme ça depuis. L'intérimaire n'a pas su nous dire ce qui s'était passé. La dernière fois qu'il l'avait vue, il l'avait déposée à un centre commercial et elle lui avait dit qu'elle le reverrait le mardi suivant. Nous avons essayé d'appeler le numéro sur sa facture, mais en vain et il n'y avait personne quand je venais. Nous nous demandions s'il lui était arrivé quelque chose. Désolé si nous avons causé des soucis.

— Ce n'est pas votre faute. Ses aides à domicile n'auraient pas dû la laisser partir seule.

S'il est difficile de trouver des gens de confiance, il faut dire aussi que ma grand-mère était douée pour convaincre ses auxiliaires que, elle, elle allait parfaitement bien et que nous, nous cherchions trop à la contrôler. À l'évidence, ils la laissaient partir en taxi tous les mardis. Bon, il ne leur avait sans doute pas échappé que c'était elle qui signait leurs chèques. Et elle était bien capable de renvoyer du personnel qui la contrariait.

La voiture rebondit sur un vieux pont de l'époque du New Deal, au garde-fou en ciment émietté et aux arches couvertes de mousse. Le chauffeur ralentit mais je ne vois aucun signe de maison ou de boîte aux lettres. Selon toute apparence, nous sommes au milieu de nulle part.

Heureuse que Oz sait précisément où il va. N'importe qui d'autre aurait raté l'intersection. Les restes à peine visibles d'une allée gravillonnée dessinent deux sillons irréguliers dans l'herbe, puis passent par-dessus un conduit d'écoulement des eaux de pluie. Juste après, un portail massif en pierre apparaît, niché sous les clématites et les mûriers. De lourdes portes en fer tordues, mesurant peut-être trois mètres de haut, s'appuient sur les branches des arbres environnants, leurs gonds rouillés et disparus depuis longtemps. Reliant les deux vantaux, une chaîne et un cadenas rouillés prêtent presque à rire. Personne n'a traversé ce portail depuis des dizaines d'années. Juste derrière, se dresse un sycomore, et ses bras musculeux passent à travers les barreaux, soulevant lentement un battant plus haut que l'autre.

— L'entrée est par là.

Oz pointe du doigt un chemin étroit menant à un porche de pierre à côté de l'entrée principale. Cette entrée, elle, sert régulièrement. Le sentier qui passe au-dessous est emprunté assez souvent pour que l'herbe de l'été ne l'ait pas complètement envahi.

— C'est par là qu'elle passait toujours.

Derrière nous, une portière claque. Je sursaute et, en jetant un coup d'œil en arrière, je me souviens que Trent est là.

Quand je me tourne de nouveau vers Oz, j'éprouve l'étrange impression que le portail aurait dû disparaître. Pouf ! Je vais me réveiller dans mon lit, à Drayden Hill, en me disant : Quel rêve étrange...

Mais le portail n'a pas disparu et le sentier attend toujours.

22

Rill

Fern se fige en plein milieu du salon. Elle est tellement tendue que je vois le moindre de ses muscles se crisper. Une seconde plus tard, elle mouille sa culotte pour la première fois depuis des semaines.

— Fern ! je lance à voix basse pour ne pas alerter Mme Sevier.

Notre nouvelle mère est si fière de Fern qu'elle nous emmène au cinéma et parle de voyages que nous ferons ensemble, et du Père Noël que nous verrons cet hiver et de ce qu'il nous apportera. Elle s'est même mis dans la tête que nous devrions tous partir en voiture pour Augusta rendre visite à sa mère. Je ne veux pas aller à Augusta, mais je ne veux pas non plus de problèmes maintenant que Mme Sevier commence à nous laisser un peu nous promener hors de sa vue.

Je me précipite vers Fern et lui enlève sa robe, ses chaussures et ses chaussettes, et je m'en sers pour éponger la flaque.

— Va vite à l'étage avant qu'elle te voie.

J'entends Mme Sevier parler à quelqu'un dans le petit bureau.

Les lèvres de Fern tremblotent et ses yeux sont replis de larmes. Elle reste là, immobile, pendant que j'enroule ses vêtements et les fourre derrière le seau à cendres, où je pourrai les récupérer plus tard.

Tout à coup, je comprends pourquoi Fern ne bouge plus. Il y a une autre voix, dans le petit bureau. Plus je m'approche, plus elle me crible d'éclats de glace, qui s'enfoncent jusqu'à mes os. Je pousse Fern vers l'escalier en lui murmurant :

— Va te cacher sous ton lit.

Fern court à l'étage et disparaît. Le souffle court, je me plaque à l'escalier et m'approche doucement de la porte ouverte du petit bureau. Dans la cuisine, Zuma met en route le luxueux mixeur. L'espace d'un instant, je n'entends plus les voix, puis elles reviennent.

— … une situation bien malheureuse, mais cela arrive, déclare Mlle Tann. Ce n'est jamais mon souhait de reprendre des enfants qui ont trouvé un bon foyer.

— Mais mon mari… les papiers… On nous a promis que nous pourrions garder les filles, répond Mme Sevier d'une voix tremblante.

Une tasse de thé tinte contre une soucoupe. Mlle Tann met une éternité à répondre.

— Et ce devrait être le cas, soupire-t-elle comme si elle compatissait à nos malheurs. Mais les adoptions ne sont pas définitives avant un an. Les familles biologiques peuvent être vraiment difficiles. La grand-mère de ces enfants a déposé une demande de garde.

Je laisse échapper un hoquet avant de plaquer ma main sur ma bouche. Nous n'avons même pas de grand-mère. Pour autant que je le sache, du moins. Les parents de Briny sont morts et Queenie n'a pas revu sa famille depuis qu'elle s'est enfuie avec Briny.

— Ce n'est pas…

Mme Sevier pousse un sanglot si violent qu'il manque la briser en deux. Elle renifle, tousse et se force à articuler quelques mots :

— Nous… nous ne pouvons pas laisser… D-Darren sera là… pour le déjeuner. S'il vous plaît… attendez un peu. Il saura ce… ce qu'il faut faire.

— Oh, par tous les cieux, j'ai peur de vous avoir bouleversée plus que nécessaire.

La voix de Mlle Tann est mielleuse, j'imagine son visage. Elle affiche le même sourire que le jour où Mme Pulnik me maintenait au sol, à genoux. Mlle Tann adore voir la peur sur le visage des gens.

— Je ne comptais pas repartir avec les filles aujourd'hui. Vous pouvez vous battre contre cette démarche absurde, évidemment. Vous le devez, même. La grand-mère n'a pas les moyens financiers de s'occuper des filles. Elles auraient une vie terrible. May et la petite Beth dépendent de vous pour leur protection. Cependant, vous devez comprendre que ce... ce travail juridique peut s'avérer... coûteux.

— C-coûteux ?

— Pour des personnes qui ont vos moyens, cela ne devrait pas être un obstacle, n'est-ce pas ? Pas quand le destin de deux enfants innocentes est en jeu. Deux enfants que vous avez appris à aimer tendrement.

— Oui, mais...

— Trois mille dollars, peut-être un peu plus. Cela devrait nous permettre d'envisager une solution à ce problème juridique.

— Trois... trois mille ?

— Peut-être quatre.

— Qu'est-ce que vous dites ?

Une autre pause, puis :

— Rien n'est plus important que votre famille, ne pensez-vous pas ?

J'entends ce sourire terrible dans la voix de Mlle Tann. Je voudrais débouler dans la pièce en hurlant la vérité. Je voudrais la pointer du doigt et crier : « Menteuse ! On n'a même pas de grand-mère ! Et j'avais trois sœurs, pas deux. Et un petit frère, et il s'appelait Gabion, pas Robby. Et vous l'avez emmené loin, comme mes sœurs. »

J'ai envie de tout raconter. Je goûte déjà les mots sur ma langue mais je ne peux pas les dire. Si je le fais, je sais ce qui se passera. Mlle Tann nous ramènera au foyer. Elle donnera Fern à quelqu'un d'autre et nous ne serons plus ensemble.

Mme Sevier renifle et toussote de plus belle.

— Bien... bien sûr, je le pense aussi, mais...

Elle éclate de nouveau en sanglots tout en s'excusant.

Une chaise craque et grince, des pas lourds, irréguliers, traversent la pièce.

— Parlez-en à votre mari. Exprimez vos sentiments les plus sincères sur la question. Dites-lui à quel point vous avez besoin de ces enfants, à quel point elles ont besoin de vous. Inutile que je voie les filles aujourd'hui. Je suis certaine qu'elles sont tout à fait heureuses avec vous. Épanouies, même.

Ses pas se rapprochent de la porte à l'autre bout du petit bureau. Je m'écarte du mur et cours à l'étage. La dernière chose que j'entends, c'est la voix de Mlle Tann qui résonne dans la maison.

— Inutile de vous lever. Je connais le chemin. J'espère avoir de vos nouvelles d'ici demain. Le temps presse.

À l'étage, je me précipite dans la chambre de Fern. Je n'essaie même pas de la tirer de sous son lit, je m'y glisse avec elle. Nous restons allongées, face à face, comme nous le faisions sur l'*Arcadie.*

— Tout va bien, murmuré-je. Je ne la laisserai pas nous reprendre. Je te le promets. Quoi qu'il arrive.

Mme Sevier passe devant notre porte. Ses sanglots se répercutent contre les murs lambrissés et le haut plafond aux corniches dorées. La porte se referme au fond du couloir, et je l'entends se jeter sur son lit et pleurer, pleurer comme elle le faisait quand je suis arrivée dans cette maison. Zuma monte et va frapper à sa porte, mais elle est verrouillée et Mme Sevier refuse de laisser entrer qui que ce soit. Elle est toujours au lit lorsque M. Sevier rentre déjeuner. Entre-temps, j'ai nettoyé Fern, je lui ai lu un livre, et elle dort profondément, son pouce dans la bouche, en serrant l'ours en peluche qu'elle appelle Gabby, comme notre petit frère.

Je tends l'oreille lorsque M. Sevier va ouvrir la porte de leur chambre. J'attends qu'il y entre pour sortir sur la pointe des pieds dans le couloir, histoire de mieux les entendre. Je n'ai pas besoin de m'approcher beaucoup pour comprendre à quel point M. Sevier est furieux après que sa femme lui a raconté ce qui s'est passé.

— C'est du chantage ! hurle-t-il. Du chantage caractérisé !

— On ne peut pas la laisser prendre les filles, Darren, l'implore Mme Sevier. Il faut faire quelque chose.

— Je refuse de laisser cette femme nous manipuler. Nous avons payé les frais d'adoption, qui étaient exorbitants, soit dit en passant, surtout la deuxième fois.

— Darren, je t'en prie.

— Victoria, si nous lui donnons satisfaction, nous n'en verrons jamais la fin.

Un objet en métal tombe au sol en cliquetant.

— Où s'arrêtera-t-elle ? reprend-il. Tu peux me le dire ?

— Je ne sais pas. Je ne sais vraiment pas. Mais nous devons faire quelque chose.

— Oh, je vais faire quelque chose, ne t'en fais pas. Cette femme ne sait pas à qui elle a à faire.

La poignée de la porte cliquette et je me précipite dans ma chambre.

— Darren, s'il te plaît. S'il te plaît, écoute-moi, l'implore sa femme. Nous irons chez ma mère, à Augusta. Dans sa propriété de Bellgrove, il y a largement la place, et cet endroit est trop grand pour elle, maintenant que mon père est parti. Les filles auront des tantes, des oncles et tous mes amis. Nous emmènerons Hoy, Zuma et Hootsie. Nous pourrons y rester aussi longtemps que nécessaire. Pour toujours, s'il le faut. Ma mère se sent seule, et Bellgrove a besoin d'une famille. C'est un endroit merveilleux, où grandir.

— Allons, Victoria, c'est ici chez nous. Les travaux de mon petit studio près du lac ont enfin commencé. Les McCamey ne sont pas les plus rapides des travailleurs, mais ils ont mis en place les piliers et le plancher, et les murs progressent rapidement. Nous ne pouvons pas laisser Georgia Tann nous chasser de notre maison, ma maison familiale, pour l'amour de Dieu !

— Bellgrove possède je ne sais combien d'hectares le long du fleuve Savannah. Nous pourrons faire construire un autre studio. Un plus grand, même. Tout ce que tu veux.

Mme Sevier parle si vite que je comprends à peine ce qu'elle dit.

— Je t'en prie, Darren, je ne peux plus vivre ici en sachant que cette femme pourrait venir toquer à notre porte n'importe quand pour nous prendre nos enfants !

M. Sevier ne répond pas. Je ferme les yeux et plante mes ongles dans mon papier peint rose velouté, attendant, espérant.

— Pas de précipitations, finit-il par dire. J'ai une réunion en ville, ce soir. Je rendrai visite à Mlle Tann pour régler ce problème en face à face, une fois pour toutes. Et là, nous verrons si elle ose maintenir ses menaces.

Mme Sevier ne proteste plus. Je l'entends qui pleure doucement, le lit qui craque, et M. Sevier qui la console.

— Allons, ma chérie. Plus de larmes. Tout va s'arranger et, si tu veux emmener les filles quelques jours à Augusta, nous prendrons les dispositions qu'il faut.

Je reste figée tandis que mon esprit passe une centaine d'idées en revue avant de s'arrêter sur l'une d'elles. Je sais ce que je dois faire. Il n'y a plus de temps à perdre. Je me précipite vers ma commode pour prendre ce dont j'ai besoin et je dévale les marches de l'escalier.

Dans la cuisine, Zuma a préparé le déjeuner ; elle a glissé la tête dans le conduit à linge sale, pour pouvoir entendre la discussion de ses employeurs. Hootsie est sans doute montée à mi-hauteur du conduit pour lui répéter tout ce qu'elle entend. Sur le plan de travail, un petit panier de pique-nique attend qu'on le descende au chantier des McCamey. En temps normal, Zuma force Hootsie à l'y emporter là-bas. Hootsie déteste y aller, et Zuma aussi. Zuma dit que les McCamey ne sont que des vermines blanches et qu'ils voleront M. Sevier à la première occasion. La seule bonne chose, c'est que Zuma et Hootsie nous haïssent moins maintenant, parce qu'elles sont trop occupées à haïr les fils McCamey et leur père.

J'attrape le panier et je sors à toute vitesse en criant :

— J'emporte ça au chantier. Je dois donner quelque chose au garçon, de toute façon.

Je disparais avant que Zuma me dise que je vais être en retard pour le déjeuner.

Je file par la porte arrière, saute les marches de la galerie et traverse le jardin aussi vite que mes jambes me le permettent, tout en regardant par-dessus mon épaule au cas où Hootsie me suivrait. Je suis soulagée de voir que ce n'est pas le cas.

Près du lac, M. McCamey ne se fait pas prier pour s'installer à l'ombre d'un arbre lorsque je lui apporte le panier. J'ai remarqué qu'il est toujours pressé de s'arrêter de travailler. S'il est obligé de mouiller sa chemise aujourd'hui, c'est parce que ses deux fils aînés ont dû aller chez des voisins pour débiter un arbre frappé par la foudre et tombé sur leur grange, avant de réparer le toit. Ils ne reviendront que dans un ou deux jours, quand ils auront fini. La seule aide de M. McCamey, pour l'instant, c'est son benjamin – il s'appelle Arney mais M. McCamey l'appelle toujours « garçon ».

Je lui adresse un signe de tête et Arney me suit dans l'allée jusqu'à un saule pleureur où nous nous sommes déjà retrouvés pour discuter. Je me glisse sous les branches et lui donne un sandwich, une pomme et deux biscuits que j'avais dissimulés dans ma poche. Arney est tout maigre, si bien que, quand je descends au chantier, je lui apporte toujours un peu de nourriture qu'il n'est pas obligé de partager avec les autres. Il en a bien besoin. Alors qu'il a un an de plus que moi, il ne fait même pas ma taille.

— Je t'ai apporté autre chose, aujourd'hui.

Je lui donne le programme du cinéma.

Il regarde la photo d'un cow-boy sur un grand cheval jaune et siffle d'admiration.

— Pour sûr, c'est joli. Dis-moi, c'était quoi l'histoire ? Y avait plein de coups de feu ?

Il s'assied et je l'imite. J'aimerais lui raconter tout le film que M. Sevier nous a emmenées voir, lui décrire le cinéma avec ses grands fauteuils en velours rouge et ses hautes tours qui ressemblent à celles d'un château de princesse. Mais je n'ai pas le temps. Pas aujourd'hui. Pas après ce qui s'est passé. Je dois convaincre Arney d'accepter ce que je lui ai demandé hier.

La lune sera pleine, cette nuit, et, sur l'eau, on y verra presque comme en plein jour. Comme les frères d'Arney sont absents, il n'y aura pas de meilleure occasion. Je ne peux pas laisser Mme Sevier nous traîner jusqu'à Augusta. Je ne peux pas laisser Mlle Tann nous ramener de force au foyer. En plus, Fern commence à prendre Mme Sevier pour sa vraie maman. Peu à peu, son esprit laisse notre vraie maman dériver au loin. Le soir, je me glisse dans la chambre de Fern et je lui parle de Queenie et de Briny, mais ça ne suffit plus. Fern oublie le fleuve et le royaume d'Arcadie. Elle oublie qui nous sommes.

Il est temps pour nous de partir.

Je lui demande :

— Alors, pour ce dont on a parlé hier... tu vas nous emmener, hein ? Ce soir. La lune se lèvera tôt et nous éclairera longtemps.

On ne vit pas toute sa vie sur le fleuve sans savoir comment naviguer grâce à la lune. Le fleuve et les bêtes qui l'habitent choisissent leur humeur en fonction de la lune.

Arney a un mouvement de recul, comme si je lui avais flanqué une gifle. Une touffe de cheveux fins auburn lui tombe sur le front et cache en partie son long nez osseux. Il secoue la tête, nerveux. Il n'a peut-être jamais eu l'intention de nous aider. Ce n'était que de belles paroles, lorsqu'il m'assurait qu'il pouvait manœuvrer le canot à moteur de son père et qu'il savait comment traverser le lac et les marais de Dedmen's Slough jusqu'au fleuve.

Je lui ai pourtant dit la vérité, pour Fern et moi. Toute l'histoire. Je lui ai même révélé nos vrais noms. Je pensais qu'il comprendrait pourquoi nous avons besoin de son aide.

Il pose les coudes sur sa salopette crasseuse, là où ses genoux pointent.

— Vous allez me manquer si vous partez, pour sûr. Toutes les deux, vous êtes les seules gentilles d'ici.

— Tu peux venir avec nous. Le vieux Zede a accueilli plein de garçons. Il t'accueillerait aussi, je parie. J'en suis sûre. Tu n'aurais plus jamais besoin de revenir ici. Tu pourrais être libre. Comme nous.

Le père d'Arney boit tous les soirs et fait travailler ses fils comme des mules, et il les bat tout le temps, surtout Arney. Hootsie a vu Arney se prendre un coup de manche de marteau sur la tempe juste parce qu'il avait apporté des clous de la mauvaise taille à son père.

— Quoi que tu décides, les perles sont pour toi, comme je te l'avais promis.

Je fouille dans ma poche, je les sors et les lui tends au creux de ma main. J'ai des remords, pour les perles. Mme Sevier me les a données le soir après le rendez-vous de Fern pour essayer ses chaussures spéciales. Elle croyait que c'était mon anniversaire, comme le mentionnaient les papiers de la Société des foyers d'accueil du Tennessee. Les Sevier pensaient que je l'avais oublié, et ils m'ont préparé une fête surprise au dîner. Et, pour une surprise, c'en était une belle. Mon anniversaire est passé depuis cinq mois et demi, et j'ai déjà un an de plus que ce qu'ils pensent. Enfin, comme je ne m'appelle pas non plus May Weathers, un anniversaire en automne ne m'embête pas plus que le reste.

Je n'ai jamais rien possédé de plus beau que ces perles, mais je suis prête à y renoncer contre Queenie, Briny et le fleuve. Sans une seconde d'hésitation.

Sans compter qu'Arney a plus besoin que moi de l'argent qu'elles peuvent valoir. La moitié du temps, ils ont du whisky, mais rien à manger, sur leur chantier.

Arney touche les perles, puis retire sa main avant de triturer des peaux sur une griffure barrant ses jointures.

— Arf... j'pourrais pas quitter ma famille. Mes frangins et le reste.

— Réfléchis-y bien. Tu vivrais avec nous sur le fleuve, je te le dis.

En vérité, les frères d'Arney sont quasiment adultes et presque aussi mauvais que leur père. Une fois fatigués d'avoir travaillé comme des chiens, ils largueront les amarres et Arney risque de mourir de faim ou de se faire battre jusqu'à finir brisé en deux.

— Briny et Queenie te trouveront un endroit où vivre, je te le promets. Ils seront tellement contents que tu nous aies ramenées, Fern et moi, qu'ils te trouveront un super endroit. Si Zede n'est plus à Mud Island, tu pourras rester avec nous sur l'*Arcadie* jusqu'à ce qu'on le recroise.

Une pointe de doute me pique le cœur. En vérité, je n'ai aucun moyen d'être sûre que Briny et Queenie sont encore amarrés au même endroit... mais je le sais. Ils attendraient l'éternité s'ils le devaient, même si les nuits se rafraîchissent, que les feuilles commencent à tomber, et que c'est le moment de descendre le fleuve vers le sud pour gagner des territoires plus chauds.

Le plus difficile, ce sera de convaincre Briny et Queenie de partir une fois que Fern et moi serons à bord de l'*Arcadie.*

Est-ce que Silas leur a dit qu'il n'y a plus que Fern et moi, que Camellia n'est plus et que Lark et Gabion ont été emmenés loin ? Est-ce qu'ils le savent ?

J'évite d'y penser, ça fait trop mal. Inutile de crier avant d'avoir mal, voilà ce que disait toujours Briny. Pour l'instant, je dois juste me concentrer sur une chose : traverser les marécages jusqu'au fleuve. De là, nous resterons près de la rive et nous ferons attention aux sillages des bateaux, aux barges... et nous garderons un œil sur les branches à la dérive, les troncs et le reste. Bien des nuits, ici, dans la maison des Sevier, je suis montée au point le plus haut de la maison, dans le belvédère, pour regarder dehors. Je ne vois pas le fleuve, de là-haut, mais je le sens. Je suis certaine d'entendre les cornes de brume et les sifflets, au loin. À l'horizon, je vois les lumières de Memphis. D'après ce que Arny m'a dit, j'imagine que les marécages qui partent de ce lac doivent déboucher sur le Mississippi quelque part entre Chickasaw Bluffs et les bancs de sable en amont de

Mud Island. Même si Arney n'en est pas tout à fait sûr, je ne dois pas me tromper de beaucoup.

Arney acquiesce, c'est un soulagement.

— Marché conclu, dit-il. Je vous emmènerai. Mais ça doit se faire ce soir. Pas moyen d'savoir quand mes frères reviendront.

— Parfait. Fern et moi, on se glissera jusqu'ici dès que la lune sera au-dessus des arbres. On te retrouvera au bateau. Assure-toi que ton père se mette de bonne heure à son whisky. Laisse-le bien manger. Ça lui donnera sommeil. Je m'assurerai que Hootsie vous apporte un repas copieux, ce soir.

Ce ne sera pas difficile. Tout ce que j'ai à faire, c'est de dire à notre « mère » que le garçon du chantier a faim et qu'il n'a pas assez à manger. Elle demandera à Zuma de préparer d'autres choses.

Mme Sevier a le cœur aussi doux que des graines de pissenlit qu'on souffle. Il est tout aussi fragile. Je ne veux pas imaginer son état après notre départ. Je ne peux pas. Queenie et Briny ont besoin de nous, et ce sont eux, nos parents. C'est aussi simple que ça. Il n'y a pas d'autres façons de voir les choses.

Il est temps pour nous de partir.

Arney acquiesce de nouveau.

— D'accord. Je s'rai au bateau mais, si on doit naviguer ensemble sur le fleuve, y a quelque chose que tu dois savoir, d'abord. Ça pourrait bien changer des trucs.

— Et c'est quoi ?

Je ravale un hoquet.

Arney soulève puis abaisse ses épaules osseuses, me décoche un regard en coin avant de lâcher le morceau :

— J'suis pas un gars.

Il défait les boutons de sa chemise, qui est presque en lambeaux. Je vois, dessous, des longueurs de mousseline sale, comme un bandage de docteur, enveloppant son torse – Arney n'est pas un garçon.

— Arney, c'est pour Arnelle, mais mon père veut que personne le sait. Les gens voudront plus me donner de travail s'ils savent.

Je suis plus que jamais certaine que Arney doit venir avec nous au sud, sur le fleuve. En plus du fait qu'il est une fille, et que ce n'est pas une vie pour elle, elle a des bleus partout sur son corps maigre.

Mais est-ce que Zede voudra d'une fille sur son bateau ?

Briny et Queenie nous laisseront peut-être la garder sur l'*Arcadie*. Si je ne sais pas encore comment, je sais que je les convaincrai.

— Peu importe que tu sois une fille, Arney. On te trouvera une place. Tiens-toi prête ce soir dès que la lune sera au-dessus des arbres.

Nous jurons croix de bois croix de fer, puis le père d'Arney l'appelle en beuglant à l'autre bout des arbres. La pause-déjeuner est terminée.

Tout l'après-midi, je me demande si Arney sera bel et bien au bateau quand Fern et moi y arriverons. Je pense que oui parce que, quand elle y réfléchira, elle verra qu'il n'y a pas grand-chose pour la retenir ici. Elle a besoin de s'enfuir sur le fleuve, tout autant que nous.

Les Sevier discutent de nouveau dans leur chambre avant que M. Sevier parte pour sa réunion à Memphis. Lorsqu'ils redescendent du premier, il porte une valisette.

— Si la réunion se prolonge, je resterai peut-être en ville, annonce-t-il avant de déposer un baiser sur la tête de Fern, puis sur la mienne, ce qu'il n'avait jamais fait.

Je serre les dents et je m'efforce de rester immobile lorsqu'il se penche vers moi. Je n'arrive pas à m'ôter M. Riggs de la tête.

— Vous trois, prenez soin de vous, dit-il avant de se tourner vers sa femme. Ne t'inquiète pas. Tout ira bien.

Zuma lui tend son chapeau lorsqu'il sort de la maison, puis nous nous retrouvons entre filles. Mme Sevier dit à Zuma et Hootsie qu'elles peuvent aller se reposer dans leur maison au-dessus de la grange. Inutile de s'embêter avec un dîner. Nous nous contenterons d'un plateau-repas froid.

Zuma nous prépare des mini-sandwichs tout mignons avant de partir.

— Une petite soirée pyjama juste entre nous. *Capitaine Minuit* passe à la radio, ce soir, déclare Mme Sevier. Et nous boirons du chocolat chaud. Ça me calmera peut-être l'estomac.

Elle s'humecte les lèvres et pose la main sur son ventre.

— Je crois que je suis barbouillée aussi, dis-je, pressée de filer à l'étage pour préparer mes affaires. ·

Parmi tous les présents des Sevier, je n'emporterai que le strict nécessaire. Ce ne serait pas correct. De toute façon, nous avons aussi des affaires sur l'*Arcadie*. Pas de jolies choses comme ici, mais tout ce dont nous avons besoin. Qu'est-ce qu'une vagabonde du fleuve ferait de robes à volants et de chaussures en cuir verni ? Les semelles qui claquent effraieraient les poissons.

— Allez faire votre toilette, les filles, et enfilez vos robes de chambre. May, tu te sentiras mieux après un bon chocolat et quelques friandises.

Du dos de la main, Mme Sevier s'essuie le front, puis se force à sourire.

— Allez. Nous allons passer une belle soirée. Entre filles.

Je prends Fern par la main et l'entraîne à l'étage.

Fern est si excitée par notre soirée avec Mme Sevier qu'elle se lave et se change à toute vitesse, au point qu'elle met sa chemise de nuit à l'envers.

Je la remets à l'endroit et lui enfile sa robe de chambre par-dessus, avant de mettre la mienne, mais, moi, je garde mes vêtements en dessous. Si Mme Sevier s'en rend compte, je lui dirai que j'avais un peu froid. Ces derniers temps, il fait frais dans la maison, le soir. Un autre signe qui nous rappelle qu'il est temps de regagner le fleuve avant que l'hiver s'installe.

J'essaie de faire comme si j'étais enchantée par cette soirée radio, alors que je suis aussi nerveuse qu'un chat quand nous mangeons nos petits sandwichs. J'en laisse tomber un sur ma robe de chambre et Mme Sevier essuie la tache à ma place.

Elle me touche le front pour voir si j'ai de la fièvre.

— Comment te sens-tu après avoir mangé un peu ?

Une seule idée m'obsède : je voudrais qu'elle soit Queenie. Je voudrais que Queenie et Briny habitent cette grande maison, et je voudrais que Mme Sevier puisse avoir des bébés les uns après les autres comme Queenie, pour qu'elle ne souffre pas de la solitude après notre départ.

Je secoue la tête en murmurant :

— Je devrais peut-être aller me coucher. Je peux emmener Fern, pour la mettre au lit.

— Ne t'embête pas.

Elle me caresse les cheveux, les prend au bout de ses doigts et les soulève de mon cou, tout comme Queenie le faisait.

— Je la ferai monter quand elle sera prête. Je suis sa maman, après tout.

Je me crispe aussitôt, soudain transie. Je le sens à peine lorsqu'elle m'embrasse sur la joue et me demande si j'ai besoin qu'elle vienne me border.

— Non... mère.

Je sors de la pièce en vitesse sans jeter ne serait-ce qu'un coup d'œil en arrière.

À l'étage, j'ai l'impression d'attendre une éternité avant que Mme Sevier vienne coucher Fern. À travers le mur, je l'entends chanter une berceuse. Je me plaque les mains sur les oreilles.

Queenie et moi, on fredonnait souvent cette comptine aux bébés :

> *Ne dis rien, ne pleure pas,*
> *Endors-toi, petit bébé.*
> *À ton réveil,*
> *Tu auras*
> *Ô merveilles,*
> *Plein de jolis poneys.*

Tout se mélange dans ma tête : l'*Arcadie* et cet endroit. Mes vrais parents et les Sevier. Queenie et mère, Briny et père. Le grand fleuve. Le lac. Le marais. De longues galeries blanches et des plus petites qui filent, filent, filent sur l'eau.

Je fais semblant de dormir lorsque Mme Sevier vient dans ma chambre et me tâte de nouveau le front. J'ai peur qu'elle essaie de me réveiller pour me demander comment je me sens, mais elle s'en va. La porte au bout du couloir se referme et je peux enfin respirer librement.

La lune se lève à peine lorsque j'enfile mon manteau, mes chaussures, m'attache un petit baluchon sur le dos et me glisse dans la chambre de Fern pour la prendre dans mes bras.

— Chhhh... Ne fais pas de bruit. Nous allons marcher jusqu'au fleuve pour essayer de voir des lucioles. Si quelqu'un nous entend, on nous empêchera d'y aller.

J'enroule ma petite sœur dans une couverture et elle se rendort sur mon épaule avant même que j'atteigne l'escalier. Sur la terrasse, il fait très sombre – j'entends des grattements dans les jardins près de la maison, sans doute un raton laveur ou un putois. Les chiens de chasse de M. Sevier se mettent à aboyer quand je m'engage sur la pelouse puis ils se taisent en me reconnaissant. Personne n'allume de lampe au-dessus de la remise. Des gouttes de rosée m'éclaboussent les jambes tandis que je me hâte vers les arbres en serrant Fern contre moi. Au-dessus des branches, la lune brille, haute, pleine, aussi clairement que la lanterne que Briny accrochait à l'*Arcadie* la nuit. La lumière nous permet de voir où nous mettons les pieds, et c'est tout ce qui compte. Nous arrivons très vite sur la berge du lac. Arney nous y attend, comme elle l'avait promis.

Nous murmurons, même si elle m'assure que son père est ivre mort à cause du whisky, comme d'habitude.

— S'il se réveille et qu'il m'appelle, y pourra même pas se relever pour voir où je suis.

Malgré tout, Arney nous fait monter en vitesse dans le bateau. Ses yeux écarquillés dessinent deux grands cercles blancs sur son visage creusé lorsqu'elle jette un coup d'œil par-dessus son épaule vers le chantier.

Elle s'attarde, une main sur le petit bateau à moteur, deux pieds sur la rive. J'ai l'impression qu'elle fixe le camp pendant une heure. Inquiète, je lui lance dans un murmure :

— Monte.

Fern se réveille un peu, dans le fond du bateau ; elle bâille, s'étire et regarde autour d'elle. Si elle comprend ce qui se passe, j'ai peur qu'elle pique une crise.

La main d'Arney se décolle du bateau jusqu'à n'y laisser que le bout de ses doigts.

— Arney.

Est-ce qu'elle envisage de nous laisser partir seules ? J'ignore comment manœuvrer le bateau à moteur et je ne connais pas le chemin à travers le marais. On se perdra dedans et on n'en ressortira jamais.

— Arney, on doit partir.

À travers les branches, je vois des ombres bouger au loin, sur la pelouse, et il me semble que des rayons lumineux dansent sur l'herbe. Ils ont disparu le temps que je me redresse pour mieux voir. Je les ai peut-être imaginés... à moins que M. Sevier ait décidé de rentrer dormir au lieu de rester en ville. Il a peut-être garé sa voiture avant de se diriger vers la maison. Il ira dans nos chambres et verra que nous sommes parties.

Je m'avance cahin-caha dans le bateau pour attraper Arney par le bras – elle sursaute comme si elle avait oublié que j'étais là. Au clair de la lune, son regard accroche le mien.

— Je sais pas si je fais bien, dit-elle. Ma famille, j'la reverrai plus jamais.

— Ils te maltraitent, Arney. Tu dois partir. Tu dois venir avec nous. Ce sera nous, ta famille. Fern, Briny, Queenie, le vieux Zede et moi.

Nous nous fixons longtemps. Elle finit par hocher la tête et pousse le bateau si vite sur le lac que je tombe sur Fern. Nous sortons les rames et pagayons un peu en laissant le vent et le courant nous entraîner vers les marais jusqu'à ce que nous soyons bien loin de la rive.

— Où... où qu'elles sont... les lucioles ? marmonne Fern.

— Chhh. Nous devons d'abord faire tout le chemin jusqu'au fleuve. Tu devrais dormir, en attendant.

Je resserre la couverture autour d'elle, lui enfile ses chaussures sur ses pieds nus pour qu'elle ne prenne pas froid et lui laisse mon baluchon comme oreiller.

— Je te réveillerai quand il sera l'heure de les regarder.

Il n'y aura pas de lucioles mais, lorsqu'elle verra l'*Arcadie*, elle ne sera pas déçue.

Arney démarre le moteur et s'assied près de la barre. Je prends ma rame et me place à l'avant pour guetter les branches flottantes.

— Allume la lampe, me conseille Arney. Il y a des allumettes dans la boîte, là.

Je m'exécute et, à peine quelques minutes plus tard, nous naviguons au milieu du grand lac clair, où les insectes nocturnes détalent à toute vitesse pour s'écarter du halo lumineux de la lanterne. Je me sens aussi libre que les oies sauvages du Canada qui passent au-dessus de nos têtes en cacardant et en éclipsant des grappes d'étoiles. Elles se dirigent dans la même direction que nous. Vers le sud du fleuve. Je les regarde passer en rêvant que je m'accroche à l'une d'elles pour qu'elle me ramène chez moi en volant.

— Il faut bien faire attention, ici, déclare Arney quand le lac s'étrécit et que les arbres se rapprochent des deux côtés. Repousse les branches, si t'en vois. Ne nous laisse pas foncer dessus.

— Je sais.

L'air frais de la nuit s'épaissit de l'odeur du marais. Je boutonne mon manteau. Les arbres recouvrent le ciel, leurs pieds larges surplombant des racines noueuses. Leurs branches se tendent vers nous comme des doigts crochus. Quelque chose griffe la coque et nous fait pencher d'un côté.

— Repousse ça loin de nous, aboie Arney. Si un tronc à la dérive fend la coque, on est foutues.

Je guette les bûches, les branches de cyprès et toutes sortes de bois flotté. Je repousse tout avec la rame, et l'eau défile doucement. Çà et là, des barques sont attachées sur la rive, des cabanes flottent sur des plateformes de bois, où des lanternes scintillent mais, dans l'ensemble, nous sommes seules. Il n'y a rien d'autre que nous et des kilomètres de marais habités par les loutres et les chats sauvages, où la mousse drape lourdement les branches. Les silhouettes des arbres évoquent des monstres dans la nuit.

Un cri de chouette retentit soudain, et Arney et moi nous baissons aussitôt. Nous l'entendons passer juste au-dessus de nos têtes.

Fern s'agite dans son sommeil, dérangée par le bruit.

Je repense aux histoires de Briny sur le vieux rougarou qui emporte les enfants dans les marécages. Même si je frissonne, je ne laisse pas Arney le voir. Ici, il n'y a pas de monstres pires que ceux qui nous attendent chez Mme Murphy.

Quoi qu'il arrive, Fern et moi, nous ne devons pas nous faire prendre.

J'observe la surface de l'eau et j'essaie de ne pas penser à ce qui pourrait se trouver dans ce marigot. Arney tourne le bateau par ici, puis par là pour suivre le canal peu à peu, comme elle me l'avait assuré.

La lune finit par se cacher, et le kérosène s'épuise dans la lanterne. La flamme crachote jusqu'à ce qu'il ne reste plus que la mèche enflammée. La brise la mouche au moment où nous nous rapprochons de la rive pour accrocher l'amarre à une branche. Mes bras et mes jambes sont lourds, comme les bûches imbibées d'eau que j'ai repoussées avec ma rame. Ils me brûlent et craquent lorsque je rampe jusqu'au centre du bateau pour me glisser sous la couverture à côté de Fern, qui a dormi presque tout le temps.

Arney nous rejoint.

— De là, c'est pas loin jusqu'au bout du marécage, dit-elle, et nous nous blottissons là, toutes les trois, transies, mouillées et épuisées.

Au loin, il me semble entendre de la musique, et je me dis que c'est un bateau-théâtre et que ça signifie que le fleuve est tout près, mais c'est peut-être juste mon imagination qui me joue des tours. Tandis que le sommeil m'emporte, je suis certaine d'entendre des bruits de bateaux et de barges au loin. Leurs cornes de brume et leurs sifflets portent dans la nuit. Je tends l'oreille pour essayer de les reconnaître. Le *Benny Slade*, le *General P.*, et un bateau à aubes avec son bruit caractéristique : *pff, clap, clap, clap, pff...*

Je suis chez moi. Enveloppée dans une berceuse que je connais par cœur. Je laisse les bruits de l'obscurité et de la nuit me pénétrer, et il n'y a plus de rêve, plus de souci nulle part. L'eau maternelle me berce doucement, gentiment, jusqu'à ce qu'il n'y ait plus rien autour de moi.

Je dors du sommeil profond d'une fille du fleuve.

Au matin, des voix me tirent de la tranquillité. Des voix... et le bruit du bois tapant du bois. Je repousse la couverture et Arney s'assied soudain de l'autre côté de Fern. On se regarde un instant, le temps de nous souvenir où nous sommes et ce que nous avons fait. Entre nous, Fern se retourne et cligne des yeux en regardant le ciel.

— J't'avais dit qu'y avait quelqu'un dans c'bateau, Remley.

Trois petits enfants noirs nous observent, perchés sur des racines de cyprès, leurs salopettes remontées au-dessus de leurs jambes maigres et boueuses.

— Y a même une fille ! lance le plus grand en tendant le menton pour me regarder de plus près tout en tapotant le bateau du bout de son harpon à grenouilles. Et y en a une petite. Des Blanches !

Les autres reculent, mais le plus grand – qui ne doit pas avoir plus de neuf ou dix ans – reste campé là, appuyé à son harpon.

— Qu'esse vous faites là ? Vous êtes perdues ?

Arney se lève et agite la main vers eux.

— Dégagez ! Vous feriez mieux de filer, sinon gare à vous.

Sa voix est plus grave, comme quand elle me parlait avant que je sache qu'elle était une fille.

— On était venues pêcher. On attend juste le matin pour recommencer. Un de vous pourrait grimper là pour défaire la corde, pour qu'on s'en aille.

Les garçons restent où ils sont et nous fixent, les yeux écarquillés.

— Allez, grouillez-vous ! lance Arney en pointant la rame vers la branche où nous sommes amarrées.

Le courant a fait bouger la barque pendant que nous dormions et la corde s'est entortillée dans les branches. On aura du mal à la défaire nous-mêmes.

Je farfouille dans le baluchon avant de brandir un biscuit. Chez les Sevier, ce n'est jamais difficile de subtiliser des pâtisseries de Zuma. J'en ai pris en douce au cours des derniers jours pour notre voyage. Maintenant, ils vont être utiles.

— Si vous le faites, je vous lancerai un biscuit.

— Où est mère ? demande Fern en se frottant les yeux.

— Chut, lui dis-je. Ne bouge pas. Plus de questions.

Je tiens le biscuit devant les garçons. Le plus petit me fait un grand sourire, lâche son harpon à grenouilles et grimpe sur la branche avec l'agilité d'un lézard. Il se débat un peu avec le nœud mais finit par le défaire. Avant que le courant nous emporte, je lance trois biscuits sur la rive.

— Pas besoin de les gaspiller comme ça, se plaint Arney.

Fern me tend les mains en se léchant les babines.

J'en donne un à ma sœur et le dernier à Arney.

— Nous aurons plein de choses à manger une fois sur l'*Arcadie*. Queenie et Briny vont être tellement contents de nous revoir qu'ils vont préparer un repas si énorme que tu n'en croiras pas tes yeux.

Depuis le début de cette aventure, je n'ai pas arrêté de promettre des choses à Arney, pour la motiver. Je vois bien qu'elle a toujours envie de rejoindre sa famille. C'est drôle comme ce à quoi on est habitué nous semble normal, même si ce n'est pas le cas.

— Tu verras, lui promets-je encore, une fois arrivées sur l'*Arcadie*, on se lancera sur le fleuve, là où personne ne pourra nous chercher d'ennuis. On ira vers le sud et le vieux Zede, il sera juste derrière nous.

Je me le répète, encore et encore et encore, tandis que nous démarrons le petit moteur pour aller nous frayer un passage jusqu'à l'embouchure du marécage, mais c'est comme s'il y avait une ligne hameçonnée en moi, qui me retenait en arrière. La ligne se tend de plus en plus, même lorsque nous tournons, et que les arbres s'ouvrent, et que je vois le fleuve, prêt à me porter chez moi. J'éprouve une inquiétude grandissante, rien à voir avec les sillages des gros bateaux qui nous ballottent de droite et de gauche alors que nous avançons doucement vers Memphis.

Quand Mud Island arrive enfin en vue, cette inquiétude me coupe carrément le souffle, et j'en viens à souhaiter qu'une barge nous fasse chavirer lorsque nous traversons le fleuve vers la lagune. Que diront Briny et Queenie en voyant qu'il ne reste plus que Fern et moi ?

La question me pèse de plus en plus, surtout lorsque nous passons devant le camp des gens du fleuve, qui est presque désert maintenant, et que je guide Arney jusqu'à la lagune où je me suis déjà rendue une centaine de fois en esprit. Je suis venue ici depuis la voiture de Mlle Tann, depuis le sous-sol de Mme Murphy, depuis le divan de la fête de présentation et depuis la chambre tout en dentelle dans la grande maison des Sevier.

J'ai du mal à y croire, même lorsque nous contournons le méandre et que l'*Arcadie* nous attend derrière, pour de vrai. Ce n'est plus un rêve.

Le bateau-maison de Zede est amarré un peu plus bas mais, plus je m'approche, plus je remarque des détails anormaux sur l'*Arcadie*. Le garde-fou est brisé. Des feuilles et des branches tombées se sont amassées sur le toit. Une fenêtre cassée fait miroiter ses crocs acérés au soleil près du tuyau du poêle. L'*Arcadie* penche sur l'eau, sa coque remonte si haut sur la rive que je me demande si on arrivera un jour à la remettre à flot.

— *Arcadie ! Arcadie !* se réjouit Fern en tapant dans ses mains avant de pointer le bateau du doigt, ses boucles dorées comme des rayons de soleil bondissant dans tous les sens.

Elle se dresse en équilibre au milieu de la barque comme seule une petite fille du fleuve peut le faire.

— *Arcadie !* Queenie ! Queenie ! crie-t-elle encore et encore tandis que nous approchons.

On dirait qu'il n'y a personne, dans le coin. Ils sont peut-être partis à la chasse ou à la pêche ce matin ? À moins qu'ils soient chez Zede ?

Mais Queenie sort rarement du bateau. Elle aime rester chez elle, à part si elle peut rendre visite à d'autres femmes, pas loin. Sauf qu'il n'y a personne, dans le coin.

— C'est là ? demande Arney, dubitative.

— Ils ne doivent pas être à la maison, pour le moment.

J'ai beau essayer de paraître sûre de moi, je ne le suis pas du tout. Un pressentiment, noir et épais, m'envahit. Queenie et Briny ne laisseraient jamais le bateau se délabrer comme ça. Briny était toujours fier de l'*Arcadie.* Il en prenait toujours soin. Même avec cinq enfants dans les pattes, Queenie maintenant notre petite maison dans un état impeccable. « Propre comme un sou neuf », comme elle disait.

L'*Arcadie* est loin d'être impeccable, maintenant. Et c'est pire encore lorsque Arney nous approche de la passerelle, puis coupe le moteur pour qu'on finisse en glissant sur l'eau. Quand j'attrape la rampe pour nous rapprocher encore, une partie me reste dans la main et je manque de tomber dans l'eau.

On vient de s'amarrer lorsque je vois Silas courir sur la berge, ses longues jambes cavalant dans le sable. Il saute par-dessus un tas de broussailles, aussi agile qu'un renard et, pendant une fraction de seconde, je revois Camellia essayant de s'échapper le jour où la police est venue.

J'ai l'impression que c'était il y a des années de ça, pas juste quelques mois.

Silas vient à ma rencontre quand je descends du bateau et me prend dans ses bras, me fait tourner et me soulève alors que ses pieds s'enfoncent dans le sable. Puis il me dépose sur le bord de la passerelle.

— Tu m'as vraiment manqué, tu sais ? dit-il. J'étais pas sûr de te revoir un jour.

— J'en étais pas sûre non plus.

Derrière moi, j'entends Arney aider Fern à descendre mais je n'arrive pas détacher mon regard de Silas. En vérité, lui aussi, il m'a vraiment manqué.

— Nous sommes rentrées à la maison. Nous avons réussi.

— Oui. Tu as réussi à ramener Fern. J'ai hâte de voir la tête de Zede !

Il me serre de nouveau et, cette fois, mes bras ne sont pas coincés par les siens. Je le serre aussi contre moi.

Ce n'est que lorsque Fern m'interroge que je me souviens que nous ne sommes pas seuls.

— Elle est où, Queenie ? demande-t-elle.

Au moment où je lâche Silas, où je recule d'un pas pour le regarder, je comprends que quelque chose ne va pas. Personne ne sort de la cabine, malgré tout le boucan que nous avons fait.

— Silas, où est Queenie ? Et Briny ?

Silas m'agrippe par les épaules. Ses yeux noirs se plantent dans les miens. Les commissures de ses lèvres tremblotent un peu.

— Votre maman, elle est morte y a trois semaines, Rill. Le docteur a dit que c'était un empoisonnement du sang, mais Zede m'a raconté qu'elle avait juste le cœur brisé. Vous lui manquiez trop.

Cette nouvelle m'éventre comme un poisson. Je me sens vidée. Ma maman n'est plus de ce monde ? Plus de ce monde, et je ne la reverrai jamais ?

— Où... où est Briny ?

Silas me tient un peu plus fort. Je vois bien qu'il a peur que, s'il me lâche, je m'effondre comme une poupée de chiffon. Et, l'espace d'un instant, je n'en suis pas loin.

— Il va plus bien depuis longtemps, Rill. Il s'est mis à boire, après vous avoir perdus, tous. C'est encore pire depuis que Queenie est morte. Cent fois pire.

23

Avery

Côte à côte, Trent et moi regardons les vieilles colonnes qui longent une dalle de pierre et de béton délabrée. Elles se dressent telles des sentinelles, de stature militaire, leurs bases perdues dans le lierre et l'herbe grasse, leurs chapiteaux ornés d'arabesques et de chérubins au teint verdi par la mousse.

Il nous faut quelques secondes pour nous rendre compte que Jonah a monté les marches pour explorer ce qui devait être jadis une galerie à étages. Les arabesques du garde-corps rouillé du premier étage s'étirent entre les colonnes, bien haut au-dessus de nos têtes, tels des galons décolorés.

— Hé, reviens là, jeune homme ! lance Trent à son fils.

Les marches ont l'air solides mais il n'y a aucun moyen de savoir si la dalle est encore stable.

Une maison coloniale se tenait là jadis, dressée sur une petite colline le long du fleuve Savannah, non loin d'Augusta. À qui appartenait-elle ? Tout près, une glacière et d'autres dépendances sont dans un même état de ruines, leurs toits de tuiles bordeaux tombant peu à peu en morceaux, d'où des poutres cassées pointent comme des os brisés.

— Qu'est-ce que ma grand-mère pouvait bien venir faire ici ?

Je n'arrive pas à imaginer mamie Judy – la femme qui râlait quand je revenais de l'écurie avec des poils de cheval sur mon pantalon et que j'avais le malheur de m'asseoir sur le canapé – dans un endroit pareil.

Tous les mardis, en plus ? Pendant des années ?

— Une chose est certaine, personne ne serait venue l'embêter, ici. Je doute que qui que ce soit connaisse l'existence de
cet endroit.

Trent s'approche des marches et attrape la main de Jonah,
qui redescend d'un pas joyeux.

— Reste à côté de papa, lapin. Je sais que ça a l'air génial,
mais il y a peut-être des serpents.

Jonah se dresse sur la pointe des pieds pour voir par-dessus
la dalle.

— Il est où, le serpent ?

— J'ai dit peut-être.

— Oh...

Je suis distraite un instant par eux deux. On dirait une photo
de magazine, la lumière vive du soleil à son zénith cascade à
travers les vieux arbres et se déverse sur eux, éclairant leurs
cheveux blonds et leurs traits similaires.

Je finis par me tourner vers les ruines de la maison. Elle
devait être imposante, en son temps.

— Eh bien, comme elle prenait un taxi plutôt que sa propre
voiture avec chauffeur pour venir ici, on peut effectivement en
déduire qu'elle ne voulait pas qu'on sache où elle allait.

Je voudrais que la vérité soit si simple, mais je ne suis pas
dupe. May nous avait parlé d'Augusta – ça ne peut pas être
une coïncidence, alors que ma grand-mère revenait ici sans
cesse. Elles sont mêlées à tout ça, toutes les deux. Nous sommes
chez May, je le sais. Ses liens avec ma grand-mère sont bien
plus profonds qu'une simple relation de travail autour d'une
histoire lointaine et tragique d'adoption.

— On dirait que le chemin continue par là.

Trent m'indique le sentier que nous avons emprunté depuis
le portail. Avec l'herbe qui a poussé au milieu et les épis des graminées qui ploient au-dessus de vieilles empreintes de pneus,
on peut à peine appeler ça une route, mais elle a visiblement
été empruntée et entretenue depuis l'été dernier. Quelqu'un
s'occupait de cet endroit jusqu'à récemment.

— Oui. Autant voir où il mène.

Pourtant, une part de moi – presque moi tout entière, en fait – a peur de le découvrir.

Nous nous engageons sur la route qui traverse ce qui devait être une pelouse. Jonah lève ses jambes autant que possible à chaque pas, pataugeant dans l'herbe haute comme si c'était des vagues sur la côte. Trent le balance en l'air avant de le prendre dans ses bras lorsque l'herbe devient trop haute et que le chemin nous entraîne sous les arbres.

Jonah pointe du doigt des oiseaux, des écureuils, des fleurs, ce qui donne un air innocent à notre expédition – une petite balade dans la campagne entre amis. Il veut que nous commentions – son père et moi – la moindre de ses trouvailles. Je fais de mon mieux, mais mon esprit file vers le pied de la colline. À travers les arbres, j'aperçois un large cours d'eau. Il scintille au soleil, ridé par le vent. Le fleuve, sans doute.

Jonah m'appelle Avry. Son père le corrige en lui disant :

— C'est Mlle Stafford. Ma famille est plutôt vieux jeu, me lance Trent avec un sourire en coin. On n'appelle pas les adultes par leurs prénoms.

— C'est mignon.

J'ai été élevée comme ça, moi aussi. Pomme d'amour m'aurait consignée dans ma chambre si j'avais oublié de donner du « monsieur » ou « madame ». La règle est restée valable jusqu'à ma sortie de l'université, lorsque je suis moi-même officiellement devenue une adulte.

Devant nous, le chemin contourne ce qui ressemble aux restes d'une clôture rouillée. Elle est tellement envahie par les clématites que je ne me rends pas compte qu'elle délimite un jardin jusqu'à ce que nous nous retrouvions presque en plein milieu. Une petite maison proprette est nichée parmi des rosiers grimpants rouges et des myrtes blanc immaculé. Située sur une petite butte dominant le fleuve, on dirait un cottage enchanté dans un conte de fées – le genre de repaire secret qui pourrait abriter une princesse en fuite ou un vieil ermite plein de sagesse qui était jadis un roi. Depuis le portail à l'avant du jardin, un chemin en caillebotis descend jusqu'à une jetée sur le fleuve.

Même si les jardins autour de la maison sont envahis par les mauvaises herbes, on voit encore qu'ils étaient naguère entretenus avec amour. Des tonnelles, des bancs, des bassins à oiseaux bordent des sentiers méticuleusement pavés. Le petit cottage se dresse sur de courts pilotis, parés à affronter une éventuelle crue. À en juger par les cadres de fenêtres en bois érodés et le toit en zinc, je dirais qu'elle a quelques dizaines d'années.

C'était donc là, la destination de ma grand-mère. Il n'est pas difficile d'imaginer qu'elle aimait venir ici. Un endroit où elle pouvait oublier ses obligations, ses soucis, ses devoirs, la réputation de la famille, l'opinion publique – tout ce que contenaient ses carnets de rendez-vous si soigneusement remplis.

— On ne se douterait pas qu'il y a une maison par ici, déclare Trent en admirant la cachette tandis que nous la contournons jusqu'à la façade, où une grande galerie fermée par des moustiquaires pointe entre les arbres.

Des rideaux de dentelle bordent les fenêtres. Un carillon chantonne dans l'air doux et délicat de midi. Des brindilles et des feuilles sur les marches confirment que personne n'est venu passer un coup de balai depuis au moins les derniers orages.

— C'est vrai.

Est-ce vraiment la maison de May Crandall, l'endroit où elle a été découverte avec le cadavre de sa sœur ?

Trent nous ouvre le portail tordu. Le battant racle le chemin pavé, protestant contre cette intrusion.

— Ça a l'air désert. Allons voir s'il y a quelqu'un.

Nous montons les marches ensemble, puis il pose Jonah sur la galerie en bois qui fait le tour du cottage tandis que la porte moustiquaire se referme derrière nous.

Sur le perron, nous frappons à la porte de la maison et attendons avant de jeter des coups d'œil à travers les rideaux de dentelle. À l'intérieur, un canapé fleuri flanqué de deux guéridons aux pieds galbés surplombés de lampes Art nouveau dénote avec l'allure humble de ce cottage en bordure du fleuve. Des peintures et des photos ornent les murs du petit salon mais, d'où je suis, je ne les vois pas bien. Tout au bout, j'aperçois une cuisine. Des portes sur le côté du salon semblent mener à des chambres et à une véranda à l'arrière.

Je me suis déplacée vers l'autre fenêtre pour y voir un peu mieux quand j'entends Trent essayer de tourner la poignée. Je m'insurge :

— Qu'est-ce que tu fabriques ?

Je jette un coup d'œil par-dessus mon épaule, m'attendant à moitié à entendre des sirènes ou, pire, à voir un fusil braqué vers nous.

Trent m'adresse un clin d'œil malicieux lorsque la porte s'ouvre.

— Je visite un bien à vendre. Je crois que quelqu'un m'a appelé pour venir faire une estimation de la maison.

Il entre sans me laisser le temps de protester. Je ne suis pas certaine que je l'aurais fait, de toute façon. Je ne peux pas partir d'ici sans en avoir appris davantage, sans découvrir ce qui se passait ici. J'ai du mal à m'imaginer comment quelqu'un d'aussi frêle que May pouvait vivre dans un endroit si isolé.

— Jonah, tu restes bien sur la galerie, hein ? Tu ne sors pas par la porte moustiquaire, ordonne-t-il en jetant un regard impérieux par-dessus son épaule.

— 'accord.

Jonah est occupé à ramasser des glands qu'un écureuil a dû faire passer dans le coin déchiré de la moustiquaire. Il les compte pendant que je suis Trent à l'intérieur.

— Un, deux, touas... sept... huit... quayante-quat'.

Le décompte se perd derrière moi lorsque je m'arrête sur le paillasson pour balayer la pièce du regard. Je ne m'attendais pas à ça. Pas de couche de poussière, pas d'insectes morts sur les appuis de fenêtre. Tout est impeccable. On a l'impression que la maison est habitée, mais les seuls bruits viennent du carillon, des oiseaux, des feuilles, de la petite voix de Jonah, et du cri d'un migrateur du fleuve.

Trent soulève une enveloppe laissée sur le comptoir de la cuisine et la tourne.

— May Crandall.

Il me montre sa preuve, que je vois à peine.

Je suis concentrée sur un tableau au-dessus de la cheminée. Les chapeaux de soleil aux couleurs vives, les robes de plage bien repassées des années soixante, les sourires, les boucles dorées soulevées par la brise iodée, le rire qu'on voit mais qu'on n'entend pas...

Je reconnais la scène, à défaut de la pause. Dans celle-ci, les quatre femmes se regardent en riant. Les petits garçons qui jouaient dans le sable ont disparu de l'arrière-plan. La photo trouvée dans le bureau de Trent Sr. était en noir et blanc, et les femmes souriaient à l'appareil photo. Le cliché qui a inspiré cette peinture avait dû être pris quelques secondes avant ou après l'autre. L'artiste a ajouté des couleurs vives. Il n'y a pas de teinte pour peindre le rire, et pourtant, cet instant saisi irradie la joie. Les femmes se tiennent par les coudes, la tête rejetée en arrière. L'une d'elles projette du bout du pied des gouttelettes d'eau de mer vers le peintre.

Je m'approche du tableau pour étudier la signature dans le coin. J'y lis *Fern*.

Une plaque de cuivre en bas du cadre porte l'inscription : *Le Jour des sœurs*.

Ma grand-mère est sur la gauche. Les trois autres, selon l'histoire qu'on a nous racontée à la maison de retraite, sont May, Lark et Fern.

Comme elles lèvent la tête, leurs visages sont exposés à la lumière et non plus à l'ombre, et elles se ressemblent vraiment comme des sœurs.

Y compris ma grand-mère.

— Ce n'est pas la seule, m'annonce Trent en pivotant pour étudier la pièce.

Partout, il y a des photos. De décennies différentes, en des lieux différents, un assortiment de cadres et de tailles variés, et toujours ces quatre mêmes femmes. Sur la jetée près du fleuve, leurs jeans remontés aux genoux, des cannes à pêche dans la main ; prenant le thé près des rosiers grimpants derrière cette petite maison ; dans des canoës rouges, les pagaies en l'air.

Trent se penche sur la table, ouvre un album photo noir défraîchi et le feuillette.

— Elles ont passé beaucoup de temps ici.

Je fais un pas vers lui.

Tout à coup, un chien aboie dehors. Nous nous figeons sur place lorsque le bruit se rapproche. Des griffes cliquettent sur les marches du perron. En quatre pas précipités, Trent a traversé la pièce pour se retrouver sur le seuil, mais pas assez vite. Un gros chien noir gronde de l'autre côté de la porte de la galerie et Jonah est pétrifié.

— Tout doux, mon gros...

Trent s'approche, attrape Jonah par le bras et le guide vers moi.

Le chien lève la tête et aboie avant de gratter en bas de la porte en essayant de fourrer son museau dans le coin déchiré de la moustiquaire.

Non loin, on entend un grondement de moteur. Une tondeuse à gazon, peut-être. Il s'approche de nous. Trent et moi, nous n'avons pas le choix, nous devons attendre. Je n'ose même pas refermer la porte de la maison derrière nous. Si le chien déchire pour de bon la moustiquaire, nous aurons besoin d'une issue de secours.

On dirait des criminels pris sur le fait. Ce que nous sommes bel et bien, à vrai dire.

Seul Jonah, qui n'a commis aucun crime, trépigne de joie. Je garde la main sur son épaule alors qu'il saute sur place pour tenter de voir ce qui fait tant de bruit.

— Oh... trateur ! Trateur ! s'écrit-il quand un homme en salopette coiffé d'un chapeau de paille apparaît sur un tracteur rouge et gris d'un âge canonique.

Une remorque à deux roues aux couleurs passées le suit, chargée d'un coupe-bordure et de quelques brindilles. Le soleil à son zénith fait briller la peau brune et tannée de l'homme lorsqu'il s'arrête au portail et coupe le moteur.

Vu de plus près, je me rends compte qu'il est plus jeune que ce que sa tenue suggère. Il doit avoir l'âge de mes parents... la soixantaine, peut-être ?

— Sammy ! gronde-t-il d'une voix grave et impérieuse lorsqu'il descend du tracteur pour rappeler le chien. Arrête ton boucan ! Tais-toi ! Viens ici !

Sammy n'en fait qu'à sa tête. Il attend que l'homme l'ait presque rejoint avant d'obéir.

L'inconnu s'arrête au milieu des marches, mais il est si grand que nous pouvons presque nous regarder dans les yeux.

— Je peux vous aider, m'sieur-dame ? demande-t-il.

Trent et moi échangeons un coup d'œil. Visiblement, ni l'un ni l'autre n'avons prévu cette éventualité.

— Nous avons discuté avec May, à la maison de retraite.

Je reconnais l'habileté d'homme d'affaires de Trent. Il présente cela comme une explication vraisemblable, alors que ce n'est pas du tout le cas.

— E-est-ce que c'est... sa... sa maison ?

Mes balbutiements nous donnent l'air encore plus coupables.

— T'as un trateur, m'sieur !

De nous trois, c'est Jonah qui fait la déclaration la plus intelligente.

— Oui, mon grand, t'as bien vu, répond l'homme qui s'est baissé, mains sur les genoux, pour parler à Jonah à travers la moustiquaire. C'était le tracteur de mon papa. Il l'a acheté tout neuf en 1958. Je le fais redémarrer quand j'ai le temps, pour rabattre les mauvaises herbes dans la ferme, ramasser les branches et jeter un œil sur ma m'man. Mes petits-enfants adorent venir avec moi. J'en ai un à la maison, en ce moment, qui doit avoir ta taille.

— Oh... fait Jonah, vraiment impressionné. J'ai troizans.

Il fait un effort pour lever les trois doigts du milieu sur une main et plier le petit doigt et le pouce.

— Ouais, Bart a pile le même âge que toi, confirme l'homme. Trois ans et demi. Il a le même nom que son papy. C'est moi.

Bart le Grand se redresse pour nous étudier, Trent et moi.

— Vous êtes de la famille de May ? Comment va-t-elle ? Ma mère m'a dit que sa sœur était morte et qu'ils avaient dû mettre Mme Crandall en maison de retraite. Et que ses petits-enfants l'avaient envoyée jusqu'à Aiken, en pensant que ce serait mieux si elle n'était si près de chez elle. C'est triste. Elle adorait cet endroit.

— Elle se porte aussi bien que possible, j'imagine, lui dis-je. Je ne crois pas qu'elle se plaise beaucoup, là-bas. Après avoir vu sa maison d'ici, je comprends pourquoi.

— Vous êtes une nièce ou une petite-fille ?

Il se focalise sur moi. Je le vois consulter son catalogue mental pour essayer de deviner qui je suis.

J'ai peur de mentir à cet homme. Je ne sais pas si May a bel et bien une petite-fille. Si ça se trouve, Bart me teste.

Un mensonge ne résoudra pas mes problèmes, de toute façon.

— Je ne... sais pas vraiment, en vérité. Vous disiez que votre mère habite près d'ici ? Je me demande si elle sait quelque chose sur les photos dans la maison et le tableau au-dessus de la cheminée ? Ma grand-mère est l'une des femmes qu'on y voit.

Bart jette un coup d'œil vers le cottage.

— Peux pas vous dire. J'suis pas rentré là-dedans depuis des années. C'est ma m'man qui s'occupait de cet endroit pendant longtemps. Avant même que la grande maison brûle quand elle a été frappée par la foudre en 1982.

— Est-ce qu'il serait possible... de lui parler ? Enfin, il ne faudrait pas que ça la dérange...

Il fait glisser son chapeau en arrière, le sourire aux lèvres.

— Vous rigolez ? Pas du tout. Elle adore qu'on vienne lui rendre visite. Mais j'espère que vous avez du temps à tuer. Ma m'man est une sacrée pipelette.

Il se penche en arrière et jette un coup d'œil au coin du cottage.

— Vous avez marché jusqu'ici depuis l'ancienne bâtisse ? Y a un chemin plus praticable de l'autre côté. Qui mène jusqu'à notre ferme. May laissait sa voiture dans le garage près de chez ma m'man.

— Oh, je ne savais pas.

Voilà qui explique l'entrée envahie par les mauvaises herbes et le chemin en mauvais état qui nous a conduits là.

— Nous sommes entrés par le portail en fer.

— Oh, bigre, vous aurez des piqûres d'aoûtat d'ici demain. Rappelez-moi de vous donner du savon anti-aoûtat de ma m'man. Elle le fait elle-même.

Mes jambes me démangent aussitôt.

— Vous allez tous monter dans ma remorque, là. Je vais vous conduire jusqu'à chez ma m'man. À moins que vous préfériez marcher ?

Je lève la tête et, tout ce que je vois dans les herbes hautes, ce sont des milliards d'aoûtats attendant de s'accrocher à moi et de me donner des démangeaisons jusqu'à la fin des temps.

Jonah ne tient déjà plus en place et tire son père par le pantalon, le doigt pointé vers le tracteur.

— Je crois qu'on va grimper derrière vous, déclare Trent.

Jonah tape dans ses mains en poussant des cris de joie.

— Allez, viens, jeune homme, lance Bart en ouvrant la moustiquaire.

Jonah lui tend les bras comme s'il était un vieil ami. Bart le fait voler dans les airs et le dépose au pied des marches, et il est clair qu'il a de l'expérience en la matière. Il doit être un papy du tonnerre.

Jonah est au paradis quand nous grimpons dans la petite remorque à deux roues, qui me rappelle le chariot à crottin que les palefreniers utilisent à Drayden Hill. Je soupçonne même cette remorque d'avoir servi pour le même usage. Des morceaux de substances douteuses rebondissent sous le tas de brindilles. Ça ne dérange pas Jonah. Il a l'air heureux comme un poisson dans l'eau tandis que nous traversons bruyamment des broussailles au bord du jardin pour suivre ce qui est clairement une piste souvent empruntée, peut-être par un quad ou une voiturette de golf.

Notre route nous éloigne du fleuve et nous entraîne vers un chemin de terre où nous tournons sur la première allée. La maison fraîchement peinte en bleu ressemble au genre d'endroit où on prendrait sa retraite. Des poules picorent dans la cour. Une vache tachetée est allongée à l'ombre d'un arbre. Des vêtements volettent nonchalamment sur plusieurs cordes à linge. Sammy bondit en avant et aboie à tue-tête pour annoncer notre arrivée.

La mère de Bart s'avance à petits pas sur le seuil, vêtue d'une robe d'intérieur, de pantoufles et d'un foulard jaune vif. Une fleur de soie assortie orne le chignon gris volumineux au sommet de sa tête. Lorsqu'elle nous voit dans la remorque, elle recule d'un pas, la main en visière au-dessus des yeux.

— Qu'est-ce que tu me ramènes là, Barthol'mew ?

Je laisse son fils lui offrir une explication, puisque je n'en ai pas.

— Ils étaient là-bas, chez Mme Crandall. Ils ont dit qu'ils l'avaient vue, à la maison de retraite.

Le menton de la femme disparaît dans les plis cirés, couleur cannelle, de son cou.

— Qui que vous dites que vous êtes ?

Je descends de la remorque avant qu'elle ordonne à son fils de nous ramener où il nous a trouvés.

— Avery.

Il n'y a que deux marches pour atteindre son perron, où je me dépêche de lui tendre la main.

— Je demandais à votre fils s'il avait des informations sur les photos et les peintures dans la maison de May. Ma grand-mère est dessus.

Le regard de la vieille dame passe entre moi et Trent, qui attend au pied des marches, pendant que Jonah inspecte le tracteur avec Bart. Un petit garçon, qui doit faire la même taille que Jonah, jaillit d'une grange voisine et court les rejoindre. Les présentations sont inutiles, mais elles sont tout de même faites en vitesse. C'est Bart le Petit.

La vieille dame reporte son attention sur moi. Elle se redresse et me dévisage longuement, comme si elle mémorisait les contours de mon visage. Est-ce que c'est mon imagination, ou est-ce qu'elle semble me reconnaître ?

— Comment vous dites que vous vous appelez ?

Je répète plus fort :

— Avery.

— Avery comment ?

— Stafford.

J'avais fait exprès de cacher cette information jusqu'à maintenant. Mais je ne veux pas partir d'ici sans réponses et, si c'est le prix à payer, ainsi soit-il.

— Vous êtes la fille de Mlle Judy ?

Mon cœur se met à palpiter si fort que le sang bat contre mes tympans.

— Sa petite-fille.

J'ai l'impression que le temps ralentit. Je n'entends plus les petites voix des garçons, ni celle de Bart le Grand, le grondement du tracteur, le caquètement des poules, le claquement de la queue de la vache qui chasse les mouches, le chant interminable d'un geai moqueur.

— Vous voulez savoir ce que c'est que cette maison, à côté. Pourquoi qu'elle y venait.

Ce n'est pas une question mais un constat, comme si cette femme attendait depuis des années, sachant que, tôt ou tard, quelqu'un viendrait la consulter.

— Oui, madame, en effet. Je pourrais interroger ma grand-mère mais, pour être franche, elle n'a plus toute sa tête. Elle oublie beaucoup de choses.

Elle secoue la tête lentement en faisant des petits *tst, tst, tst* avec sa langue. Puis elle se concentre de nouveau sur moi et dit :

— Ce dont l'esprit ne se souvient pas, le cœur se rappelle. L'amour, la chose la plus forte de toutes. Plus forte que tout le reste. Vous voulez en savoir plus sur les sœurs.

Ma réponse n'est qu'un murmure :

— S'il vous plaît. Oui. Dites-moi.

— Ce n'est pas à moi de vous révéler ce secret.

Elle pivote, avance vers sa maison d'un pas traînant et, alors que je me crois congédiée, un coup d'œil rapide jeté par-dessus son épaule me détrompe. On me demande de la suivre.

On m'ordonne.

Je m'arrête sur le seuil et j'attends, pendant qu'elle ouvre un secrétaire en chêne et en sort un crucifix en fer-blanc cabossé. Elle prend les trois feuilles de papier qui étaient glissées en dessous – des feuilles chiffonnées, arrachées à un calepin jaune. Même si elles ont été froissées avant d'être lissées, elles ne semblent pas particulièrement vieilles et ne datent certaine-ment pas de la même époque que l'objet en fer-blanc embossé.

— J'ai juste pris ça pour les sauvegarder, explique la dame âgée.

Elle me tend le crucifix et les papiers séparément.

— Cette croix était à Queenie, y a très longtemps. Mlle Judy a écrit le reste. C'est son histoire, mais elle a jamais écrit la suite. Les sœurs, elles ont décidé qu'elles l'emporteraient dans leur tombe, j'imagine. Moi, je me suis dit qu'un jour quelqu'un pourrait bien venir demander. Les secrets, c'est pas sain. Les secrets, c'est pas sain, même quand ils sont vieux. Parfois, les plus vieux sont les plus pires. Emmenez votre grand-mère voir Mlle May. Le cœur se rappelle. Il se rappelle qui il aime.

Je baisse les yeux vers la croix, la fait tourner dans ma main, puis je déplie les feuilles jaunes. Je reconnais l'écriture. C'est celle de ma grand-mère. J'ai parcouru suffisamment de ses car-nets pour en être certaine.

— Asseyez-vous, ma fille.

La mère de Bart m'entraîne vers un fauteuil à oreilles. Je m'y effondre plus que je ne m'y assieds. Sur la première page, on peut lire :

Prélude

Le 3 août 1939
Baltimore, Maryland

La date de naissance de ma grand-mère et la ville où elle est née.

Mon histoire débute lors d'une nuit d'août caniculaire, en un lieu où mon regard ne se posera jamais. La pièce ne prend vie que dans mon imagination. Je me la figure le plus souvent comme une grande salle. Les murs sont blancs et propres, les draps amidonnés aussi craquants qu'une feuille morte. La suite privée est aménagée avec un raffinement extrême...

Je remonte le temps en flottant, déboulant des années, des décennies en arrière, glissant dans l'espace jusqu'à une chambre d'hôpital en août 1939, vers une petite vie qui vient au monde et le quitte aussitôt, au milieu du sang et du chagrin, vers une jeune mère épuisée qui s'enfonce dans un sommeil béni.

J'entends des conversations murmurées entre hommes importants. Un grand-père qui, malgré toute sa fortune et sa position, ne peut pas sauver son minuscule petit-enfant.

C'est un homme important... un sénateur, peut-être ?

Il ne peut pas sauver sa fille. Sauf si...

« Je connais une femme, à Memphis... »

S'ensuit un choix désespéré.

C'est là que se termine l'histoire écrite.

Et où débute une autre histoire. La saga d'une enfant aux cheveux blonds qui, si le récit sordide de Georgia Tann est fiable, est arrachée à sa mère juste après sa naissance. Des papiers falsifiés sont signés, ou alors on dit juste à la jeune mère épuisée que sa fille est mort-née. Le bébé disparaît dans les bras de Georgia et est remise en secret à une famille qui l'attendait ardemment, qui la revendiquera comme sienne et enfouira son terrible secret.

La petite fille minuscule devient Judy Myers Stafford.

Voilà la vérité que mon cœur poursuivait depuis le jour où j'ai vu la photo passée sur la table de nuit de May et où j'ai été frappée par la ressemblance.

Cette photo, c'est Queenie et Briny. Ce ne sont pas juste des gens hantant les souvenirs de May Crandall. Ce sont aussi mes arrière-grands-parents. Des gens du fleuve.

J'aurais pu en être une, moi aussi, si le hasard n'avait pas décidé d'un retournement inimaginable.

La mère de Bart vient se placer près de moi. Elle s'assied sur le bras du fauteuil et me frotte le dos en me tendant un mouchoir devant mes larmes abondantes.

— Oh, ma chérie... Mon enfant. La meilleure des choses, c'est de savoir. Je leur dis toujours ça, mieux vaut savoir qui t'es. Qui on est au fond de nous. Y a pas d'autre bonne façon de vivre. Mais c'est pas à moi de décider.

Je sais pas combien de temps je reste là, tandis que la vieille dame me tapote le dos et me réconforte pendant que je contemple tous les obstacles qui ont tenu les enfants de l'*Arcadie* loin les uns des autres. Je pense à la façon dont May a expliqué ses choix. « La première fois que nous avons été réunies, nous étions déjà des jeunes femmes avec nos vies, nos maris, nos enfants. Nous avons choisi de ne pas faire intrusion dans nos existences respectives. Savoir que les autres se portaient bien, ça nous suffisait... »

En vérité, ça ne suffisait pas. Même les remparts de la réputation, de l'ambition, de la position sociale ne pouvaient contenir l'amour entre sœurs, ce lien formidable qui les unissait. Tout à coup, ces barrières qui les ont poussées vers des doubles vies, dans des lieux de rencontre secrets, semblent presque aussi cruelles que les barrières initiales qu'avaient été leurs adoptions monnayées, leurs papiers falsifiés et leurs séparations forcées.

— Emmenez votre grand-mère voir sa sœur.

Une main tremblante serre la mienne.

— Il reste qu'elles deux. Les deux seules sœurs. Dites-leur que Hootsie elle a dit qu'elles doivent être qui elles sont – il est grand temps.

24

Rill

Le cri de l'engoulevent tente de m'arracher à mon rêve, mais je le repousse et m'y accroche. Dans ce rêve, nous sommes tous à bord de l'*Arcadie*... Briny et Lark, Fern et Gabion. Nous descendons le grand Mississippi en plein milieu, comme si le fleuve tout entier nous appartenait, et à nous seuls. Le ciel est dégagé, il fait beau, et il n'y a pas un remorqueur, pas une barge ni un bateau à aubes en vue.

Nous sommes libres. Nous sommes libres, et nous laissons le fleuve nous porter vers le sud. Loin, très loin de Mud Island et de tout ce qui s'y est passé.

Silas et Zede sont avec nous. Ainsi que Camellia et Queenie.

C'est pour ça que je sais que rien de tout cela n'est vrai.

J'ouvre les yeux, repousse la couverture et, l'espace d'un instant, je suis perdue, aveuglée par le soleil. C'est le milieu de la journée, pas la nuit. Je me rends compte alors que je suis roulée en boule dans la barque avec Fern, et nous nous sommes blotties sous les bâches effilochées, pas sous une couverture. La barque est attachée à l'arrière de l'*Arcadie*, prisonnière. C'est le seul endroit où nous pouvons nous reposer dans la journée sans craindre que Briny nous tombe dessus.

L'engoulevent crie de plus belle. C'est Silas, je le sais. Je le guette dans les sous-bois mais il s'est bien caché.

Quand je me tortille pour sortir de sous la bâche, Fern se réveille et m'attrape par la cheville. Depuis que nous sommes revenues à l'*Arcadie*, elle a peur de rester seule ne serait-ce qu'un instant. Elle ne sait jamais quand Briny va la pousser si brusquement qu'elle tombera par terre ou la prendre dans ses bras et la serrer si fort qu'elle ne pourra plus respirer.

Je réponds à l'engoulevent pendant que Fern se met à genoux pour scruter les bois.

— Chhh, je lui murmure.

Quand nous sommes allées en douce dans la barque ce matin, Briny traînait dans le coin avec une bouteille de whisky. Il dort sans doute sur le pont, maintenant. Mais je n'en suis pas sûre à cent pour cent.

— Mieux vaut éviter que Briny découvre que Silas est ici.

Fern hoche la tête et s'humecte les lèvres. Son estomac gargouille. Elle se doute que Silas va nous apporter à manger. Sans Silas, le vieux Zede et Arney, on serait mortes de faim, après trois semaines passées sur l'*Arcadie*. Briny n'a guère besoin de manger. Il ne se nourrit plus que de whisky, maintenant.

Je soulève la bâche pour Fern en lui disant :

— Retourne là-dessous un instant.

Si Briny voit Silas et se met en colère, je ne veux pas que Fern soit dans le coin.

Je dois la décrocher de moi de force pour la remettre sous la bâche, mais elle y reste sagement.

Silas attend dans les broussailles. Il me serre fort et je me mords la lèvre pour m'empêcher de pleurer. Nous nous éloignons un peu, mais pas trop, pour que je puisse tout de même entendre Fern si elle m'appelle.

— Ça va ? me demande-t-il quand nous nous asseyons sous un arbre.

Je hoche la tête.

— Mais la pêche n'a rien donné, ce matin.

Même si je ne veux pas lui demander ouvertement de la nourriture, j'espère bien qu'il en a apporté dans le petit baluchon qu'il tient à la main.

Il me tend un paquet pas plus gros que deux poings, ce qui est déjà énorme. Les réserves de Zede sont au plus bas et il doit aussi nourrir Arney. Elle s'est installée sur son bateau, où elle sera en sécurité. Zede voulait que nous y allions aussi, Fern et moi, mais je sais que Briny ne nous fera pas de mal.

— Quelques galettes d'avoine et un peu de poisson salé. Une pomme que vous pourrez partager.

Appuyé sur ses mains, Silas se penche en arrière, inspire en fixant le fleuve à travers les sous-bois.

— Briny va mieux aujourd'hui ? Il a retrouvé la raison ?

— Un peu.

Je ne sais pas si c'est vrai ou si je veux juste que ce le soit. La plupart du temps, Briny traîne dans le bateau, boit et beugle la nuit. Puis il cuve dans la journée.

— Zede a dit qu'il allait pleuvoir, ce soir.

J'ai vu les signes, moi aussi. Ça m'inquiète.

— Ne reviens pas dénouer les cordes en cachette, d'accord ? Pas encore. Bientôt, peut-être. Dans quelques jours, je pense que Briny sera prêt.

Voilà trois semaines que nous restons sur la rive face à Mud Island, alors que le froid s'installe. Même si Silas et Zede ont prévenu Briny que la police n'aurait aucun mal à nous retrouver ici, Briny refuse de laisser qui que ce soit défaire les amarres. Il a tiré sur Silas et a failli lui emporter la main pour avoir essayé. Il a aussi tiré sur la pauvre Arney. Je lui avais donné des habits de Queenie, et Briny s'était mis dans la tête qu'elle était vraiment Queenie, et il était furieux contre elle car elle était morte.

— Il faut attendre encore un peu, dis-je d'un ton implorant à Silas.

Il se frotte l'oreille comme si ce n'était pas ce qu'il voulait entendre.

— Tu devrais prendre Fern et venir avec moi sur le bateau de Zede. Quand nous partirons vers le canal principal, on verra bien si Briny refusera toujours de venir.

— Encore quelques jours. Briny ira mieux. Il a un peu perdu la tête, c'est tout. Ça va passer.

J'espère que j'ai raison mais, en vérité, Briny ne veut pas laisser Queenie, et Queenie est enterrée sur la rive du Mississippi, non loin d'ici. Un prêtre est venu faire une bénédiction, m'a dit Zede. Je ne savais pas que ma maman était catholique. Avant de vivre chez les Sevier, je ne savais même pas ce que cela voulait dire. Zuma porte une petite croix comme celle accrochée au mur de notre bateau. Elle la tenait et lui parlait parfois, tout comme Queenie le faisait, mais pas en polonais. Cela ne dérangeait pas les Sevier, car ils étaient baptistes.

Je me dis que, dans un sens ou dans l'autre, c'est réconfortant de savoir que ma mère a été enterrée comme il faut et qu'un prêtre est venu dire des prières sur sa tombe.

— Zede veut que tu dises à Briny que, dans quatre jours au plus, nous larguerons les amarres et, si Briny ne veut pas venir, il vous enlèvera, Fern et toi, de l'*Arcadie*. Vous descendrez vers le sud avec nous.

La voix de Briny retentit soudain tout près de la rive :

— C'est qui qu'est là ?

Sa voix est empesée par les restes de whisky. Il a dû nous entendre parler.

— Qui qu'est là, là-bas, dans les broussailles ? répète-t-il en fonçant bruyamment à travers les sous-bois et l'herbe sèche.

J'attrape le baluchon, le fourre sous ma robe et pousse Silas pour qu'il s'en aille. Je laisse Briny tituber seul sous les arbres et je file à la barque où je récupère Fern pour l'emmener sur le bateau.

Briny nous trouve dans la cabine quand il finit par revenir. Je fais comme si je venais de frire les galettes. Il ne remarque même pas que le poêle n'est pas allumé.

— J'ai presque fini de préparer le repas, dis-je en remplissant les assiettes avec des gestes exagérés. Tu as faim ?

Il cligne des yeux, prend Fern dans ses bras, s'assied à table et la serre fort. Elle m'observe, pâle, effrayée.

Ma gorge se serre tellement que j'ai l'impression qu'on m'étrangle. Comment vais-je dire à Briny que Zede n'attendra pas plus de quatre jours ?

Je n'y arrive pas, alors je lance :

— Des galettes d'avoine, du poisson salé et des tranches de pomme.

Je pose la nourriture sur la table et Briny remet Fern sur sa chaise. L'espace d'un instant, on pourrait croire que tout est normal. Que nous prenons tous les jours un repas correct ensemble. Briny me sourit et ses yeux noirs, fatigués, me rappellent Camellia.

Ma sœur me manque, même si nous nous chamaillions tout le temps. Sa dureté, sa détermination me manquent. Sa façon de ne jamais céder.

— Zede dit que, dans quatre jours, les courants seront bons et qu'il faudra prendre le fleuve. Vers le sud, où la pêche est bonne et le temps plus doux. Il dit que c'est le moment.

Briny pose un coude sur la table, se frotte les yeux et secoue la tête lentement. Comme il marmonne, je ne comprends que ses derniers mots :

— ... pas sans Queenie.

Il se lève, se dirige vers la porte, attrape sa bouteille de whisky vide au passage. Un instant plus tard, le bruit des rames m'apprend qu'il s'éloigne à bord de la barque.

Je tends l'oreille jusqu'à ce que je ne l'entende plus et, dans le silence qui suit, j'ai l'impression que le monde s'écroule autour de moi. Quand j'étais chez Mme Murphy, puis dans la maison des Sevier, je me disais que, si je pouvais seulement retourner à l'*Arcadie,* tout redeviendrait comme avant. Je pensais que je redeviendrais comme avant, mais je comprends maintenant que je me racontais des histoires, juste pour tenir le coup, jour après jour.

En vérité, au lieu de tout arranger, notre retour à l'*Arcadie* a rendu tout le reste réel. Camellia n'est plus. Lark et Gabion sont très loin. Queenie est enterrée dans une tombe de fortune, et le cœur de Briny l'y a suivi. Le whisky lui a fait perdre la raison, et il ne veut pas la retrouver.

Pas même pour moi. Pas même pour Fern. Nous ne suffisons pas.

Fern vient se blottir sur mes genoux, et je la serre fort. Nous attendons jusqu'au soir un signe de Briny, mais personne ne rentre. Il est sans doute parti en ville se faire un peu d'argent au billard pour se racheter à boire.

Je finis par border Fern sur sa couchette et me glisse dans la mienne où j'attends que le sommeil vienne. Il n'y a même pas un livre pour me tenir compagnie. Tout ce qui pouvait acheter du whisky a déjà été troqué.

La pluie commence à tomber avant que je m'endorme, et toujours aucun signe de Briny.

Je le retrouve en rêve. Nous sommes tous ensemble, et tout est parfait. Briny joue de l'harmonica pendant que nous pique-niquons sur le sable près de la berge. Nous cueillons des pâquerettes et goûtons le nectar du chèvrefeuille. Gabion et Lark pourchassent des petites grenouilles jusqu'à en remplir tout un pot.

— Elle est belle comme une reine, pas vrai, ta maman ? demande Briny. Et du coup, tu es quoi, toi ? La princesse Rill du royaume d'Arcadie, pardi !

Quand je me réveille, j'entends Briny dehors, mais il n'y a pas de musique. Il hurle au cœur de l'orage. La sueur plaque le drap à ma peau, si bien que je dois le décoller de moi pour m'asseoir. Ma bouche est sèche et pâteuse, et mes yeux ne veulent pas s'accomoder. Il fait aussi noir que dans un four. La pluie crépite sur le toit. La chaudière à bois a été remplie et le registre de la cheminée a dû être ouvert en grand, parce que le feu crépite et siffle, et qu'il fait une chaleur épouvantable dans le bateau.

Dehors, sur le pont, Briny jure comme un charretier. Une lanterne illumine un instant la fenêtre. Je saute sur mes pieds pour me lever mais le bateau gîte comme un fou et me refait tomber sur la toile à matelas. L'*Arcadie* penche complètement d'un côté.

Fern roule par-dessus la barrière de sa couchette et s'affale par terre.

Tout à coup, je comprends... nous ne sommes plus amarrés à la berge. Nous sommes sur l'eau.

Silas et Zede sont venus couper la corde après le retour de Briny. Voilà ma première conclusion. Il est là, dehors, à hurler, parce qu'il est furieux contre eux.

Aussitôt, je change d'avis. Ils ne nous lanceraient pas à la dérive en pleine nuit. C'est trop dangereux, avec les troncs qui flottent, les bancs de sable et les sillages des gros bateaux et des barges. Silas et Zede le savent.

Briny aussi, mais il a à moitié perdu la boule. Il n'essaie pas de nous ramener vers la berge. Il met au défi le fleuve de nous prendre.

— Vas-y, espèce de scélérat ! s'époumone-t-il, tel le capitaine Achab dans *Moby Dick*. Essaie de m'avoir ! Viens me chercher ! Allez !

Le tonnerre gronde. Un éclair fuse. Briny maudit le fleuve. Il rit.

La lanterne disparaît derrière la fenêtre, puis commence à monter l'échelle sur le côté du bateau tandis que Briny grimpe sur le toit.

Je traverse tant bien que mal la pièce pour vérifier que Fern n'a rien et la remettre sur sa couchette.

— Reste là. Reste là et ne bouge pas sauf si je t'appelle.

Elle m'agrippe par la chemise de nuit et m'implore d'une voix enrouée :

— Nooon.

Depuis que nous sommes de retour sur l'*Arcadie*, elle est morte de peur la nuit.

— Tout va bien se passer. Je crois que les amarres se sont détachées, c'est tout. Briny essaie sans doute de nous ramener à la rive.

Je la laisse dans son lit et me dirige vers la porte. L'*Arcadie* est ballottée tandis que j'avance en trébuchant, et j'entends le klaxon d'un remorqueur, les craquements, les cliquètements de coques de barge et je sais que des vagues plus hautes encore nous attendent. Je tends la main vers la porte et m'y accroche juste à temps. L'*Arcadie* se soulève sur une crête, avant de basculer violemment pour redescendre la vague. Le bois glisse entre mes doigts et des échardes se plantent sous la peau. Je tombe vers l'avant, j'atterris sur le pont, dans le froid. Le bateau, lui, bascule vers l'arrière et se laisse entraîner par le courant en tourbillonnant.

Non, non ! Pitié, non !

L'*Arcadie* se redresse comme s'il m'avait entendue. Il chevauche la vague suivante en restant bien droit.

— Tu crois que tu me peux m'avoir ? Tu crois que tu peux me prendre ? hurle Briny depuis son perchoir.

Une bouteille se brise et des éclats dégringolent du toit, scintillant dans la pluie nocturne et la lumière du remorqueur. On dirait qu'il neige. Puis ils tombent dans l'eau noire avec une série de *plic*.

Je crie :

— Briny, on doit rejoindre la rive ! Briny, il faut s'arrimer !

Mais le klaxon du remorqueur et l'orage noient mes paroles.

Quelque part, un homme hurle des jurons et des mises en garde. Une sirène d'alerte résonne. L'*Arcadie* monte sur une haute vague et s'y tient en équilibre comme une danseuse sur la pointe des pieds.

Puis il donne de la bande lorsqu'il bascule de l'autre côté. De l'eau glacée passe par-dessus le pont.

Nous nous retrouvons en travers du fleuve.

Le projecteur du remorqueur nous balaie avant de s'arrêter sur nous.

Un tronc fonce droit vers notre proue – un arbre géant à la dérive, brandissant encore ses racines pleines de terre. Je le vois juste avant que la lumière ne glisse plus loin. Je cherche à tâtons la gaffe pour le repousser, mais elle n'est pas à sa place. Je ne peux rien faire à part m'enrouler autour du poteau à l'entrée de la cabine et hurler à Fern de se cramponner en regardant l'arbre nous percuter, ses racines s'ouvrant autour de l'*Arcadie* comme des doigts, qui m'agrippent la cheville, se tournent et tirent de toutes leurs forces.

Dans la cabine, Fern crie mon nom.

— Accroche-toi bien ! De toutes tes forces !

L'arbre tire et craque, fait tournoyer l'*Arcadie* comme une toupie, l'entraîne dans la direction opposée avant de se libérer et de nous laisser gîter dans le courant. Les vagues déferlent sur nous et s'engouffrent dans la cabine.

Mes pieds glissent sous moi.

L'*Arcadie* gémit. Des clous sautent. Des poutres craquent.

La coque percute un obstacle dur, le poteau m'est presque arraché des mains et me voilà qui m'envole dans la pluie. J'ai le souffle coupé. Tout devient noir.

Je perçois des bruits de bois brisé, des cris, le tonnerre lointain.

L'eau est froide, et pourtant, j'ai chaud. Je vois une lumière et, à l'intérieur, ma maman. Queenie me tend la main et je lui tends la mienne mais, juste avant que je puisse l'atteindre, le fleuve m'écarte d'elle, me tirant par la taille.

Je donne des coups de pied, je me démène et me revoilà à la surface. Je vois l'*Arcadie* sous les projecteurs du remorqueur. Je vois un bateau à moteur qui s'approche de nous. J'entends des sifflets et des cris. Mes jambes sont trop raides et je suis transie jusqu'aux os.

L'*Arcadie* est coincée de biais contre un énorme tas de bois flotté. Le Mississippi semble vouloir l'engloutir comme la gueule d'un dragon géant, avalant peu à peu sa poupe.

— Fern !

Ma voix se perd dans l'eau et le bruit. Je nage de toutes mes forces, je sens le tourbillon et le courant qui veulent m'entraîner lorsque j'arrive devant l'amas de débris. Le tourbillon essaie de me tirer en arrière, mais je l'affronte, me hisse sur le tas de bois, le traverse sans perdre l'équilibre jusqu'au pont et grimpe à quatre pattes jusqu'à la cabine.

La porte tombe vers l'intérieur quand je l'ouvre.

— Fern ! Fern ! Fern ! Réponds-moi !

La fumée étrangle ma voix, le poêle à bois s'est renversé. Des braises rouges roulent partout sur le sol. Elles grésillent sur le parquet mouillé et sifflent sous mes pieds.

Tout est sens dessus dessous, et je n'y vois rien. Je vais d'abord dans la mauvaise direction, près de la table au lieu de la couchette de Fern. Le couvre-lit en sacs de farine de Briny et Queenie flotte devant moi comme une baleine colorée, portant une flammèche sur son dos. Tout près, des flammes remontent le long des rideaux.

— Fern !

Est-ce qu'elle est partie ? Est-ce qu'elle est tombée dans le fleuve ? Est-ce que Briny l'a déjà fait sortir ?

Une vague déferle à l'intérieur, s'empare des braises rouges et les chasse par la porte. Elles sautent et gémissent dans leur agonie.

— Riiiiill ! J'suis là ! Là !

Le faisceau du projecteur glisse sur nous, s'engouffre par la fenêtre en un long cercle lent. Je vois le visage de ma sœur, terrifiée, les yeux écarquillés, sous son lit. Elle tend les bras vers moi, puis, aussitôt que je l'ai prise par la main et que je tente de la tirer, l'eau nous attrape toutes les deux. Une chaise glisse vers nous, me cogne fort dans le dos et me fait tomber par terre. De l'eau déferle sur mon visage et mes oreilles. Je m'accroche à Fern de toutes mes forces.

La chaise bascule. J'attrape ma sœur, trébuche et crapahute à travers la cabine jusqu'à la porte.

Le faisceau de lumière entre de nouveau. Je vois la photo de Briny et de Queenie sur le mur, et la croix de Queenie juste en dessous.

Je ne devrais pas, pourtant, je coince Fern contre le mur avec ma cuisse pour attraper la photographie et la croix de ma mère, que je passe par le col de ma chemise de nuit et que je coince dans l'élastique de mes sous-vêtements. Ces objets me rentrent dans la peau quand nous remontons le pont jusqu'à la balustrade, que nous enjambons pour gagner le tas de bois flotté, où nous crapahutons par-dessus les branches, les planches de bois et les troncs. Aussi rapides que des souris. On a fait ça toute notre vie.

Mais nous en savons assez toutes les deux pour comprendre qu'un tas de bois flotté n'est pas un endroit sûr. Même lorsque nous arrivons à l'autre bout, je sens encore la chaleur du feu.

Je tiens la main de Fern, me tourne et regarde vers l'*Arcadie*
avant de lever la main pour me protéger les yeux. Des flammes
s'enroulent autour de la cabine et s'étirent vers le ciel, dévorant
le toit, les murs et le pont, rongeant l'*Arcadie* jusqu'à l'os, la
dépossédant de sa beauté. Des cendres volent dans les airs. Elles
montent, montent, montent en tourbillonnant et fusent dans
toutes les directions comme un million de nouvelles étoiles.

Refroidies par la pluie, elles retombent et se déposent sur
notre peau. Fern pousse un cri lorsqu'une cendre atterrit,
encore tiède, sur elle. Je l'attrape par le col de la chemise de
nuit, m'accroupis et la plonge dans l'eau en lui disant de s'agrip-
per très fort au tas de bois mort. Ici, le courant est trop fort
pour qu'on puisse nager jusqu'à la berge. Quand je la ressors,
elle claque des dents et son visage pâlit.

Le tas de bois commence à brûler. Le feu va bientôt se frayer
un passage jusqu'à nous.

Un nom s'arrache soudain de ma bouche :

— Briny !

Il est là, quelque part. Il a sans doute réussi à quitter le
bateau. Il va nous sauver.

N'est-ce pas ?

— Accrochez-vous ! hurle quelqu'un, mais ce n'est pas la
voix de notre père. Accrochez-vous. Ne bougez pas !

Un réservoir explose sur l'*Arcadie.* Des flammèches jaillissent
vers le ciel et retombent partout. L'une d'elles se pose sur mon
pied et la douleur me transperce de part en part. Je hurle, j'agite
le pied, puis plonge ma jambe dans l'eau sans lâcher Fern.

Le tas de débris s'ébranle. Il brûle à des dizaines d'endroits,
maintenant.

— On y est presque ! lance l'homme.

Un petit bateau apparaît dans l'obscurité, tandis que deux
hommes du fleuve au visage caché par des capuches rament
de toutes leurs forces.

— Ne lâchez pas, surtout. Ne lâchez pas !

Les branches craquent. Des troncs gémissent et sifflent. Le
tas de bois mort glisse sur le fleuve sur quelques dizaines de

centimètres. L'un des hommes dans le canot de sauvetage prévient l'autre qu'ils se feront submerger si le tas cède.

Ils s'approchent tout de même, nous font monter en vitesse dans la barque et nous jettent des couvertures avant de ramer de plus belle.

— Est-ce qu'il y avait quelqu'un d'autre sur le bateau ? Une ou plusieurs personnes ? veulent-ils savoir.

— Mon papa, dis-je dans une quinte de toux. Briny, Briny Foss.

Rien n'est plus rassurant que la terre ferme sous nos pieds lorsqu'ils nous déposent sur la berge et repartent à la recherche de Briny. Je prends Fern sur mes genoux, contre moi, sous ma couverture, la photo et la croix de Queenie entre nous. Nous frémissons, nous frissonnons en regardant l'*Arcadie* brûler jusqu'à ce que le tas de débris se disloque et emporte ce qu'il en reste avec lui.

Fern et moi, nous nous levons et avançons au bord de l'eau pour regarder le royaume d'Arcadie disparaître peu à peu dans le fleuve. Pour finir, il n'en reste plus rien. Plus une trace. Comme s'il n'avait jamais existé.

Dans la lumière grise de l'aube qui pointe à l'est, je vois les hommes et les bateaux. Ils cherchent, encore et encore et encore. Ils hèlent, les faisceaux de leurs lampes balaient le fleuve, ils rament.

Il me semble voir quelqu'un debout, plus bas sur la berge. Un ciré claque autour de ses genoux. Il ne bouge pas, n'appelle pas, ne fait pas signe vers les lumières. Il se contente de fixer le fleuve, où la vie que nous connaissions s'est fait engloutir.

Est-ce que c'est Briny ?

Les mains en coupe autour de ma bouche, je l'appelle. Ma voix porte dans la brume matinale et son écho résonne plusieurs fois.

Dans l'une des barques, un sauveteur se tourne vers moi.

Quand je plisse de nouveau les yeux pour scruter la rive, je ne vois presque plus l'homme en ciré. Il se tourne et marche vers les arbres jusqu'à ce que les ombres de l'aurore l'enveloppent.

Je l'ai peut-être imaginé.

Je fais quelques pas pour crier son nom, encore et encore. Ma voix résonne, puis meurt au loin.

— Rill !

Quand on me répond enfin, ce n'est pas depuis la rive. Ce n'est pas la voix de Briny.

Un petit canot à moteur s'approche de la berge sablonneuse et Silas en saute avant même que la *Jenny* s'arrête. Il tire l'amarre derrière lui et court vers moi pour me prendre dans ses bras. Je m'accroche à lui en pleurant.

— Tu vas bien ! Tu vas bien ! souffle-t-il dans mes cheveux, me serrant si fort que le cadre de la photo et la croix de Queenie me rentrent profondément dans la peau. Zede, Arney et moi, on a eu la peur de notre vie en voyant que l'*Arcadie* était plus là.

— Briny a tranché les amarres, cette nuit. Je me suis réveillée, et le bateau était sur le fleuve.

Je raconte le reste en sanglotant – Briny sur le toit disant n'importe quoi, la barge qui nous a évités de peu, notre collision avec le tas de bois flotté, le feu, ma fuite sur le fleuve, ma vision de Queenie, mon retour à la surface, pour regrimper à bord de l'*Arcadie* alors que le fleuve le dévorait.

— Des hommes nous ont tirées du tas de bois avant qu'il se désagrège, dis-je pour conclure notre triste histoire, frissonnant dans le froid. Ils sont repartis chercher Briny.

Je ne dis pas à Silas que je l'ai vu et que, au lieu de venir nous chercher, il s'est éloigné.

Si je ne le dis à personne, ce ne sera jamais vrai. Ce ne sera jamais comme ça que le royaume d'Arcadie a pris fin.

Silas m'écarte de lui un instant pour me regarder des pieds à la tête.

— Mais vous êtes saines et sauves. Toutes les deux, vous êtes en un seul morceau. Que tous les saints soient loués ! Zede et Arney vont nous rejoindre avec le bateau dès que possible. On retrouvera Briny. Vous resterez tous avec nous. Nous irons là où il fait chaud, où la pêche est bonne, et...

Il continue à me dire comment Zede et Briny ramasseront des planches et d'autres pièces de bois sur les rives pour nous construire un nouveau bateau. Une nouvelle *Arcadie*. Ce sera un nouveau départ, et nous voyagerons toujours ensemble, à partir de maintenant et jusqu'à la fin des temps.

Mon esprit voudrait ajouter des couleurs à ses images, mais il ne le peut pas. Le bateau de Zede est trop petit pour nous tous et Briny est parti. Zede est trop vieux pour vivre sur le fleuve encore longtemps. Trop vieux pour élever Fern. Ma sœur est trop petite.

Accrochée à ma jambe, elle se faufile sous la couverture et tire ma chemise de nuit.

— 'veux voir maman, renifle-t-elle.

Ses doigts frôlent presque le bord de la photo de Queenie, pourtant, je sais que ce n'est pas à elle qu'elle pense.

Je regarde Silas droit dans les yeux tandis que les premiers rayons du soleil frappent son visage. Mon cœur se serre si fort que ça brûle. J'aimerais que nous soyons plus âgés. Suffisamment âgés. J'aime Silas. Je le sais.

Mais j'aime aussi Fern. Je l'ai aimée en premier. Elle est tout ce qu'il me reste de ma famille.

Un peu plus loin sur la rive, les recherches pour retrouver Briny ralentissent sous le soleil matinal. Dans un instant, les secouristes verront qu'il n'y a plus d'espoir de repêcher un autre survivant. Ils viendront nous chercher, Fern et moi.

— Silas, tu dois nous emmener loin d'ici. Tout de suite.

Je m'écarte de lui pour m'approcher du canot à moteur en traînant Fern derrière moi.

— Mais... Briny...

— Nous devons partir. Avant que les hommes ne reviennent. Ils nous ramèneront au foyer.

Tout à coup, Silas comprend. Il sait que j'ai raison. Il nous fait monter dans le bateau et nous nous éloignons en silence jusqu'à ce que nous soyons suffisamment loin pour que personne ne remarque le bruit du moteur. Nous longeons la rive opposée aux entrepôts de coton, aux quais, à Mud Island et à tout Memphis. Quand nous arrivons à notre petite lagune, je dis à Silas que je veux qu'il nous ramène au bateau de Zede juste pour lui dire au revoir.

Je dois accompagner Fern plus haut sur le fleuve, en espérant que les Sevier accepteront de la reprendre. Ce n'est pas sa faute si nous sommes parties. Ce n'est pas elle qui a eu l'idée de voler des choses. Mais moi. Ce qui s'est passé n'avait rien à voir avec Fern.

Avec un peu de chance, ils la laisseront revenir... s'ils n'ont pas déjà pris une autre petite fille du foyer. Et même si c'est le cas, ils garderont peut-être Fern quand même. Ils lui promettront peut-être de l'aimer un peu et de la protéger de Mlle Tann.

Ce qui m'arrivera ensuite, aucun moyen de le savoir. Les Sevier ne voudront plus de moi, c'est sûr – moi, la menteuse, la voleuse. Je ne peux pas laisser Mlle Tann me retrouver. Je pourrais peut-être chercher du travail dans le coin, mais les temps sont durs. Je ne peux pas retourner au fleuve. Le vieux Zede n'a pas les moyens de nourrir la moindre bouche supplémentaire, mais ce n'est pas la vraie raison.

La vraie raison, c'est que je dois être près de ma sœur. Depuis sa naissance, c'est comme si nos cœurs étaient cousus ensemble. Je serais incapable de respirer dans un monde où elle ne serait pas près de moi.

Je dis à Silas ce que j'attends de lui. Il secoue la tête et, plus j'en parle, plus son visage s'allonge.

— Prends soin d'Arney, lui dis-je enfin. Elle n'a nulle part où retourner. Sa famille la maltraitait. Trouve-lui du travail, d'accord ? Le labeur ne lui fait pas peur.

Silas regarde filer le courant, pas moi.

— D'accord.

Silas et Arney se marieront peut-être dans quelques années, pensé-je.

Mon cœur se serre de plus belle.

Tout ce que j'espérais de la vie, je ne l'aurai jamais. Le chemin qui m'a conduite ici est inondé. Il n'y a pas de retour possible. C'est la véritable raison pour laquelle, quand nous trouvons le bateau de Zede, je lui dis que les Sevier seront ravis de nous reprendre, Fern et moi.

— J'ai juste besoin que Silas nous ramène au lac.

Je ne veux pas que Zede vienne. J'ai peur qu'il ne nous laisse pas partir au dernier moment.

Il jette un coup d'œil vers la porte ouverte de la cabine de son bateau, comme s'il se demandait s'il pouvait nous garder tous pour de bon.

— Chez les Sevier, Fern a plein de beaux habits, de jolis jouets. Et des pastels. Moi, je vais bientôt recommencer l'école.

Ma voix tremble et je me force à déglutir pour la stabiliser.

Lorsque le regard de Zede se tourne vers moi, j'ai l'impression qu'il ne me voit déjà plus.

Fern lui tend les bras, il la soulève et pose sa tête sur celle de ma sœur.

— Petite puce, sanglote-t-il avant de m'attirer contre lui pour nous serrer toutes les deux fort dans ses bras.

Il sent la cendre, le poisson, le pétrole, le fleuve. Des odeurs familières.

— Si vous avez besoin de moi un jour, faites passer le mot sur le fleuve.

J'acquiesce mais, quand il nous relâche, nous savons tous les deux que ce sont des adieux. Le fleuve est vaste.

La tristesse ronge son visage. Il se passe les mains sur la figure comme pour la chasser, puis hoche la tête, les lèvres pincées, avant de déposer Fern dans la *Jenny* pour que nous puissions partir.

— Y faut que j'vienne aussi, vous connaissez pas les marais, déclare Arney. Sauf que je resterai pas là-bas. Je vais ramener le bateau de mon père et l'amarrer quelque part, pas loin. Tu pourras lui dire où le trouver. Je veux rien lui devoir.

Sans attendre de réponse, elle va chercher le petit canot à moteur. Même après tout ce que sa famille lui a infligé, elle se demandait comment ils allaient se débrouiller sans leur barque.

Je ne pleure pas lorsque nous repartons. Le moteur Waterwitch lutte pour remonter le courant mais nous finissons par arriver à l'embouchure du marais. Les arbres se referment derrière nous lorsque nous nous y engageons et je jette un dernier coup d'œil en arrière. Je laisse le fleuve emporter une part de moi-même.

Les restes de Rill Foss.

Rill Foss, princesse du royaume d'Arcadie. Le roi n'est plus, le royaume non plus.

Rill Foss doit mourir avec lui.

Je suis May Weathers, à présent.

25

Avery

— Et c'est là que se termine mon histoire.

Les yeux bleus de May, embués, humides, m'observent de l'autre côté de la petite table éclairée par une lampe basse, dans une alcôve de la maison de retraite.

— Est-ce que tu es contente de connaître la vérité ? Ou bien n'est-ce qu'un fardeau ? Je me suis toujours demandé comment vous le prendriez, vous, les jeunes de la nouvelle génération. Je pensais ne jamais le savoir.

— Je crois... que c'est un peu des deux.

Même après avoir pris une semaine pour réfléchir à tout ça après notre visite du cottage et de la ferme de Hootsie, je lutte encore pour intégrer cette histoire à la mienne.

J'ai pesé sans fin les mises en garde d'Elliot, m'avertissant que je joue avec le feu – et que le passé devrait rester dans le passé. Les révélations stupéfiantes qui ont découlé de mon voyage près du fleuve Savannah ne l'ont pas fait changer d'avis. « Pense aux répercussions, Avery. Il y a des gens qui... ne verraient plus ta famille de la même façon. »

Par « des gens », j'ai l'impression qu'il veut dire « Bitsy ».

Le plus triste, c'est que Bitsy ne serait pas la seule. Si toute cette histoire devenait publique, impossible d'anticiper les implications que cela aurait sur notre avenir politique, notre réputation, le nom même des Stafford.

Même si les temps ont changé, les vieilles doctrines ont la vie dure. Si le monde devait découvrir que les Stafford ne sont pas vraiment ce que nous avons prétendu être, les conséquences seraient...

Je n'arrive même pas à l'imaginer.

Et cela m'effraie au plus haut point mais, en vérité, je supporte encore moins l'idée que ma grand-mère et sa sœur finissent leurs vies séparées l'une de l'autre. Au bout du compte, je dois savoir que j'ai agi au mieux pour mamie Judy.

— Une fois ou deux, j'ai envisagé de le dire à mes petits-enfants, m'apprend May. Mais ils ont leurs vies. Après la mort de mon fils, leur mère s'est remariée avec un homme qui avait déjà des enfants. Ce sont de jeunes gens formidables qui élèvent leur propre progéniture au milieu d'un tas d'oncles, de tantes et de cousins. C'est un peu pareil avec les enfants de mes sœurs. Lark s'était mariée avec un homme d'affaires qui s'était bâti un empire en construisant des centres commerciaux. Fern avait épousé un éminent docteur d'Atlanta. À elles deux, elles ont eu huit enfants, deux douzaines de petits-enfants et, bien sûr, des arrière-petits-enfants. Ils ont tous réussi, dans la vie, ils sont heureux et... occupés. Qu'est-ce qu'une vieille histoire pourrait leur apporter qu'ils n'ont pas déjà ?

May me dévisage, me regarde vaciller sur la ligne de démarcation qui est passée de sa génération à la mienne.

— Est-ce que tu partageras cette histoire avec ta famille ? me demande-t-elle.

Je déglutis avec peine, en guerre contre moi-même.

— Je le dirai à mon père. C'est sa décision plus que la mienne. Mamie Judy est sa mère.

Je ne sais pas du tout comment mon père prendra cette information, ni ce qu'il en fera.

— Une part de moi-même pense que Hootsie a raison. La vérité, c'est toujours la vérité. Elle a de la valeur.

— Hootsie... grommelle-t-elle. C'est comme ça qu'elle me remercie, après que je lui ai vendu ce bout de terrain à côté de l'ancienne propriété de ma grand-mère pour que Ted et elle puissent y construire leur ferme. Après toutes ces années, elle dévoile mes secrets.

— Je pense vraiment qu'elle l'a fait pour votre bien. Elle voulait que je comprenne le lien entre ma grand-mère et toi. Elle pensait à vous deux.

May chasse cette idée d'un geste de la main comme une mouche bourdonnant autour de sa tête.

— Pff ! Hootsie est une mêle-tout. Elle a toujours été comme ça. C'est d'ailleurs aussi pour ça que je suis restée chez les Sevier, finalement. Quand nous sommes arrivés à leur maison, Silas m'avait presque convaincue de prendre le fleuve avec lui. Sur la berge, il m'a attrapée par les épaules pour m'embrasser. C'était mon premier baiser.

Elle glousse, ses joues rosissent et ses yeux pétillent comme ceux d'une enfant. J'entrevois un instant la fille de douze ans sur la berge du lac.

— « Je t'aime, Rill, qu'il m'a dit. Je t'attendrai ici une heure. J'attendrai que tu reviennes. Je peux prendre soin de toi, Rill. C'est vrai. » Je savais qu'il me faisait des promesses intenables. Quelques mois seulement plus tôt, c'était un vagabond qui sautait de train en train, clandestinement, pour tenter de survivre. S'il y avait une chose que j'avais apprise en observant Briny et Queenie, c'est qu'on ne vit pas d'amour et d'eau fraîche. L'amour ne suffit pas à protéger une famille.

Sourcils froncés, elle hoche la tête, comme pour approuver sa propre conclusion.

— Vouloir et pouvoir, ce sont deux choses bien différentes. J'imagine que, d'une certaine façon, je savais que Silas et moi n'étions pas faits pour être ensemble. Pas alors que nous étions si jeunes, du moins. Pourtant, quand j'ai commencé à remonter l'allée avec Fern, tout ce que je voulais, c'était rebrousser chemin vers ce garçon brun et retourner au fleuve. Je l'aurais peut-être fait sans Hootsie. Elle a choisi à ma place, sans me laisser le temps de me décider. Mon plan, c'était de me glisser jusqu'à l'orée des bois et de m'y cacher, le temps de m'assurer que les Sevier acceptaient de reprendre Fern. J'étais morte de peur qu'on me surprenne, qu'on me renvoie au foyer, ou loin dans une maison de correction pour mauvaises filles, ou même en prison. Mais Hootsie était dehors, à déterrer des tubercules pour sa mère et, dès qu'elle nous a vues en bas, près du jardin, elle est partie en hurlant. Presque aussitôt, Zuma, Hoy, M. et Mme Sevier dévalaient la colline, les chiens en tête. Je n'avais nulle part où m'enfuir, alors je suis restée là et j'ai attendu que le pire arrive.

Elle marque une pause et je me retrouve en équilibre au bord du précipice où elle m'a laissée.

— Et qu'est-ce qui s'est passé ?

— J'ai appris qu'il ne faut pas forcément être née dans une famille pour être aimée par elle.

— Alors, ils ont accepté que tu reviennes ?

Une esquisse de sourire tiraille sa bouche.

— Oui, ils m'ont acceptée. Papa Sevier, et Hoy et les autres hommes nous avaient cherchées dans les marais pendant des semaines. Ils savaient qu'on avait dû partir par bateau avec Arney. Lorsque nous sommes revenues, ils avaient perdu tout espoir de nous retrouver.

Elle rit doucement.

— Même Zuma et Hootsie nous ont serrées dans leurs bras, ce jour-là, tant elles étaient contentes de nous voir en vie.

— Et vous avez vécu heureuses avec les Sevier, ensuite ?

— Ils se sont montrés compréhensifs, après ce que nous avions fait, quand ils ont appris la vérité pour l'*Arcadie.* Ou du moins ce que j'avais réussi à leur en révéler. J'avais décidé de ne jamais leur dire qu'il y avait d'autres enfants, en plus de Fern et moi. J'imagine que, dans mon cœur de fille de douze ans, j'avais encore honte de ne pas avoir réussi à protéger Camellia, Lark et Gabion. Je craignais que les Sevier ne m'aiment plus s'ils l'apprenaient. Ils avaient bon cœur – ils étaient patients et gentils. Ils m'ont appris à trouver la musique.

— La musique ?

Elle tend la main vers moi pour me serrer les doigts.

— Oui, la musique, ma chérie. Vois-tu, il y a une chose que j'ai apprise en suivant les traces de papa Sevier en grandissant. La vie n'est guère différente du cinéma. Chaque scène a sa propre musique, et la musique est créée pour cette scène précise, elle s'y entrelace d'une façon qui nous échappe. Que nous aimions de tout notre cœur la mélodie d'un jour passé ou que nous imaginions la chanson d'un jour à venir, nous devons danser sur la musique du présent, sans quoi nous serons toujours à contretemps, à chanceler dans un écho qui ne correspond pas à l'ici et le maintenant. J'ai laissé partir le chant du fleuve et j'ai découvert la musique de cette grande maison. J'ai trouvé de la place pour une nouvelle vie, une nouvelle mère pour qui je comptais, un nouveau père qui m'a appris patiemment non seulement la musique, mais surtout à faire confiance. C'était l'homme le plus gentil que j'aie jamais connu. Oh, ce ne fut jamais comme l'*Arcadie*, bien sûr, pourtant, c'était une vie agréable. Nous étions aimées, choyées et protégées.

Un soupir soulève ses épaules puis la quitte.

— À me voir maintenant, on croirait que je n'ai jamais compris le secret... Mais cette musique-ci, la musique de la vieillesse... n'est pas faite pour danser. Elle est si... solitaire. Nous sommes un fardeau pour tout le monde.

Je repense à ma grand-mère, à sa maison déserte, à sa chambre dans la maison de retraite, à son incapacité à me reconnaître, la plupart du temps. Les larmes me montent aux yeux. La musique de la vieillesse est bien dure à écouter, lorsqu'elle se joue pour quelqu'un qu'on aime. Je me demande si ma grand-mère reconnaîtra May, lorsqu'elles seront enfin réunies. May acceptera-t-elle seulement de me suivre ? Je ne lui ai pas encore demandé. Trent attend dans le couloir. Il est venu en voiture depuis Edisto. Après avoir discuté des différentes possibilités, nous avons décidé qu'il valait mieux que je parle d'abord seule à seule avec May.

— Est-ce que tu as revu Silas ?

La question semble sortir de nulle part. Pourtant, je sais que je la lui pose parce que je pense à Trent... et au récit du premier amour de May. Bizarrement, j'y pense souvent, ces derniers temps. Le sourire de Trent, ses blagues idiotes, sa proximité, même sa simple voix au téléphone m'émeut, parfois. Le fait

405

qu'il se fiche complètement de savoir ce que mon histoire familiale a pu être ou ce que je décide d'en révéler me touche d'une façon qui me prend au dépourvu. Je ne sais même pas comment décrire ce sentiment, ni comment l'inclure dans ma vie.

Je sais seulement que je ne peux pas l'ignorer.

L'expression de May me transperce. Comme si elle creusait et suivait les veines de mes émotions jusqu'à mon âme.

— Je l'ai souhaité de tout mon cœur, mais certains souhaits ne se réalisent jamais. Papa Sevier nous a fait déménager jusqu'à Augusta pour nous protéger de Georgia Tann. Comme notre famille y était assez connue, il devait penser qu'elle n'oserait pas s'attaquer à lui par-delà les frontières de l'État. Silas et le vieux Zede ne pouvaient pas nous trouver. Je n'ai jamais su ce qui leur était arrivé. La dernière fois que j'ai vu Silas, c'était à travers les mèches de cheveux de ma nouvelle mère tandis qu'elle me serrait contre elle. Il est resté à l'orée des bois, où je m'étais tenue un instant plus tôt, puis il a tourné les talons pour regagner l'eau. Je ne l'ai jamais revu.

Elle secoue doucement la tête.

— Je me suis toujours demandé ce qu'il était devenu. Il valait peut-être mieux que je ne le sache pas. Je m'habituais à une nouvelle vie, un nouveau monde, un nouveau nom. En revanche, j'ai eu des nouvelles d'Arney, des années plus tard. Une lettre est arrivée de nulle part. Ma mère me l'avait mise de côté quand je suis rentrée à la maison à la fin du trimestre universitaire. Je m'étais toujours dit qu'Arney et Silas se marieraient un jour, mais non. Zede avait trouvé un travail pour Arney dans une laiterie, peu après notre départ. Même si ses patrons la faisaient travailler dur, ils étaient justes avec elle. Elle a fini par se faire embaucher dans une usine de production de bombardiers et par épouser un soldat. Ils vivaient à l'étranger quand elle m'a écrit, et elle était ravie de voir le monde. Jamais elle n'aurait cru avoir ce genre d'opportunité, dans la vie.

Aujourd'hui encore, cette histoire la fait sourire.

— Je suis contente que les choses aient bien tourné pour elle, après une enfance si difficile, dis-je.

Étant donné que May a quatre-vingt-dix ans et que Arney était plus âgée qu'elle, il est peu probable qu'elle soit toujours en vie, mais j'éprouve tout de même un certain soulagement. L'histoire de May a rendu Arney et Silas, et tous les autres habitants du fleuve, très vivants pour moi.

— En effet, confirme-t-elle avec un signe de tête. Elle a allumé en moi un feu qui a continué à brûler pour toutes les jeunes ingénues dont les play-boys de Hollywood profitaient. J'en ai rencontré tellement durant mes années là-bas... et je me faisais un devoir de les aider – je leur offrais un endroit où dormir ou une épaule pour s'épancher. Cela arrivait très souvent, des filles qui se retrouvaient dans des situations terribles. Je repensais sans cesse aux mots qu'Arney m'avait écrits au bas de sa lettre.

— Qu'est-ce qu'elle disait ?

— Que je l'avais sauvée.

May se tamponne le coin de l'œil.

— Évidemment, c'était faux. Nous nous sommes sauvées mutuellement. Sans elle pour me ramener jusqu'au fleuve, sans ce qui s'est passé sur l'*Arcadie*, je n'aurais jamais pu laisser partir Briny et Queenie, et le fleuve. Arney m'a permis d'avancer. C'est ce que je lui ai répondu.

— J'imagine que cela signifiait beaucoup pour elle.

— Les gens n'entrent jamais par accident dans nos vies.

— C'est vrai.

De nouveau, je pense à Trent. De nouveau, je me sens déchirée entre mes propres sentiments, et les espoirs et projets que ma famille a toujours eus pour moi. Des projets auxquels j'avais toujours cru adhérer.

— Arney et moi, nous sommes restées en contact au fil des années, poursuit May tandis que je m'efforce de me reglisser dans son histoire et d'oublier mes inquiétudes concernant le reste de la journée. C'était une femme remarquable. Son mari et elle ont fondé leur propre entreprise de construction lorsqu'ils sont rentrés au pays. Elle travaillait avec lui, au côté des autres hommes, et elle tenait le coup. J'imagine que ces maisons étaient aussi solides qu'il était possible de les faire. Elles nous survivront à tous.

— Je n'en doute pas.

May se tourne vers moi d'un air résolu et se penche de façon presque intime, comme si elle voulait me révéler un secret.

— Le passé d'une femme ne prédit pas nécessairement son avenir. Elle peut danser sur une musique nouvelle si elle le choisit. Sa propre musique. Pour en entendre l'air, elle doit juste s'arrêter de parler. À elle-même, je veux dire. Nous essayons toujours de nous persuader d'un tas de choses.

Je suis frappée par la profondeur de ses paroles. Sent-elle que, depuis notre visite au cottage sur le fleuve, depuis que j'ai appris la vérité sur ma grand-mère, j'ai remis toute ma vie en question ?

Je ne veux blesser personne, mais je souhaite trouver ma propre musique. May m'a convaincue que c'était possible. Ce qui m'amène au motif réel de ma visite à la maison de retraite.

— Je me demandais si tu voudrais bien m'accompagner quelque part, cet après-midi, dis-je finalement.

— Et puis-je savoir où ? dit-elle en se levant déjà de son fauteuil, les deux mains sur les accoudoirs.

— Est-ce que tu accepterais quand même de venir si je ne te le dis pas à l'avance ?

— Est-ce que c'est hors de ces murs sordides ?

— Oui.

Elle est étonnamment alerte lorsqu'elle se met sur ses pieds.

— Dans ce cas, j'imagine que je me moque de savoir où nous allons. Je suis tout à toi. Tant que tu ne m'emmènes pas à un meeting politique, cela dit. Je hais la politique.

— Non, rien de politique, lui promets-je en riant.

— Parfait.

Nous sortons dans le couloir, côte à côte, May poussant son déambulateur avec une vitesse surprenante. Je m'attends presque à ce qu'elle le jette de côté pour se mettre à courir vers la porte.

— Trent attend dehors pour nous y conduire.

— Le bel homme aux yeux bleus ?

— Oui, celui-là même.

— Oh, j'ai vraiment hâte d'y être.

Elle baisse la tête, soucieuse, vers son T-shirt et son pantalon en coton aux allures de pyjama.

— Je ne suis pas très bien habillée. Je devrais peut-être me changer ?

— Je pense que tu seras très bien comme ça.

Elle n'insiste pas lorsque nous passons devant sa chambre. En fait, elle s'attarde juste le temps de prendre son sac à main.

Trent se lève de son fauteuil lorsque nous arrivons dans le hall. Il me sourit et lève le pouce dans le dos de May lorsqu'elle informe la dame de l'accueil que nous la faisons sortir tout l'après-midi. Elle me tend son déambulateur et opte pour le bras de Trent quand nous franchissons la porte. Je n'ai plus qu'à plier l'appareil et à le ranger dans le coffre pendant que Trent installe May dans la voiture. Heureusement, j'ai une certaine expérience avec ce genre de chose.

May raconte son histoire à Trent pendant le trajet – toute son histoire, pas seulement les morceaux qu'elle nous avait confiés après notre premier jour de fouilles dans le cabanon derrière la maison de Trent à Edisto. Trent croise mon regard à intervalles réguliers dans le rétroviseur et secoue la tête, impressionné et triste. Il est difficile de croire que, il n'y a pas si longtemps encore, les orphelins étaient à peine plus que du bétail.

May est tellement perdue dans son récit, ou tellement charmée par Trent, qu'elle ne remarque pas où nous allons. Ce n'est que lorsque nous nous rapprochons d'Augusta qu'elle se penche vers la fenêtre en soupirant.

— Vous me ramenez chez moi. Vous auriez dû me le dire. J'aurais enfilé mes baskets.

Trent jette un coup d'œil vers les chaussons plats de May.

— Ça ira, la rassure-t-il. Votre voisin a tondu la pelouse.

— Il est vrai que Hootsie a élevé les enfants les plus gentils qui soient. Même si c'est dur à croire. Elle était si mauvaise... Je me suis chamaillée avec elle plus qu'avec mes sœurs.

Trent sourit.

— Après avoir fait sa connaissance, je n'ai aucun mal à le croire.

Il a discuté avec Hootsie de notre visite d'aujourd'hui. Bart et elle ont remué ciel et terre pour la rendre possible.

May remarque la différence lorsque nous passons devant la maison de Hootsie : sur le chemin de la ferme, la route a été entièrement dégagée, du bois jusqu'au cottage. Nous nous garons sur du gravier fraîchement répandu devant le portail.

— Qui a fait tout cela ?

May regarde la pelouse tout juste tondue, les jardins impeccables, la véranda et les fauteuils qui attendent derrière la moustiquaire.

— J'avais peur que vous ne soyez pas capable de marcher jusqu'ici, lui expliqué-je. Cela semblait le plus pratique. J'espère que cela ne vous dérange pas.

En guise de réponse, elle s'essuie les yeux, les lèvres pressées, tremblantes.

— Je me disais que vous voudriez revenir plus souvent, ensuite. Ma grand-mère a un abonnement avec la compagnie de taxis. Ils connaissent le chemin.

— Je ne suis pas certaine... qu'on me laisse venir, murmure-t-elle. La maison de retraite... Je ne veux pas non plus qu'ils appellent mes petits-enfants et qu'ils les embêtent avec ça.

— J'en ai parlé avec un ami, un homme qui préside une association militant pour les droits des seniors. Je pense qu'on pourra vous aider sur certaines questions. Vous n'êtes pas prisonnière dans cet établissement, May. Ils essaient juste d'assurer votre sécurité.

Je la laisse digérer ces informations. Nous pourrons discuter plus tard des suggestions d'Andrew Moore – il voudrait entre autres proposer à May de faire du bénévolat pour l'association, afin que sa vie retrouve du sens. Andrew est un homme remarquable, plein d'idées. Je crois que May l'apprécierait.

Pour l'instant, elle est trop émerveillée par la vue pour parler d'autre chose. Elle pose la tête contre la vitre du siège passager et ne parvient plus à contenir ses larmes.

— Oh... oh, je suis chez moi. Je pensais ne jamais plus revoir ma maison.

— Hootsie et sa petite-fille l'ont entretenue pour vous.

— Mais... je n'ai pas pu la payer... depuis...

Les larmes interrompent ses paroles.

— Depuis qu'ils m'ont emmenée.

— Elle dit que cela ne la dérange pas.

J'ouvre ma portière pendant que Trent contourne la voiture. J'ajoute :

— Elle vous aime beaucoup, vous savez.

— Elle a dit ça ?

— Eh bien, non, mais c'est évident.

May pousse un soupir sceptique et, une fois encore, j'entrevois la malice d'une fille du fleuve.

— Vous m'avez fait craindre que Hootsie ait perdu la boule, me lance-t-elle, un sourire en coin, avant de laisser Trent l'aider à sortir de voiture. Hootsie et moi, nous ne nous sommes jamais fait de cadeaux. Ce serait dommage de gâcher cela maintenant en devenant sentimentales.

Je regarde à travers les arbres les ruines de la maison coloniale lorsque je me lève et m'étire. J'ai du mal à appréhender l'évolution de la relation de ces deux femmes, au fil des années.

— Tu pourras le dire à Hootsie en personne, si tu veux. Elle va passer tout à l'heure. Je lui ai demandé de nous laisser un peu de temps seuls, d'abord.

May me jette une œillade suspicieuse tout en avançant vers le portail, la main lovée au creux du coude de Trent.

— Qu'est-ce que vous comptiez faire, ici ? Je vous ai tout raconté, cette fois-ci. Vous connaissez toute l'histoire.

Au loin, j'entends déjà le moteur d'une voiture, sur l'allée menant à la ferme. May ne l'a pas encore remarqué, ce qui vaut sans doute mieux. Je pensais la faire entrer dans le cottage et l'y installer. Mais le planning va être plus serré que prévu. C'est bien ma mère, ça, d'arriver en avance, même si elle n'a aucune idée de là où elle va ni de ce qui l'attend.

— J'ai demandé à mes parents de venir.

Je n'ai pas trouvé de meilleurs moyens de les faire croire à cette histoire que de la leur montrer. Sinon, j'ai peur qu'ils pensent que j'ai complètement perdu la raison.

— Le sénateur ? articule May, horrifiée, avant de se tapoter les cheveux.

Trent tente d'attirer May vers le portail, mais elle s'accroche au poteau comme un enfant qu'on emmène chez le médecin pour une piqûre.

— Dieu du ciel ! Je t'ai demandé si j'avais besoin de me changer. Je ne peux pas le rencontrer dans cette tenue.

Je sens toutes mes bonnes intentions se heurter aux murailles de l'étiquette et rien ne peut détruire ce genre de remparts. J'ai eu toutes les peines du monde à convaincre mes parents d'adhérer à mon plan mystérieux de cet après-midi. Je leur ai dit que c'était pour faire une faveur à une amie, sauf que ma mère repère un mensonge à des kilomètres. Elle sonnera l'alerte rouge dès qu'elle arrivera ici, surtout vu l'étrangeté de la requête et ce lieu reculé.

Pourtant, mon plan va réussir, que les différents protagonistes le veuillent ou non et, en mon for intérieur, je sais que je l'ai organisé ainsi exprès. J'avais peur que, en m'y prenant autrement, je manque de courage.

— Eh bien, dépêchez-vous ! lance soudain May, qui tire sur le bras de Trent et manque le faire tomber. Il me reste plein de vêtements dans mes armoires. J'y trouverai une tenue correcte.

À travers les arbres, je vois la voiture blanche de la compagnie de taxis.

— Nous n'avons pas le temps. Ils sont au bout de la route.

Les narines de May se dilatent.

— Est-ce que Hootsie était au courant de tout ça ?

— Oui et non, mais c'était mon idée. S'il te plaît. Fais-moi confiance. Je pense vraiment que ce sera mieux pour tout le monde.

Après cette rencontre, soit nous serons plus proches que jamais, soit May ne voudra plus me parler.

— Je crois que je vais m'évanouir.

May s'affaisse contre Trent. Je ne sais pas si c'est du cinéma ou non.

Trent passe son bras autour de ses épaules, prêt à la soutenir.

— Et si je vous guidais jusqu'à la maison ?

Elle se laisse entraîner, trop sonnée pour protester.

J'attends au portail. Quand la limousine s'arrête, ma mère sort de son côté sans même attendre qu'Oz vienne lui ouvrir la portière. Pomme d'amour est folle de rage.

— Avery Judith Stafford, dis-moi immédiatement ce qui se passe ici ! J'étais certaine que le conducteur était perdu ou que nous avions été kidnappés !

À voir son visage rouge et brillant de sueur, il est évident qu'elle bouillonne de colère depuis des kilomètres, qu'elle s'est sans doute plainte à mon père, sans parler de ce pauvre Oz, qui a dû s'en prendre plein la tête alors que, s'il s'est trouvé mêlé à tout cela, c'est uniquement parce qu'il connaît le chemin.

— Je t'ai appelée sur ton portable au moins quinze fois. Pourquoi tu n'as pas décroché ?

— Je crois qu'il n'y a pas de réseau, par ici.

J'ignore complètement si c'est vrai. J'ai laissé mon téléphone éteint toute la matinée. Si Pomme d'amour ne pouvait pas me joindre pour annuler ou modifier ce que nous avions prévu, elle n'avait pas le choix, elle était obligée de venir. Pomme d'amour ne manque jamais un engagement.

— Allons, les filles... lance mon père, plus accommodant.

Contrairement à ma mère, il aime les chemins cahoteux de campagne. Maintenant que les saignements intestinaux ont été stoppés par la chirurgie laparoscopique, ses analyses sanguines sont meilleures et il a repris des forces. De nouveau en pleine possession de ses moyens, il est de taille à affronter ses adversaires sur la question des chaînes de maisons de retraite. Il a commencé une campagne de démenti. Il rassemble aussi un comité de soutien pour un projet de loi évitant que les propriétaires des maisons de retraite ne se servent de sociétés-écrans pour éviter de payer les dommages et intérêts.

Il couve le fleuve d'un regard intéressé.

— C'était une charmante promenade dominicale. Il y avait longtemps que nous n'étions pas venus dans la région d'Augusta. Si j'avais su, j'aurais apporté ma canne à pêche et le reste de mon matériel.

Il me sourit et je repense aussitôt nos moments passés ensemble, à mes visites de petite fille à son bureau, à nos virées à la pêche peu fructueuses, jusqu'au bal de fin d'année, à la remise des diplômes... et plus récemment, aux briefings, aux réunions stratégiques et aux déplacements publics.

— Ce n'est pas si souvent qu'elle nous demande quelque chose, Pomme d'amour, ajoute-t-il en me glissant un clin d'œil. Au contraire de ses sœurs.

Il veut me rassurer, me faire comprendre que, quoi que nous ayons prévu aujourd'hui, il est partant. Cela me rappelle tout ce que j'ai à perdre, dans cette histoire – et, au premier chef, la préférence de mon père. Oui, je suis sa fille préférée. J'ai toujours été sa petite merveille.

Comment prendra-t-il le fait que, pendant des semaines, j'ai fureté en douce, j'ai déterré des informations que ma grand-mère avait gardées secrètes pour protéger l'héritage des Stafford ?

Que se passera-t-il ensuite, quand je leur dirai que cette exploration a changé ma vie ? Je ne veux pas vivre comme ma grand-mère. Je veux pouvoir être qui je suis vraiment, au fond de moi. Cela pourrait ou non signifier que la dynastie politique des Stafford s'arrêtera après mon père. Avec un peu de chance, son état de santé lui permettra de continuer longtemps. Sur pied, il arrivera à vaincre cette controverse autour des maisons de retraite et il en sortira de bonnes choses. J'en suis persuadée.

Je serai là pour l'aider de toutes les façons possibles mais, à dire vrai, je ne suis pas prête pour me présenter à une élection. Je n'ai pas assez d'expérience en la matière. Je n'ai pas gagné le droit de le faire. Ce poste ne devrait pas m'être proposé juste parce que je suis qui je suis. Je veux gagner ma légitimité à l'ancienne. Je veux prendre le temps d'avoir une compréhension globale des dossiers – et tous, pas juste quelques sujets – et de me forger ma propre opinion. Si jamais mon tour vient un jour, je me présenterai grâce à mon propre mérite, pas en tant que la fille de mon père. En attendant, Andrew Moore m'a signalé que l'Association de défense des droits des seniors qu'il dirige cherche un bon avocat. Le salaire est sans doute très bas, mais ce n'est pas le sujet. Si je veux m'aventurer dans les eaux boueuses de la vie politique, c'est le genre d'endroit par lequel une personne normale commencerait, et je suis une bonne avocate.

Est-ce que mon père comprendra ?

Est-ce qu'il m'aimera toujours ?

Bien sûr. Quelle question. Il a toujours été un père, avant tout. Je sais que c'est vrai. Oui, il y aura des conséquences, et nous y survivrons. Comme toujours.

— Avery, je refuse que ta grand-mère sorte de voiture dans cet endroit.

Le regard de Pomme d'amour glisse sur le petit cottage, le fleuve au pied de la colline, les arbres trop grands qui penchent au-dessus du toit du porche. Elle croise les bras et se frotte les biceps.

— Pomme d'amour, susurre mon père pour l'amadouer, tout en m'adressant un sourire indulgent. Avery ne nous aurait pas fait venir jusqu'ici sans une bonne raison.

Il se penche près d'elle, glisse un bras autour de sa taille et lui chatouille le point sensible qu'il est le seul à connaître. C'est son arme secrète.

— Arrête ! lance-t-elle en réprimant un sourire.

Le regard qu'elle braque sur moi est beaucoup moins joyeux.

— Avery, pour l'amour du ciel, est-ce que tout cela était vraiment nécessaire ? Pourquoi tant de mystères ? Pourquoi venir ici dans une limousine ? Et pourquoi faillait-il obligatoirement que nous traînions ta pauvre grand-mère ? Sortir de Magnolia Manor est très perturbant pour elle. Ensuite, elle a du mal à retrouver ses repères.

— Je voulais voir si elle se souvient de quelque chose.

— Je doute qu'elle se souvienne de cet endroit.

— De quelqu'un, en fait.

— Enfin, elle ne peut pas connaître quelqu'un qui habite ici, Avery. Je crois qu'il vaut mieux que...

— Maman, je te demande juste d'entrer là, avec moi. Mamie Judy est déjà venue. Je suis sûre qu'elle va s'en souvenir.

— Est-ce que quelqu'un compte me faire sortir un jour ? s'impatiente ma grand-mère dans la voiture.

Oz nous regarde. Mon père hoche la tête. Il a peur que, s'il lâche Pomme d'amour, elle s'enfuie aussi sec.

Devant le portail, je prends ma grand-mère par le bras et nous remontons l'allée ensemble. Malgré son déclin mental, mamie Judy n'a que soixante-dix-huit ans et se déplace encore très bien. Sa démence n'en paraît que plus injuste.

Je l'observe pendant notre avancée. Son visage s'éclaire un peu plus à chaque pas. Son regard file ici et là, s'attardant un instant sur les rosiers grimpants, les azalées, le banc près du fleuve, la vieille clôture en bois, la glycine, une clématite, un bassin à oiseaux en bronze arborant deux statues de petites filles jouant dans l'eau.

— Oh, murmure-t-elle. Oh, comme j'aime cet endroit... Il y avait longtemps, non ?

— Je crois, dis-je.

— Ça me manquait... ça me manquait tellement...

Ma mère et mon père hésitent au sommet des marches du perron, nous regardent tour à tour, ma grand-mère et moi, en clignant des yeux, bouche bée. Pomme d'amour est dans une situation qu'elle ne contrôle pas et, de ce fait, elle déteste déjà cette journée, quoi qu'il puisse arriver.

— Avery Judith, tu ferais mieux de t'expliquer.

— Maman ! dis-je sèchement, et Pomme d'amour a un mouvement de recul car je ne lui ai jamais parlé sur ce ton, même en trente ans. Laisse mamie Judy voir ce dont elle se souvient.

Une main posée sur l'épaule de ma grand-mère, je la guide jusqu'au seuil, puis à l'intérieur. Elle s'arrête un instant, ses yeux s'accommodant au changement de luminosité.

Je l'observe pendant qu'elle inspecte les lieux, les photos, le tableau au-dessus de la cheminée.

Il lui faut un moment avant de se rendre compte qu'il y a quelqu'un dans la pièce.

— Oh, oh... May ! dit-elle aussi naturellement que si elles s'étaient vues hier.

— Judy.

May tente de se lever du canapé mais il est trop mou et, comme elle n'arrive pas à se mettre sur ses pieds, elle tend les bras à sa sœur. Trent, qui s'apprêtait à l'aider, recule.

Ma grand-mère se hâte de traverser la pièce. Je la laisse faire seule. Les larmes aux yeux, May lève un peu plus les bras, en tendant et en pliant les doigts pour appeler sa sœur. Mamie Judy, qui bien souvent ne sait plus comment se comporter avec les gens, n'hésite pas un instant. Comme si c'était la chose la plus naturelle au monde, elle se penche et prend May dans ses bras. Elle partage l'accolade tremblante du vieil âge. May ferme les yeux, le menton niché sur l'épaule de sa sœur. Elles s'accrochent l'une à l'autre jusqu'à ce que ma grand-mère, épuisée, se laisse tomber dans le fauteuil près du canapé. Elles se tiennent la main au-dessus de la table basse. Elles se dévisagent comme s'il n'y avait personne d'autre dans la pièce.

— J'ai cru que je ne te reverrai jamais, avoue May.

Le sourire radieux de ma grand-mère semble tout ignorer des obstacles qui les séparaient.

— Tu sais que je viendrai toujours. Le mardi. Le jour des sœurs. Où est passée Fern, aujourd'hui ? demande-t-elle en pointant du doigt une chaise à bascule près de la fenêtre.

May soulève leurs mains jointes et les secoue un peu.

— Fern n'est plus là, ma chérie. Elle est décédée dans son sommeil.

— Fern ?

Les épaules de ma grand-mère s'affaissent et ses yeux s'embuent. Une larme suinte au coin de son œil et glisse le long de son nez.

— Oh... Fern.

— Il ne reste plus que nous deux, maintenant.

— Lark est avec nous.

— Lark est morte il y a cinq ans. Le cancer, tu te rappelles ?

Mamie Judy s'affaisse un peu plus, écrase une autre larme.

— Bon sang, j'avais oublié. Je n'ai plus toute ma tête, tu sais.

— Peu importe, la rassure May en couvrant leurs doigts joints de sa main libre. Tu te souviens de la première semaine que nous avons passée ensemble, à Edisto ? demande-t-elle avec un signe de tête vers le tableau au-dessus de la cheminée. C'était beau, non ? Toutes les quatre, réunies ? Fern adorait cet endroit.

— Oui, c'était beau.

Mamie Judy approuve. Je ne sais pas si elle se souvient vraiment ou si elle essaie juste d'être polie, mais elle sourit au tableau et, tout à coup, son esprit semble s'éclaircir.

— Tu nous as donné les bracelets libellules. Trois libellules, en souvenir des trois que nous n'avons jamais revus. Camellia, Gabion et mon frère jumeau. Nous célébrions l'anniversaire de Camellia, l'après-midi où tu nous les as donnés, non ? Camellia était la libellule aux yeux d'onyx.

La lumière du souvenir illumine les yeux de ma grand-mère. L'amour des sœurs réchauffe son sourire.

— Dis donc, nous étions de vraies beautés, à cette époque.

— Oui, en effet. Nous avions toutes les jolis cheveux de maman, mais tu as été la seule à hériter de son doux visage. Si je ne savais pas que c'est toi, sur cette peinture, je pourrais croire que c'était notre maman qui était là, avec nous.

Derrière moi, ma mère siffle entre ses dents :

— Mais qu'est-ce qui se passe ici ?

Je sens la chaleur émaner de son corps. Elle transpire. Or, Pomme d'amour ne transpire jamais.

— Nous devrions peut-être ressortir.

J'essaie d'entraîner mes parents sur la galerie. Mon père n'a pas l'air d'avoir envie de sortir de la pièce. Il est trop occupé à fixer les photos, à tenter de comprendre ce que tout cela signifie. Est-ce que, quelque part en lui, il a retrouvé le souvenir des absences inexpliquées de sa mère ? Est-ce qu'il se rappelle être sur l'arrière-fond de ce tableau ? A-t-il toujours soupçonné que sa mère était davantage que la femme qu'il connaissait ?

À l'autre bout de la pièce, Trent m'adresse un hochement de tête juste avant que je referme la porte derrière nous. Grâce à son encouragement, je me sens forte, capable, confiante. Il est de ceux qui croient que la vérité doit être révélée, quelle qu'elle soit. Hootsie et lui ont cela en commun.

— Vous devriez vous asseoir avant de m'écouter, dis-je à mes parents.

À contrecœur, Pomme d'amour s'assied au bord d'un fauteuil à bascule. Mon père choisit la balancelle à deux places et adopte une posture qui m'indique qu'il s'attend à une révélation grave et déplaisante. Penché en avant, les pieds bien à plat, les coudes sur les genoux, les doigts en clocher devant son menton. Quelle que soit la situation, il est prêt à l'analyser et à évaluer les dégâts.

— Laissez-moi parler sans m'interrompre. Ne me posez par de questions avant la fin, d'accord ?

Sans attendre de réponse, j'inspire un bon coup et je commence l'histoire.

Mon père écoute attentivement, derrière son masque stoïque habituel. Ma mère finit par s'avachir dans son fauteuil à bascule, le poignet sur le front.

À la fin de mon récit, un silence pesant s'installe. Personne ne sait quoi dire. Il est évident que mon père ne se doutait absolument de rien, même si quelque chose dans son expression m'indique qu'il comprend enfin quelques détails du comportement de sa mère.

— Comment... comment sais-tu que tout cela est vrai ? Cette... cette femme... peut-être que...

Ma mère laisse sa phrase en suspens, regarde vers la fenêtre du cottage. Elle pense à ce qu'elle a entendu à l'intérieur, aux photos sur les murs.

— Je ne comprends vraiment pas comment c'est possible.

Mon père souffle au-dessus de ses doigts joints, sourcils grisonnants froncés. Lui, il sait que c'est possible, même s'il veut que cela ne le soit pas. Mais je lui ai dit ce que Trent et moi avons appris à propos de la Société des foyers d'accueil du Tennessee, et je vois bien que ce n'était pas une nouvelle pour lui ou ma mère. Ils avaient dû entendre parler du scandale ou voir les téléfilms reproduisant la vie dans les célèbres orphelinats de Georgia Tann.

— Je ne... Ma mère ? marmonne mon père. Est-ce que mon père le savait ?

— Je ne pense pas que quiconque était au courant. Mamie Judy et ses sœurs étaient déjà adultes lorsqu'elles se sont retrouvées. May m'a dit qu'elles ne voulaient pas s'immiscer dans les vies les unes des autres. Étant donné que les archives étaient scellées pour empêcher les familles biologiques de retrouver leurs membres, c'est un miracle que quatre d'entre elles ont été réunies.

— Mon Dieu... souffle-t-il en secouant la tête comme pour réarranger ses idées, pour les hiérarchiser. Ma mère avait un frère jumeau ?

— À sa naissance, oui. Elle l'a cherché pendant des années mais elle n'a jamais pu découvrir ce qui lui était arrivé – s'il est mort ou s'il a survécu et été adopté.

Mon père pose son menton sur ses mains. Il lève les yeux vers les arbres.

— Dieu du ciel...

Je sais ce qu'il pense. J'ai retourné ces idées dans tous les sens depuis que j'ai appris la vérité. Toute la semaine, j'ai hésité entre emporter ce secret dans ma tombe... et libérer la vérité, quoi qu'il advienne. Au bout du compte, j'en suis arrivée à cette conclusion : mon père mérite de savoir qui il est. Ma grand-mère mérite de passer le temps qu'il lui reste au côté de sa sœur.

Les cinq enfants du fleuve qui ont souffert aux mains de la Société des foyers d'accueil méritent que leurs histoires traversent le temps. Sans un étrange coup du sort, la mère de mon père aurait grandi sur un bateau de fortune, parmi des gens ordinaires, au milieu de la pauvreté de la Grande Dépression.

Elle n'aurait pas fréquenté la haute société, elle n'aurait pas pu rencontrer mon grand-père et encore moins l'épouser.

Nous ne serions pas des Stafford.

Ma mère se reprend un peu, relève le menton et tend le bras pour dénouer les mains de mon père et en prendre une dans la sienne.

— C'est du passé. Inutile de se torturer avec cela maintenant, Wells. Il n'y aucune raison d'en parler à qui que ce soit.

Sur ces mots, elle me glisse un regard en coin – une mise en garde.

Je me retiens de bondir. Pour moi, il n'y a pas de retour en arrière possible.

— Papa, c'est à toi de décider de la suite. Tout ce que je demande, c'est que mamie Judy puisse profiter de sa sœur... quel que soit le temps qu'il leur reste. Elles ont passé toute leur vie à se cacher du monde, pour notre bien. Elles méritent d'être en paix, maintenant.

Mon père embrasse les doigts de ma mère, les replie entre les siens et hoche la tête. Il nous dit silencieusement qu'il réfléchira longuement à tout cela et prendra ses propres décisions.

Pomme d'amour se penche vers moi.

— Et pour cet... l'homme qui est à l'intérieur ? Est-ce qu'on peut lui faire confiance pour... disons... ne pas se servir de ces informations ? Avec l'élection sénatoriale l'année prochaine, il n'y a rien que Cal Fortner aimerait davantage qu'un scandale familial pour distraire les électeurs des vrais problèmes.

Je suis soulagée qu'elle regarde automatiquement mon père, et pas moi, en évoquant la prochaine élection. Je sens que la vie retrouve son ancien équilibre et j'en suis contente. Ce sera plus facile de leur dire qu'il n'y aura pas de mariage politiquement avantageux dans notre jardin à la saison des azalées. Je ne suis pas encore prête à aborder le sujet, mais j'y viendrai.

À voir May et ma grand-mère ensemble, je suis plus sûre que jamais d'avoir pris la bonne décision. Plus sûre de moi, aussi.

— Vous n'avez pas à vous inquiéter pour Trent. Il ne ferait jamais une chose pareille. C'est un ami. Sans son grand-père, les sœurs de mamie Judy ne l'auraient jamais retrouvée. Elle n'aurait jamais appris la vérité sur son passé.

À son expression, je devine que ma mère aurait préféré qu'il en soit ainsi. Le visage de mon père, lui, exprime un autre point de vue.

— J'aimerais parler un instant à May Crandall.

La mâchoire de Pomme d'amour tombe un peu. Puis elle referme la bouche, se redresse et hoche la tête. Quel que soit le chemin choisi par mon père, elle sera à ses côtés. Mes parents ont toujours fonctionné ainsi.

— Je crois que May en serait ravie. Nous pouvons vous laisser seuls, tous les quatre, pour qu'elle puisse vous raconter son histoire.

L'entendre de la bouche de May, avec ses propres mots, achèvera de convaincre mon père, je l'espère. C'est notre histoire familiale.

— Tu peux rester, suggère ma mère, hésitante.

— Je préfère vous laisser ensemble.

En vérité, je veux me retrouver seule avec Trent. Je sais qu'il meurt d'impatience de savoir comment mes parents ont pris la nouvelle. Il n'arrête pas de me regarder à travers la fenêtre.

Il est visiblement soulagé lorsque nous nous levons pour rentrer dans le cottage. À l'intérieur, ma grand-mère évoque un voyage en bateau sur le fleuve. Elle en parle comme s'il avait eu lieu la veille. Apparemment, May avait acheté un canot à moteur, à une époque. Mamie Judy rit en les décrivant toutes les quatre à la dérive sur le fleuve car le moteur refusait de démarrer.

Mon père s'approche d'un pas hésitant d'un fauteuil et regarde sa mère comme s'il la voyait pour la première fois. Ce qui est vrai, en un sens. La femme dont il se souvient n'était qu'une actrice jouant un rôle, du moins en partie. Pendant toutes les années qui ont suivi le jour où ses sœurs l'ont retrouvée, il y a eu deux femmes dans le corps de Judy Stafford. L'une d'elles est épouse de sénateur. L'autre est une fille du fleuve.

Dans ce petit cottage, à la faveur d'un nouveau jour des sœurs, les deux se fondent en une seule.

Trent est plus que soulagé de quitter les lieux avec moi. Je lui suggère une petite promenade :

— Allons vers le sommet de la colline. Je voulais prendre quelques photos des ruines de la maison coloniale... juste au cas où elle s'effondrerait avant qu'on ait le temps de revenir.

Trent me sourit, puis nous passons le portail et laissons les jardins du cottage derrière nous.

— Je doute qu'elle s'effondre un jour.

Nous suivons le sentier jusqu'à l'orée des bois. Je pense à Rill Foss, devenant May Weathers, toutes ces années plus tôt.

Avait-elle pu imaginer la vie qu'elle vivrait ?

Les rayons du soleil me réchauffent lorsque nous traversons un champ pour nous lancer à l'assaut de la colline. C'est une journée magnifique – de celles qui suggèrent un changement de saison imminent. L'ombre des restes de l'ancienne demeure glisse sur l'herbe et donne à la structure imposante l'air d'être de nouveau solide. Mes mains tremblent lorsque je sors mon téléphone pour prendre quelques photos. Ce n'est pas la vraie raison qui m'a poussée à vouloir venir ici. Et cette raison exigeait que je m'éloigne du cottage... et des oreilles indiscrètes.

À présent, les mots me manquent... ou le courage. Au lieu de quoi, je prends un nombre insensé de photos. Mais ma ruse ne peut pas durer indéfiniment.

Je déglutis pour calmer mes palpitations soudaines, j'essaie de prendre mon courage à deux mains.

Trent me devance.

— Tu n'as plus ta bague, constate-t-il, les yeux pleins de questions, quand je me tourne vers lui.

Je baisse la tête vers ma main, je repense à tout ce que j'ai appris depuis que j'ai accepté la demande en mariage d'Elliot, avant de retourner en Caroline du Sud pour faire mon devoir.

J'ai l'impression que c'était une autre vie, la musique d'une autre femme.

— Elliot et moi avons longuement discuté. Il n'approuve pas ma décision de réunir ma grand-mère et May, et il ne l'approuvera sans doute jamais, mais ce n'est pas tout. Je crois que nous savions tous les deux depuis un moment que nous fonctionnons mieux en amis qu'en couple. Nous nous connaissons depuis des années, nous partageons beaucoup de bons souvenirs, pourtant, il y a... quelque chose qui nous manque. Je pense que cela explique pourquoi nous avons évité d'arrêter une date pour la cérémonie ou de faire de vrais projets. Ce mariage était plus voulu par nos familles que par nous, en fait. Peut-être que, quelque part, nous l'avons toujours su.

J'observe Trent tandis qu'il scrute nos ombres sur l'herbe, sourcils froncés, contemplatif.

Mon cœur tressaute, puis palpite. Les secondes me semblent collantes, poisseuses, comme ralenties. Est-ce que Trent est sur la même longueur d'onde que moi ? Et si ce n'était pas le cas ?

Pour commencer, il doit penser à son fils, si jeune.

Ensuite, je ne sais pas vraiment où je vais, dans la vie. En travaillant pour l'ADDS, je pourrai prendre le temps de découvrir qui je veux être. J'aime réparer des injustices. C'est sans doute pour ça que j'ai creusé si profondément pour découvrir l'histoire de May, pour ça que j'ai amené ma grand-mère et May ici cet après-midi.

Aujourd'hui, une vieille injustice a été réparée, autant que possible, après tant d'années.

J'en tire une certaine satisfaction mais, maintenant, mon incertitude concernant Trent l'éclipse. Quelle est sa place dans le futur que je commence à peine à m'imaginer ? Sa famille et la mienne sont si différentes...

Un rayon de soleil éclaire ses yeux lorsqu'il se tourne vers moi. Ils sont du bleu des eaux profondes et, pour la première fois, je comprends que nous ne sommes peut-être pas si différents que nous le semblons. Nous partageons un riche héritage. Nous sommes des enfants du fleuve, tous les deux.

— Est-ce que cela me donne le droit de te prendre la main ?

Il me sourit, les sourcils haussés, dans l'expectative.

— Oui. Sans aucun doute.

Il tourne sa paume vers le ciel et j'y glisse la mienne.

Ses doigts se referment sur les miens en un cercle chaud et fort, et nous grimpons la colline, le dos tourné aux ruines d'une vie révolue.

Vers une vie pleine de promesses.

26

May Crandall
De nos jours

Notre histoire débute par une nuit d'août caniculaire, dans une chambre blanche stérile où une unique décision fatidique est prise sur les ruines insensées du chagrin. Mais notre histoire ne s'arrête pas là. Elle n'a pas encore pris fin.

Changerais-je le cours de nos vies si je le pouvais ? Aurais-je passé ma vie à pianoter sur un bateau-théâtre ou à bêcher la terre en tant que femme de fermier, ou à attendre qu'un marin rentre à la maison et s'installe près de moi devant un petit feu de cheminée chaleureux ?

Est-ce que j'échangerais le fils que j'ai eu pour un autre, pour d'autres enfants, pour une fille qui me réconforterait durant ma vieillesse ? Renoncerais-je aux maris que j'ai aimés et enterrés, à la musique, les symphonies, les lumières de Hollywood, les petits-enfants et arrière-petits-enfants qui vivent loin de moi et qui pourtant ont mes yeux ?

Je réfléchis à tout cela, assise sur le banc de bois, la main de Judy dans la mienne tandis que nous partageons un autre jour des sœurs. Ici, dans les jardins de Magnolia Manor, nous pouvons fêter le jour des sœurs quand bon nous semble. Il n'est pas compliqué de quitter ma chambre, de traverser le couloir contigu et de dire à l'employée :

— Je crois que je vais emmener Judy, ma bonne amie, faire une petite promenade. Oh, oui, bien sûr, je ne manquerai pas de la ramener à l'unité de soins de la mémoire. Vous savez bien que je le fais toujours.

Parfois, ma sœur et moi rions de notre ruse.

— En fait, nous sommes sœurs, pas amies, lui rappelé-je. Il ne faut pas leur dire. C'est notre secret.

— Je ne dirai rien, promet-elle avec son doux sourire. Mais les sœurs sont aussi des amies. Des amies spéciales.

Nous évoquons nos nombreuses aventures, vécues lors des jours des sœurs des années passées, et elle me supplie de lui raconter ce dont je me souviens de Queenie, de Briny et de notre vie sur le fleuve. Je lui raconte les jours, les saisons passées avec Camellia, Lark, Fern et Gabion, sans oublier Silas et le vieux Zede. Je lui parle de lagunes tranquilles et de courants violents, du ballet des libellules de la mi-été, et des eaux gelées qui permettent de marcher sur l'eau l'hiver. Ensemble, nous voyageons sur le fleuve comme si nous y étions. Nous levons nos visages vers le soleil et nous filons encore et encore jusque chez nous au royaume d'Arcadie.

D'autres jours, ma sœur ne voit en moi rien d'autre qu'une voisine de chambre dans ce vieux manoir. Mais l'amour entre sœurs n'a pas besoin de mots. Il ne dépend pas de souvenirs, d'objets du passé, de preuves. Il accompagne le moindre battement de notre cœur. Il est omniprésent, comme notre pouls.

— Ne sont-ils pas adorables ? me lance Judy en me montrant du doigt un jeune couple qui parcourt les allées du jardin, près du lac, main dans la main. C'est vrai qu'ils vont bien ensemble.

Je tapote doucement le bras de Judy.

— C'est ta petite-fille. J'imagine qu'elle est venue te voir. Et elle a amené son soupirant. Il est bel homme, celui-ci. Je le lui ai dit, la première fois que je les ai vus ensemble, qu'il fallait le garder. Je sais reconnaître une flamme, entre deux personnes.

— Oh, ma petite-fille, bien sûr !

Judy fait comme si elle s'en souvenait depuis le début. Certains jours, ça aurait pu être le cas. Mais pas aujourd'hui.

— Et son prétendant, ajoute-t-elle en plissant les yeux. J'ai du mal à me rappeler les noms, en ce moment. Ma sotte mémoire, vois-tu...

— Avery.

— Bien sûr... Avery.

— Et Trent.

— Nous connaissions un Trent, jadis, non ? C'était un homme charmant. Il a vendu les terres autour du cottage d'Edisto, je crois.

— Oui, en effet. C'est son petit-fils qui remonte l'allée vers nous, avec Avery.

— Eh bien, ça alors !

Judy agite la main avec enthousiasme et Avery lui fait signe en retour. Son soupirant et elle disparaissent un instant derrière la tonnelle. Ils ne réapparaissent pas aussi vite qu'on aurait pu s'y attendre.

Judy se couvre la bouche en gloussant :

— Dis donc !

— En effet, soupiré-je en pensant aux amours perdues et à d'autres qui ne furent jamais. Nous, les Foss, nous avons toujours été du genre passionné. J'imagine que cela ne changera jamais.

— Et je l'espère bien ! renchérit Judy.

Nous tombons dans les bras l'une de l'autre – douce embrassade entre sœurs – et rions de nos propres secrets.

Note de l'auteur

Alors que vous vous apprêtez à refermer ce livre, vous vous demandez peut-être : Mais qu'est-ce qui est vrai, dans cette histoire ? Si vous voulez creuser davantage l'histoire vraie des « fermes à bébés », des orphelinats, des changements dans les procédures d'adoption, de Georgia Tann et du scandale autour de la Société des foyers d'accueil du Tennessee de Memphis, vous trouverez d'excellentes informations dans *Pricing the Priceless Child*, de Viviana A. Zelizer (1985), *Babies For Sale : The Tennessee Children's Home Adoption Scandal* de Linda Tollett Austin (1993), *Alone in the World : Orphans and Orphanages in America* de Catherine Reef (2005) et *The Baby Thief : The Untold Story of Georgia Tann, the Baby Seller Who Corrupted Adoption* de Barbara Bisantz Raymond (2007), qui contient aussi des interviews de plusieurs victimes de Georgia Tann. Pour un aperçu du scandale lorsqu'il a éclaté, voir le rapport original du gouverneur Gordon Browning sur la branche du comté de Shelby de la Société des foyers d'accueil du Tennessee (*Report to Governor Gordon Browning on Shelby County Branch, Tennessee Children's Home Society*), qui est disponible sur le réseau des bibliothèques publiques américaines. On y trouve aussi beaucoup d'articles de journaux et de magazines traitant du scandale à l'époque et des réunions de famille dans les années qui ont suivi, ainsi que des reportages dans les émissions *60 minutes*, *Unsolved Mysteries*, sans oublier le documentaire *Deadly Women* de la chaîne Investigation Discovery. Toutes ces sources se sont révélées des matériaux de recherche inestimables.

La fratrie Foss et l'*Arcadie* ont pris vie à partir de l'argile de mon imagination et des eaux boueuses du Mississippi. Même si Rill, son frère et ses sœurs n'existent que dans ces pages, leurs expériences reflètent celles rapportées par des enfants arrachés à leurs familles des années vingt jusqu'à la fin des années cinquante.

L'histoire vraie de Georgia Tann et de la branche du comté de Shelby de la Société des foyers d'accueil du Tennessee est un paradoxe triste et bizarre. Il ne fait aucun doute que l'organisation a sauvé de nombreux enfants dans des situations déplorables et dangereuses, ou a parfois simplement recueilli des enfants non désirés pour les placer dans des foyers aimants. De même, il ne fait aucun doute non plus que de nombreux enfants ont été arrachés à des parents aimants sans raison, et leurs familles biologiques désespérées ne les ont le plus souvent jamais revus. Des récits de survivants confirment que des mères aux bras vides ont pleuré leurs enfants disparus pendant des décennies et que nombre de ces enfants ont été placés dans des structures d'accueil où ils étaient traités comme des objets, négligés, battus, voire violés.

Des mères célibataires, des parents indigents, des femmes dans des hôpitaux psychiatriques, et ceux qui cherchaient de l'aide par le biais des services sociaux et des maternités étaient des cibles privilégiées. Les mères biologiques étaient trompées, on leur faisait signer des papiers alors qu'elles étaient encore sous sédatifs, on leur disait qu'elles devaient confier temporairement la garde de leurs enfants pour qu'ils bénéficient d'un traitement médical adapté, ou on leur disait simplement que leurs nouveau-nés étaient morts. Des enfants ayant connu l'enfer de ces orphelinats – ceux qui étaient assez âgés pour se souvenir de leur ancienne vie – ont rapporté avoir été arrachés du seuil de leur maison, du bord de la route pendant qu'ils allaient à l'école et, oui, du pont de bateaux, sur le fleuve. De façon générale, si vous étiez pauvres et si vous viviez, séjourniez ou passiez dans les environs de Memphis, vos enfants étaient en danger.

Les blonds comme la fratrie Foss étaient particulièrement populaires dans le système de Georgia Tann et étaient souvent ciblés par des « guetteurs » qui travaillaient dans des dispensaires de santé ou autres cliniques publiques. La plupart des habitants de la ville, bien qu'ignorant ses méthodes, avaient entendu parler de son travail. Pendant des années, les gens guettaient les publicités portant des photos d'adorables enfants et bébés, soulignées de slogans du genre : « Il n'attend que vous », « Vous voulez un vrai cadeau de Noël, bien vivant ? » et « George veut jouer à la balle, mais il a besoin d'un papa ». Georgia Tann a été nommée « mère de l'adoption moderne » et fut même consultée par Eleanor Roosevelt sur la question du bien-être des enfants. Aux yeux du grand public, c'était juste une femme maternelle qui voulait bien faire en vouant sa vie à sauver des enfants dans le besoin. Parce qu'elle célébrait le fait que des familles fortunées et connues aient recours à l'adoption, elle a contribué à populariser cette démarche et à dissoudre la croyance répandue voulant que les orphelins fussent indésirables et tarés de naissance. Les exemples notoires de Georgia incluaient des figures politiques telles qu'Herbert Lehman, le gouverneur de New York, et des célébrités de Hollywood comme June Allyson et son mari Dick Powell, ainsi que Joan Crawford. Des anciens employés des foyers de Tann de Memphis murmuraient qu'on avait enlevé jusqu'à sept enfants en même temps à la faveur de la nuit, pour des livraisons dans un nouveau foyer en Californie, New York et d'autres États. Lorsqu'on l'interrogeait sur ses méthodes, Georgia vantait sans honte aucune les vertus qu'il y avait à prendre des enfants à leurs parents trop démunis, incapables de les élever correctement, pour les placer chez des personnes de « haut rang ».

Vu de notre époque, il est difficile d'imaginer comment Georgia Tann et son réseau ont réussi à opérer à si large échelle pendant des décennies, et comment elle trouvait des employés prêts à fermer les yeux en permanence sur le traitement inhumain réservé aux enfants dans les orphelinats et autres foyers non conventionnés, comme celui où Rill et les autres atterrissent. Pourtant, tout cela est bel et bien arrivé. À un moment donné, le U.S. Children's Bureau a envoyé un inspecteur à Memphis pour enquêter sur l'explosion du taux de mortalité infantile de la ville. En 1945, une épidémie de dysenterie a causé la mort de quarante ou cinquante enfants confiés aux soins de Georgia Tann, malgré les efforts d'un médecin qui fournissait bénévolement ses services. Georgia, de son côté, prétendit que seuls deux enfants avaient succombé à la maladie. Sous la pression, l'État a voté une loi obligeant chaque foyer d'accueil du Tennessee a être conventionné. Cependant, cette nouvelle législation incluait une sous-section prévoyant une exemption pour toutes les pensions employées par l'agence de Georgia Tann.

Si la Mme Murphy de cette histoire et son foyer relèvent de la fiction, les expériences vécues là-bas par Rill ont été inspirées par celles racontées par des survivants. Ils sont aussi nombreux ceux qui, par maltraitance, négligence, maladie ou mauvais suivi médical, n'ont pas survécu pour raconter leurs histoires. Ce sont les victimes silencieuses d'un système non régulé motivé par la cupidité et l'appât du gain. On estime entre cinq et six cents le nombre d'enfants ayant simplement disparu sous la responsabilité de Georgia Tann. Des milliers d'autres ont disparu dans des adoptions à but lucratif au cours desquelles les noms, les dates de naissance et les dossiers médicaux ont été modifiés pour empêcher les familles biologiques de retrouver leurs enfants.

Au vu de ces statistiques épouvantables, on aurait pu croire que le règne de Georgia Tann finirait dans une tempête médiatique mêlant révélations publiques, enquêtes policières et action juridique. Si *Les Enfants du fleuve* était une œuvre de pure fiction, c'est la fin que j'aurais écrite, avec des scènes témoignant d'une justice rapide et implacable. Malheureusement, tel ne fut pas le cas. La carrière de Georgia dans le monde de l'adoption ne s'arrêta pas avant 1950. Lors d'une conférence de presse au mois de septembre de cette année-là, le gouverneur Gordon Browning évita de parler de la tragédie humaine déchirante pour se concentrer sur l'argent – Mlle Tann, expliqua-t-il, s'était enrichie illégalement à hauteur d'un million de dollars (l'équivalent approximatif de dix millions de dollars de nos jours), tout en étant l'employée de la Société des foyers d'accueil du Tennessee. Malgré la révélation de ses crimes, Georgia était, à ce moment-là, hors d'atteinte de la justice. Quelques jours après la conférence de presse, elle mourut chez elle d'un cancer de l'utérus, contre lequel elle avait refusé tout traitement. Un article de presse fut publié face à sa notice nécrologique en une du journal local. Les foyers de son réseau furent fermés et un enquêteur fut nommé, mais il se retrouva bien vite bloqué par des gens puissants ayant des secrets, des réputations et, parfois, des adoptions, à préserver.

Tandis que la fermeture des foyers donna aux familles biologiques accablées de chagrin des raisons d'espérer, cet espoir leur fut bien vite arraché. Des magistrats et de puissants hommes politiques firent passer des lois pour légaliser même les plus discutables de ces adoptions, avant de sceller les archives. Des vingt-deux pupilles qui restaient sous la responsabilité de Georgia Tann au moment de sa mort, seules deux – qui avaient déjà été rejetées par leurs familles d'adoption – furent restituées à leurs familles biologiques. Des milliers d'autres familles ne surent jamais ce qu'il était arrivé à leurs enfants. Pour l'opinion publique, ces enfants étaient passés de la misère à un monde privilégié, et ils étaient mieux où ils étaient, quelles qu'aient pu être les circonstances de leurs adoptions.

Même si certains enfants adoptés, certains frères et sœurs, certaines familles biologiques ont pu se retrouver grâce à des bouts de souvenirs emboîtés les uns dans les autres, des documents subtilisés aux dossiers des tribunaux et grâce à l'assistance de détectives privés, les dossiers de Georgia Tann n'auront été ouverts à ses victimes qu'en 1995. Pour bien des parents biologiques et des enfants adoptés, qui ont pleuré leurs pertes toutes leurs vies durant, c'était simplement trop tard. Pour d'autres, ce fut le début de réunions de famille reportées depuis trop longtemps et l'opportunité de raconter enfin leurs propres histoires.

S'il y a une leçon prédominante à retenir de l'histoire des enfants Foss et du scandale réel de la Société des foyers d'accueil du Tennessee, c'est que les bébés et les enfants, quel que soit le recoin du monde où ils naissent, ne sont pas des produits, des objets ou des ardoises vierges, comme Georgia Tann aimait à présenter ses pupilles ; ce sont des êtres humains, avec leur propre histoire, leurs propres besoins, leurs propres espoirs et leurs propres rêves.

Remerciements

Les personnages de roman sont un peu comme les gens dans la vraie vie – quels que soient leurs humbles débuts, leurs trajectoires sont façonnées par la famille, les amis, les voisins, les collègues et tout un tas de connaissances. Certains les encouragent même, certains les guident, certains leur offrent un amour inconditionnel, certains leur enseignent des choses, certains les poussent à être à la hauteur de leur potentiel. Cette histoire, comme la plupart des histoires, doit son existence à un éventail d'individus uniques et généreux.

Avant tout, je remercie ma famille de m'avoir soutenue pendant toutes ces années d'écriture, même quand cela incluait des nuits blanches, des emplois du temps de folie et des raids dans la cuisine pour y manger ce qui n'avait pas encore été dévoré. Cette année, je remercie particulièrement mon fils aîné d'être tombé amoureux et d'avoir enfin ajouté une fille à notre famille. Un mariage est non seulement une distraction formidable pour oublier un instant les corrections, l'écriture, la réécriture et d'autres corrections sur le texte en cours mais, en plus, j'ai enfin quelqu'un dans mon entourage qui m'accompagne à des rencontres littéraires, et avec qui je peux papoter à l'aller et au retour.

Merci à ma mère d'avoir été mon assistante officielle, ainsi qu'une première lectrice fabuleuse. Tout le monde n'a pas la chance d'avoir une aide capable de vous dire quand votre coupe de cheveux ou votre dernier chapitre a besoin d'un petit ravalement. Merci à ma chère belle-mère de m'avoir aidée à faire en sorte que la prochaine génération de Wingate sache comment raconter une bonne histoire le soir autour de la table. Merci aussi à mes parents et amis, proches et lointains, pour leur amour, leur aide et leur hospitalité lorsque je voyage. Vous êtes les meilleurs.

Je remercie particulièrement mes amis – presque – membres – de la famille, surtout Ed Stevens pour son aide documentaire et ses encouragements constants, et Steve et Rosemary Fitts pour nous avoir hébergés sur l'île d'Edisto. S'il existe un meilleur endroit qu'Edisto pour effectuer un voyage de recherches, je ne l'ai pas encore découvert. Merci également à la fabuleuse équipe qui m'a aidée dans les premières relectures et pour l'organisation de la tournée de signatures : Duane Davis, Mary Davis, Virginia Rush et, enfin, ma merveilleuse tata Sandy qui a un sens de la narration formidable et un sens de l'humour tout aussi bon. Merci à Kathie Bennet et Susan Zurenda, de *Magic Time Literary*, d'avoir organisé des tournées incroyables par le passé, d'avoir soutenu ce livre dès ses balbutiements et d'avoir œuvré avec enthousiasme pour qu'il voie le jour.

Côté publication, je ne remercierai jamais assez mon agente fabuleuse, Elisabeth Weed, de m'avoir encouragée à écrire ce livre, puis d'avoir accompli un travail d'expert afin de trouver la maison d'édition parfaite. Merci à l'éditrice extraordinaire Susanna Porter de m'avoir poussée à approfondir les expériences des enfants de la famille Foss et le voyage d'Avery dans son passé familial caché. Merci à l'équipe éditoriale formidable derrière ce livre : Kara Welsh, Kim Hovey, Jennifer Hershey, Scott Shannon, Susan Corcoran, Melanie DeNardo, Kristin Fassler, Debbie Aroff, Lynn Andreozzi, Toby Ernst, Beth Pearson et Emily Hartley. Les mots me manquent pour vous dire à quel point je vous apprécie tous personnellement, comme la façon dont vous avez mis cette histoire sur le marché avec tant de soins. Toute ma gratitude va également aux maquettistes, à la fabrication, au service marketing et au service de presse. Merci d'avoir mis tous vos talents au service de cette aventure. Sans votre travail, les histoires prendraient littéralement la poussière sur des étagères, inconnues de tous, lues par personne. Vous mettez les livres en relation avec leurs lecteurs et, ce faisant, vous connectez les gens les uns aux autres. Si les livres peuvent changer le monde, alors ceux d'entre vous qui aident à les mettre au monde sont les agents du changement.

Je finirai par remercier les nombreux lecteurs qui ont partagé des voyages passés et qui partagent aujourd'hui celui-ci. Je vous chéris. Je chéris le temps que nous passons ensemble à travers ces histoires. Merci d'avoir choisi ce livre. Merci d'avoir recommandé mes livres précédents à des amis, de les avoir suggérés à des clubs de lecture et de prendre le temps de m'envoyer des petits mots d'encouragement par e-mail, Facebook et Twitter. Je suis reconnaissante envers tous ceux qui lisent ces histoires, et aussi envers les libraires qui les conseillent avec tant de dévotion. Comme M. Rogers, ce célèbre animateur d'émissions pour enfants, l'a dit un jour : « Cherchez ceux qui aident. Vous trouverez toujours des gens qui viennent aider. »

Vous, mes amis, vous m'aidez au jour le jour.

Et, pour cela, je vous remercie du fond du cœur.

Les Escales

Chantel Acevedo
Lointaines merveilles

Rabih Alameddine
Les Vies de papier

Jeffrey Archer
Seul l'avenir le dira
Les Fautes de nos pères
Des secrets bien gardés
Juste retour des choses
Plus fort que l'épée
Le temps est venu

M.J. Arlidge
Am stram gram
Il court, il court, le furet
La Maison de poupée
Au feu, les pompiers

Jami Attenberg
La Famille Middlestein
*Mazie, sainte patronne des fauchés
et des assoiffés*
L'Âge de raison

Laura Barnett
Quoi qu'il arrive

Fatima Bhutto
Les Lunes de Mir Ali

Daria Bignardi
Accords parfaits

Jenna Blum
Les Chasseurs de tornades

Blanca Busquets
Un cœur en silence

Chris Carter
Le Prix de la peur

Hannah Michell
Dissidences

Derek B. Miller
Dans la peau de Sheldon Horowitz

Fernando Monacelli
Naufragés

Julia Montejo
Une vie à t'écrire

Juan Jacinto Munoz Rengel
Le Tueur hypocondriaque

Idra Novey
Le jour où Beatriz Yagoda s'assit dans un arbre

Chibundu Onuzo
La Fille du roi araignée

Gunilla Linn Persson
Par-delà les glaces

Ismet Prcić
California Dream

Paola Predicatori
Mon hiver à Zéroland

Dorit Rabinyan
Sous la même étoile

Raffaela Romagnolo
La Masnà

Paolo Roversi
La Ville rouge

Sandip Roy
Bien comme il faut

Eugen Ruge
Quand la lumière décline
Le Chat andalou

Amy Sackville
Là est la danse

William Shaw
Du sang sur Abbey Road

Anna Shevchenko
L'Ultime Partie

Liad Shoham
Tel-Aviv Suspects
Terminus Tel-Aviv
Oranges amères

Priscille Sibley
Poussières d'étoiles

Marina Stepnova
Les Femmes de Lazare
Leçons d'Italie

Daniel Torday
Le Dernier exploit de Poxl West

Karen Viggers
La Mémoire des embruns
La Maison des hautes falaises
Le Murmure du vent

Stella Vretou
Les Souliers vernis rouges

A.J. Waines
Les Noyées de la Tamise

Cecily Wong
Comme un ruban de soie rouge

Pour en savoir plus
sur l'actualité des Escales,
vous pouvez consulter notre site Internet
www.lesescales.fr
et nous suivre sur les réseaux sociaux

 Editions Les Escales

 @LesEscales

 @LesEscales